Therapeutic Potential of Silver Nanoparticles (AgNPs)

Therapeutic Potential of Silver Nanoparticles (AgNPs)

Guest Editor

Goreti Pereira

MDPI Basel • Beijing • Wuhan • Barcelona • Belgrade • Novi Sad • Cluj • Manchester

Guest Editor
Goreti Pereira
Chemistry Department and
CESAM
University of Aveiro
Aveiro
Portugal

Editorial Office
MDPI AG
Grosspeteranlage 5
4052 Basel, Switzerland

This is a reprint of the Special Issue, published open access by the journal *Pharmaceuticals* (ISSN 1424-8247), freely accessible at: https://www.mdpi.com/journal/pharmaceuticals/special_issues/42C23JT873.

For citation purposes, cite each article independently as indicated on the article page online and as indicated below:

Lastname, A.A.; Lastname, B.B. Article Title. *Journal Name* **Year**, *Volume Number*, Page Range.

ISBN 978-3-7258-4751-8 (Hbk)
ISBN 978-3-7258-4752-5 (PDF)
https://doi.org/10.3390/books978-3-7258-4752-5

Contents

About the Editor vii

Preface ix

Tiarpa Thongwattana, Ronnakorn Chaiyo, Khanittha Ponsanti, Benchamaporn Tangnorawich, Patcharee Pratumpong, Surachet Toommee, et al.
Synthesis of Silver Nanoparticles and Gold Nanoparticles Used as Biosensors for the Detection of Human Serum Albumin-Diagnosed Kidney Disease
Reprinted from: *Pharmaceuticals* **2024**, *17*, 1421, https://doi.org/10.3390/ph17111421 1

Iris Xiaoxue Yin, Veena Wenqing Xu, Grace Yuchan Xu, Ollie Yiru Yu, John Yun Niu and Chun Hung Chu
Synthesis and Application of Silver Nanoparticles for Caries Management: A Review
Reprinted from: *Pharmaceuticals* **2024**, *17*, 1264, https://doi.org/10.3390/ph17101264 17

Hafez Al-Momani, Muhannad I. Massadeh, Muna Almasri, Dua'a Al Balawi, Iman Aolymat, Saja Hamed, et al.
Anti-Bacterial Activity of Green Synthesised Silver and Zinc Oxide Nanoparticles against *Propionibacterium acnes*
Reprinted from: *Pharmaceuticals* **2024**, *17*, 255, https://doi.org/10.3390/ph17020255 31

Sindy Magri Roque, Ana Carolina Furian, Marcela Kim Takemoto, Marta Cristina Teixeira Duarte, Rafaela Durrer Parolina, Adriano Luís Roque, et al.
Biosynthesis and Characterization of Silver Nanoparticles and Simvastatin Association in Titanium Biofilms
Reprinted from: *Pharmaceuticals* **2024**, *17*, 1612, https://doi.org/10.3390/ph17121612 53

Liaqat Ali, Nisar Ahmad, Muhammad Nazir Uddin, Mostafa A. Abdel-Maksoud, Hina Fazal, Sabiha Fatima, et al.
Immobilization of Silver Nanoparticles with Defensive Gum of *Moringa oleifera* for Antibacterial Efficacy Against Resistant Bacterial Species from Human Infections
Reprinted from: *Pharmaceuticals* **2024**, *17*, 1546, https://doi.org/10.3390/ph17111546 71

Tehmina Khan, Ali Umar, Zakia Subhan, Muhammad Saleem Khan, Hafeeza Zafar Ali, Hayat Ullah, et al.
Therapeutic Potential of Novel Silver Carbonate Nanostructures in Wound Healing and Antibacterial Activity Against *Pseudomonas chengduensis* and *Staphylococcus aureus*
Reprinted from: *Pharmaceuticals* **2024**, *17*, 1471, https://doi.org/10.3390/ph17111471 95

Ayşe Baran, Erdal Ertaş, Mehmet Fırat Baran, Aziz Eftekhari, Zübeyir Gunes, Cumali Keskin, et al.
Green-Synthesized Characterization, Antioxidant and Antibacterial Applications of CtAC/MNPs-Ag Nanocomposites
Reprinted from: *Pharmaceuticals* **2024**, *17*, 772, https://doi.org/10.3390/ph17060772 113

Mohammed Ali Abdel-Rahman, Khalid S. Alshallash, Ahmed M. Eid, Saad El-Din Hassan, Mutaz Salih, Mohammed F. Hamza and Amr Fouda
Exploring the Antimicrobial, Antioxidant, and Antiviral Potential of Eco-Friendly Synthesized Silver Nanoparticles Using Leaf Aqueous Extract of *Portulaca oleracea* L.
Reprinted from: *Pharmaceuticals* **2024**, *17*, 317, https://doi.org/10.3390/ph17030317 130

Muhammad Asif, Wajeeha Iqbal, Muhammad Fakhar-e-Alam, Zahid Hussain, Malik Saadullah, Mudassir Hassan, et al.
Synthesis and Characterization of Chemically and Green-Synthesized Silver Oxide Particles for Evaluation of Antiviral and Anticancer Activity
Reprinted from: *Pharmaceuticals* **2024**, *17*, 908, https://doi.org/10.3390/ph17070908 . . . . **149**

Paras Dayma, Nisha Choudhary, Daoud Ali, Saud Alarifi, Pravin Dudhagara, Kuldeep Luhana, et al.
Exploring the Potential of Halotolerant Actinomycetes from Rann of Kutch, India: A Study on the Synthesis, Characterization, and Biomedical Applications of Silver Nanoparticles
Reprinted from: *Pharmaceuticals* **2024**, *17*, 743, https://doi.org/10.3390/ph17060743 . . . . **162**

Gulamnabi Vanti, Naresh Poondla, Prasath Manogaran, Nagappa Teradal, Veeresh S, Ram Kaulgud and Mahantesh Kurjogi
Synthesis and Characterization of Multifunctional Chitosan–Silver Nanoparticles: An In-Vitro Approach for Biomedical Applications
Reprinted from: *Pharmaceuticals* **2024**, *17*, 1229, https://doi.org/10.3390/ph17091229 . . . . **190**

Ibtissam Laib, Boutlilis Djahra Ali, Ali Alsalme, David Cornu, Mikhael Bechelany and Ahmed Barhoum
Therapeutic Efficacy of *Helianthemum lippii* Extract and Silver Nanoparticles Synthesized from the Extract against Cadmium-Induced Renal Nephrotoxicity in Wistar Rats
Reprinted from: *Pharmaceuticals* **2024**, *17*, 982, https://doi.org/10.3390/ph17080982 . . . . **204**

Ludmila Rudi, Inga Zinicovscaia, Liliana Cepoi, Tatiana Chiriac, Dmitrii Grozdov and Alexandra Kravtsova
The Impact of Silver Nanoparticles Functionalized with Spirulina Protein Extract on Rats
Reprinted from: *Pharmaceuticals* **2024**, *17*, 1247, https://doi.org/10.3390/ph17091247 . . . . **229**

Sodiq Kolawole Lawal, Samuel Oluwaseun Olojede, Babatunde Adebola Alabi, Kafalotse Sylvia Dithole, Samuel Thopho Matula, Edwin Coleridge Naidu, et al.
Evaluation of Hippocampal Microanatomy and Neuro-Biomarkers Following Administration of Silver Nanoparticles Conjugated with Tenofovir Disoproxil Fumarate in Experimental Diabetic Rats
Reprinted from: *Pharmaceuticals* **2024**, *17*, 1635, https://doi.org/10.3390/ph17121635 . . . . **246**

About the Editor

Goreti Pereira

Goreti Pereira obtained a PhD in Sciences, with Specialty in Chemistry (2012), from the University of Minho (Portugal). In October 2022, she joined the Department of Chemistry and CESAM of the University of Aveiro (UA, Portugal) as an assistant researcher.

Her research focuses on developing quantum dots (QDs) and metallic nanoparticles (NPs) prepared in aqueous media for biomedical and environmental applications. These include diagnostic tools, therapeutic agents, sensors, and catalysts. Her research has been also focused on minimizing the environmental impact of the preparation of QDs and NPs, applying synthetic procedures aligned with green chemistry principles.

Preface

Silver nanoparticles (AgNPs) have rapidly emerged as one of the most promising nanomaterials in modern biomedicine. Initially recognized for their potent antimicrobial properties, these versatile nanoparticles are now revealing an impressive range of therapeutic applications, from anticancer strategies to alternative antimicrobials, and biosensor platforms. These novel approaches take advantage of the AgNPs' size, shape, and surface-dependent physical and chemical characteristics.

This reprint aims to showcase the high-impact research published in the MDPI Pharmaceuticals Special Issue titled "Therapeutic Potential of Silver Nanoparticles (AgNPs)", which includes 14 contributions. These articles provide a comprehensive overview of current innovations in the field. These works present interdisciplinary perspectives, from nanotechnology to pharmacology, also covering environmental sustainability issues.

Within this reprint, readers will find strategies for novel green synthesis and routes to produce eco-friendly AgNPs, as well as insights into their antimicrobial, antioxidant, and anticancer effects. Several contributions include both in vitro and in vivo studies, offering a valuable bridge between laboratory formulation and potential clinical application.

This reprint is intended for researchers, clinicians, and students with an interest in the therapeutic application of AgNPs. The aim is to inspire new research directions and foster continued collaboration across different scientific disciplines. Finally, I would like to express my gratitude to all the contributing authors for their valuable work.

Goreti Pereira
Guest Editor

pharmaceuticals

MDPI

Article

Synthesis of Silver Nanoparticles and Gold Nanoparticles Used as Biosensors for the Detection of Human Serum Albumin-Diagnosed Kidney Disease

Tiarpa Thongwattana [1], Ronnakorn Chaiyo [2], Khanittha Ponsanti [2], Benchamaporn Tangnorawich [2,3], Patcharee Pratumpong [2,3], Surachet Toommee [4], Ratchapol Jenjob [5], Su-Geun Yang [5,6], Yardnapar Parcharoen [3,7], Sitakan Natphopsuk [3,7,*] and Chiravoot Pechyen [1,3,*]

1 Department of Materials and Textile Technology, Faculty of Science and Technology, Thammasat University, Pathum Thani 12120, Thailand

2 Department of Physics, Faculty of Science and Technology, Thammasat University, Pathum Thani 12120, Thailand

3 Thammasat University Center of Excellence in Modern Technology and Advanced Manufacturing for Medical Innovation, Thammasat University, Pathum Thani 12120, Thailand

4 Industrial Arts Program, Faculty of Industrial Technology, Kamphaeng Phet Rajabhat University, Kamphaeng Phet 62000, Thailand

5 BK21 FOUR Program in Biomedical Science and Engineering, Department of Biomedical Science, Inha University College of Medicine, Incheon 22212, Republic of Korea

6 Inha Institute of Aerospace Medicine, Inha University College of Medicine, Incheon 22332, Republic of Korea

7 Chulabhorn International College of Medicine, Thammasat University, Pathum Thani 12120, Thailand

* Correspondence: sitakan@tu.ac.th (S.N.); cpechyen@tu.ac.th (C.P.)

Abstract: Background/Objectives: This study aims to develop a screen-printed carbon electrode (SPCE) modified with silver nanoparticles (AgNPs) and gold nanoparticles (AuNPs) for the detection of human serum albumin (HSA). The objectives include utilizing green synthesis methods for nanoparticle production and evaluating the electrochemical performance of the modified electrodes. **Methods:** AgNPs and AuNPs were synthesized using Phulae pineapple peel extract (PPA) as a reducing agent. The nanoparticles were characterized using UV-visible spectrophotometry (UV-vis), Fourier transform infrared spectroscopy (FTIR), X-ray diffraction (XRD), and transmission electron microscopy (TEM). The electrochemical performance of AgNP/SPCE and AuNP/SPCE was assessed by cyclic voltammetry (CV) studies, and the electrodes were functionalized with anti-HSA antibodies for HSA detection. **Results:** Characterization revealed spherical nanoparticles ranging from 10 to 30 nm. Both AgNP/SPCE and AuNP/SPCE demonstrated improved electrochemical performance compared to bare SPCEs. The modified sensors could detect serum albumin concentrations from 10 to 400 μg/mL, with high correlation values of 0.97 and 0.99 for AgNPs and AuNPs, respectively. **Conclusions:** This research demonstrates the potential of using agricultural waste for green synthesis of nanoparticles and highlights the application of AgNPs and AuNPs in developing sensitive biosensing platforms for the detection of human serum albumin.

Keywords: silver nanoparticles; gold nanoparticles; green synthesis; Phulae pineapple; human serum albumin (HSA); carbon screen-printed electrode

1. Introduction

Human serum albumin (HSA) is a critical protein found in blood plasma, serving as an important biomarker for kidney health. When HSA leaks into urine due to kidney damage, it indicates the presence of microalbumin, a significant early warning sign of kidney disease. This condition is characterized by urinary albumin excretion levels from 30–300 mg/day from a 24 h urine collection or 30–300 mg/L from a random or first-morning urine sample [1–3]. Traditional analytical methods for measuring microalbumin, including fluorescence immunoassays [4,5], radioimmunoassays [6], high-performance liquid chromatography (HPLC) [7], and others [8–13], often present challenges such as high costs, prolonged analysis times, low sensitivity, and complex pre-treatment procedures [14].

Electrochemical biosensors have emerged as a promising alternative due to their high sensitivity, stability, low detection limits, cost-effectiveness, and ease of use [15,16]. As a result, there has been a growing interest in the development of electrochemical biosensors for albumin measurement [17–25]. Metal nanoparticles, particularly silver (Ag) and gold (Au), are widely used in constructing electrochemical sensors due to their excellent electrical conductivity, catalytic properties, and biocompatibility [26,27]. While these nanoparticles can be synthesized using physical or chemical methods, such approaches often involve high costs, significant energy consumption, and the use of toxic solvents, posing environmental and health risks [28]. In contrast, biological or green synthesis methods are environmentally friendly, cost-effective, and safe, utilizing plant extracts as reducing agents [29,30]. Previous studies have demonstrated the potential of various plant components, including fruits, seeds, and peels, in the synthesis of AgNPs [31,32] and AuNPs [33–35].

Thailand, being a tropical country, produces a diverse range of fruits, with pineapple being one of its major agricultural products. The 'Phulae' variety of pineapple, known for its unique taste and crisp texture, is highly sought after both domestically and internationally [36,37]. Despite being considered agricultural waste, pineapple peels are rich in bioactive compounds that can facilitate the reduction of metal ions and stabilize the resulting nanoparticles [38–41].

This study aims to synthesize AgNPs and AuNPs using an eco-friendly biological method that not only addresses the issue of agricultural waste but also enhances the value of such waste products. Specifically, we employ Phulae pineapple peel extract as both the reducing and stabilizing agent in the synthesis of these nanoparticles. The synthesized nanoparticles are subsequently used to modify electrodes designed for electrochemical biosensing applications. We investigate the electrochemical response of the modified electrodes through cyclic voltammetry (CV) and assess their performance as highly sensitive biosensors for the detection of HSA using square-wave voltammetry (SWV).

2. Results and Discussion

2.1. Characterization of AgNPs and AuNPs Synthesized Using PPA

The initial indicator showing that PPA was an effective agent for the synthesis of AgNPs and AuNPs was the visual color change that occurred after PPA was added to the solution. The color of the AgNP solution changed to orange-brown (Figure 1a), indicating that AgNPs were formed by the reduction of silver ions (Ag^+) into silver particles (Ag^0). The samples show an optical absorption band peak ranging from 440–460 nm (Figure 1c) [42–44]. Similarly, the color of the AuNP solution changed to purple (Figure 1b), indicating that AuNPs were formed by the reduction of gold ions (Au^{3+}) into gold particles (Au^0). The samples show an optical absorption band peak ranging from 540–580 nm (Figure 1d) [45–47]. These typical characteristic absorption bands for metallic Ag and Au nanoclusters were due to surface plasmon resonance (SPR).

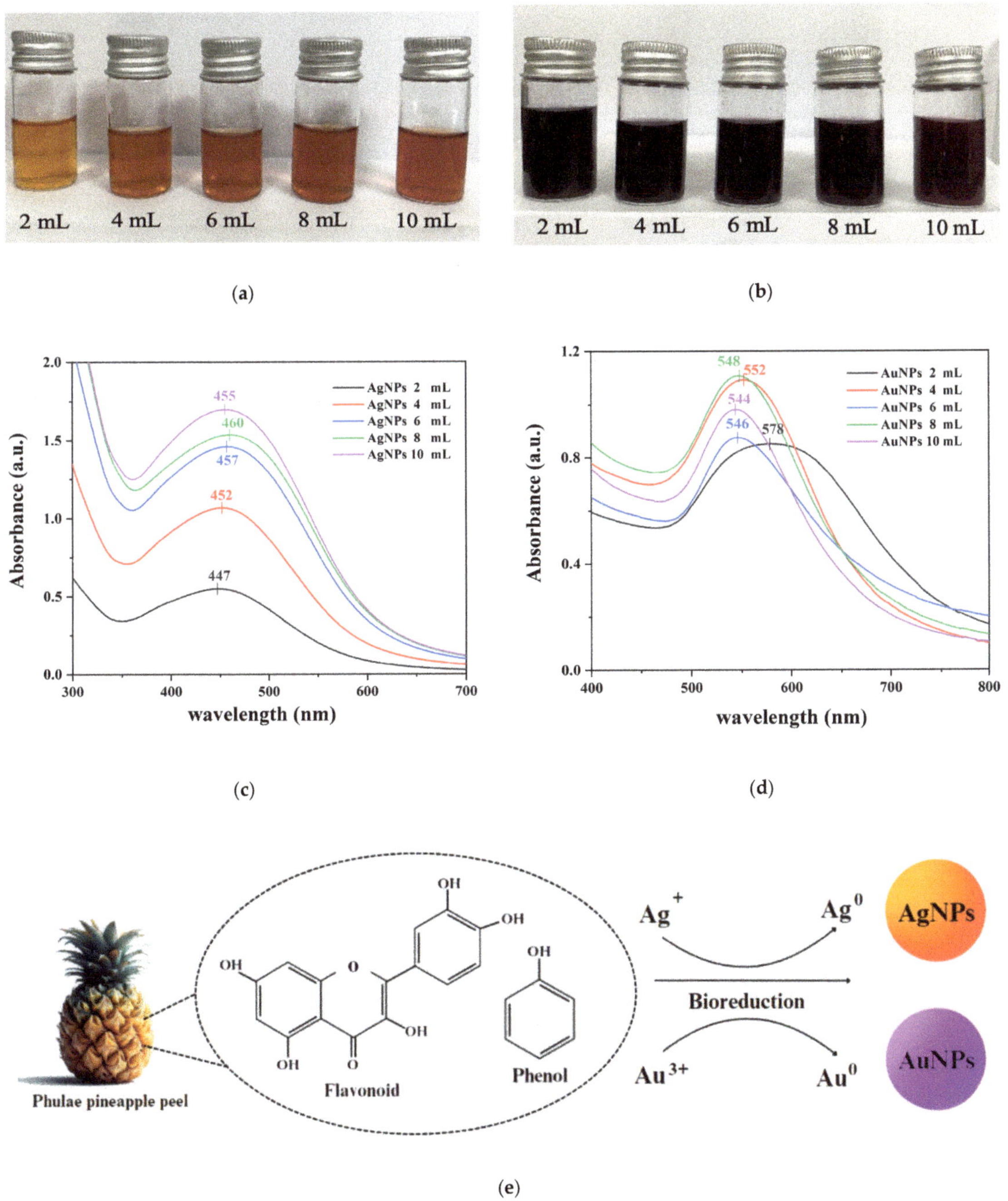

Figure 1. Photographs show the color changes in the solution of (**a**) AgNPs and (**b**) AuNPs formed at different PPA quantities. UV-vis absorption spectra of biosynthesized (**c**) AgNPs and (**d**) AuNPs at different PPA quantities. (**e**) Mechanism of AgNP and AuNP formation using PPA.

The XRD patterns of the crystalline structures of biosynthesized AgNPs and AuNPs using PPA at different PPA quantities are shown in Figure 2a,b. Both have XRD peaks at 2θ degrees that are evident approximately at 38°, 44°, 64°, and 77°, which correspond to the (111), (200), (220), and (311) planes of a face-centered cubic (FCC) structure. These peaks agree with standard report values from the Joint Committee on Powder Diffraction Standards (JCPDS): JCPDS No. 04-0783 for Ag [48–50], and JCPDS No. 04-0784 for Au [51,52]. However, some other peaks observed in the diffraction pattern, marked by asterisks* in Figure 2a, were detected at 2θ degrees of 28°, 32°, 54°, and 57°. These peaks could indicate the presence of Ag_2O and AgO. It is assumed that these peaks are related to residual reducing agents" or might be due to phytochemicals in the extract involved in the reduction of silver ions and stabilization process of AgNPs [40,53–57].

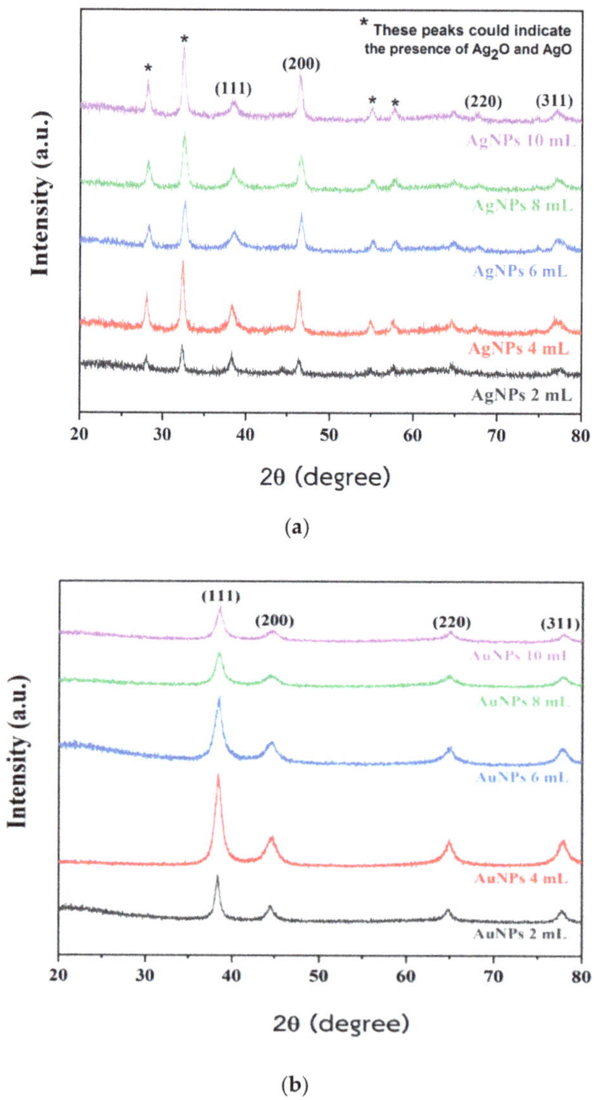

Figure 2. XRD pattern of biosynthesized (**a**) AgNPs and (**b**) AuNPs at different PPA quantities.

FTIR was performed to identify the functional groups on Phulae pineapple peel, which are involved in the reduction of metallic ions and the stabilization of nanoparticles, and the results are shown in Figure 3a–c. The FTIR spectra of Phulae pineapple peel exhibited characteristic peaks at around 3715, 2980, 1297, 1045, and 827 cm^{-1}. In the spectra of synthesized nanoparticles, these bands shift to around 3725, 2988, 1365, 1040, and 825 cm^{-1} for AgNPs, and 3700, 2986, 1290, 1050, and 827 cm^{-1} for AuNPs. The peak at 3725–3700 cm^{-1} could be due to the stretching vibration of O-H [58,59]. The peak at 2988–2980 cm^{-1} was assigned to alkane C-H stretching vibrations [60]. The peak at 1365–1290 cm^{-1} was assigned to C-H bending [61]. The peak at 1050–1040 cm^{-1} was assigned to the stretching and deformation of aromatic C-O groups [62]. The peak at 827–825 cm^{-1} was assigned to illustrate the angular deformation of aromatic hydrogen [63]. All the aforementioned vibration bands are caused by the presence of phytochemical substances present in Phulae pineapple peel, which contains functional groups that may have aided the reduction and stability of the nanoparticles.

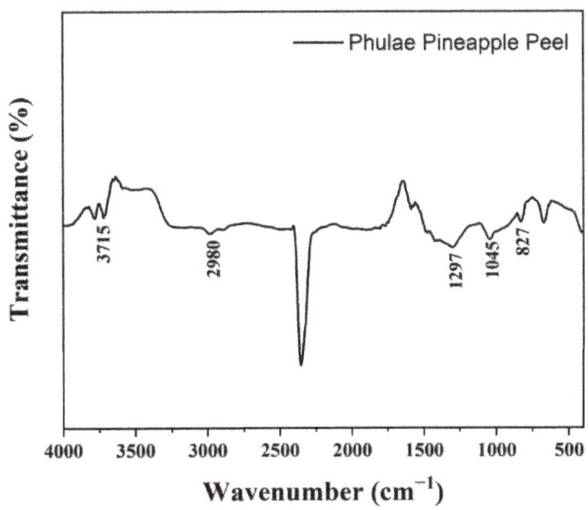

(a)

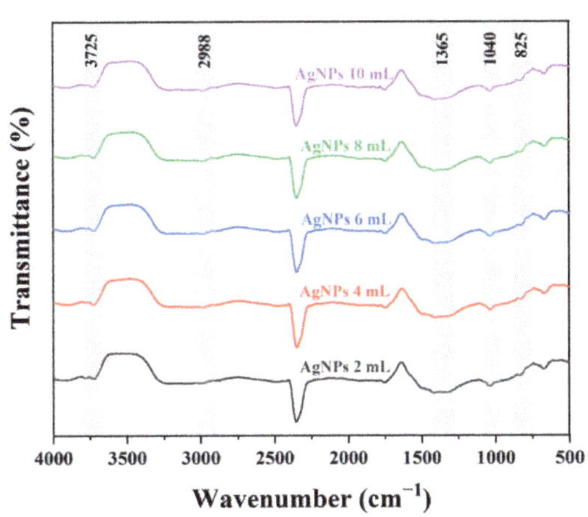

(b)

Figure 3. *Cont.*

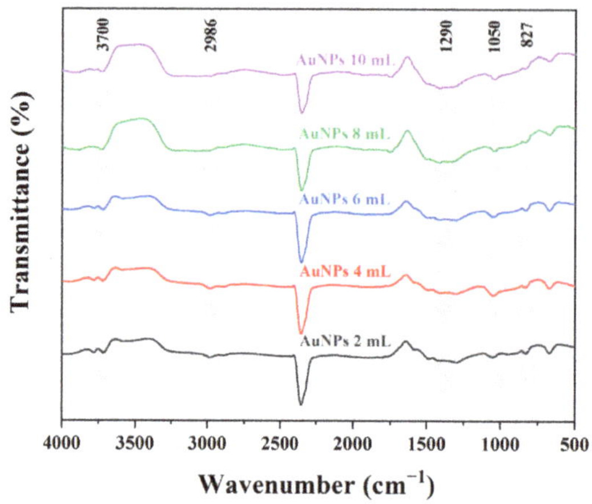

(c)

Figure 3. FTIR spectra of (**a**) Phulae pineapple peel, (**b**) AgNPs, and (**c**) AuNPs at different PPA quantities.

TEM images reveal that AgNPs and AuNPs synthesized using PPA predominantly exhibit spherical morphologies, as shown in Figure 4. TEM imaging revealed that the average particle size for AgNPs and AuNPs was between 10 and 30 nm. The average particle sizes of AgNPs and AuNPs synthesized with 10 mL and 6 mL PPA quantities are the smallest overall.

Zeta potential is a measure of the effective electric charge on the surface of a nanoparticle; it is often used to analyze the stability of colloidal solutions. The range for stable and unstable suspensions are frequently defined as −30 mV to 30 mV, which means that particles having zeta potentials less than −30 mV or greater than 30 mV are typically considered stable. If an unstable nanoparticle suspension has a zeta potential value greater than −15 mV, it indicates a suspension at the threshold of agglomeration and the formation of larger particles. Coagulation or flocculation is most rapid when the zeta potential is 0 mV ± 3 mV [64,65]. The zeta potential values of AgNPs and AuNPs synthesized using PPA at different PPA quantities (Figure 5) are in the range of −20.7 to −0.3 mV and −12.7 to −0.5 mV, respectively. The colloidal solution of both AgNPs and AuNPs was found to be stable for 1 week, and all particles were not settled down to the bottom (no aggregate). AgNPs precipitated rapidly at 6 and 8 mL PPA quantities, as did AuNPs at 4 and 10 mL PPA quantities. On the contrary, AgNPs at PPA quantities of 10 mL and AuNPs at PPA quantities of 6 mL have the slowest sedimentation without aggregate. It may be inferred that quantities of 10 mL for AgNPs and 6 mL for AuNPs have the greatest colloid solution stability.

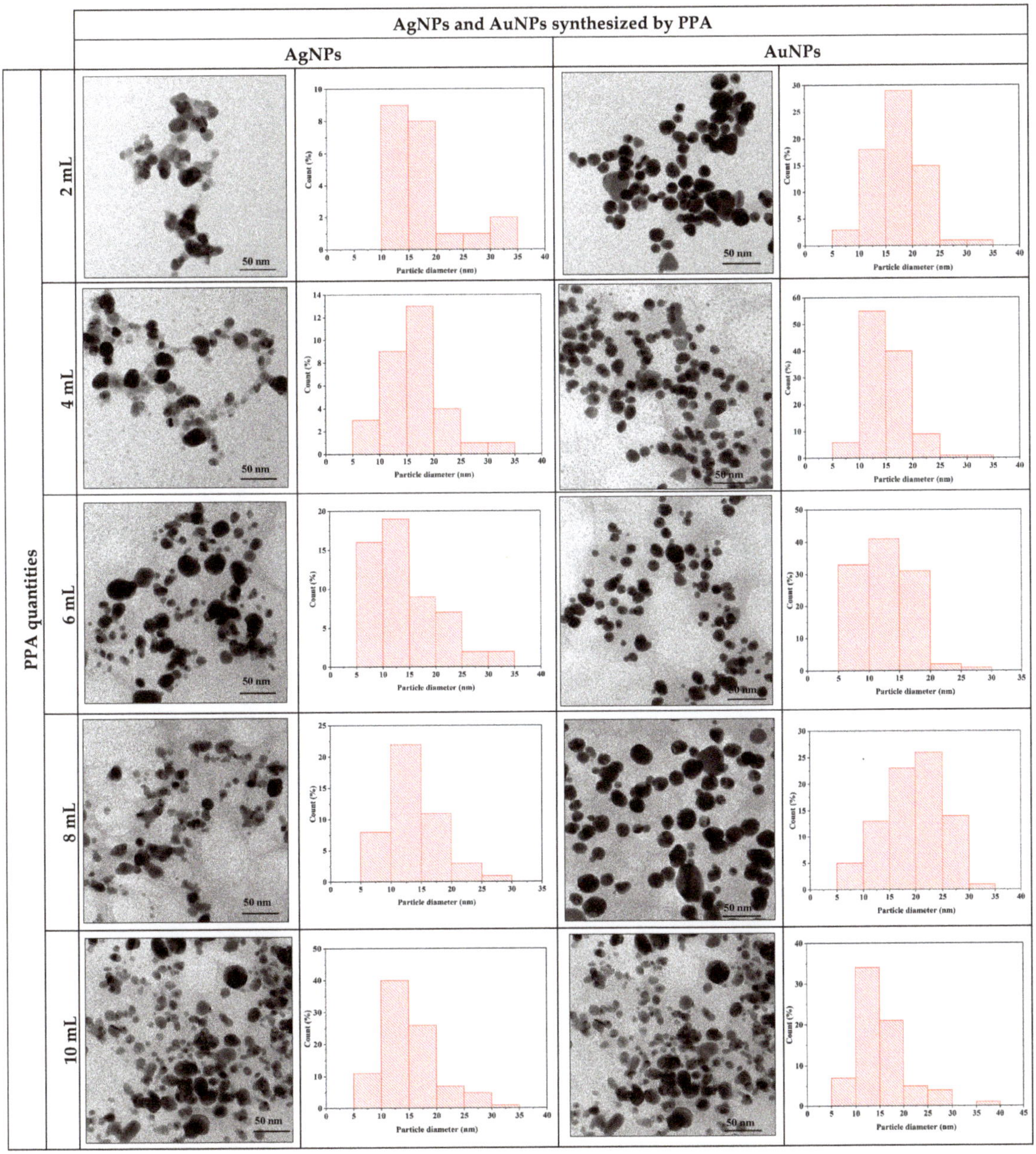

Figure 4. TEM image of biosynthesized AgNPs and AuNPs at different PPA quantities.

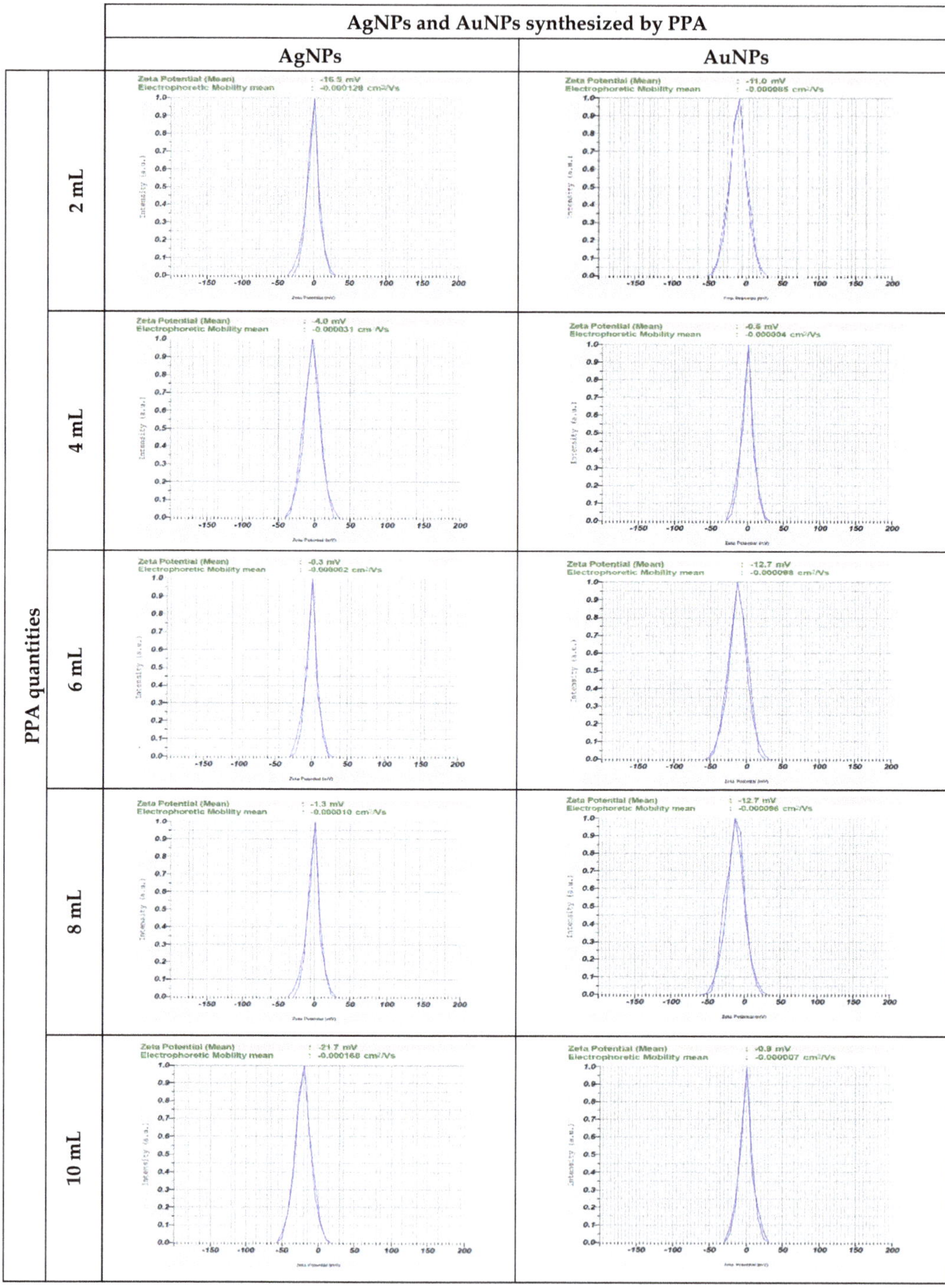

Figure 5. Zeta potential values of biosynthesized AgNPs and AuNPs at different PPA quantities.

2.2. Electrochemical Properties of AgNPs and AuNPs Modified Electrodes

The electrochemical properties of both bare screen-printed carbon electrodes (SPCE) and modified electrodes (AgNPs/SPCE and AuNPs/SPCE) were evaluated by comparing their electrochemical responses using cyclic voltammetry (CV) in a potassium chloride (KCl) solution with a 5 mM concentration of the redox probe $[Fe(CN)_6]^{3-/4-}$. The CV curves depicted in Figure 6a,b demonstrate that both the bare SPCEs and the modified electrodes exhibit reversible redox reactions, indicative of effective electron transfer at the electrode surfaces. The peak currents observed for the AgNPs/SPCE electrodes, prepared with 10 mL of phosphoric acid (PPA), and AuNPs/SPCE electrodes, prepared with 6 mL of PPA, were significantly higher than those recorded for the bare SPCE [66]. This enhancement can be attributed to several factors: firstly, the incorporation of nanoparticles increases the effective surface area of the electrodes, allowing for greater accessibility for the redox probe to the electrode surface. Secondly, the nanoparticles serve as catalytic sites that facilitate more efficient electron transfer processes. The morphology of the nanoparticles, as confirmed by transmission electron microscopy (TEM), indicates the presence of small, well-dispersed particles, which enhances the electroactive surface area. Additionally, the stability of the zeta potential values suggests that the modified electrodes maintain a favorable dispersion of nanoparticles, contributing to their electrochemical activity. These findings highlight the potential of using AgNPs and AuNPs to enhance the electrochemical performance of modified electrodes, paving the way for their application in the detection of biomolecules, such as human serum albumin (HSA). Prior to detection, antibodies can be immobilized on the AgNPs/SPCE and AuNPs/SPCE, as outlined in Section 3.7.

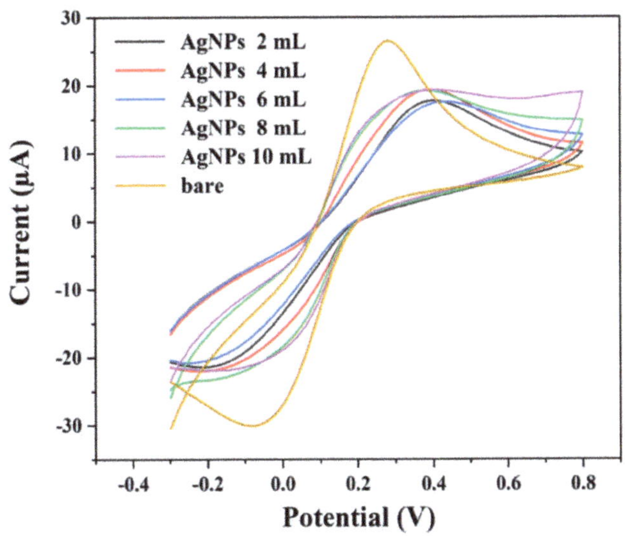

(a)

Figure 6. *Cont.*

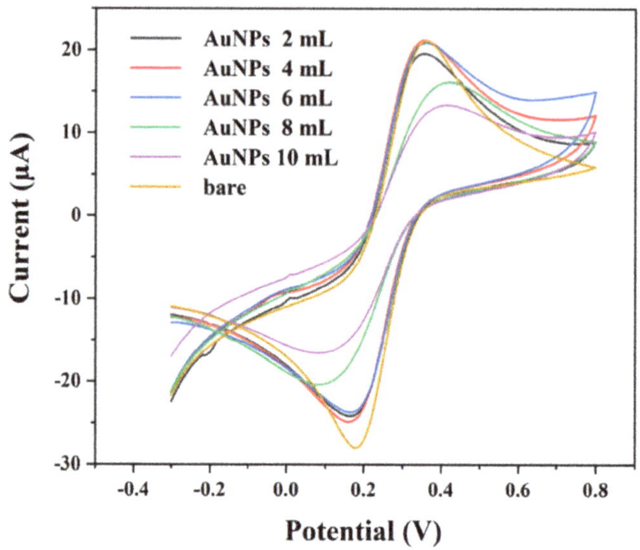

(b)

Figure 6. CV curves of bare SPCE with (**a**) AgNPs/SPCE and (**b**) AuNPs/SPCE. The scan rate is 0.1 Vs^{-1} in 5 mM $K_3Fe\ (CN)_6$ and 5 mM KCl in PBS (pH 7.4).

2.3. Electrochemical Detection of HSA

For the detection of human serum albumin (HSA), we used square-wave voltammetry (SWV) measurements, which are more sensitive than CV and are applicable to the qualitative determination of analyte concentrations. The different concentrations of HSA responses on the AgNP/SPCE/antibody HSA and AuNP/SPCE/antibody HSA electrodes are shown in Figure 7a,b, Within the investigated potential range (0–0.7 V), measurements revealed a peak position for the oxidation of HSA at −0.29 V. The graph shows that the concentration of HSA increased, but the position of the oxidation peak did not change, and it was found that current is related to the concentration of solution in detection. Figure 7c,d show a linear relationship between the peak current and HSA concentration obtained (HSA concentration of 10–400 μm/mL), with the linear regression equation being defined by Y = 0.03609X + 15.17787 (R^2 = 0.97468) for AgNP/SPCE/antibody HSA electrodes and Y = 0.01735X + 14.11654 (R^2 = 0.99221) for AuNP/SPCE/antibody HSA electrodes. Hence, the relative current measured in SWV demonstrated conclusively that HSA detection was successful.

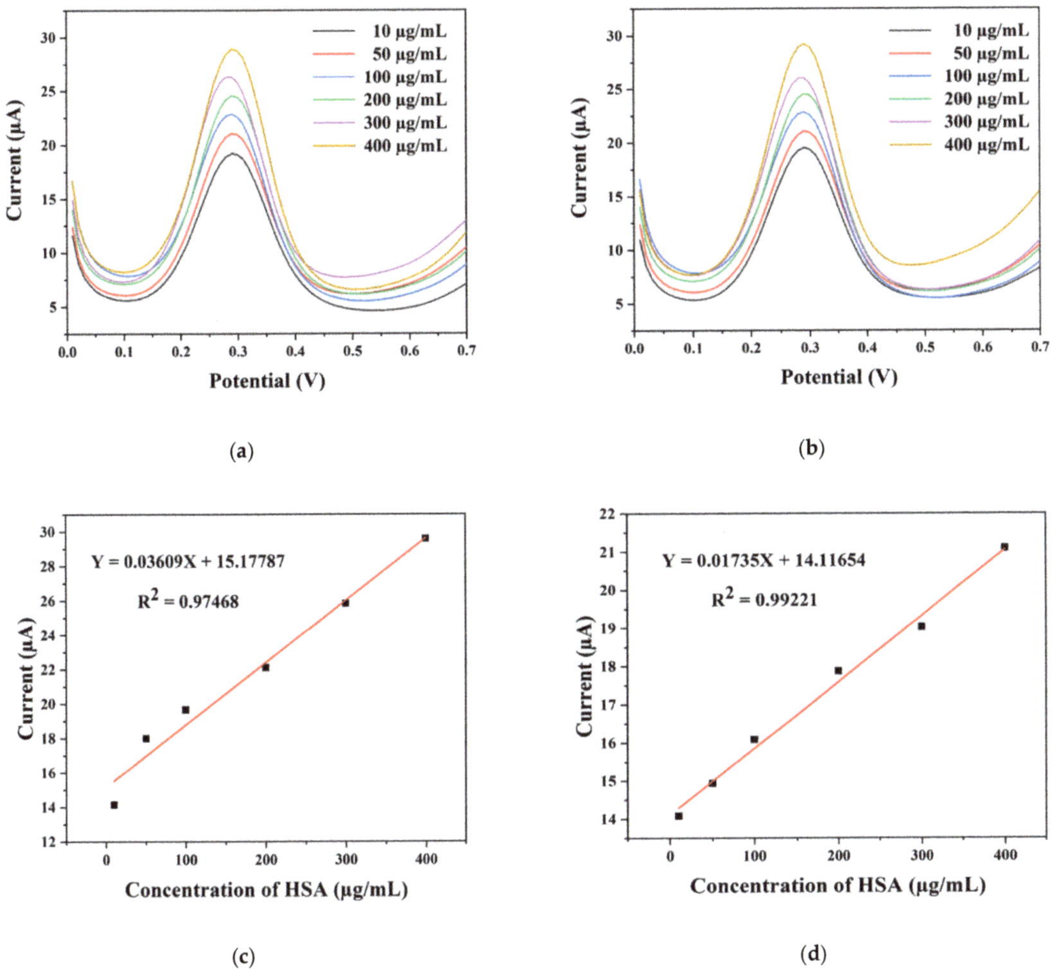

Figure 7. SWV curves of (**a**) AgNP/SPCE/antibody HSA and (**b**) AuNP/SPCE/antibody HSA for detection of different HSA concentrations (10–400 µm/mL). The relationship between the current vs. HSA concentrations for (**c**) AgNP/SPCE/antibody HSA and (**d**) AuNP/SPCE/antibody HSA.

3. Materials and Methods

3.1. Materials

Hydrogen tetrachloroaurate (III) hydrate ($HAuCl_4 \cdot 3H_2O$, 99.9%), anti-human serum albumin antibody, and human serum albumin (HSA) were purchased from Sigma Aldrich. Silver nitrate ($AgNO_3$, 99.9%) was purchased from QRëC. Phosphate buffer (0.1 M PBS, pH 7.4) was purchased from Apsalagen Co., Ltd. Screen-printed carbon electrodes (SPCE) and potassium ferricyanide ($K_3[Fe(CN)_6]$) were purchased from Quasense Co., Ltd., Thailand. Phulae pineapple was purchased from Iyara Market in Pathumthani Province, Thailand.

3.2. Preparation for Phulae Pineapple Peel Extract (PPA)

To obtain the fruit peel extract, Phulae pineapple peels were washed and cut into smaller pieces, and then were divided into two portions. For the first portion, 20 g of peel was added to 100 mL of deionized water (DI) and boiled. From the moment it started boiling, we waited for about 45–60 min and left it to cool fully covered. After that, the peel was removed by filtration to afford the extract. The peel extract was stored at 4 °C prior to use. For the second portion, it was dried at 80 °C. After drying completely, we crushed the pineapple peel and put it in a humidity chamber to be analyzed using FTIR to verify the presence of any phytochemicals in the plant extract.

3.3. Synthesis of Nanoparticles

AgNPs were synthesized by mixing 50 mL of $AgNO_3$ solution with a concentration of 3 mM with 2, 4, 6, 8, and 10 mL of PPA. The reaction mixture was magnetically stirred at 60 °C for 1 h, with the formation of AgNPs being observed by a color change to orange-brown. AuNPs were synthesized by mixing 27 mL of $HAuCl_4{\cdot}3H_2O$ solution with a concentration of 1 mM with 2, 4, 6, 8, and 10 mL of PPA. The reaction mixture was magnetically stirred at 100 °C for 15 min, with the formation of AuNPs being observed by a color change to purple. Both samples were taken to undergo UV-vis analysis, and the solution was centrifuged at 10,000 rpm for 15 min to remove any excess reagents and silver ions. The supernatant was discarded, and the resulting pellet was washed with doubly distilled water and then again centrifuged. This process was repeated three times. Subsequently, the purified pellets of synthesized AgNPs and AuNPs were dried at 80 °C in a vacuum oven before analysis by XRD and FTIR.

3.4. Characterization of Synthesized Nanoparticles

The optical absorbance nanoscale of the formed AgNPs and AuNPs was confirmed using UV-vis spectrophotometry (Thermo Scientific, GENESYS 10S UV-Vis) spanning a 300–800 nm wavelength range. The X-ray diffraction (XRD) patterns of crystalline structures were measured using a powder X-ray diffractometer (Bruker, D2 PHASER) equipped with CuKα radiation (1.54 Å) in the range of 20–80° in 2θ angles with a scan speed of 2°/min, voltage of 30 kV, and current of 10 mA. To detect organic functional groups contained in powdered Phulae pineapple peel samples and on the surface of nanoparticles, Fourier transform infrared spectrophotometer (FTIR) examinations were performed throughout a 4000–400 cm^{-1} range (Shimadzu, IRSpirit). The samples were prepared as KBr disks. Morphology was investigated using a transmission electron microscope (TEM) (JEOL, JEM-2010). The sample was dispersed in water at a controlled temperature of 25 °C, with the scattering angle set to 90° and the viscosity of the dispersion medium fixed at 0.89 mPa.s (Horiba, Nanopartica sz-100).

3.5. Measurements of Electrochemical Responses

Electrochemical experiments were performed using a PalmSens 4 with the PSTrace software 5.9 instrument. A screen-printed carbon electrode (SPCE) consists of three electrodes: the working electrode, a reference electrode (Ag/AgCl), and a counter electrode (carbon bases). Cyclic voltammetry (CV) and square-wave voltammetry (SWV) were used to measure the responses of the modified electrodes.

3.6. Preparation of Electrodes Modified with Nanoparticles

The electrode was prepared by dropping 3 µL of nanoparticles onto a screen-printed carbon electrode (SPCE) at the working electrode, which was then dried for 10 min at 40 °C (or at room temperature until it dried) before being used in detection experiments. The electrochemical response of modified electrodes, namely, AgNPs/SPCE and AuNPs/SPCE, was investigated using cyclic voltammetry (CV) with the following parameters: they were measured from 0.4–0.8 V at a scan rate of 0.1 V s^{-1} in 5 mM $K_3Fe\ (CN)_6$ and 5 mM KCl in PBS (pH 7.4).

3.7. Procedure for Detection of HSA

Select the electrode in Section 3.6 that provides the highest electric current signal. Coat the working electrode with 2 µL of the serum albumin antibody and then allow it to dry at room temperature (also called AgNPs/SPCE/antibody (HSA) and AuNPs/SPCE/antibody (HSA)).

Next, prepare human albumin solutions at 10, 50, 100, 200, 300, and 400 μg/mL, mix with electrolyte, and drop 5 μL onto AgNPs/SPCE/antibody (HSA) and AuNPs/SPCE/antibody (HSA) electrodes. Subsequently, the response was evaluated using square-wave voltammetry (SWV) at a frequency of 10.0 Hz and an amplitude of 0.05 V, with a measurement range of 0.0 to 0.7 V.

4. Conclusions

This study illustrates the feasibility and efficacy of electrochemical methods combined with AgNP- and AuNP-modified electrodes for sensitivity, high stability, good analytical performance, and specific HSA detection. This will lead to the development of efficient and inexpensive diagnostic tools for various kinds of diseases and health conditions.

Author Contributions: Conceptualization, K.P., B.T., P.P., S.T., R.J., S.-G.Y., Y.P., S.N. and C.P.; investigation, T.T. and R.C.; methodology, T.T., R.C., B.T. and P.P.; project administration, S.N. and C.P.; supervision, S.N. and C.P.; writing—original draft, T.T. All authors have read and agreed to the published version of the manuscript.

Funding: The research team would like to thank the Thammasat University Research Fund for granting the "Thammasat University Research Fund" (TUFT 72/2566).

Institutional Review Board Statement: Not applicable.

Informed Consent Statement: Not applicable.

Data Availability Statement: The datasets generated and/or analyzed during the current study are not publicly available but are available from the corresponding author upon reasonable request.

Acknowledgments: The research team appreciates the Graduate Development Scholarship (NRCT) from The National Research Council of Thailand for funding this research. In addition, for the provision of the facilities, tools, and equipment used in this research, we thank Rajamangala University of Technology Thanyaburi and Thammasat University.

Conflicts of Interest: The authors declare that they have no known competing financial interests or personal relationships that could have appeared to influence the work reported in this paper.

References

1. Tsai, J.Z.; Chen, C.J.; Settu, K.; Lin, Y.F.; Chen, C.L.; Liu, J.T. Screen-printed carbon electrode-based electrochemical immunosensor for rapid detection of microalbuminuria. *Biosens. Bioelectron.* **2016**, *77*, 1175–1182. [CrossRef] [PubMed]
2. Lin, S.Y.; Lin, C.Y. Electrochemically-functionalized CNT/ABTS nanozyme enabling sensitive and selective voltammetric detection of microalbuminuria. *Anal. Chim. Acta* **2022**, *1197*, 339517. [CrossRef] [PubMed]
3. Tseng, C.-C.; Ko, C.-H.; Lu, S.-Y.; Yang, C.-E.; Fu, L.-M.; Li, C.-Y. Rapid electrochemical-biosensor microchip platform for determination of microalbuminuria in CKD patients. *Anal. Chim. Acta* **2021**, *1146*, 70–76. [CrossRef]
4. Wang, H.; Wang, J.; Ma, G.; Zhou, J.; Du, L.; Wu, H.; Zhang, X.; He, Y.; Zhou, J. TICT-based turn-on deep-red fluorescent probe for endoplasmic reticulum targeted detection of serum albumin in kidney diseases. *Chem. Eng. J.* **2023**, *464*, 142551. [CrossRef]
5. Chawjiraphan, W.; Apiwat, C.; Segkhoonthod, K.; Treerattrakoon, K.; Pinpradup, P.; Sathirapongsasuti, N.; Pongprayoon, P.; Luksirikul, P.; Isarankura-Na-Ayudhya, P.; Japrung, D. Sensitive detection of albuminuria by graphene oxide-mediated fluorescence quenching aptasensor. *Spectrochim. Acta Part A Mol. Biomol. Spectrosc.* **2020**, *231*, 118128. [CrossRef] [PubMed]
6. Benesch, J.; Askendal, A.; Tengvall, P. Quantification of adsorbed human serum albumin at solid interfaces: A comparison between radioimmunoassay (RIA) and simple null ellipsometry. *Colloids Surf. B Biointerfaces* **2000**, *18*, 71–81. [CrossRef]
7. Magliano, D.J.; Polkinghorne, K.R.; Barr, E.L.M.; Su, Q.; Chadban, S.J.; Zimmet, P.Z.; Shaw, J.E.; Atkins, R.C. HPLC-detected albuminuria predicts mortality. *J. Am. Soc. Nephrol.* **2007**, *18*, 3171–3176. [CrossRef]
8. Shi, M.; Duan, X.; Zheng, X.; Lu, D.; Ge, Y.; Zhang, N.; Liu, Y.; You, J.; Xue, H.; Yin, L. Quantification of human serum albumin by combining chymotrypsin/trypsin digestion coupled with LC-MS/MS technique. *Anal. Biochem.* **2023**, *680*, 115316. [CrossRef] [PubMed]
9. Brede, C.; Hop, B.; Jørgensen, K.; Skadberg, Ø. Measurement of glycated albumin in serum and plasma by LC-MS/MS. *Scand. J. Clin. Lab. Investig.* **2016**, *76*, 195–201. [CrossRef]
10. Markó, L.; Molnár, G.A.; Wagner, Z.; Koszegi, T.; Matus, Z.; Mohás, M.; Kuzma, M.; Szijártó, I.A.; Wittmann, I. Analysis of microalbuminuria with immunonephelometry and high performance liquid chromatography. Evaluation of new criteria. *Orvosi Hetil.* **2008**, *149*, 59–67. [CrossRef]
11. Jiang, Z.; Huang, Y.; Liang, A.; Pan, H.; Liu, Q. Resonance scattering detection of trace microalbumin using immunonanogold probe as the catalyst of Fehling reagent–glucose reaction. *Biosens. Bioelectron.* **2009**, *24*, 1674–1678. [CrossRef] [PubMed]

12. Liao, B.-Y.; Chang, C.-J.; Wang, C.-F.; Lu, C.-H.; Chen, J.-K. Controlled antibody orientation on Fe_3O_4 nanoparticles and CdTe quantum dots enhanced sensitivity of a sandwich-structured electrogenerated chemiluminescence immunosensor for the determination of human serum albumin. *Sens. Actuators B Chem.* **2021**, *336*, 129710. [CrossRef]
13. Murtaza, G.; Rizvi, A.S.; Irfan, M.; Li, L.; Qu, F. Determination of glycated albumin in serum and saliva by capillary electrophoresis utilizing affinity of 3-acrylamido phenylboronic acid selected by virtual screening and molecular docking. *J. Chromatogr. A* **2021**, *1636*, 461793. [CrossRef] [PubMed]
14. Saeed, U.; Fatima, B.; Hussain, D.; Ashiq, R.; Naeem Ashiq, M.; Najam-ul-Haq, M. CoTe nanorods based electrochemical sensor for quantitative detection of albumin from chronic kidney disease patients. *J. Electroanal. Chem.* **2022**, *906*, 115999. [CrossRef]
15. Fatoni, A.; Numnuam, A.; Kanatharana, P.; Limbut, W.; Thavarungkul, P. A novel molecularly imprinted chitosan-acrylamide, graphene, ferrocene composite cryogel biosensor used to detect microalbumin. *Analyst* **2014**, *139*, 6160–6167. [CrossRef]
16. Tayyab Raza Naqvi, S.; Rasheed, T.; Naeem Ashiq, M.; Najam ul Haq, M.; Majeed, S.; Fatima, B.; Nawaz, R.; Hussain, D.; Shafi, S. Fabrication of iron modified screen printed carbon electrode for sensing of amino acids. *Polyhedron* **2020**, *180*, 114426. [CrossRef]
17. Taleat, Z.; Khoshroo, A.; Mazloum-Ardakani, M. Screen-printed electrodes for biosensing: A review (2008–2013). *Microchim. Acta* **2014**, *181*, 865–891. [CrossRef]
18. Stanković, V.; Đurđić, S.; Ognjanović, M.; Antić, B.; Kalcher, K.; Mutić, J.; Stanković, D.M. Anti-human albumin monoclonal antibody immobilized on EDC-NHS functionalized carboxylic graphene/AuNPs composite as promising electrochemical HSA immunosensor. *J. Electroanal. Chem.* **2020**, *860*, 113928. [CrossRef]
19. Shaikh, M.O.; Srikanth, B.; Zhu, P.-Y.; Chuang, C.-H. Impedimetric Immunosensor Utilizing Polyaniline/Gold Nanocomposite-Modified Screen-Printed Electrodes for Early Detection of Chronic Kidney Disease. *Sensors* **2019**, *19*, 3990. [CrossRef]
20. Omidfar, K.; Dehdast, A.; Zarei, H.; Sourkohi, B.K.; Larijani, B. Development of urinary albumin immunosensor based on colloidal AuNP and PVA. *Biosens. Bioelectron.* **2011**, *26*, 4177–4183. [CrossRef]
21. Ghosh Dastidar, M.; Murugappan, K.; RNisbet, D.; Tricoli, A. Simultaneous electrochemical detection of glycated and human serum albumin for diabetes management. *Biosens. Bioelectron.* **2024**, *246*, 115876. [CrossRef] [PubMed]
22. Choosang, J.; Thavarungkul, P.; Kanatharana, P.; Numnuam, A. AuNPs/PpPD/PEDOT:PSS-Fc modified screen-printed carbon electrode label-free immunosensor for sensitive and selective determination of human serum albumin. *Microchem. J.* **2020**, *155*, 104709. [CrossRef]
23. Lai, S.-Y.; Liu, J.-T.; Chen, C.-J.; Tsai, J.-Z. Detecting human serum albumin using screen-printed carbon electrode by cyclic voltammetry. *J. Microbiol. Immunol. Infect.* **2015**, *48* (Suppl. 1), S82. [CrossRef]
24. Shaikh, M.O.; Zhu, P.Y.; Wang, C.C.; Du, Y.C.; Chuang, C.H. Electrochemical immunosensor utilizing electrodeposited Au nanocrystals and dielectrophoretically trapped PS/Ag/ab-HSA nanoprobes for detection of microalbuminuria at point of care. *Biosens. Bioelectron.* **2019**, *126*, 572–580. [CrossRef] [PubMed]
25. Zhang, G.; Yu, Y.; Guo, M.; Lin, B.; Zhang, L. A sensitive determination of albumin in urine by molecularly imprinted electrochemical biosensor based on dual-signal strategy. *Sens. Actuators B Chem.* **2019**, *288*, 564–570. [CrossRef]
26. Smith, B.R.; Gambhir, S.S. Nanomaterials for In Vivo Imaging. *Chem. Rev.* **2017**, *117*, 901–986. [CrossRef]
27. Mahobiya, S.K.; Balayan, S.; Chauhan, N.; Rosario, W.; Kuchhal, N.K.; Islam, S.S.; Jain, U. Fabricating a rapid and low-cost electrochemical biosensor with imprints of glycated albumin molecules to detect diabetes using bimetallic Au-Pt nanoparticles on µSPE. *Appl. Surf. Sci. Adv.* **2023**, *16*, 100425. [CrossRef]
28. Thakkar, K.N.; Mhatre, S.S.; Parikh, R.Y. Biological synthesis of metallic nanoparticles. *Nanomedicine* **2010**, *6*, 257–262. [CrossRef]
29. Mittal, A.K.; Chisti, Y.; Banerjee, U.C. Synthesis of metallic nanoparticles using plant extracts. *Biotechnol. Adv.* **2013**, *31*, 346–356. [CrossRef]
30. Nande, A.; Raut, S.; Michalska-Domanska, M.; Dhoble, S.J. Green Synthesis of Nanomaterials Using Plant Extract: A Review. *Curr. Pharm. Biotechnol.* **2021**, *22*, 1794–1811.
31. Alabdallah, N.M.; Hasan, M.M. Plant-based green synthesis of silver nanoparticles and its effective role in abiotic stress tolerance in crop plants. *Saudi J. Biol. Sci.* **2021**, *28*, 5631–5639. [CrossRef] [PubMed]
32. Rodríguez-Félix, F.; Graciano-Verdugo, A.Z.; Moreno-Vásquez, M.J.; Lagarda-Díaz, I.; Barreras-Urbina, C.G.; Armenta-Villegas, L.; Olguín-Moreno, A.; Tapia-Hernández, J.A. Trends in Sustainable Green Synthesis of Silver Nanoparticles Using Agri-Food Waste Extracts and Their Applications in Health. *J. Nanomater.* **2022**, *2022*, 8874003. [CrossRef]
33. Nadaf, S.J.; Jadhav, N.R.; Naikwadi, H.S.; Savekar, P.L.; Sapkal, I.D.; Kambli, M.M.; Desai, I.A. Green synthesis of gold and silver nanoparticles: Updates on research, patents, and future prospects. *OpenNano* **2022**, *8*, 100076. [CrossRef]
34. Balkrishna, A.; Rohela, A.; Kumar, A.; Mishra, S.; Arya, V.; Kala, V.; Thakur, N.; Thakur, N.; Kumari, A.; Khan, N. Elucidating the Role of Plant Extracts Mediated Gold Nanoparticles as Smart Antimicrobials: Two-Way Attack. *J. Nanomater.* **2023**, *2023*, 4085090. [CrossRef]
35. Ashique, S.; Afzal, O.; Khalid, M.; Faruque Ahmad, M.; Upadhyay, A.; Kumar, S.; Garg, A.; Ramzan, M.; Hussain, A.; Altamimi, M.A.; et al. Biogenic nanoparticles from waste fruit peels: Synthesis, applications, challenges and future perspectives. *Int. J. Pharm.* **2023**, *643*, 123223.
36. Thu, S.L.; Tam, H.L.M.; Tongdeesoontorn, W.; Suthiluk, P. Quality changes and volatile compounds in fresh-cut 'phulae' pineapple during cold storage. *Curr. Appl. Sci. Technol.* **2017**, *17*, 162–171.
37. Techavuthiporn, C.; Boonyaritthongchai, P.; Supabvanich, S. Physicochemical changes of 'Phulae' pineapple fruit treated with short-term anoxia during ambient storage. *Food Chem.* **2017**, *228*, 388–393. [CrossRef]

38. Mahardika, D.P.; Yusrita, E.; Surya, A.; Juariah, S. Phytogenic silver nanoparticle (AgNP) from *Ananas comosus* (L) Merr. peel extract to inhibiting the pathogen resistance. *J. Phys. Conf. Ser.* **2021**, *1811*, 012124. [CrossRef]
39. Agnihotri, S.; Sillu, D.; Sharma, G.; Arya, R.K. Photocatalytic and antibacterial potential of silver nanoparticles derived from pineapple waste: Process optimization and modeling kinetics for dye removal. *Appl. Nanosci.* **2018**, *8*, 2077–2092. [CrossRef]
40. Das, G.; Patra, J.K.; Debnath, T.; Ansari, A.; Shin, H.S. Investigation of antioxidant, antibacterial, antidiabetic, and cytotoxicity potential of silver nanoparticles synthesized using the outer peel extract of *Ananas comosus* (L.). *PLoS ONE* **2019**, *14*, e0220950. [CrossRef]
41. Basavegowda, N.; Sobczak-Kupiec, A.; Malina, D.; Yathirajan, H.S.; Keerthi, V.R.; Chandrashekar, N.; Dinkar, S.; Liny, P. Plant Mediated Synthesis of Gold Nanoparticles Using Fruit Extracts of *Ananas comosus* (L.) (Pineapple) And Evaluation of Biological Activities. *Adv. Mater. Lett.* **2013**, *4*, 332–337. [CrossRef]
42. Hamdiani, S.; Shih, Y.-F. A Green Method for Synthesis of Silver-Nanoparticles-Diatomite (AgNPs-D) Composite from Pineapple (*Ananas comosus*) Leaf Extract. *Indones. J. Chem.* **2021**, *21*, 740. [CrossRef]
43. Huq, M.; Ashrafudoulla, M.; Rahman, M.M.; Balusamy, S.; Akter, S. Green Synthesis and Potential Antibacterial Applications of Bioactive Silver Nanoparticles: A Review. *Polymers* **2022**, *14*, 742. [CrossRef]
44. Ahmad, N. Green Synthesis of Silver Nanoparticles Using Extracts of Ananas comosus. *Green Sustain. Chem.* **2012**, *02*, 141–147. [CrossRef]
45. Pechyen, C.; Ponsanti, K.; Tangnorawich, B.; Ngernyuang, N. Waste fruit peel—Mediated green synthesis of biocompatible gold nanoparticles. *J. Mater. Res. Technol.* **2021**, *14*, 2982–2991. [CrossRef]
46. Alikhani, N.; Hekmati, M.; Karmakar, B.; Veisi, H. Green synthesis of gold nanoparticles (Au NPs) using Rosa canina fruit extractand evaluation of its catalytic activity in the degradation of organic dye pollutants of water. *Inorg. Chem. Commun.* **2022**, *139*, 109351. [CrossRef]
47. Kumari, P.; Meena, A. Green synthesis of gold nanoparticles from Lawsoniainermis and its catalytic activities following the Langmuir-Hinshelwood mechanism. *Colloids Surf. A Physicochem. Eng. Asp.* **2020**, *606*, 125447. [CrossRef]
48. Jaffar, S.S.; Saallah, S.; Misson, M.; Siddiquee, S.; Roslan, J.; Lenggoro, W. Green Synthesis of Flower-Like Carrageenan-Silver Nanoparticles and Elucidation of Its Physicochemical and Antibacterial Properties. *Molecules* **2023**, *28*, 907. [CrossRef]
49. Ning, T.; Luo, Y.; Liu, P.; Lu, A. A novel Ag nanoparticles purification method and the conductive ink based on the purified Ag nanoparticles for printed electronics. *J. Nanoparticle Res.* **2022**, *24*, 15. [CrossRef]
50. Vamshi, B.S.; Sharma, V.; Ahmad, W.; Kumar, V.; Sharma, S.; Joshi, N.C.; Hussain, A.; Kohli, D.; Shabaaz Begum, J.P.; Kumar, S. Green Synthesis of Silver Nanoparticles Generated by the Photoionization Process for Anti-biofilm Application. *Catal. Lett.* **2023**, *154*, 2151–2161. [CrossRef]
51. Alharbi, N.; Bhakyaraj, K.; Gopinath, K.; Govindarajan, M.; Kumaraguru, S.; Mohan, S.; Periyannan, K.; Km, S.; Khaled, J.; Benelli, G. Gum-Mediated Fabrication of Eco-Friendly Gold Nanoparticles Promoting Cell Division and Pollen Germination in Plant Cells. *J. Clust. Sci.* **2017**, *28*, 507–517. [CrossRef]
52. Gautam, P.; Kumar, S.; Singh, R.; Shyanti, R.; Swaroop, S.; Ram, B.; Chauhan, A. Biologically Synthesized Gold Nanoparticles using *Ocimum sanctum* (Tulsi Leaf Extract) Induced Anti-Tumor Response in a T Cell Daltons Lymphoma. *J. Cell Sci. Ther.* **2017**, *8*, 6. [CrossRef]
53. Rautela, A.; Rani, J.; Debnath, M. Green synthesis of silver nanoparticles from *Tectona grandis* seeds extract: Characterization and mechanism of antimicrobial action on different microorganisms. *J. Anal. Sci. Technol.* **2019**, *10*, 5. [CrossRef]
54. Willian, N.; Syukri, S.; Zulhadjri, Z.; Pardi, H.; Arief, S. Marine plant mediated green synthesis of silver nanoparticles using mangrove *Rhizophora stylosa*: Effect of variable process and their antibacterial activity. *F1000Res* **2021**, *10*, 768. [CrossRef] [PubMed]
55. Mondal, A.; Yadav, D.; Mitra, S.; Mukhopadhyay, K. Biosynthesis of Silver Nanoparticles Using Culture Supernatant of *Shewanella* sp. ARY1 and Their Antibacterial Activity. *Int. J. Nanomed.* **2020**, *15*, 8295–8310. [CrossRef]
56. Yang, H.; Ren, Y.-y.; Wang, T.; Wang, C. Preparation and antibacterial activities of Ag/Ag+/Ag3+ nanoparticle composites made by pomegranate (*Punica granatum*) rind extract. *Results Phys.* **2016**, *6*, 299–304. [CrossRef]
57. Poadang, S.; Yongvanich, N.; Phongtongpasuk, S. Synthesis, Characterization, and Antibacterial Properties of Silver Nanoparticles Prepared from Aqueous Peel Extract of Pineapple, Ananas comosus. *Chiang Mai Univ. J. Nat. Sci.* **2017**, *16*, 2. [CrossRef]
58. Tadesse, M.; Kasaw, E.; Lübben, J. Valorization of Banana Peel Using Carbonization: Potential Use in the Sustainable Manufacturing of Flexible Supercapacitors. *Micromachines* **2023**, *14*, 330. [CrossRef]
59. El-Nafaty, U.; Misau, I.; Abdulsalam, S. Biosorption and Kinetic Studies on Oil Removal from Produced Water Using Banana Peel. *Civ. Environ. Res.* **2013**, *3*, 125–136.
60. Klinbumrung, A.; Panya, R.; Pung-Ngama, A.; Nasomjai, P.; Saowalakmeka, J.; Sirirak, R. Green synthesis of ZnO nanoparticles by pineapple peel extract from various alkali sources. *J. Asian Ceram. Soc.* **2022**, *10*, 755–765. [CrossRef]
61. Rosales, E.; Escudero-Curiel, S.; Pazos, M.; Sanromán, M. Sustainable Removal of Cr(VI) by Lime Peel and Pineapple Core Wastes. *Appl. Sci.* **2019**, *9*, 1967. [CrossRef]
62. Machmudah, S.; Shiddiqi, Q.; Karisma, A.; Widiyastuti, W.; Diono, W.; Kanda, H.; Winardi, S.; Goto, M. Subcritical Water Extraction of Xanthone from Mangosteen (Garcinia mangostana Linn) Pericarp. *J. Adv. Chem. Eng.* **2015**, *5*, 1000117. [CrossRef]
63. Sengar, A.S.; Sunil, C.K.; Rawson, A.; Venkatachalapathy, N. Identification of volatile compounds, physicochemical and techno-functional properties of pineapple processing waste (PPW). *J. Food Meas. Charact.* **2022**, *16*, 1146–1158. [CrossRef]

64. Raut, R.W.; Mendhulkar, V.D.; Kashid, S.B. Photosensitized synthesis of silver nanoparticles using *Withania somnifera* leaf powder and silver nitrate. *J. Photochem. Photobiol. B Biol.* **2014**, *132*, 45–55. [CrossRef]
65. Pechyen, C.; Ponsanti, K.; Tangnorawich, B.; Ngernyuang, N. Biogenic synthesis of gold nanoparticles mediated by *Spondias dulcis* (Anacardiaceae) peel extract and its cytotoxic activity in human breast cancer cell. *Toxicol. Rep.* **2022**, *9*, 1092–1098. [CrossRef]
66. Le Nhat Trang, N.; Thi Nguyet Nga, D.; Hoang, V.T.; Ngo, X.D.; Tuyet Nhung, P.; Le, A.T. Bio-AgNPs-based electrochemical nanosensors for the sensitive determination of 4-nitrophenol in tomato samples: The roles of natural plant extracts in physicochemical parameters and sensing performance. *RSC Adv.* **2022**, *12*, 6007–6017. [CrossRef]

pharmaceuticals

MDPI

Review

Synthesis and Application of Silver Nanoparticles for Caries Management: A Review

Iris Xiaoxue Yin, Veena Wenqing Xu, Grace Yuchan Xu, Ollie Yiru Yu, John Yun Niu and Chun Hung Chu *

Faculty of Dentistry, University of Hong Kong, Hong Kong, China; irisxyin@hku.hk (I.X.Y.); u3008489@connect.hku.hk (V.W.X.); gracexu1@connect.hku.hk (G.Y.X.); ollieyu@hku.hk (O.Y.Y.); niuyun@hku.hk (J.Y.N.)
* Correspondence: chchu@hku.hk

Abstract: Silver nanoparticles have unique physical, chemical, and biological properties that make them attractive for medical applications. They have gained attention in dentistry for their potential use in caries management. This study reviews the different synthesis methods of silver nanoparticles and the application of them for caries management. Silver nanoparticles are tiny silver and are typically less than 100 nanometres in size. They have a high surface area-to-volume ratio, making them highly reactive and allowing them to interact with bacteria and other materials at the molecular level. Silver nanoparticles have low toxicity and biocompatibility. Researchers have employed various methods to synthesise silver nanoparticles, including chemical, physical, and biological methods. By controlling the process, silver nanoparticles have defined sizes, shapes, and surface properties for wide use. Silver nanoparticles exhibit strong antibacterial properties, capable of inhibiting a broad range of bacteria, including antibiotic-resistant strains. They inhibit the growth of cariogenic bacteria, such as *Streptococcus mutans*. They can disrupt bacterial cell membranes, interfere with enzyme activity, and inhibit bacterial replication. Silver nanoparticles can inhibit biofilm formation, reducing the risk of caries development. Additionally, nano silver fluoride prevents dental caries by promoting tooth remineralisation. They can interact with the tooth structure and enhance the deposition of hydroxyapatite, aiding in repairing early-stage carious lesions. Silver nanoparticles can also be incorporated into dental restorative materials such as composite resins and glass ionomer cements. The incorporation can enhance the material's antibacterial properties, reducing the risk of secondary caries and improving the longevity of the restoration.

Keywords: silver nanoparticles; caries; nanoparticles synthesis; antimicrobial properties

1. Introduction

Dental caries, also known as tooth decay, is a chronic illness caused by various factors, such as cariogenic microorganisms, fermentable carbohydrates, tooth surfaces, and the passage of time [1]. Enamel is the hardest substance in human tissue. It still can undergo dissolution in acidic oral environments, leading to the destruction of tooth structure and the formation of dental caries.

Dental caries is the most prevalent chronic oral disease and the fourth most expensive to treat worldwide, according to the World Health Organisation [2]. Dental caries is hard in terms of self-limitation. If left untreated, dental caries can advance, causing discomfort, infection, and tooth loss. Fortunately, preventive strategies have been considerably progressed in recent decades. Various dental materials, including metals, ceramics, polymers, and hybrids, are employed for caries management [3–5].

Nanotechnology has revealed potential in the development of anti-caries agents through the utilisation of nanoparticles [6]. Nanoparticles are tiny particles with sizes ranging from 1 nm to 100 nm [7]. They possess unique physical properties, such as homogeneity, conductivity, or distinctive optical properties, which make them desirable in the fields of biology and material science.

The biomedical activities of nanoparticles differ from those of regular size due to their high surface area-to-volume ratios [8]. The development of nanoparticles for medical care is a critical aspect of nanotechnology applications. The use of nanoparticles has had a significant impact on people's health and daily lives over the past decades.

Among the various types of nanoparticles, silver nanoparticles have exhibited substantial potential in biomedical applications [9]. Silver nanoparticles can enhance medical imaging by providing more detailed visual representations of cellular processes, aiding in medical diagnostics by serving as molecular contrast agents, and improving drug delivery by increasing solubility and bioavailability [10–12]. In cancer therapies, silver nanoparticles can eliminate drug-resistant tumour cells and enhance the effectiveness of treatment by targeting and transporting anticancer medications specifically to tumour tissues [13].

Silver nanoparticles are also recognised for their exceptional antimicrobial properties, low toxicity, and cost-effectiveness. They can be used at low doses and do not promote microbial resistance [14]. Various antimicrobial actions have been proposed to explain the reason for the excellent antibacterial effect of silver nanoparticles [15]. Silver nanoparticles release silver ions that penetrate microbial membranes, causing disruption to DNA replication and protein synthesis. Respiratory enzymes may also be activated by silver ions, which can result in cell lysis. Silver nanoparticles can accumulate in the pits of cell walls and denature the cell envelopment. Additionally, they can infiltrate microbial cell walls and cytoplasmic membranes, resulting in the destruction of both the cell wall and cytoplasmic membrane [16].

Researchers have investigated using silver nanoparticles to improve the antimicrobial effect of dental materials for clinical use [17]. For caries management, researchers have developed silver nanoparticles using various synthesis strategies. The synthesised silver nanoparticles have shown enormous potential in managing dental caries by preventing biofilm formation and regulating the balance between demineralisation and remineralisation.

Silver nanoparticles enhance dental adhesives and orthodontic brackets for preventing enamel caries, a common orthodontic treatment complication [18]. Incorporating silver nanoparticles into restorative materials can effectively prevent secondary caries, a prevalent factor contributing to restoration failure. Nonetheless, a thorough investigation of silver nanoparticles synthesised for caries management is required. The objective of this study is to present a succinct review of silver nanoparticles synthesised for caries management.

2. Synthesis of Silver Nanoparticles

Researchers have employed various methods to synthesise silver nanoparticles, which can be divided into chemical, physical, and biological synthesis methods. The chemical reduction method is the most prevalent method to synthesise silver nanoparticles for caries management. Reducing agents, such as sodium borohydride, ascorbic acid, or citric acid, reduce silver ions to silver nanoparticles.

Researchers are also exploring physical and biological methods, such as laser ablation and green synthesis using plant extracts or microorganisms, as alternative approaches [19]. Controlling the process allows for low-cost synthesis of homogenous silver nanoparticles with controlled size, morphology, and function for dental applications. Table 1 summarises the advantages and disadvantages of chemical, physical, and biological synthesis methods for developing silver nanoparticles.

Table 1. Chemical, biological, and physical synthesis methods for silver nanoparticles for caries management.

Methods (Ref.)	Reaction Conditions	Advantages	Disadvantages
Chemical Methods (*Common methods to synthesise silver nanoparticles*)			
Chemical reduction [20]	• Silver precursors • Reducing agents • Stabilising agents	• High yield • Simple and low-cost method	• Toxic chemicals • Low purity • Toxic byproducts
Cryochemical synthesis [21]	• Silver precursors • Reducing agents • Stabilising agents • Low temperature	• Narrow size distribution • Little particle agglomeration	• Specialised equipment • Time-consuming process • Low yield
Electrochemical reduction [22]	• Silver precursors • Reducing agents • Stabilising agents • Electrodes	• Precise control over particle size • Precise control over particle shape • High yield • Simple and low-cost method	• Toxic chemicals • Wide size distribution • Low purity
Sonochemical synthesis [23]	• Silver precursors • Reducing agents • Stabilising agents • Ultrasound irradiation	• Narrow size distribution • High yield	• Specialised equipment • High energy consumption • Risk of agglomeration
Photoinduced reduction [24]	• Silver precursors • Reducing agents • Stabilising agents • Light irradiation	• Simple and low-cost method • Precise control over particle size • Precise control over particle shape • High purity of nanoparticles	• Toxic chemicals • Low yield
Thermal decomposition [25]	• Silver complex • Reducing agents • Stabilising agents • High temperature • Inert gas atmosphere	• Simple and low-cost method • High purity of nanoparticles • Narrow size distribution • High yield	• High energy consumption • Toxic byproducts • Limited size control
Biological Method (*alternative method to synthesise silver nanoparticles*)			
Bio-reduction [26,27]	• Silver precursors • Bio-reducing agents • Bio-stabilising agents	• Environmentally friendly • Sustainability • Biocompatible and non-toxic.	• Low yield • Limited size control
Physical Methods (*Less frequently used methods to synthesise silver nanoparticles*)			
Laser ablation [19]	• Silver bulk • Laser irradiation	• High purity of nanoparticles • Narrow size distribution • No chemical reducing agents	• High energy consumption • Specialised equipment • Low yield
Evaporation-condensation [28]	• Silver precursors • Organic solvents • High temperature • Vacuum conditions	• Low-cost method • High yield	• Wide size distribution • Low purity
Electrical irradiation [29]	• Silver precursors • Electrical current	• High yield • Narrow size distribution • No chemicals reducing agents	• High energy consumption • Specialised equipment • Potential toxic byproduct

Table 1. *Cont.*

Methods (Ref.)	Reaction Conditions	Advantages	Disadvantages
Gamma irradiation [30]	• Silver precursors • Gamma irradiation	• High yield • Narrow size distribution • No chemicals reducing agents	• High energy consumption • Specialised equipment • Risk of radiation hazards
Lithography [31]	• Silver precursors • Photoresist • Developer • Photolithography • Etching • UV irradiation	• Precise control of particle size • Precise control of particle shape • High purity of nanoparticles • Narrow size distribution	• Specialised equipment • Time-consuming process • Low yield

2.1. Chemical Methods

Chemical methods are one of the most common ways to synthesise silver nanoparticles due to their simple operation [32]. To synthesise silver nanoparticles, chemical methods use water or organic solvents. This procedure typically uses three primary constituents, including silver precursors, reducing agents, and stabilising/capping agents [33]. For the chemical synthesis of silver nanoparticles, silver nitrate commonly serves as a silver precursor due to its desirable characteristics, including its low cost. Various chemical reducing agents can reduce silver ions to silver nanoparticles, such as sodium citrate, ascorbate, sodium borohydride, and elemental hydrogen [34]. The reduction of silver salts essentially consists of two stages: nucleation and subsequent growth. Silver ions receive electrons from reducing agents and are subsequently converted to metallic form. The metallic silver then agglomerates to form silver nanoparticles. Thus, chemical methods are basically a "bottom-up" approach to synthesising silver nanoparticles. Utilising protective agents is crucial for stabilising dispersive nanoparticles during the synthesis process [35]. The stabilising agents absorb onto or bind to the surfaces of nanoparticles, protecting them from aggregation. Surfactants with various functionalities, such as thiols, amines, acids, and alcohols, can cap on the surfaces of silver nanoparticles to enhance their stability and protect them from sedimentation, agglomeration, or losing their defining surface characteristics [36].

Chemical methods have a significant advantage in terms of high yield in contrast to physical methods. Chemical methods require more practical and convenient apparatus compared to physical and biological methods [10]. Nevertheless, the produced nanoparticles may not achieve the anticipated level of purity, as their surfaces were detected to be contaminated with chemicals. Furthermore, the production of silver nanoparticles with precisely determined sizes is challenging, necessitating an additional procedure to avoid particle aggregation. Moreover, the chemical substances employed in the production of silver nanoparticles, including citrate, borohydride, and thio-glycerol, are toxic and hazardous [37,38].

To address the shortcomings of traditional chemical reduction methods, researchers developed alternative methods, such as cryochemical synthesis, electrochemical reduction, sonochemical synthesis, photoinduced reduction, and thermal decomposition methods. Cryochemical synthesis is a method using low-temperature chemical processes to develop nanomaterials [21]. The low-temperature condition minimises the potential for oxidation or other chemical reactions and produces silver nanoparticles with a high degree of purity. Electrochemical reduction is a technique reducing silver ions to silver nanoparticles at the electrode surface by potentiostatic or galvanostatic polarisation [22]. Adjusting electrochemical parameters allows for large-scale production of silver nanoparticles, with control over nanoparticle size and shape.

Sonochemical synthesis uses ultrasound to generate acoustic cavitation in liquid, which leads to high pressure and temperature followed by a high rate of cooling [23].

It can synthesise shape- and size-selective nanoparticles. Photoinduced reduction uses different light sources, such as ultraviolet, white, blue, cyan, green, and orange light, to initiate the reduction reaction of silver ions [24]. This method allows for precise control of the reaction kinetics and results in highly uniform nanoparticles. Furthermore, the photoinduced method has the ability to transform silver nanospheres into triangular silver nanocrystals [39]. Thermal decomposition uses high temperatures to decompose the silver complex to produce silver nanoparticles [25]. It is an efficient technique for the large-scale production of silver nanoparticles.

Researchers have used chemical methods to synthesise silver nanoparticles on graphene oxide. These silver nanoparticle composites are chemically stable and exhibit antibacterial activity against cariogenic bacteria. They inhibit the progression of enamel caries [20]. Chemically synthesised silver nanoparticles can be combined with fluoride to form nano silver fluoride. Studies have reported that nano silver fluoride inhibited cariogenic bacteria and prevented early childhood caries [40,41]. Furthermore, researchers incorporated chemically synthesised silver nanoparticles into resin composites and glass ionomer cement. They used fissure sealant containing silver nanoparticles to inhibit demineralisation and promote remineralisation [42]. Researchers also coated the chemically synthesised silver nanoparticles on orthodontic brackets to prevent enamel caries [43].

2.2. Biological Methods

To address the chemical methods' limitations, biological methods have emerged as viable alternatives. Biological methods, which avoid the involvement of toxic and hazardous chemicals in the synthesis process of silver nanoparticles, have received significant attention in the last decade [44]. The biochemical-mediated synthesis of silver nanoparticles has demonstrated its simplicity, cost-effectiveness, reliability, and environmental friendliness [45]. The synthesis of silver nanoparticles with controllable sizes was achieved by employing biological materials such as bacteria, fungi, plant extracts, and small biomolecules. Studies have reported the biological synthesis of silver nanoparticles using green, cost-effective, and biocompatible methods without the use of toxic chemicals. Bacteria such as *Pseudomonas stutzeri*, *Lactobacillus strains*, and *Bacillus licheniformis* can be used as biomaterials to produce silver nanoparticles [46–48]. The formation of silver nanoparticles can occur on the surface of the cytoplasmic cell membrane, inside the cytoplasm, and outside of the cells. It might be because of the bio-reduction of the silver ions by enzymes in the cytoplasm and on the cytoplasmic membrane [45].

It is possible for the silver nuclei that are synthesised outside of the cell wall to enter the cell and combine into larger-sized nanoparticles. Fungi have also been investigated for the synthesis of silver nanoparticles, for example, *Fusarium oxysporum* and *Aspergillus flavus* [49]. The bio-reduction of the silver ions takes place on the surface of the fungi. Proteins play a role in the formation and stabilisation of silver nanoparticles. The plant extracts from green tea, alfalfa, lemongrass, and geranium are abundant in polyphenols and flavonoids. They can be reductants to reduce silver ions, as well as scaffolds to direct the formation of silver nanoparticles [26,27,50]. Biologically synthesised silver nanoparticles using plant extracts may have stronger antibacterial properties than chemically synthesised silver nanoparticles using reductants such as sodium borohydride [51]. Plant extracts exhibit antibacterial properties against cariogenic bacteria. They can synergistically inhibit bacteria with silver nanoparticles. Additionally, plant extracts can stabilise and prevent the aggregation of silver nanoparticles, maintaining the antibacterial properties [52].

Researchers have also used biopolymers, proteins/enzymes, amino acids, and polysaccharides to synthesise silver nanoparticles [53]. These biomaterials allow researchers to control the shape, size, and homogeneity of nanoparticles. The advantages of biological methods include a wide variety of biological resources, reduced time required, high density, stability, and the promising solubility of synthesised nanoparticles in aqueous solutions. Importantly, they are ecologically and financially sustainable with minimal toxicity.

Researchers have synthesised silver nanoparticles using tea extract as a bio-reducing agent, which can impede biofilm formation on dentine surfaces [26]. They have also synthesised nano silver fluoride using glucose. The nano silver fluoride can promote dentine remineralisation [54]. Furthermore, researchers have synthesised silver nanoparticles on an orthodontic elastomeric module using plant extract to prevent enamel caries. This orthodontic elastomeric module can inhibit cariogenic bacteria without compromising physical properties [55].

2.3. Physical Methods

Physical methods for synthesising silver nanoparticles include laser ablation, evaporation-condensation, electrical irradiation, gamma irradiation, and lithography. Laser ablation and evaporation-condensation are the commonly used physical methods for nanoparticle synthesis. Without chemical reagents in solution, laser ablation of bulk silver can produce silver nanoparticles [19]. This approach enables the preparation of pure and uncontaminated metal colloids for subsequent applications. The evapouration-condensation method involves the evapouration of a silver-containing solution followed by the condensation of the vapour to form silver nanoparticles [28]. This method can produce high-purity silver nanoparticles because there are no reducing or stabilising agents during the synthesis process. Although laser ablation and evapouration-condensation have the benefit of not requiring hazardous reducing or stabilising agents, both methods have drawbacks such as low yield, high energy consumption, and a lack of uniform distribution. Electrical irradiation uses high-energy electrical discharges to produce plasma, which then interacts with a silver-containing solution to produce silver nanoparticles [29]. This method can yield silver nanoparticles efficiently, but it requires the use of toxic gases. Gamma irradiation uses high-energy gamma rays to reduce silver ions to form nanoparticles [30]. The lithography method uses lithographic techniques to selectively deposit silver onto specifically patterned areas [31].

Physical methods have been less frequently used to synthesise silver nanoparticles for caries management. Researchers have used the evapouration-condensation method to synthesise silver nanoparticle-loaded amorphous calcium phosphate. They incorporated nanocomposite into dental adhesive to prevent secondary caries [56].

3. Silver Nanoparticles Application for Caries Management

Silver nanoparticles have the potential to manage dental caries. Researchers have utilised silver nanoparticles in toothpaste to prevent caries [57]. The combined use of silver nanoparticles and fluoride can remineralise and halt enamel and dentine caries [58]. Silver nanoparticles have been incorporated into restorative materials, including filling resins and adhesives, to inhibit secondary caries [59,60]. The addition of silver nanoparticles into glass ionomer cements can prevent dental caries [61]. According to a clinical trial, a dental sealant containing silver nanoparticles was more effective than a conventional sealant in preventing enamel caries in the first permanent molars [42]. In addition, orthodontic brackets were coated with silver nanoparticles to guard against enamel caries [62]. Researchers have also incorporated silver nanoparticles into the resin of orthodontic materials, including adhesives, elastomeric ligatures, and removable retainers, to prevent caries. Glass ionomers with silver nanoparticles can prevent enamel caries as orthodontic cements.

Researchers have applied silver nanoparticles to teeth to prevent dental caries because silver nanoparticles inhibit bacterial growth and biofilm formation (Figure 1). Moreover, silver nanoparticles can infiltrate and lodge into dentinal tubules without aggregation on the dentine surface [63]. They can remain in the dentine structure as a stable and continuous source of silver ions to prevent bacterial invasion. The depth of silver nanoparticles' infiltration increases with longer exposure times and smaller nanoparticle size. This mechanism explains the long-term anti-caries effectiveness of silver nanoparticles reported in clinical trials [40].

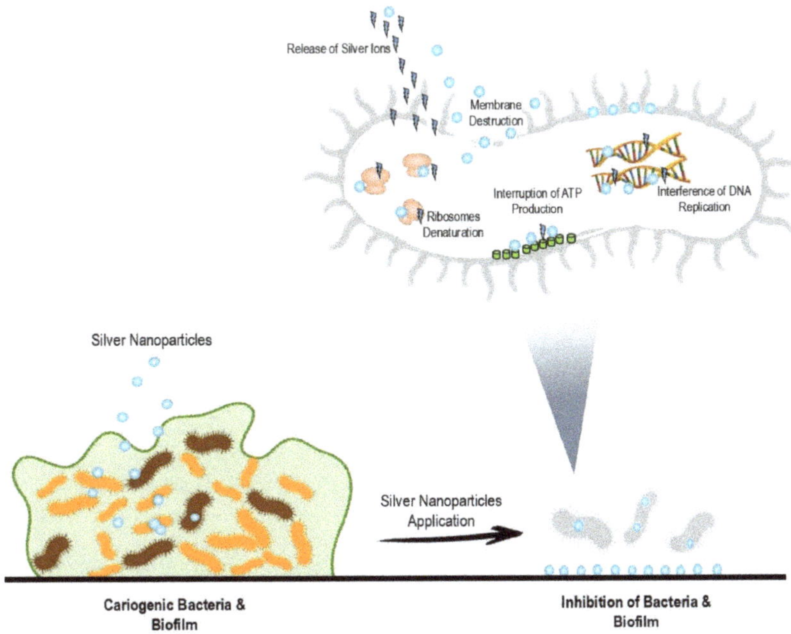

Figure 1. The inhibitory effects of silver nanoparticles on bacterial growth and biofilm formation.

Glass ionomer cement is a commonly used restorative material that releases fluoride for remineralisation. Nevertheless, cariogenic bacteria can invade when microleakage occurs between the tooth and glass ionomer cement interface [64]. The fluoride released from glass ionomer cement is insufficient to suppress bacterial growth. Therefore, researchers have incorporated silver nanoparticles into glass ionomer cement to reduce biofilm formation and prevent secondary caries. Additionally, glass ionomer cement exhibits inferior wear resistance because of voids in the cement matrix. These voids can act as stress raisers and eventually weaken the mechanical properties of the glass ionomer cement. The incorporation of silver nanoparticles into glass ionomer cement can reduce voids. Silver nanoparticles improve the packing of particles within the cement matrix, leading to a more homogeneous and denser structure. Moreover, silver nanoparticles can occupy the empty spaces between the large glass particles and provide an additional bonding site. Researchers have found that silver nanoparticle-containing glass ionomer cement has improved flexural and compressive strengths [65]. The concentration of silver nanoparticles in glass ionomer cement can affect the interaction of glass ionomer cement with the tooth structure. Several studies have shown that using less than 0.5% silver nanoparticles in glass ionomer cement improves its mechanical properties. When the concentration exceeds 0.5%, silver nanoparticles can affect the bond strength of glass ionomer cement with the tooth [65].

Resin composite is another commonly used restorative material with favourable aesthetic and adhesive properties. However, the polymerisation shrinkage of resin composite adversely affects the longevity of restoration. It causes interfacial defects and the marginal microleakage of resin composite [66]. Resin composite lacks antibacterial properties. Thus, biofilm can form on resin composite resulting in secondary caries. The incorporation of silver nanoparticles into resin composite provides antibacterial properties without compromising the mechanical properties. Silver nanoparticles can be well dispersed in the bond interfaces of resin composite without agglomeration. Moreover, silver nanoparticles less than 20 nm in size could infiltrate and occlude dentinal tubules [67]. Silver nanoparticles can also prevent the destruction of bond strength by reducing acid produced by bacteria.

3.1. Effect of Silver Nanoparticles on Cariogenic Bacteria

Silver nanoparticles have antibacterial properties against cariogenic bacteria, including *Streptococcus*, *Lactobacillus*, and *Pseudomonas*. *Streptococcus mutans* is the most common cariogenic bacterium found in carious lesions [68]. It is associated with the initiation and development of caries. This bacterium is the most used bacteria for examining the antibacterial efficacy of silver nanoparticles in caries therapy. Silver nanoparticles kill cariogenic bacteria in all studies. However, the findings regarding the minimum inhibitory concentration of silver nanoparticles against cariogenic bacteria varied in different studies [6].

Bacteria gather inside the extracellular matrix to form biofilm. Biofilms can augment the resistance of microbes to antimicrobial drugs by obstructing the transit of drugs. Consequently, the inhibitory impact of biofilm adherence is essential for assessing the antibacterial properties of silver nanoparticles. Single-species biofilm is commonly employed to examine the inhibition properties of silver nanoparticles because of its stability and operational simplicity [26]. Nonetheless, single-species biofilm significantly differs from dental biofilm in vivo. The dental biofilm is a complex biological system consisting of more than 1000 bacterial species [69]. Therefore, some researchers have suggested using the extraction of various microorganisms and the extracellular matrix from patients to culture the microcosm. It can convincingly replicate the intricacy and diversity of the biological biofilm found in the human oral cavity. Therefore, researchers have frequently selected the microcosm model to investigate the antibacterial impact of silver nanoparticles [70].

Researchers have also demonstrated the antimicrobial effect of silver nanoparticles against oral microcosms. Silver nanoparticles can decrease the metabolic activity, lactic acid production, and glucosyltransferase gene expression of biofilm [26,71]. While the microcosm model is unable to completely replicate the real-life oral environment, an in-situ model remains essential for assessing the effectiveness of anti-biofilm measures. Thus, some studies use animal tests or clinical trials to determine the authentic antimicrobial efficiency of silver nanoparticles.

Different antibacterial actions have been suggested, even though the exact mechanism of silver nanoparticles' antibacterial effects has not been fully revealed (Figure 1). Silver nanoparticles can continuously release silver ions. Silver ions can increase the permeability of the cell membrane and destroy the bacteria envelopment [72]. After silver ions enter the cell membrane, they can deactivate respiratory enzymes and inhibit adenosine triphosphate production. Furthermore, silver ions suppress deoxyribonucleic acid replication and then impact protein synthesis. Silver nanoparticles can eradicate bacteria on their own in addition to releasing silver ions. Silver nanoparticles can anchor and accumulate in the pits of the cell wall [73]. Additionally, the cell membrane becomes denatured when silver nanoparticles accumulate on it. Silver nanoparticles penetrate bacterial cell walls and cause structural damage in the cell membrane due to the nanoscale size of silver nanoparticles.

The antibacterial properties of silver nanoparticles against cariogenic bacteria are dependent on their specific properties. The silver nanoparticles of smaller sizes have a stronger antibacterial effect against cariogenic bacteria [74]. Due to their higher surface-to-volume ratios, smaller silver nanoparticles have a higher propensity to release silver ions. The increased release of silver ions from silver nanoparticles promotes their inhibition effect against the bacteria. Moreover, silver nanoparticles can penetrate dentinal tubules and adhere to their walls. The smaller the silver nanoparticles, the deeper their penetration. The penetration of silver nanoparticles into dentinal tubules may explain their long-term antibacterial effect on dentine surfaces. Furthermore, capping agents have an impact on the anti-cariogenic bacterial activity of silver nanoparticles [75]. The surface modification of silver nanoparticles by capping agents alters the dissolving efficiency of the nanoparticles. The positively charged silver nanoparticles exhibit a significant level of bacterial activity against *Streptococcus mutans* [76]. The cellular membranes of cariogenic bacteria such as *Streptococcus mutans* are negatively charged. Cariogenic bacteria attract positively charged silver nanoparticles due to their mutual electrostatic attraction. Silver nanoparticles effectively suppress both gram-positive and gram-negative bacteria. Generally, gram-positive bacteria are more resistant to silver nanoparticles than gram-negative bacteria [77,78]. Gram-negative bacteria have an outer cell membrane. It serves as a barrier to inhibit the entry of antibiotics into the cells. However, silver nanoparticles can pass through this barrier because of their nanoscale. Silver nanoparticles can disrupt the outer membrane and increase permeability. Furthermore, gram-positive bacteria have a thicker peptidoglycan layer in their cell wall to reduce damage induced by silver nanoparticles.

The formation of biofilm is rapid in the oral environment. The biofilm can significantly hinder the movement of silver nanoparticles. Thus, biofilm can protect bacteria from impact. Research indicates that bacterial viability can be preserved in biofilm after the treatment of silver nanoparticles. Although, at the same concentration, silver nanoparticles can eliminate all planktonic bacteria [17]. Because of its complicated architecture, the biofilm is tolerant of silver nanoparticles. Silver nanoparticles of different sizes, shapes, and synthesis methods have diverse diffusion coefficients. The mobility of silver nanoparticles in biofilm is closely related to their diffusion coefficients [79]. The diffusion coefficient is negatively correlated with the particle's size. Silver nanoparticles of large sizes find it harder to penetrate biofilm than those of small sizes. Transport through biofilm can be significantly hindered for particles larger than 50 nm. The surface charge and modification of silver nanoparticles can influence their diffusion in biofilm by causing absorption and aggregation. The biofilm can electrostatically interact with charged silver nanoparticles and hinder their penetration of biofilm [80]. Meanwhile, the increased concentration of silver nanoparticles in materials improved their antibacterial properties.

3.2. *Effects of Silver Nanoparticles on Enamel and Dentine*

Silver nanoparticles can inhibit tooth demineralisation under acidic or cariogenic conditions. Researchers have found that silver nanoparticles can make the carious lesion on sound enamel shallower during biofilm challenging. In addition, enamel with artificial caries treated with silver nanoparticles increased in terms of microhardness. Thus, the topical use of silver nanoparticles reduced mineral loss and prevented dental caries on both sound and demineralised enamel [81]. This inhibition effect on demineralisation can be attributed to the suppression of acid production in biofilm by silver nanoparticles. In dentine caries, collagen exposure occurs after the dissolution of mineral content. Silver nanoparticles can protect exposed collagen [82]. The exposed collagen is subject to degradation by bacterial collagenases, as well as proteinases present in saliva and the dentine matrix. Silver nanoparticles can deactivate these enzymes for the conservation of dentine collagen. Then, the conserved collagen can promote remineralisation by acting as a framework for mineral crystal formation. A study using a chemical model found that silver nanoparticles increased the microhardness of enamel caries [83]. Silver nanoparticles have the capability to infiltrate carious lesions and adhere to hydroxyapatite crystals. Moreover, the released silver ions from silver nanoparticles can produce insoluble silver chloride on dental hard tissue [58]. The insoluble silver chloride and precipitated silver nanoparticles raise the mineral density of enamel and dentine.

Even though silver nanoparticles have a positive effect on dental hard tissue, fluoride has a more promising remineralising effect than silver nanoparticles do. Fluoride has been widely used for caries management in practice. Fluoride can react with calcium ions and hydrogen phosphate ions to produce fluorapatite and fluorhydroxyapatite. These chemicals exhibit greater resistance to acidity compared to hydroxyapatite. Therefore, the combination use of silver nanoparticles and fluoride (nano silver fluoride) can enhance the remineralising effect of tooth structure [58]. The microhardness of sound enamel treated with nano silver fluoride is comparable to that of sodium fluoride-treated enamel. Nano silver fluoride also exhibited efficacy on enamel with carious lesions. Nano silver fluoride exhibited a stronger effect on arresting enamel caries than sodium fluoride in the microhardness test. However, optic coherence tomography is unable to distinguish the variation in mineral composition between decayed enamel treated with nano silver fluoride and sodium fluoride. A clinical investigation showed that nano silver fluoride is as efficient at preventing dental cavities in children as silver diamine fluoride [84]. While nano silver fluoride did not show a significant staining effect on a carious lesion, silver diamine fluoride dyed it black. Moreover, the use of silver nanoparticles in restorative materials prevented demineralisation. A resin with silver nanoparticles increased the microhardness of dentine caries after acid challenge [85]. In addition, a clinical trial demonstrated that dental sealant containing silver nanoparticles effectively reduced mineral loss in children's molars. Nevertheless, some studies did not specify the precise amounts of silver nanoparticles used in their investigations. Therefore, further investigation is required to examine the optimal concentrations of silver nanoparticles for caries prevention.

4. Potential Risk

Despite the potential benefits of using silver nanoparticles to prevent dental caries, some risks and concerns need to be addressed. High concentrations of silver nanoparticles can lead to inflammation, oxidative stress, and cell damage [86]. Researchers have explored the nontoxic and low-toxic range of silver nanoparticles' concentrations to safely use. The size, surface charge, and functionalisation of silver nanoparticles can influence their toxicity. It is crucial to optimise the silver nanoparticles' size and surface modification to ensure safety and biocompatibility. To minimise toxicity, researchers have developed silver nanoparticles using capping agents. Capped silver nanoparticles displayed lower toxicity than uncapped silver nanoparticles when used on human cells. The widespread use of silver nanoparticles may also raise concerns about their potential environmental impact. Silver nanoparticles can enter the environment through wastewater systems, leading to the accumulation of silver in water bodies, soil, and organisms [86]. The long-term effects of this accumulation on ecosystems and human health are still unknown. To minimise their environmental impact, it is essential to develop strategies for the safe disposal and recycling of dental materials containing silver nanoparticles.

5. Conclusions

Silver nanoparticles inhibit bacteria growth and biofilm formation and hence impede the demineralisation of enamel and dentine. Researchers have synthesised silver nanoparticles using chemical, physical, and biological methods for caries management. They incorporated silver nanoparticles into topical fluoride agents and restorative dental materials for caries prevention.

Author Contributions: Conceptualization, I.X.Y. and C.H.C.; methodology, I.X.Y. and V.W.X.; investigation, I.X.Y. and G.Y.X.; data curation, I.X.Y. and O.Y.Y.; writing—original draft preparation, I.X.Y.; writing—review and editing, I.X.Y. and J.Y.N.; supervision, C.H.C. All authors have read and agreed to the published version of the manuscript.

Funding: This study was supported by the Health and Medical Research Fund (HMRF 19180782 and 22210782) from the Food and Health Bureau of the Hong Kong Government.

Institutional Review Board Statement: Not applicable.

Data Availability Statement: Not applicable.

Conflicts of Interest: The authors declare no conflicts of interest.

References

1. Manji, F.; Dahlen, G.; Fejerskov, O. Caries and periodontitis: Contesting the conventional wisdom on their aetiology. *Caries Res.* **2018**, *52*, 548–564. [CrossRef] [PubMed]
2. Peres, M.A.; Macpherson, L.M.; Weyant, R.J.; Daly, B.; Venturelli, R.; Mathur, M.R.; Listl, S.; Celeste, R.K.; Guarnizo-Herreño, C.C.; Kearns, C. Oral diseases: A global public health challenge. *Lancet* **2019**, *394*, 249–260. [CrossRef] [PubMed]
3. Niu, J.Y.; Yin, I.X.; Wu, W.K.K.; Li, Q.-L.; Mei, M.L.; Chu, C.H. Antimicrobial peptides for the prevention and treatment of dental caries: A concise review. *Arch. Oral Biol.* **2021**, *122*, 105022. [CrossRef]
4. Nizami, M.Z.I.; Xu, V.W.; Yin, I.X.; Yu, O.Y.; Chu, C.-H. Metal and metal oxide nanoparticles in caries prevention: A review. *Nanomaterials* **2021**, *11*, 3446. [CrossRef]

5. Zhang, O.L.; Niu, J.Y.; Yin, I.X.; Yu, O.Y.; Mei, M.L.; Chu, C.H. Bioactive materials for caries management: A literature review. *Dent. J.* **2023**, *11*, 59. [CrossRef]
6. Yin, I.X.; Zhao, I.S.; Mei, M.L.; Li, Q.; Yu, O.Y.; Chu, C.H. Use of silver nanomaterials for caries prevention: A concise review. *Int. J. Nanomed.* **2020**, *15*, 3181–3191. [CrossRef] [PubMed]
7. Khan, I.; Saeed, K.; Khan, I. Nanoparticles: Properties, applications and toxicities. *Arab. J. Chem.* **2019**, *12*, 908–931. [CrossRef]
8. McNamara, K.; Tofail, S.A. Nanoparticles in biomedical applications. *Adv. Phys. X* **2017**, *2*, 54–88. [CrossRef]
9. Yaqoob, A.A.; Ahmad, H.; Parveen, T.; Ahmad, A.; Oves, M.; Ismail, I.M.I.; Qari, H.A.; Umar, K.; Mohamad Ibrahim, M.N. Recent Advances in Metal Decorated Nanomaterials and Their Various Biological Applications: A Review. *Front. Chem.* **2020**, *8*, 341. [CrossRef]
10. Xu, L.; Wang, Y.-Y.; Huang, J.; Chen, C.-Y.; Wang, Z.-X.; Xie, H. Silver nanoparticles: Synthesis, medical applications and biosafety. *Theranostics* **2020**, *10*, 8996. [CrossRef]
11. Aslan, N.; Ceylan, B.; Koç, M.M.; Findik, F. Metallic nanoparticles as X-Ray computed tomography (CT) contrast agents: A review. *J. Mol. Struct.* **2020**, *1219*, 128599. [CrossRef]
12. Tang, L.; Mei, Y.; Shen, Y.; He, S.; Xiao, Q.; Yin, Y.; Xu, Y.; Shao, J.; Wang, W.; Cai, Z. Nanoparticle-mediated targeted drug delivery to remodel tumor microenvironment for cancer therapy. *Int. J. Nanomed.* **2021**, *16*, 5811–5829. [CrossRef] [PubMed]
13. Oves, M.; Ahmar Rauf, M.; Aslam, M.; Qari, H.A.; Sonbol, H.; Ahmad, I.; Sarwar Zaman, G.; Saeed, M. Green synthesis of silver nanoparticles by *Conocarpus Lancifolius* plant extract and their antimicrobial and anticancer activities. *Saudi J. Biol. Sci.* **2022**, *29*, 460–471. [CrossRef] [PubMed]
14. Dos Santos, E.M.P.; Martins, C.C.B.; de Oliveira Santos, J.V.; da Silva, W.R.C.; Silva, S.B.C.; Pelagio-Flores, M.A.; Galembeck, A.; Cavalcanti, I.M.F. Silver nanoparticles–chitosan composites activity against resistant bacteria: Tolerance and biofilm inhibition. *J. Nanopart. Res.* **2021**, *23*, 196. [CrossRef]
15. Mikhailova, E.O. Silver nanoparticles: Mechanism of action and probable bio-application. *J. Funct. Biomater.* **2020**, *11*, 84. [CrossRef]
16. Hamida, R.S.; Ali, M.A.; Goda, D.A.; Redhwan, A. Anticandidal potential of two cyanobacteria-synthesized silver nanoparticles: Effects on growth, cell morphology, and key virulence attributes of *Candida albicans*. *Pharmaceutics* **2021**, *13*, 1688. [CrossRef]
17. Yin, I.X.; Zhang, J.; Zhao, I.S.; Mei, M.L.; Li, Q.; Chu, C.H. The antibacterial mechanism of silver nanoparticles and its application in dentistry. *Int. J. Nanomed.* **2020**, *15*, 2555–2562. [CrossRef]
18. Alam, M.K.; Alsuwailem, R.; Alfawzan, A.A. Antibacterial activity and bond strength of silver nanoparticles modified orthodontic bracket adhesive: A systematic review and meta-analysis of in-vitro and in-vivo studies. *Int. J. Adhes. Adhes.* **2022**, *113*, 103040. [CrossRef]
19. Rafique, M.; Rafique, M.S.; Kalsoom, U.; Afzal, A.; Butt, S.H.; Usman, A. Laser ablation synthesis of silver nanoparticles in water and dependence on laser nature. *Opt. Quantum Electron.* **2019**, *51*, 179. [CrossRef]
20. Wu, R.; Zhao, Q.; Lu, S.; Fu, Y.; Yu, D.; Zhao, W. Inhibitory effect of reduced graphene oxide-silver nanocomposite on progression of artificial enamel caries. *J. Appl. Oral. Sci.* **2018**, *27*, e20180042. [CrossRef]
21. Sergeev, G.B. Cryochemistry of metal nanoparticles. *J. Nanopart. Res.* **2003**, *5*, 529–537. [CrossRef]
22. Treshchalov, A.; Erikson, H.; Puust, L.; Tsarenko, S.; Saar, R.; Vanetsev, A.; Tammeveski, K.; Sildos, I. Stabilizer-free silver nanoparticles as efficient catalysts for electrochemical reduction of oxygen. *J. Colloid Interface Sci.* **2017**, *491*, 358–366. [CrossRef] [PubMed]
23. Vinoth, V.; Wu, J.J.; Asiri, A.M.; Anandan, S. Sonochemical synthesis of silver nanoparticles anchored reduced graphene oxide nanosheets for selective and sensitive detection of glutathione. *Ultrason. Sonochem.* **2017**, *39*, 363–373. [CrossRef] [PubMed]
24. Maduraimuthu, V.; Ranishree, J.K.; Gopalakrishnan, R.M.; Ayyadurai, B.; Raja, R.; Heese, K. Antioxidant activities of photoinduced phycogenic silver nanoparticles and their potential applications. *Antioxidants* **2023**, *12*, 1298. [CrossRef] [PubMed]
25. Hosseinpour-Mashkani, S.M.; Ramezani, M. Silver and silver oxide nanoparticles: Synthesis and characterization by thermal decomposition. *Mater. Lett.* **2014**, *130*, 259–262. [CrossRef]
26. Yin, I.X.; Yu, O.Y.; Zhao, I.S.; Mei, M.L.; Li, Q.-L.; Tang, J.; Chu, C.-H. Developing biocompatible silver nanoparticles using epigallocatechin gallate for dental use. *Arch. Oral Biol.* **2019**, *102*, 106–112. [CrossRef]
27. Logeswari, P.; Silambarasan, S.; Abraham, J. Synthesis of silver nanoparticles using plants extract and analysis of their antimicrobial property. *J. Saudi Chem. Soc.* **2015**, *19*, 311–317. [CrossRef]
28. Sakono, N.; Ishida, Y.; Ogo, K.; Tsumori, N.; Murayama, H.; Sakono, M. Molar-fraction-tunable synthesis of Ag–Au Alloy Nanoparticles via a dual evaporation–condensation method as supported catalysts for CO oxidation. *ACS Appl. Nano Mater.* **2023**, *6*, 3065–3074. [CrossRef]
29. Kang, H.S.; Kim, B.; Park, J.H.; Kim, H.W.; Koo, Y.H.; Bae, H.B.; Park, C.; Lee, B.C. Size control technology of silver nanoparticles using electron beam irradiation. *Bull. Korean Chem. Soc.* **2013**, *34*, 3899–3902. [CrossRef]
30. Afify, T.; Saleh, H.; Ali, Z. Structural and morphological study of gamma-irradiation synthesized silver nanoparticles. *Polym. Compos.* **2017**, *38*, 2687–2694. [CrossRef]
31. Kabusure, K.M.; Piskunen, P.; Yang, J.; Kataja, M.; Chacha, M.; Ojasalo, S.; Shen, B.; Hakala, T.K.; Linko, V. Optical characterization of DNA origami-shaped silver nanoparticles created through biotemplated lithography. *Nanoscale* **2022**, *14*, 9648–9654. [CrossRef] [PubMed]

32. Vishwanath, R.; Negi, B. Conventional and green methods of synthesis of silver nanoparticles and their antimicrobial properties. *Curr. Res. Green Sustain. Chem.* **2021**, *4*, 100205. [CrossRef]
33. Patil, S.; Ganeshpurkar, A.; Shrotriya, S.; Sawant, P.; Mulgund, S. Small size silver nanoparticles loaded with glycoside rich portion of *Boerhavia Diffusa* Linn. promotes wound healing: In-silico and in-vivo studies. *Colloids Surf. B Biointerfaces* **2023**, *230*, 113483. [CrossRef] [PubMed]
34. Nguyen, N.P.U.; Dang, N.T.; Doan, L.; Nguyen, T.T.H. Synthesis of silver nanoparticles: From conventional to 'modern' methods—A review. *Processes* **2023**, *11*, 2617. [CrossRef]
35. Rónavári, A.; Bélteky, P.; Boka, E.; Zakupszky, D.; Igaz, N.; Szerencsés, B.; Pfeiffer, I.; Kónya, Z.; Kiricsi, M. Polyvinyl-pyrrolidone-coated silver nanoparticles—The colloidal, chemical, and biological consequences of steric stabilization under biorelevant conditions. *Int. J. Mol. Sci.* **2021**, *22*, 8673. [CrossRef]
36. Guerrini, L.; Alvarez-Puebla, R.A.; Pazos-Perez, N. Surface modifications of nanoparticles for stability in biological fluids. *Materials* **2018**, *11*, 1154. [CrossRef]
37. Monchi, M. Citrate pathophysiology and metabolism. *Transfus. Apher. Sci.* **2017**, *56*, 28–30. [CrossRef]
38. Khatoon, U.T.; Velidandi, A.; Rao, G.N. Sodium borohydride mediated synthesis of nano-sized silver particles: Their characterization, anti-microbial and cytotoxicity studies. *Mater. Chem. Phys.* **2023**, *294*, 126997. [CrossRef]
39. An, J.; Tang, B.; Ning, X.; Zhou, J.; Xu, S.; Zhao, B.; Xu, W.; Corredor, C.; Lombardi, J.R. Photoinduced shape evolution: From triangular to hexagonal silver nanoplates. *J. Phys. Chem. C* **2007**, *111*, 18055–18059. [CrossRef]
40. Santos, V.E., Jr.; Vasconcelos Filho, A.; Targino, A.G.; Flores, M.A.; Galembeck, A.; Caldas, A.F., Jr.; Rosenblatt, A. A new "silver-bullet" to treat caries in children—Nano silver fluoride: A randomised clinical trial. *J. Dent.* **2014**, *42*, 945–951. [CrossRef]
41. Targino, A.G.; Flores, M.A.; dos Santos Junior, V.E.; de Godoy Bené Bezerra, F.; de Luna Freire, H.; Galembeck, A.; Rosenblatt, A. An innovative approach to treating dental decay in children. A new anti-caries agent. *J. Mater. Sci. Mater. Med.* **2014**, *25*, 2041–2047. [CrossRef] [PubMed]
42. Salas-López, E.K.; Pierdant-Pérez, M.; Hernández-Sierra, J.F.; Ruíz, F.; Mandeville, P.; Pozos-Guillén, A.J. Effect of silver nanoparticle-added pit and fissure sealant in the prevention of dental caries in children. *J. Clin. Pediatr. Dent.* **2017**, *41*, 48–52. [CrossRef]
43. Jasso-Ruiz, I.; Velazquez-Enriquez, U.; Scougall-Vilchis, R.J.; Morales-Luckie, R.A.; Sawada, T.; Yamaguchi, R. Silver nanoparticles in orthodontics, a new alternative in bacterial inhibition: In vitro study. *Prog. Orthod.* **2020**, *21*, 24. [CrossRef] [PubMed]
44. Qayyum, S.; Oves, M.; Khan, A.U. Obliteration of bacterial growth and biofilm through ROS generation by facilely synthesized green silver nanoparticles. *PLoS ONE* **2017**, *12*, e0181363. [CrossRef] [PubMed]
45. Poulose, S.; Panda, T.; Nair, P.P.; Theodore, T. Biosynthesis of silver nanoparticles. *J. Nanosci. Nanotechnol.* **2014**, *14*, 2038–2049. [CrossRef]
46. Bachii, S.A.; Abd-Al Sahib, W.H. Preparation and characterization of silver nanoparticles biosynthesis by *Pseudomonas stutzeri* environmental bacteria isolated from oil fields and their antimicrobial activity. *Sci. J. Med. Res.* **2021**, *5*, 7–15.
47. Naseer, Q.; Xue, X.; Wang, X.; Dang, S.; Din, S.; Jamil, J. Synthesis of silver nanoparticles using *Lactobacillus bulgaricus* and assessment of their antibacterial potential. *Braz. J. Biol.* **2021**, *82*, e232434. [CrossRef]
48. Kalishwaralal, K.; Deepak, V.; Ramkumarpandian, S.; Nellaiah, H.; Sangiliyandi, G. Extracellular biosynthesis of silver nanoparticles by the culture supernatant of *Bacillus licheniformis*. *Mater. Lett.* **2008**, *62*, 4411–4413. [CrossRef]
49. Durán, N.; Marcato, P.D.; Alves, O.L.; De Souza, G.I.; Esposito, E. Mechanistic aspects of biosynthesis of silver nanoparticles by several *Fusarium oxysporum* strains. *J. Nanobiotechnol.* **2005**, *3*, 8. [CrossRef]
50. Oves, M.; Rauf, M.A.; Qari, H.A. Therapeutic Applications of Biogenic Silver Nanomaterial Synthesized from the Paper Flower of *Bougainvillea glabra* (Miami, Pink). *Nanomater.* **2023**, *13*, 615. [CrossRef]
51. Majoumouo, M.S.; Sibuyi, N.R.S.; Tincho, M.B.; Mbekou, M.; Boyom, F.F.; Meyer, M. Enhanced Anti-Bacterial Activity of Biogenic Silver Nanoparticles Synthesized from *Terminalia mantaly* Extracts. *Int. J. Nanomed.* **2019**, *14*, 9031–9046. [CrossRef] [PubMed]
52. Urnukhsaikhan, E.; Bold, B.E.; Gunbileg, A.; Sukhbaatar, N.; Mishig-Ochir, T. Antibacterial activity and characteristics of silver nanoparticles biosynthesized from *Carduus crispus*. *Sci. Rep.* **2021**, *11*, 21047. [CrossRef] [PubMed]
53. Lateef, A.; Ojo, S.; Azeez, M.; Asafa, T.; Yekeen, T.; Akinboro, A.; Oladipo, I.; Gueguim-Kana, E.; Beukes, L. Cobweb as novel biomaterial for the green and eco-friendly synthesis of silver nanoparticles. *Appl. Nanosci.* **2016**, *6*, 863–874. [CrossRef]
54. Soekanto, S.A.; Fadillah, F.; Nuraisiya, P.; Gultom, F.; Sarwono, A.T. The potential of several fluoride-based varnishes as remineralization agents: Morphological studies, dentin surface hardness, and crystallinity tests. *Int. J. Appl. Pharm.* **2017**, *9*, 60–66. [CrossRef]
55. Hernández-Gómora, A.E.; Lara-Carrillo, E.; Robles-Navarro, J.B.; Scougall-Vilchis, R.J.; Hernández-López, S.; Medina-Solís, C.E.; Morales-Luckie, R.A. Biosynthesis of Silver Nanoparticles on Orthodontic Elastomeric Modules: Evaluation of Mechanical and Antibacterial Properties. *Molecules* **2017**, *22*, 1407. [CrossRef]
56. Keskar, M.; Sabatini, C.; Cheng, C.; Swihart, M.T. Synthesis and characterization of silver nanoparticle-loaded amorphous calcium phosphate microspheres for dental applications. *Nanoscale Adv.* **2019**, *1*, 627–635. [CrossRef] [PubMed]
57. Ahmed, O.A.K.; Sibuyi, N.R.S.; Fadaka, A.O.; Maboza, E.; Olivier, A.; Madiehe, A.M.; Meyer, M.; Geerts, G. Prospects of using gum Arabic silver nanoparticles in toothpaste to prevent dental caries. *Pharmaceutics* **2023**, *15*, 871. [CrossRef]
58. Zhao, I.S.; Yin, I.X.; Mei, M.L.; Lo, E.C.M.; Tang, J.; Li, Q.; So, L.Y.; Chu, C.H. Remineralising dentine caries using sodium fluoride with silver nanoparticles: An in vitro study. *Int. J. Nanomed.* **2020**, *15*, 2829–2839. [CrossRef]

59. Zhang, N.; Melo, M.A.; Chen, C.; Liu, J.; Weir, M.D.; Bai, Y.; Xu, H.H. Development of a multifunctional adhesive system for prevention of root caries and secondary caries. *Dent. Mater.* **2015**, *31*, 1119–1131. [CrossRef]
60. Yang, Y.; Ding, Y.; Fan, Y.; Ren, L.; Tang, X.; Meng, X. Application of silver nanoparticles in situ synthesized in dental adhesive resin. *Int. J. Adhes. Adhes.* **2021**, *108*, 102890. [CrossRef]
61. Chen, J.; Zhao, Q.; Peng, J.; Yang, X.; Yu, D.; Zhao, W. Antibacterial and mechanical properties of reduced graphene-silver nanoparticle nanocomposite modified glass ionomer cements. *J. Dent.* **2020**, *96*, 103332. [CrossRef] [PubMed]
62. Espinosa-Cristóbal, L.F.; López-Ruiz, N.; Cabada-Tarín, D.; Reyes-López, S.Y.; Zaragoza-Contreras, A.; Constandse-Cortéz, D.; Donohué-Cornejo, A.; Tovar-Carrillo, K.; Cuevas-González, J.C.; Kobayashi, T. Antiadherence and antimicrobial properties of silver nanoparticles against *Streptococcus mutans* on brackets and wires used for orthodontic treatments. *J. Nanomater.* **2018**, *2018*, 9248527. [CrossRef]
63. de Andrade, M.C.M.; Rosenblatt, A.; Galembeck, A. Silver nanoparticles penetration in dentin: Implications for long-term caries arrestment. *Materialia* **2022**, *24*, 101489. [CrossRef]
64. Nasr, R.A.; Saber, H. MicroTensile Bond Strength of Glass Ionomer Cement to Silver Fluoride and Potassium Iodide-Treated Carious Primary Dentin. *Egypt. Dent. J.* **2020**, *66*, 815–827. [CrossRef]
65. Abed, F.M.; Kotha, S.B.; AlShukairi, H.; Almotawah, F.N.; Alabdulaly, R.A.; Mallineni, S.K. Effect of different concentrations of silver nanoparticles on the quality of the chemical bond of glass ionomer cement dentine in primary teeth. *Front. Bioeng. Biotechnol.* **2022**, *10*, 816652. [CrossRef]
66. Boruziniat, A.; Gharaee, S.; Shirazi, A.S.; Majidinia, S.; Vatanpour, M. Evaluation of the efficacy of flowable composite as lining material on microleakage of composite resin restorations: A systematic review and meta-analysis. *Quintessence Int.* **2016**, *47*.
67. Wang, J.; Jiang, W.; Liang, J.; Ran, S. Influence of silver nanoparticles on the resin-dentin bond strength and antibacterial activity of a self-etch adhesive system. *J. Prosthet. Dent.* **2022**, *128*, 1363.e1–1363.e10. [CrossRef] [PubMed]
68. Forssten, S.D.; Björklund, M.; Ouwehand, A.C. Streptococcus mutans, caries and simulation models. *Nutrients* **2010**, *2*, 290–298. [CrossRef]
69. Marsh, P.; Zaura, E. Dental biofilm: Ecological interactions in health and disease. *J. Clin. Periodontol.* **2017**, *44*, S12–S22. [CrossRef]
70. Cheng, L.; Weir, M.D.; Xu, H.H.; Antonucci, J.M.; Lin, N.J.; Lin-Gibson, S.; Xu, S.M.; Zhou, X. Effect of amorphous calcium phosphate and silver nanocomposites on dental plaque microcosm biofilms. *J. Biomed. Mater. Res. Part B Appl. Biomater.* **2012**, *100*, 1378–1386. [CrossRef]
71. Mohamad Hanafiah, R.; Abd Ghafar, S.A.; Lim, V.; Musa, S.N.A.; Yakop, F.; Hairil Anuar, A.H. Green synthesis, characterisation and antibacterial activities of strobilanthes crispus-mediated silver nanoparticles (SC-AGNPS) against selected bacteria. *Artif. Cells Nanomed. Biotechnol.* **2023**, *51*, 549–559. [CrossRef] [PubMed]
72. Wang, L.; Periyasami, G.; Aldalbahi, A.; Fogliano, V. The antimicrobial activity of silver nanoparticles biocomposite films depends on the silver ions release behaviour. *Food Chem.* **2021**, *359*, 129859. [CrossRef] [PubMed]
73. Khalandi, B.; Asadi, N.; Milani, M.; Davaran, S.; Abadi, A.J.N.; Abasi, E.; Akbarzadeh, A. A review on potential role of silver nanoparticles and possible mechanisms of their actions on bacteria. *Drug Res.* **2017**, *11*, 70–76. [CrossRef] [PubMed]
74. Pérez-Díaz, M.A.; Boegli, L.; James, G.; Velasquillo, C.; Sánchez-Sánchez, R.; Martínez-Martínez, R.-E.; Martínez-Castañón, G.A.; Martinez-Gutierrez, F. Silver nanoparticles with antimicrobial activities against *Streptococcus mutans* and their cytotoxic effect. *Mater. Sci. Eng. C* **2015**, *55*, 360–366. [CrossRef] [PubMed]
75. Ahmed, O.; Sibuyi, N.R.S.; Fadaka, A.O.; Madiehe, M.A.; Maboza, E.; Meyer, M.; Geerts, G. Plant extract-synthesized silver nanoparticles for application in dental therapy. *Pharmaceutics* **2022**, *14*, 380. [CrossRef]
76. Abbaszadegan, A.; Ghahramani, Y.; Gholami, A.; Hemmateenejad, B.; Dorostkar, S.; Nabavizadeh, M.; Sharghi, H. The effect of charge at the surface of silver nanoparticles on antimicrobial activity against gram-positive and gram-negative bacteria: A preliminary study. *J. Nanomater.* **2015**, *2015*, 720654. [CrossRef]
77. Mohanbaba, S.; Gurunathan, S. Differential biological activities of silver nanoparticles against Gram-negative and Gram-positive bacteria: A novel approach for antimicrobial therapy. In *Nanobiomaterials in Antimicrobial Therapy*; Elsevier: Amsterdam, The Netherlands, 2016; pp. 193–227.
78. More, P.R.; Pandit, S.; Filippis, A.; Franci, G.; Mijakovic, I.; Galdiero, M. Silver Nanoparticles: Bactericidal and Mechanistic Approach against Drug Resistant Pathogens. *Microorganisms* **2023**, *11*, 369. [CrossRef]
79. Peulen, T.-O.; Wilkinson, K.J. Diffusion of nanoparticles in a biofilm. *Environ. Sci. Technol.* **2011**, *45*, 3367–3373. [CrossRef]
80. Joshi, A.S.; Singh, P.; Mijakovic, I. Interactions of gold and silver nanoparticles with bacterial biofilms: Molecular interactions behind inhibition and resistance. *Int. J. Mol. Sci.* **2020**, *21*, 7658. [CrossRef]
81. Aldhaian, B.A.; Balhaddad, A.A.; Alfaifi, A.A.; Levon, J.A.; Eckert, G.J.; Hara, A.T.; Lippert, F. In vitro demineralization prevention by fluoride and silver nanoparticles when applied to sound enamel and enamel caries-like lesions of varying severities. *J. Dent.* **2021**, *104*, 103536. [CrossRef]
82. Sayed, M.; Hiraishi, N.; Matin, K.; Abdou, A.; Burrow, M.F.; Tagami, J. Effect of silver-containing agents on the ultra-structural morphology of dentinal collagen. *Dent. Mater.* **2020**, *36*, 936–944. [CrossRef] [PubMed]
83. Scarpelli, B.B.; Punhagui, M.F.; Hoeppner, M.G.; Almeida, R.S.C.d.; Juliani, F.A.; Guiraldo, R.D.; Berger, S.B. In vitro evaluation of the remineralizing potential and antimicrobial activity of a cariostatic agent with silver nanoparticles. *Braz. Dent. J.* **2017**, *28*, 738–743. [CrossRef] [PubMed]

84. Quritum, M.; Abdella, A.; Amer, H.; El Desouky, L.M.; El Tantawi, M. Effectiveness of nanosilver fluoride and silver diamine fluoride in arresting early childhood caries: A randomized controlled clinical trial. *BMC Oral Health* **2024**, *24*, 701. [CrossRef] [PubMed]
85. Firouzmandi, M.; Vasei, F.; Giti, R.; Sadeghi, H. Effect of silver diamine fluoride and proanthocyanidin on resistance of carious dentin to acid challenges. *PLoS ONE* **2020**, *15*, e0238590. [CrossRef]
86. León-Silva, S.; Fernández-Luqueño, F.; López-Valdez, F. Silver nanoparticles (AgNP) in the environment: A review of potential risks on human and environmental health. *Water Air Soil Pollut.* **2016**, *227*, 306. [CrossRef]

pharmaceuticals MDPI

Article

Anti-Bacterial Activity of Green Synthesised Silver and Zinc Oxide Nanoparticles against *Propionibacterium acnes*

Hafez Al-Momani [1,*], Muhannad I. Massadeh [2], Muna Almasri [2], Dua'a Al Balawi [3], Iman Aolymat [4], Saja Hamed [5], Borhan Aldeen Albiss [6], Lugain Ibrahim [3], Hadeel Al Balawi [3] and Sameer Al Haj Mahmoud [7]

1 Department of Microbiology, Pathology and Forensic Medicine, Faculty of Medicine, The Hashemite University, Zarqa 13133, Jordan

2 Department of Biology and Biotechnology, Faculty of Science, The Hashemite University, Zarqa 13115, Jordan; massadeh@hu.edu.jo (M.I.M.); monaalmasri23@yahoo.com (M.A.)

3 Faculty of Applied Medical Sciences, The Hashemite University, Zarqa 13133, Jordan

4 Department of Anatomy, Physiology and Biochemistry, Faculty of Medicine, The Hashemite University, Zarqa 13133, Jordan; imank@hu.edu.jo

5 Department of Pharmaceutical & Pharmaceutical Technology, Faculty of Pharmaceutical Sciences, The Hashemite University, Zarqa 13133, Jordan; hamedsh@hu.edu.jo

6 Nanotechnology Institute, Jordan University of Science & Technology, Irbid 22110, Jordan; baalbiss@just.edu.jo

7 Department of Basic Medical Science, Faculty of Medicine, Al-Balqa' Applied University, AL-Salt 19117, Jordan; sameer.alhaj@bau.edu.jo

* Correspondence: hafez@hu.edu.jo

Abstract: *Propionibacterium acnes* plays a critical role in the development of acne vulgaris. There has been a rise in the number of patients carrying *P. acnes* strains that are resistant to antibiotics. Thus, alternative anti-microbial agents are required. Zinc oxide (ZnO-NPs) and silver (Ag-NPs) nanoparticles can be used against several antibiotic-resistant bacteria. The impact of Ag-NPs and ZnO-NPs against two clinical strains of *P. acnes*, P1 and P2, and a reference strain, NCTC747, were investigated in this research. A chemical approach for the green synthesis of Ag-NPs and ZnO-NPs from *Peganum harmala* was employed. The microtiter plate method was used to examine the effects of NPs on bacterial growth, biofilm development, and biofilm eradication. A broth microdilution process was performed in order to determine minimal inhibitory (MIC) concentrations. Ag-NPs and ZnO-NPs had a spherical shape and average dimensions of 10 and 50 nm, respectively. MIC values for all *P. acnes* strains for Ag-NPs and ZnO-NPs were 125 μg/mL and 250 μg/mL, respectively. Ag-NP and ZnO-NP concentrations of 3.9- 62.5 μg/mL and 15–62.5 μg/mL significantly inhibited the growth and biofilm formation of all *P. acnes* strains, respectively. ZnO-NP concentrations of 15–62.5 μg/mL significantly inhibited the growth of NCTC747 and P2 strains. The growth of P1 was impacted by concentrations of 31.25 μg/mL and 62.5 μg/mL. Biofilm formation in the NCTC747 strain was diminished by a ZnO-NP concentration of 15 μg/mL. The clinical strains of *P. acnes* were only affected by ZnO-NP titres of more than 31.25 μg/mL. Established *P. acne* biofilm biomass was significantly reduced in all strains at a Ag-NP and ZnO-NP concentration of 62.5 μg/mL. The findings demonstrated that Ag-NPs and ZnO-NPs exert an anti-bacterial effect against *P. acnes*. Further research is required to determine their potential utility as a treatment option for acne.

Keywords: acne vulgaris; biofilm; *Propionibacterium acne*; silver; zinc oxide; nanoparticles

1. Introduction

The human dermis is a particularly vulnerable structure which may allow a range of bacteria to gain entry into the body [1]. Acne vulgaris is one of the most frequently arising skin pathologies in young adults aged between 11 and 30 years, and typically affects 50.9% of females and 42.5% of males [2,3]. The presentation of acne can be affected by numerous factors, including hormone titres and variations in keratinisation, as well as altered inflammatory or immune activity [4,5]. It has been recognised that the degree of inflammation may be influenced by the reaction of the host to the bacterium, *P. acnes*, formerly known as *Corynebacterium acne* [6], which liberates free fatty acids as a result of sebaceous triglyceride metabolism [7]. The latter cause irritation of the follicular wall and neighbouring dermal layer. *P. acnes* also produces exoenzymes and chemoattractants which target neutrophils [5,7]. It has been demonstrated that diminishing the bacterial population of *P. acnes* on the skin can be a successful treatment [8].

Antibiotics are frequently used topically and orally to treat acne [9]. According to data from multiple studies, the percentage of patients who have *P. acnes* strains that are resistant to one or more medications has dramatically increased in recent years [10–14]. This may be due to the fact that cells of *P. acnes* present within the pilosebaceous unit develop and form a biofilm [15]. Genome sequencing of *P. acnes* shows three distinct clusters of genes that encode enzymes involved in the extracellular polysaccharide production necessary for biofilm formation [6]. The most significant property of biofilm, and the main contributor to persistent infections, is its resistance to anti-microbial drugs and to elements of the human immune system [16–18]. In the treatment of acne, the use of nanoparticles (NPs) is a promising method with which to overcome bacterial resistance [19,20].

NPs exhibit considerable potential for use as anti-bacterial treatments, offering a broad spectrum of activity and appearing resilient to the development of bacterial resistance to their anti-microbial effects. These therapeutic properties arise as a result of their small size and consequent high surface/volume ratio, which enable NPs to interact with bacterial membranes [21]. Both organic and inorganic NPs exist; examples include liposomes or metallic NPs, respectively. These two types of NPs have been successfully utilised for a number of clinical disorders, with metallic NPs demonstrating the greatest therapeutic potential [22]. The latter have a range of effects on a number of bacteria which exhibit resistance to multiple conventional anti-bacterial agents [23]. There is therefore considerable interest in exploiting metallic NPs in both biomedical and pharmaceutical domains [24,25].

The most widely studied metal NPs are silver (Ag) NPs (Ag-NPs). Although Ag ions and substances based on Ag exhibit extreme toxicity to a number of bacteria, the metal's anti-bacterial properties are markedly improved when Ag-NPs are utilised, owing to the resulting surface area augmentation [26–28]. Anti-microbial properties have also been demonstrated in metallic oxide NPs, e.g., zinc oxide NPs (ZnO-NPs) [22]. The latter have been investigated in detail owing to their specific physiochemical characteristics, as they exhibit effects which counter bacterial infection, malignancy, and inflammation [29,30]. Earlier studies have shown that when used at specific doses, ZnO-NPs may be of value for use as clinical anti-bacterial agents [31,32].

The biomedical and anti-bacterial characteristics of NPs are, in general, a consequence of the techniques and chemicals used for their manufacture and formulation, e.g., temperature, concentration, and the reducing agent and solvent utilised [33,34]. A green synthesis strategy has been applied to generate NPs that exhibit biocompatibility and biodegradability which make them suitable for various biomedical applications [35]. This environmentally friendly, sustainable, and dependable method of manufacture also circumvents the creation of undesirable or noxious by-products [36–38]. Plant extracts have been studied in depth for use in this process owing to their ability to enhance NP monodispersity. They contain a range of biomolecules, such as phenolics, polysaccharides, flavones, terpenoids, alkaloids, proteins, amino acids, enzymes, and alcoholic compounds, which can function as reducing and capping agents, the latter contributing to the stability and controlling the configuration of the produced NPs [39,40].

A member of the Zygophyllaceae family, harmala (*P. harmala*), is recognised for its medicinal properties. Its 5 mm diameter seeds are black in colour, globular in shape, and have a spicy taste and nut-like scent. They are frequently used as a condiment in cooking. Clinically, they have been utilised therapeutically for conditions including back pain, bronchospasm, colic, and jaundice, and to promote menstruation [41,42]. The activity of *P. harmala* against disease-inducing pathogens, such as bacteria, fungi, and viruses, has also been documented [42,43]. It has been hypothesised in this research paper that the pharmacological properties of Ag-NPs and ZnO-NPs synthesised using *P. harmala* seed extract as a reducing agent could be used to generate potent cosmeceutical products that could be utilised as acne treatments. The effects of Ag-NPs and ZnO-NPs on the growth and biofilm formation of *P. acnes* have therefore been examined in this study.

2. Methods

2.1. Propionibacterium Acne Strains and Culture Conditions

Two clinical strains of *P. acnes* were acquired from the Prince Hamza Hospital and identified by their analytical profile index (BioMerieux, Marcy-l'Etoile, France). A reference strain, NCTC747, was also used in this study. *P. acnes* strains were cultured in tryptic soy broth (TSB) at 37 °C under anaerobic conditions using an OXOID anaerobic jar and AnaeroGen atmosphere generation systems. Written informed consent was obtained from the patients whose clinical isolates were obtained, and all ethical guidelines were properly observed. The ethics service committees from both Hashemite University and the Prince Hamza Hospital granted ethical approval for this case study (reference number 5/3/2020/2021).

2.2. Green Synthesis of Silver and Zinc Oxide Nanoparticles

2.2.1. Preparation of Aqueous *P. Harmala* Seed Extract

The first researcher obtained whole *P. harmala* plants from their own farm in the Abbin region of Ajloun Governorate in September 2023. The identification of the *P. harmala* seeds was verified by comparing them to the sample at the herbarium of Jerash University's Faculty of Agriculture and confirmed by the Assistant Professor of Agriculture. A voucher specimen (AM/2023/01/002) was then stored at the herbarium within the Plant Protection Department at Jerash University in Jordan. The harvesting of *P. harmala* followed institutional, national, and international guidelines and laws.

After being fully dried at room temperature and cleaned with double-distilled water (Sigma-Aldrich, Darmstadt, Germany), the *P. harmala* seeds were machine-ground into a coarse powder. A total of 5 g of powder was combined with 50 mL of double-distilled water and heated to 75 °C for 90 min before being filtered twice through Whatman filter paper. Using microfiltration through a 0.22 mm syringe membrane filter, a clear aqueous extract with a pH of 6.4 at 25 °C was obtained.

2.2.2. Determination of Total Phenolic and Total Flavonoid Content in the *P. harmala* Extract

The Folin–Ciocalteu technique [44] was utilised in order to quantify the phenolic compounds, i.e., secondary metabolites from plants characterised by their ability to scavenge radicals as result of their redox potentials [45], in the extract of *P. harmala*. This investigation involves phenolic moiety oxidation following the addition of Folin–Ciocalteu reagent, which comprises phosphomolybdic and phosphotungstic acids [46]. Following the published method by Singleton, Orthofer, et al. [44] with some modifications, 100 µL Folin–Ciocalteu reagent was combined with 20 µL *P. harmala* extract. A total of 300 µL 25% sodium carbonate solution was admixed after 10 min. The absorbance of the solution was then determined at a wavelength of 765 nm. This experiment was performed in triplicate and the mean absorbance value was calculated. Solutions of gallic acid of strengths 0–500 mg/L were utilised to determine the calibration curve. Data are expressed as gallic acid equivalents (GAE) per 100 gm extract.

The number of flavonoids within the sample were also established using spectrophotometry. The technique used relied on the production of a flavonoid–aluminium complex [47], which demonstrated maximum absorption at a wavelength of 430 nm. A calibration was constructed using quercetin. A total of 1 mL of both extracts of *P. harmala* and 2% aluminium chloride methanolic solution were admixed, and then incubated for 10 min in ambient conditions. The solution's absorbance was quantified at the above wavelength. Data are expressed as quercetin equivalents (QE) per 100 gm extract.

2.2.3. Green Synthesis of Silver and Zinc Oxide Nanoparticles

Ag-NPs were produced by heating a 50 mL solution of 3 mM $AgNO_3$ to 80 °C in a 100 mL foil-lined Erlenmeyer flask and stirring it constantly at 1100 rpm. A 4 mL aqueous *P. harmala* seed extract solution was applied using a micropipette at a rate of 34 µL/min. The colour of the solution changed from orange to dark brown immediately as the Ag-NPs started to form. Ag-NPs are created through the reduction of silver ions, and this process was observed using ultraviolet (UV) spectrophotometry, which measured the absorbance of the reaction medium in the 300–800 nm wavelength range. Centrifugation was performed for 15 min at 10,000 rpm to purify the synthesised Ag-NPs. The supernatant was placed in a dry, clean container to enable particles to settle further, after which centrifugation was performed repeatedly using a cooling microfuge. This enabled the Ag-NPs to be dried, purified, and characterised.

In order to produce ZnO-NPs, 50 mL aqueous zinc sulphate heptahydrate solution ($ZnSO_4{\cdot}7H_2O$, ACS reagent, 99%, Sigma-Aldrich, St. Louis, MO, USA) was combined with 5 mL aqueous yellow seed extract solution from *P. harmala*. The mixture was then agitated at room temperature for 10 min, creating a pale-yellow solution. After a thorough washing process, the obtained NP solutions were centrifuged at 4500 rpm for 15 min and then dried at 80 °C for 7–8 h. Before usage, the crude pellets were resuspended in sterile double-distilled water, filtered through a 0.2 µm filter, and stored in the dark at a temperature of 4 °C. Once they had been dispersed in sterile, double-distilled water and centrifuged three times, the suspended particles were filtered. This resulted in the formation of ZnO-NPs.

2.3. *Characterisation of Zinc Oxide and Silver Nanoparticles*

2.3.1. X-ray Diffraction

An X-ray diffractometer (XRD-6000, Shimadzu, Kyoto, Japan)), equipped with a copper K-α radiation source with a wavelength of 0.154 nm, was employed to measure the X-ray diffraction (XRD) spectra of the nanoparticles. The sample holder was 2 cm long and 0.5 mm wide.

2.3.2. Analysis of Particle Sizes

A Malvern Zetasizer Nano ZS90 (Malvern Ltd., Malvern, UK) was used to measure particle sizes. The stock suspensions were diluted in distilled water. In order to guarantee temperature homogeneity, particle samples were allowed to equilibrate at 25 °C for 5 min before duplicate tests, including three separate trials, were performed. The viscosity and refractive index values of the solution used were 0.8872 cP and 1.59, respectively. The tests and experiments were performed at the Nanotechnology Institute at Jordan University of Science and Technology.

2.3.3. Ultraviolet–Visible Spectroscopy

UV–visible (UV-Vis) spectroscopy (UV-1900, Shimadzu, Kyoto, Japan) was used to track the bioreduction of the $AgNO_3$ salt solution and to examine the production of the Ag-NPs and ZnO-NPs using *P. harmala* seed aqueous extract. Double-distilled water was employed as a control. All spectrophotometric analyses were carried out inside a quartz cuvette with a path length of 1 cm. The surface plasmon resonance (SPR) of the NPs was measured using a wavelength range of 800–200 nm.

2.3.4. Scanning Electron Microscopy

In order to examine the surface size and characteristics of the biosynthesised NPs, a scanning electron microscope (SEM) was employed. A fine 4 nm layer of gold was applied to the surface of the samples, after which they were evaluated using a low vacuum of 50 Pa and 3 KV, which had a working distance of 8–10 mm.

2.4. *Anti-Acne Effect of Synthesised Silver and Zinc Oxide Nanoparticles*

2.4.1. Agar Well Diffusion Approach

In order to determine the efficacy of the Ag-NPs and ZnO-NPs against *P. acnes*, the agar well diffusion technique was applied. During this experiment, a single colony from each strain was incubated under ideal anaerobic conditions for 72 h at 37 °C. This led to the generation of a standardised culture, 1.5×10^8 CFU/mL, of each bacterium. Following incubation, a spectrophotometer, measuring optical density (OD) at a wavelength of 600 nm, was used to adjust the culture turbidity to 0.5 MFU. Sterile cotton swabs were used to distribute 100 µL of the previously generated standardised culture for each bacterium onto the Mueller–Hinton agar plates. Wells of 6 mm were punched into the agar plates containing the bacterial lawn, into which 40 µL of each 250 µg/mL NP solution was poured. The plates were kept for 10 min at room temperature so as to allow the NPs to diffuse into the agar bacterial lawn. The positive and negative controls were double-distilled, and then antibiotic discs containing doxycycline were added. Following incubation of each plate in the previously recommended ideal conditions, a growth inhibition zone was determined and measured. Each experiment was performed twice.

2.4.2. Determination of Minimum Inhibitory and Bactericidal Concentrations Using the Broth Microdilution Method

The minimum bactericidal concentration (MBC), i.e., the lowest concentration of anti-microbial agent needed to kill microorganisms, and the minimum inhibitory concentration (MIC), i.e., the lowest concentration of anti-microbial agent required to prevent microbial growth, were determined in this experiment. According to Clinical and Laboratory Standards Institute procedure, under ideal conditions, a single colony of the *P. acnes* bacterial strains should be used to create a standardised *P. acnes* culture.

Culture turbidity was adjusted to the 0.5 MFU standard by applying a spectrophotometer to measure the absorbance. This was then diluted with sterile Mueller–Hinton Broth (MHB) so as to create a standard inoculum strength (10^5 CFU/mL) over a 15 min period. Subsequently, 180 µL of sterile MHB was added to 96-well plates; 200 µL of Ag-NPs and ZnO-NPs stock solutions (1000 µg/mL) were placed into the first well. Subsequently, with each progressive well up until the ninth well, two-fold serial dilutions were performed with up and down mixing in order to produce NP solution concentrations of 1.9, 3.9, 7.8, 15.625, 31.25, 62.5, 125, 250, and 500 µg/mL.

A total of 20 µL from earlier bacteria standard cultures was added to each of the wells with the exception of wells 10 and 12, which were kept in place in order to maintain media sterility. The 96-well *P. acnes* plates underwent anaerobic incubation for 72 h at 37 °C. The lowest NP concentration, where there was no visible growth in the wells, was the MIC endpoint. The MBC endpoint was considered to have been reached when 99.9% of the bacteria had been killed in the presence of the lowest NP concentration. This was achieved by evaluating the volume of bacteria present on agar plates before and after incubation. The experiments were repeated twice.

2.4.3. Bacterial Growth Assays

Various titres of Ag-NPs and ZnO-NPs were studied to assess their impact on bacterial growth and biofilm development using 96-well, flat-bottomed, transparent, and sterile microtiter plates (BD Falcon Franklin Lakes, NJ, USA). For the growth assay, 180 µL aliquots of TSB were used to prepare standardised suspensions of *P. acnes* cultures; the latter were added to 20 µL bacterial aliquots suspended in TSB and 200 µL of either Ag-NPs or ZnO-NPs, i.e., 200 µL of 125 g/mL in the first well, which was then double-diluted to concentrations ranging from 0.79 µg/mL to 62.5 µg/mL. Each test was carried out three times.

Control wells were also employed, with positives containing *P. acnes* and TSB, and negatives containing only TSB. The samples were then subjected to anaerobic incubation in the dark at 37 °C and shaken for 72 h. After the incubation process was completed, the total cell numbers at different NP concentrations were determined by measuring the optic density (OD) at 600 nm (OD600, Infinite® 200 PRO NanoQuant, TECAN, Austria). In order to calculate the final cell growth value, the average reading from each well containing *P. acnes* was subtracted from the average reading of the wells without *P. acnes* (blanks) at the relevant Ag-NP concentration. The total cell growth measured was that for all cells, i.e., biofilm-associated and planktonic. At the end of the incubation period, 100 µL of the culture was spread over a nutrient agar plate and incubated at 37 °C for 72 h under anaerobic conditions using an OXOID anaerobic jar.

2.4.4. Quantitative Determination of Biofilm Formation via Microtiter Plate Assessments

A spectrophotometric method was used to compute the total biofilm biomass, counting bacterial cells and extracellular polymeric substances (EPSs) [48]. Similar to the procedure used for the growth assay, after a 72 h incubation period without shaking, the wells were then shaken and washed with 250 µL sterile phosphate buffer saline in order to eliminate any bacteria that had not adhered to the wells.

A total of 200 µL 99% methanol was used to fix the microorganisms in each well. Before being emptied and given time to dry, the initial plates were allowed to stand for 15 min, following which they were stained for 5 min using 200 µL 2% Hucker crystal violet, a stain that is suitable for Gram-staining the contents of each individual well. The wells were cleaned three times in 200 µL of sterile water to eliminate any remaining staining material. Care was taken not to disturb the biofilm with each wash. Following another period of drying, the cell-bound dye on the plates was redissolved in 33% (*v*/*v*) glacial acetic acid at a rate of 160 µL per well.

An automated reader (ICN Flow Titertek Multiscan Plus McLean, VA, USA)) was used to determine the OD of each well. The measurements were taken three times, i.e., before the samples were incubated (OD, 600 nm), during sample incubation at the growth evaluation stage (OD, 600 nm), and after the biofilm assay had been created (OD, 570 nm). A ratio of 570:600 was selected in order to normalise the quantity of biofilm that had developed in comparison to the rate of bacterial development. An OD value that was negative was shown as 0. Each test was carried out three times. A cut-off value (ODc) was confirmed, which was three standard deviations (SDs) higher than the mean OD of the negative control, i.e., ODc = average OD of negative control + 3SDs of negative control. Based on the OD, the isolates were assigned to one of four categories, i.e., non-biofilm producer (OD < ODc), weak biofilm producer (ODc < OD < 2ODc), moderate biofilm producer (2ODc < OD < 4ODc), and strong biofilm producer (4ODc < OD).

2.4.5. Microtiter Biofilm Eradication Test

A process combining crystal violet (CV) staining with a tetrazolium dye was used to evaluate the effects of both Ag-NPs and ZnO-NPs on already formed biofilms. As cellular nicotinamide adenine dinucleotide and hydrogen drives the creation of colourful formazan salts, tetrazolium salts are frequently used as reagents in biological tests to assess the metabolic behaviour of living cells [49]. Various tetrazolium-based dyes, therefore, have been utilised to identify and to evaluate biofilms [50]. In this work, triphenyl tetrazolium chloride (TTC) was employed as a metabolic marker of bacterial survival and biofilm development.

In order to create biofilms, standardised bacterial suspensions were prepared. Seventy-two-hour cultures of each *P. acnes* strain were carried out on 2 different 96-well plates, using TSB at a concentration of 0.5 MFU. Aliquots of 20 µL of the bacterial suspension were introduced to 250 µL aliquots of TSB, containing no Ag-NPs, to produce biofilms. Ultimately, this produced a 270 µL volume in the microtiter well. The plates were incubated anaerobically for 72 h at 37 °C to promote biofilm attachment and growth. Two wells were placed on separate, parallel microtiter plates for each concentration that was tested; one was stained with CV, and TTC was added to the other.

The media were taken off the plates over the next three days, after which the plates were placed upside down on sterile paper and left to dry for 15 min at room temperature. Subsequently, a multi-channel pipette was used to remove the planktonic and unattached cells from each well, and the remaining biofilm was rinsed three times in 150 μL new, sterile media. Any excess rinsing material was aspirated out of each well before 200 μL of fresh MHB containing NP concentrations ranging from 0.97 μg/mLto 62.5 μg/mL was added. The plates were then incubated at 37 °C for 72 h. Following incubation, the planktonic cells and media were removed, the planktonic growth was estimated, and the remaining biomass was rinsed three times in distilled water.

An enzyme-linked immunosorbent assay microplate reader was then used to obtain the OD600 values of each plate, which were documented before and after incubation. The combined results from the three different biological replicate results were averaged out.

As mentioned previously, the second plate was stained with TCC. Microplates were incubated at 37 °C for 6 h after adding 40 μL 0.2 mg/mL TCC, dissolved in deionised water, to the wells of the *P. acnes*, which had been treated with various Ag-NP concentrations for 72 h. Results from a minimum of three replicates were averaged. Once treatment had been performed, the mean OD490 values for each biofilm were measured [51].

2.5. Statistical Analysis

The experimental findings were presented as the mean standard error of the mean of at least three replicates. One-way analysis of variance (ANOVA) was used to assess differences between samples and controls where pertinent. The OD values from the microtiter plate tests with and without Ag-NP treatment at different dilutions were compared using the Mann–Whitney U test or Kruskal–Wallis test followed by post hoc Dunn's multiple comparisons. Significant p values were determined to be less than 0.05. GraphPad Instat 6.0 software was used to analyse the data.

3. Results

3.1. Determination of Total Phenolic and Flavonoid Content

The Folin–Ciocalteu method determined that the samples had a total phenolic content of 8.11 ± 1.7 mg GAE/100 mg extract. Spectrophotometric analysis following the colorimetric aluminium chloride assay revealed a total flavonoid content in the samples of 0.76 ± 0.12 mg QE/100 mg extract.

3.2. Nanoparticle Characterisation

3.2.1. Ultraviolet–Visible Spectroscopy

During their preparation, the formation of Ag-NPs causes a colour change in the reaction mixture from orange to dark brown, indicating $AgNO_3$ reduction in the Ag-NPs. During the preparation of the ZnO-NPs, the solution mixture of $ZnSO_3$ and *P. harmala* seed extract changed from light brown to yellowish-black in colour, indicative of the formation of ZnO-NPs (Supplementary Figure S1).

The green synthesised Ag-NPs and ZnO-NPs were characterised using a UV-Vis spectrophotometer in the wavelength range 800–200 nm. As both Ag-NPs and ZnO-NPs are direct bandgap semiconductors, with a wide bandgap of ~3.37 eV between the conduction and the valence bands [52], the electron jump from the valence band to the conduction band generates an absorption peak between 450 and 500 nm, and between 350 and 450 nm, respectively. The UV-Vis spectrum shows a large absorption peak at approximately 460 nm for Ag-NPs, and at 399 nm for ZnO-NPs (Figure 1).

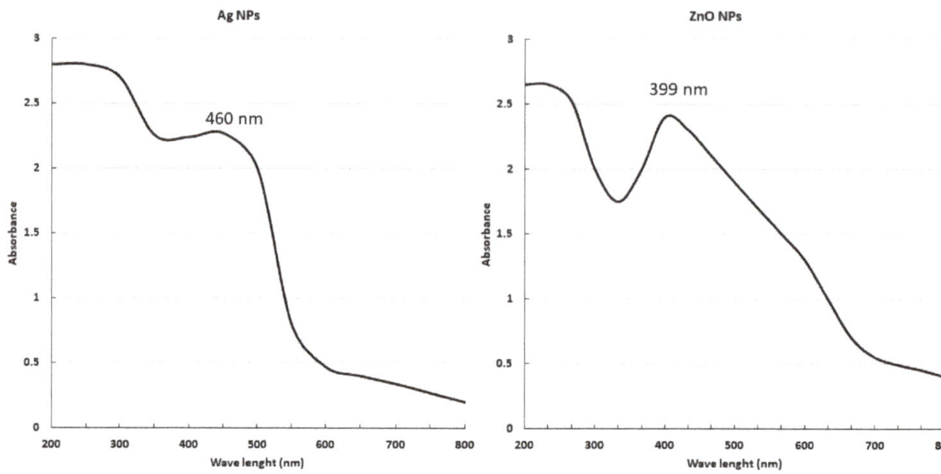

Figure 1. Characterisation of NPs by ultraviolet–visible spectroscopy.

3.2.2. Scanning Electron Microscopy

The size and surface morphology of the nanoparticles were assessed using SEM. Figure 2A reveals the morphological characteristics of the Ag-NPs; they have an average particle size of approximately 10 nm, are of a uniform spherical shape, and do not aggregate. The size histograms of the Ag-NPs are displayed in Figure 2B and show that the main particle sizes for the Ag-NPs produced in this experiment were 10.9 ± 2.7 nm.

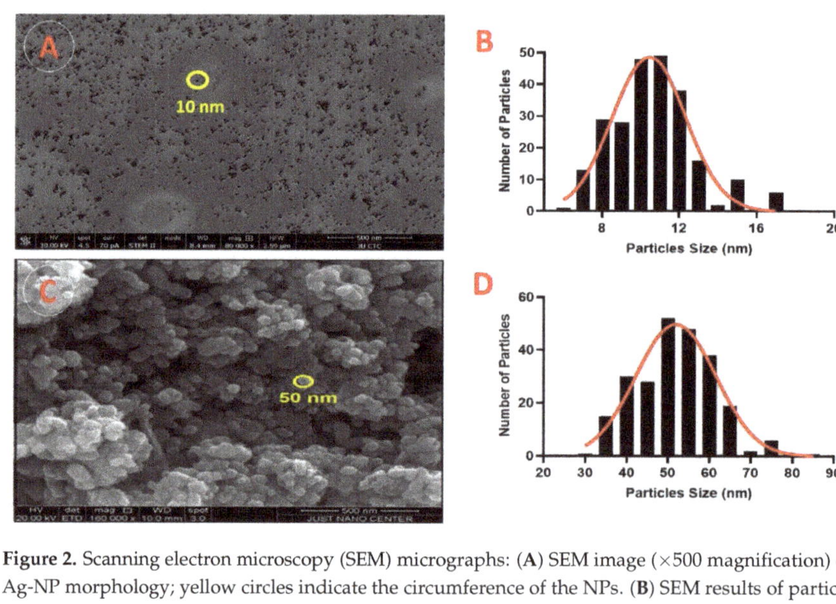

Figure 2. Scanning electron microscopy (SEM) micrographs: (**A**) SEM image (×500 magnification) of Ag-NP morphology; yellow circles indicate the circumference of the NPs. (**B**) SEM results of particle size distribution of Ag-NPs. (**C**) SEM image (×500 magnification) of ZnO-NP morphology; yellow circles indicate the circumference of the NPs. (**D**) SEM results of particle size distribution of ZnO-NPs.

The SEM images of the ZnO-NPs demonstrated that these NPs were uniformly shaped and sized, measuring, on average, 50 nm (Figure 2C). Figure 2D displays the size histograms for the ZnO-NPs; these have a main particle size of 49.8 ± 12.6 nm.

3.2.3. X-ray Diffraction

The samples were left at an ambient temperature of 24.85 °C in order to investigate the formation of crystalline phases in the synthesised Ag-NPs and ZnO-NPs using copper K-α radiation, with a wavelength of 1.5406 Å in the (2θ) range from 10 to 80.

The Ag-NPs showed four peaks at the 2θ values, 38.2901, 44.5583, 64.8185, and 77.4383 (Figure 3A). These were considered to represent the Ag metal and the corresponding Ag plane values of hkl, which are (111), (200), (220), and (311), respectively. The diffractogram (Figure 1) and the Joint Committee on Powder Diffraction Standards (JCPDS), silver file No. 04-0783, were compared and demonstrated the face-centred cubic configuration of the Ag-NPs. The Scherrer equation [53] was applied to compute the Ag-NPs' particle dimension, which was determined to be in the region of 13.9 nm.

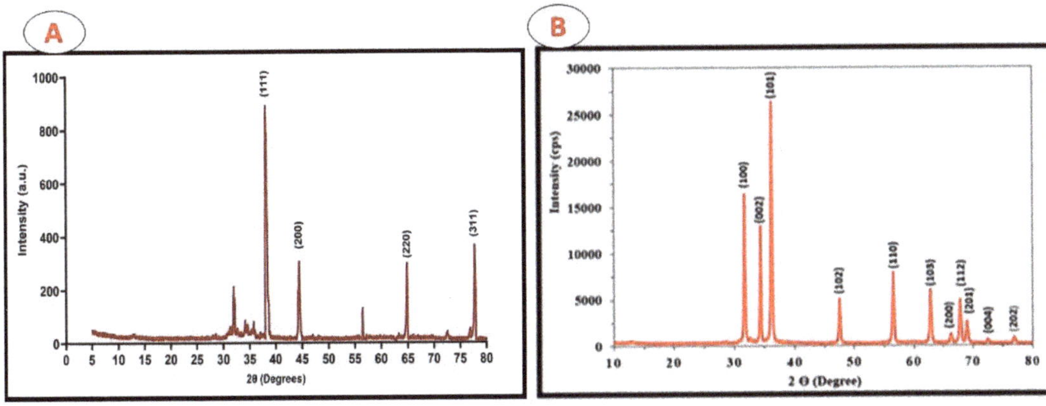

Figure 3. X-ray diffraction showing crystalline phases of the synthesised Ag-NPs (**A**) and ZnO-NPs (**B**).

In the ZnO-NP sample, the Miller indices h, k, and l, i.e., (100), (002), (101), (102), (110), (103), (200), (112), (201), (004), and (202) [JCPDS No. 36-1451], were associated with the typical hexagonal wurtzite ZnO-NP architecture reflecting the orientation of the crystals. The dimensions of the latter were shown to be 44 nm by entering the dominant peaks of diffraction, essentially 101, into the Debye–Scherrers equation. These results confirm that the Ag-NPs and ZnO-NPs produced were of a high quality, containing no contaminants within the crystalline configuration.

3.2.4. Particle Size and Zeta Potential Analysis

Dynamic light scattering demonstrated mean Ag-NP particle dimensions to be 22 nm (Figure 4A) and mean ZnO-NP particle size to be 48 nm (Figure 4B). The electrical potential which arises as a result of the relative motions of the NP and solvent at the solid–liquid interface is referred to as the zeta potential. The electrical potential and the surface charge influence NP stability. The Ag-NPs were determined to have a zeta potential of −25.3 Mv (Figure 4C); the zeta potential of the ZnO-NPs was −34.7 Mv (Figure 4D).

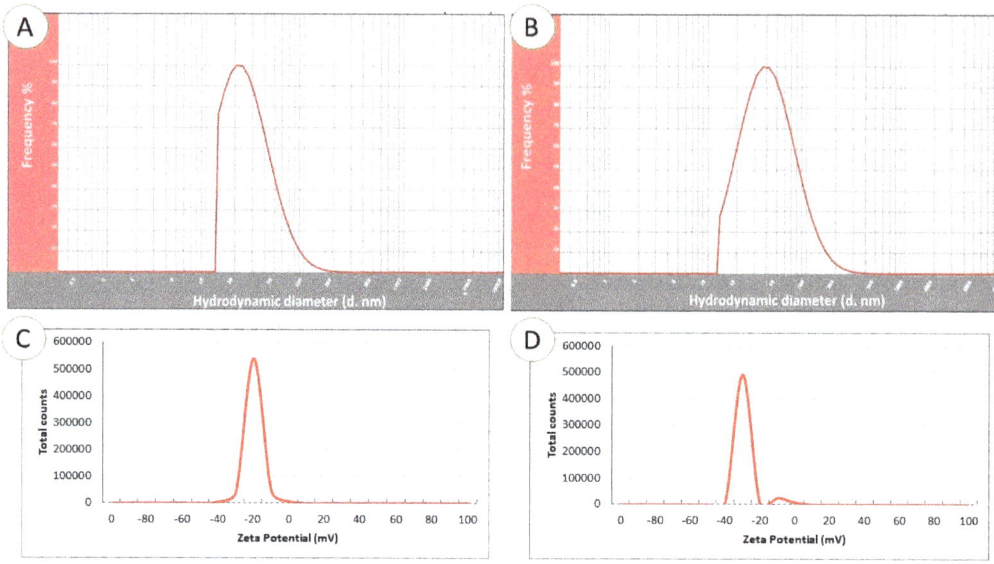

Figure 4. Dynamic light scattering (DLS) spectrum showing the particle size distribution of Ag-NPs (**A**) and ZnO-NPs (**B**). Zeta potential analysis of Ag-NPs (**C**) and ZnO-NPs (**D**).

3.3. Anti-Bacterial Activity of Silver and Zinc Oxide Nanoparticles against P. acnes

3.3.1. Well Diffusion Assay

Both Ag-NPs and ZnO-NPs showed encouraging anti-microbial properties when tested in the presence of all of the *P. acnes* strains under investigation (Table 1). After taking into account the inhibitory zones, the *P. acnes* reference strain, NCTC747, showed the maximum sensitivity towards Ag-NPs, with an inhibition zone of 13.2 ± 0.8 mm. P1 and P2 measurements were 11.7 ± 0.8 mm and 11.5 ± 0.5 mm, respectively. For NCTC747, P1, and P2, the mean inhibition zone measurements using ZnO-NPs were 11.0 ± 1.0, 9.7 ± 1.2 mm, and 9.7 ± 0.6 mm, respectively.

Table 1. Impact of Ag-NPs and ZnO-NPs on *P. acnes* strains as demonstrated by the well diffusion assay. The average ± standard deviation scores from three experiments were used to determine each value in the table. Positive control, 30 μg doxycycline; negative control, distilled water.

	Zone of Inhibition (mm)			
	Ag-NPs (250 μg/mL)	**ZnO-NPs (250 μg/mL)**	**Positive Control**	**Negative Control**
P. acnes NCTC747	13.2 (0.8)	11(1.0)	16.7 (0.3)	0.0
P1	11.7 (0.8)	9.7(1.2)	13.0 (0.5)	0.0
P2	11.0 (0.5)	9.7(0.6)	14.0 (0.5)	0.0

There was a significant larger zone of inhibition created by the Ag-NPs in relation to NCTC747 (t(df) = 7.778 (4.00), p = 0.001) and P2 strains (t(df) = 7.348 (4.00), $p < 0.001$) (Figure 5A). The ZnO-NPs showed a larger zone of inhibition compared to the positive control: NCTC (t(df) = 7.707 (4.00), $p < 0.001$); P1 (t(df) = 4.588(4.00), $p = 0.003$); P2 (t(df) = 9.827(4.00), $p < 0.001$) (Figure 5B).

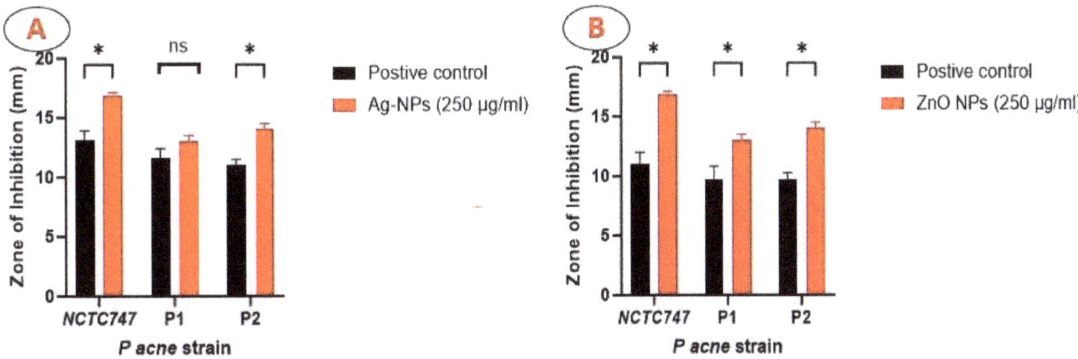

Figure 5. Bar graph showing the diameter of the zone of inhibition produced by Ag-NPs (**A**) and ZnO-NPs (**B**) at a concentration of 250µg/mL, compared to the positive control (30 µg doxycycline).* statistically significant with $p < 0.01$, ns (not statistically significant).

3.3.2. Minimal Inhibitory and Bactericidal Concentrations for Silver and Zinc Oxide Nanoparticles

After a 72 h incubation period in anaerobic conditions at 37 °C, turbidity was evident in the test tubes containing *P. acnes* strains at doses from 3.9 µg/mL to 62.5 µg/mL of Ag-NPs, indicating bacterial growth. There was no sign of turbidity in the test tubes containing the studied strains with Ag-NP concentrations of 125 µg/mL and 250 µg/mL, demonstrating that bacterial growth had been inhibited. Two brain heart infusion agar plates were inoculated, one with the suspension from the tube containing a concentration of 125 µg/mL, and the other from the tube containing 250 µg/mL. The plates were incubated for 72 h. The Ag-NPs were considered bactericidal since there was no bacterial growth on either plate; the MIC and MBC values were both 125 µg/mL. The MIC and MBC values for the ZnO-NPs were both 250 µg/mL.

3.3.3. Inhibitory Effect of Silver and Zinc Oxide Nanoparticles on Planktonic Growth and Biofilm Formation of *P. acnes*

P. acnes strains were incubated with different concentrations (0.97–62.5 µg/mL) of Ag-NPs and ZnO-NPs for 72 h (Figure 6). Bacterial growth was identified and compared to the growth of the controls. Ag-NP concentrations >3.9 µg/mL inhibited the growth of all *P. acnes* strains after 72 h ($F(10, 11) = 24.85$, $p < 0.0001$) (Figure 6A).

ZnO-NP concentrations of 15–62.5 µg/mL inhibited growth in two *P. acnes* strains, i.e., NCTC747 and P2 ($p < 0.05$). The P1 strain was impacted by concentrations of 31.25 µg/mL and 62.5 µg/mL ($F(10, 11) = 36.27$, $p < 0.0001$). Lower Zn-NP concentrations showed a trend towards negatively affecting growth for all strains, but this failed to reach statistical significance (Figure 6B).

Figure 7 illustrates the use of the spreading method to determine the anti-microbial activities of the Ag-NPs and ZnO-NPs at concentrations of 62.5 µg/mL and 3.9 µg/mL against *P. acne* in comparison to the control samples.

Based on the findings of the microtiter plate tests, it can be concluded that the NCTC747 strain was an intermediate biofilm producer, and that the remaining strains were strong biofilm producers (Supplementary Table S1).

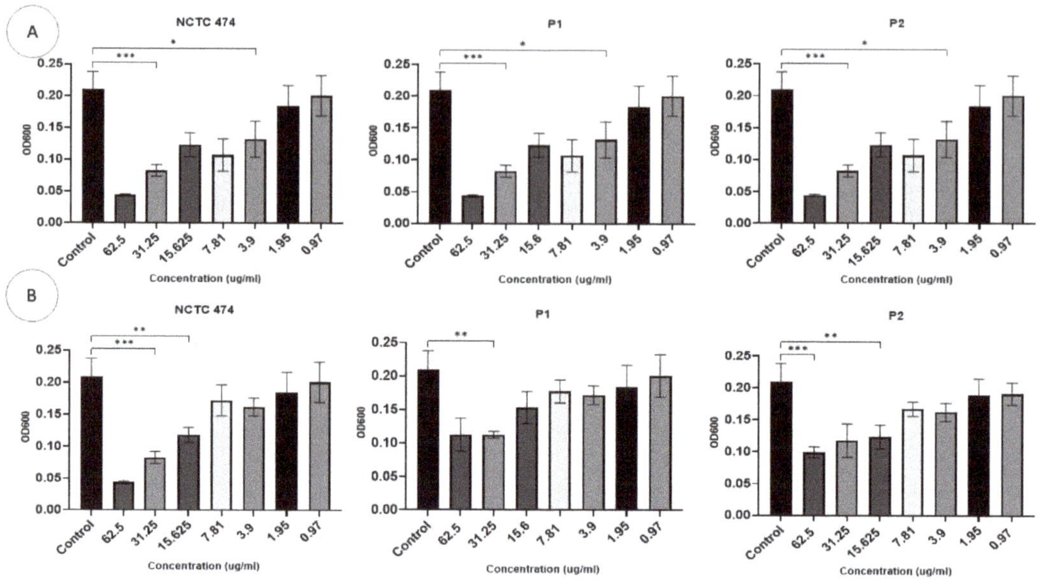

Figure 6. The effect of different concentrations (0.97–62.5 g/mL) of Ag-NPs (**A**) and ZnO-NPs (**B**) on the growth of *P. acne* strains after a 72 h incubation period. The OD at 600 nm is represented on the *Y*-axis. Data are calculated as mean ± standard deviation. Asterisks are used to denote the different *p* values as calculated by one-way analysis of variance (ANOVA): *** $p < 0.0001$, ** $p < 0.001$, and * $p < 0.01$.

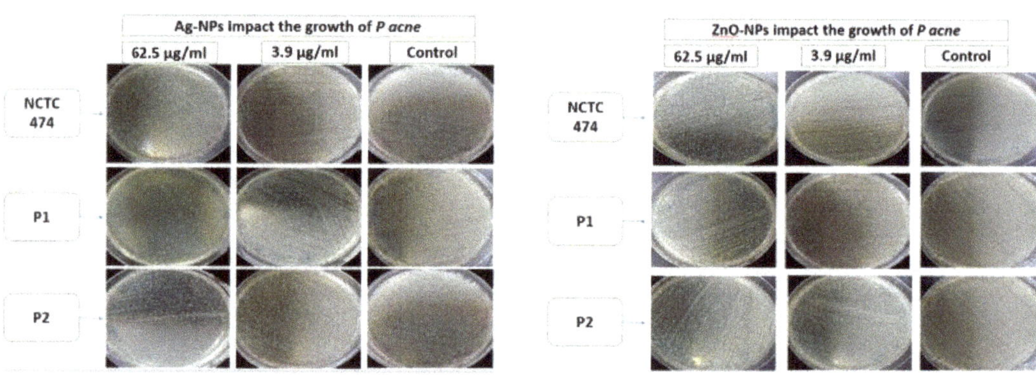

Figure 7. Anti-bacterial activity of Ag-NPs and ZnO-NPs at concentrations of 62.5 µg/mL and 3.9 µg/mL using the spreading method with respect to NCTC747, P1, and P2 strains.

Biofilm formation was reduced by the incorporation of Ag-NPs at concentrations of ≥15.6 µg/mL in the NCTC747 strain ($F (7, 8) = 7.703$, $p < 0.0001$). The P1 and P2 strains were only impacted by concentrations >15.6 µg/mL (Figure 8A). Biofilm formation in the NCTC747 strain was influenced by a ZnO-NP concentration of 15 µg/mL ($F (1.731, 10.39) = 16.12$, $p = 0.0009$). The clinical strains of *P. acnes* were only affected by ZnO-NP titres >31.25 µg/mL (Figure 8B).

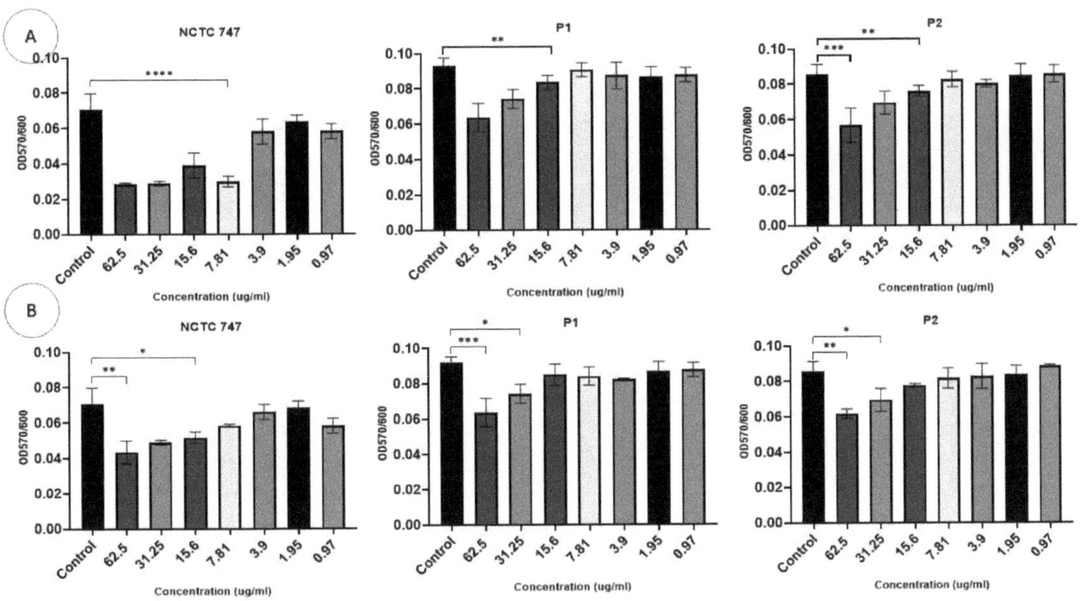

Figure 8. Effects of different concentrations (0.97–62.5 g/mL) of Ag-NPs (**A**) and ZnO-NPs (**B**) on biofilm development for the *P. acnes* strains following a 72 h incubation. The biomass was stained using the crystal violet process. Data are calculated as mean ± standard deviation. Asterisks are used to mark the different *p* values as calculated by one-way analysis of variance (ANOVA): **** $p < 0.0001$, *** $p < 0.0001$, ** $p < 0.001$, and * $p < 0.01$.

3.3.4. Inhibitory Effect of Silver and Zinc Oxide Nanoparticles on Established *P. acne* Biofilm

In the experiments that evaluated the impact of Ag-NPs on two-day-old pre-formed biofilms, a larger concentration of Ag-NPs was necessary for the eradication of a CV-stained *P. acnes* biomass. CV staining was significantly reduced in all strains at a Ag-NP concentration >31.25 µg/mL. The metabolic activity of the cells in the pre-formed biofilms was largely influenced by Ag-NPs at concentrations ≥15.6 µg/mL ($F (10, 66) = 29.27$, $p < 0.0001$) (Figure 9A). Using Ag-NP doses of 15.625–62.5 µg/mL significantly decreased the metabolic activity of each strain (Figure 9A).

The eradication assays that were used to evaluate the treatment of pre-formed biofilms demonstrated an overall reduction in biofilm biomass in all strains exposed to ZnO-NPs compared to the controls ($F (20, 66) = 9.148$, $p < 0.0001$), although this effect was not consistent. Concentrations of 31.25 µg/mL and 62.5 µg/mL significantly decreased CV staining in the *P. acnes* biomass of the NCTC747 strain. Concentrations of 62.5 µg/mL also decreased CV staining in P1 and P2 strains (Figure 9B).

The metabolism of the pre-formed biofilm community of *P. acne* strains incubated with Ag-NPs was inhibited ($F (7, 8) = 6.741$, $p = 0.0076$). Concentrations of ≥15.6 µg/mL of either Ag-NPs or ZnO-NPs were needed to inhibit the metabolic activity of all *P. acnes* strains (Figure 10A,B).

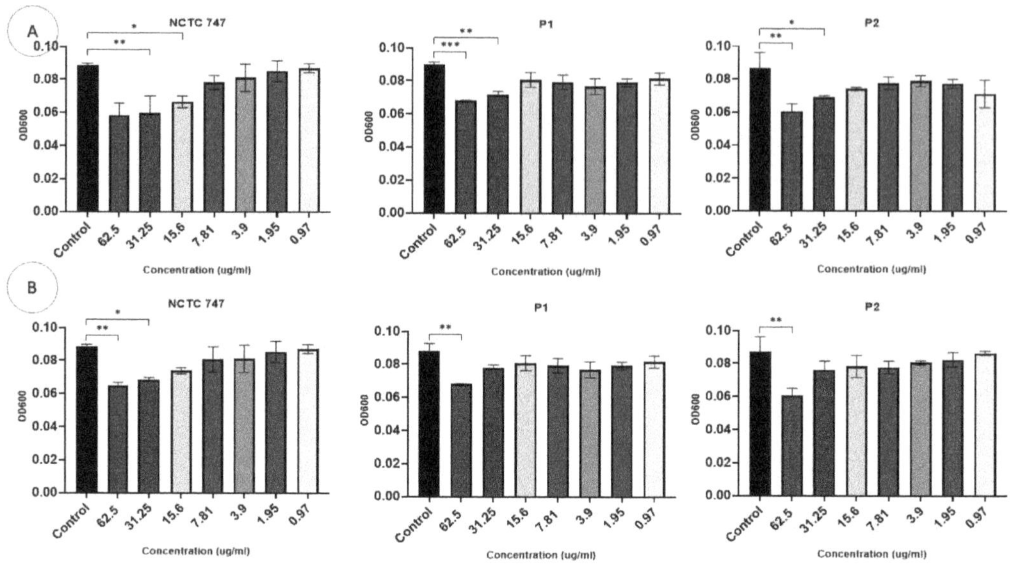

Figure 9. Impacts of different concentrations (0.97–62.5 µg/mL) (X-axis) of Ag-NPs (**A**) and ZnO-NPs (**B**) on biofilm eradication in the *P. acne* strains, NCTC747, P1, and P2, using CV staining after a 72 h incubation period and measuring OD at 600 nm (Y-axis). *** $p < 0.0001$, ** $p < 0.001$, and * $p < 0.01$.

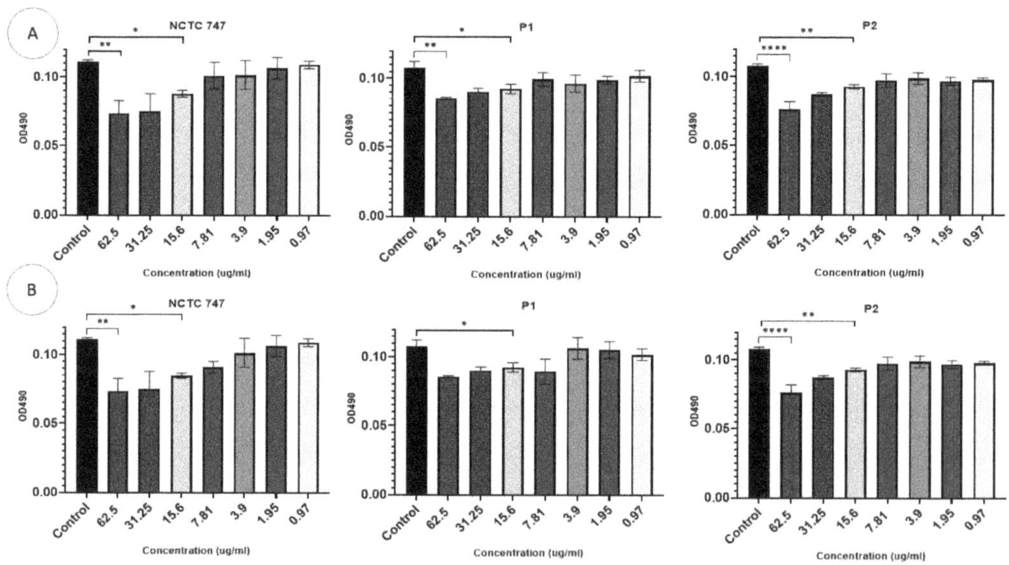

Figure 10. Impacts of different (A) Ag-NP and (B) ZnO-NP concentrations (0.97–62.5 µg/mL) (X-axis) on biofilm eradication of the *P. acne* strains, NCTC747, P1, and P2, using TCC staining after a 72 h incubation period and measuring OD at 490 nm (Y-axis). **** $p < 0.0001$, ** $p < 0.001$, and * $p < 0.01$.

4. Discussion

P. acnes is one of the most abundant bacteria present on human skin. Although acne is not a contagious condition, an earlier study has highlighted the involvement of *P. acnes*, a Gram-positive bacterium, which resides on the pilosebaceous unit [54]. The continuous therapeutic application of antibiotics can cause them to become ineffective against *P.*

acnes owing to the development of antibiotic resistance [10–12,55]. Employing NPs as a treatment for *P. acnes* may have clinical utility considering the increasing emergence of bacteria demonstrating resistance to traditional antibiotics. The aim of this study was to observe the anti-microbial properties of Ag-NPs and ZnO-NPs in relation to the growth of *P. acnes*. Three strains were investigated, i.e., two *P. acnes* clinical isolates, and the reference strain, NCTC747.

In this research, NPs were manufactured in conjunction with a seed extract obtained from *P. harmala*. The latter provided an economical source of both reducing and capping agents, which stabilise the NPs produced, facilitate the use of an environmentally friendly green synthesis approach, and restrict the toxic by-products and chemical waste substances created by chemical production methods [56,57].

In this study, the presence of both phenolic compounds and flavonoids was demonstrated in the extract produced from *P. harmala*. As secondary metabolites, phenolic compounds are characterised by their redox potentials which facilitate their ability to scavenge radicals and confer an antioxidant action which enables them to be utilised as reducing agents, hydrogen donors, and singlet oxygen quenchers, as well as for the chelation of metals [58]. Flavonoids, saponins, tannins, compounds reducers, volatile oils, anthraquinones, triterpenes, sterols, and alkaloids have been demonstrated in extract of *P. harmala* [59]. Therapeutic properties have been attributed to several of the chemical substances present [42,60]. The spectrum of phytochemical components found in plants reflects their practically unrestricted capacity to manufacture aromatic compounds and their derivatives. The latter have frequently been utilised by healers for their pain-relieving and antiseptic properties, as well as their activity against malaria and bacterial pathogens [61].

In the current study, green synthesised Ag-NPs and ZnO-NPs were produced using *P harmala* extracts, which function as both reducing and stabilising agents [62]. The formation of NPs was evidenced by the alteration in colour of the silver nitrate solution, transitioning from a brightly coloured orange to a deep reddish-brown colour for AgNPs, and from a light brown colour to a yellowish-black colour for ZnO-NPs. The results were consistent with earlier research [63,64].

The production of NPs was confirmed using UV–visible spectroscopy, which proved to be an effective way to confirm the synthesis of NPs [65]. The Ag-NPs and ZnO-NPs exhibited absorption peaks at around 460 and 399 nm, respectively; this is related to SPR in the case of AgNPs and due to the transition from valence band to conduction band in ZnO-NPs. The results obtained were consistent with the research conducted by Singh, Kim [66], and Pryshchepa and Pomastowski [67], which indicated that AgNPs and ZnO-NPs exhibited spectral bands within the range from 450 to 500 nm and from 350 to 450 nm, respectively. Upon comparing our findings with the prior results, it was discovered that both Ag-NPs and ZnO-NPs were successfully created.

The Ag-NPs exhibited a lower particle size compared to the ZnO-NPs, along with a more limited range of particle sizes. This observation was supported by the computed standard deviation (SD) obtained from the measurement of particle sizes. The DLS results validated the analysis of UV spectra for both AgNPs and ZnO-NPs.

The X-ray diffraction (XRD) peaks exhibited a strong correlation with the crystalline structure of Ag-NPs and ZnO-NPs. The examination revealed the degree of purity in the manufacturing of nanoparticles. The diffraction peak positions exhibited an identical pattern to that observed in the JCPDS.

The stability of NPs is governed by their zeta potential values [68]. These values indicate that the surface of the NPs has a negative charge, allowing them to disperse in the medium with a high level of stability. Particles with zeta potential values ranging from +35 to −35 mV are classified as a stable suspension, according to reports [69]. This suggests that our NPs were in a state of stability. Therefore, the presence of negative charges prevents the agglomeration of particles by creating an electric repulsion force between molecules with identical negative charges. This force stabilises the particles in their colloidal solution [70].

The SEM data validated the production of NPs and demonstrated their approximately spherical morphology and consistent dimensions.

The data revealed in this investigation show that the Ag-NPs and ZnO-NPs produced using this green synthesis technique could have significant anti-bacterial properties, as indicated specifically by the MIC and MBC values obtained via the broth microdilution method. It was observed that at low concentrations, both types of NPs were biocidal and effective against the anaerobic bacterium, *P. acnes*. Additionally, a disc diffusion anti-microbial activity assay demonstrated relatively high anti-bacterial activity in comparison to doxycycline, based on the size of the inhibition zones. Numerous investigations have documented the strong anti-bacterial activity of Ag-NPs and ZnO-NPs [71–74]. This arises because the small particle size creates a high surface/volume ratio, which allows NPs to permeate membranes more effectively and consequently to disturb bacterial metabolism and cell structure [75]. Despite the fact that both Ag-NPs and ZnO-NPs demonstrated powerful anti-microbial actions in the assays evaluating growth and MIC, in general, the effectiveness of the Ag-NPs was superior with respect to the three *P. acne* strains as a lower concentration proved to be efficacious.

Interestingly, this study's findings also revealed that Ag-NPs and ZnO-NPs have a dose-dependent effect, which prevents the development of *P. acnes*-related biofilms in vitro. It has been demonstrated that established biofilms degrade when exposed to Ag-NPs and ZnO-NPs, despite the fact that many anti-microbials are less effective at killing bacteria enmeshed in biofilms [76]. *P. acnes* has also been shown to be more resistant to antibiotics when it is present as a biofilm rather than in the planktonic development phase [77,78].

A number of researchers have proposed that biofilm is predominantly disrupted as a result of Ag-NPs attaching to the EPS matrix. Recognition of the bacterial membrane peptidoglycan moieties leads to physical disruption, the liberation of ions, and the synthesis of reactive oxygen species (ROS), thereby generating oxidative stress and injuring chromosomal material [79]. The administration of Ag-NPs leads to alterations in the morphology in the structure of the biofilm, e.g., the creation of irregularities on the cell surface which infer the presence of cell lysis [80], cell wall disturbances, corrugation damage to the membrane, polarisation, and permeability variations within the membrane, and the generation of a specific EPS matrix which encompasses the strains of the organism [81]. Bacterial membrane breaches may also occur as a result of electrostatic bond formation with Ag-NPs, enabling them to pass through into the established biofilm [82].

The mechanisms responsible for the anti-bacterial actions of ZnO-NPs remain unclear. It has been postulated that NPs may injure the membrane of bacteria through perforation, penetration, or cellular uptake. Cytoplasmic contents may consequently escape and lead to cellular demise [83,84]. Following internalisation, the production of ROS may be promoted by ZnO-NPs, or Zn ions may be liberated which cause injury to genetic material, mitochondria, proteins, or other key cellular constituents essential for bacterial viability [85,86]. If NPs become associated with the membrane of bacteria, the NP–cell wall interface becomes a site for ROS manufacture. This process is promoted by irradiation with light and is the principal mode of bactericidal activity [87]. ROS produced and accrued precipitate oxidative stress-induced plasma membrane injury. The larger surface area of smaller NPs enables a higher concentration of ROS to be generated in proximity to the cell wall and consequently enhances the bactericidal effect [19].

Our findings show that the metabolic activity of the strains of *P. acnes* was diminished following the addition of both ZnO-NPs and Ag-NPs; the liberation of Ag and Zn ions could underlie this observation [88,89]. The inhibition of such cellular activities would inevitably lead to impaired bacterial cell function. Consequently, the free metal ions cause the demise of the bacterial cell via toxicity [90,91].

The current results demonstrate a higher efficacy of the Ag-NPs, in comparison to ZnO-NPs, in suppressing biofilm development or destroying biofilm. The Ag-NPs had larger growth inhibition diameters but were of a smaller dimension than the ZnO-NPs. Typically, the anti-bacterial or biomedical characteristics of NPs reflect the production technique and conditions, e.g., the reducing agent used and temperature, as well as the strength applied and their dimensions [33,34]. The identical reducing agent for each NP type was utilised for this study, and so the anti-biofilm and anti-bacterial properties observed may be partially a result of NP dimension disparity [92]. For the NPs that are of a greater dimension, they form clusters at the outer membrane of bacterial pathogens, and ROS manufacture forms the principal anti-microbial mechanism, the latter being able to injure the bacterial membrane [93]. The greater surface area of smaller NPs facilitates a higher degree of ROS production and, consequently, a more potent anti-bacterial effect [94]. Earlier studies have shown that NPs of smaller dimensions congregate in proximity to pathogens [92]. Consequently, their anti-microbial effect is enhanced as ROS are generated adjacent to the bacterial membrane. The ability of NPs to breach cell membranes and to enter the cell also facilitates the catastrophic intracellular manufacture of ROS, thereby promoting smaller NPs to a state of higher bactericidal efficacy [92].

Ions are liberated from the surface of intracellular NPs and become bound to key cell constituents and nutrients, resulting in a cytotoxic effect [95]. Although the true mechanism through which NPs negatively impact bacteria merits additional study, the current findings suggest that the dimension of the NPs is a factor governing their bactericidal activity. ZnO-NPs, with a spherical morphology and diameter of 6 nm, were demonstrated to have greater efficacy than 55 nm long ZnO nanorods when tested against *E. Coli* and *S. aureus* according [96].

Despite the fact that Ag-NPs and ZnO-NPs are promising anti-bacterial tools, concern remains regarding their adverse event profile in humans. The likelihood of cytotoxicity following their use has retarded their development for inclusion in chemotherapy regimens [97]. One study utilised the neutral red uptake test to determine the toxic profile of a spectrum of Ag-NP titres in HeLa cell lines [98]. At strengths of $\leq$120 μg/mL, no toxicity was demonstrated, but at 240 μg/mL, cytotoxicity was seen. This is a higher titre of Ag-NPs and ZnO-NPs than that investigated in the current study. Experiments performed on in vitro human cell cultures have identified toxic effects for Ag-NPs within the dose spectrum 10–100 μg/mL [99,100]. In the current study, bacterial inhibition was observed at lower does than those reported as toxic, which implies that there is the potential for the safe use of low concentrations of NPs.

To the best of the authors' knowledge, large research studies have not yet been performed which have investigated the possible utility of NPs in the treatment of infection with *P. acnes*. A limitation of the current work was that only two strains of *P. acnes* were studied, and so only preliminary data could be presented. Additional studies are therefore required, for instance, to assess the impact of using NPs either admixed with or containing conventional anti-bacterial agents. The current study presents some basic data which substantiate the use of NPs against biofilms of *P. acnes*. This is highly pertinent to the ongoing difficulties created by the emergence of resistance to traditional anti-microbial agents and their control worldwide.

To date, unlike the issue with conventional antibiotics, there has been no emergence of bacterial resistance to NPs despite extended periods of exposure. The biocidal effects of NPs appear to focus on a number of loci within bacterial cells and therefore offer a broad activity spectrum. This may underlie the failure of bacteria to show resistance despite prolonged applications. The technique used for preparing Ag-NPs and ZnO-NPs was simple, eco-friendly, and cost-effective, and thus, the method is suitable for commercial upscaling. However, further studies are required to determine the safety of these green synthesised NPs in order to enable these agents to become established as a treatment for use in vivo. Further research is recommended.

It can be concluded that dilute titres of Ag-NPs and ZnO-NPs could have anti-bacterial effects and also exhibit anti-biofilm activity in the context of either de novo created or well-established biofilms. They therefore could have the potential to be an efficacious constituent in dermo-cosmetic therapies for acne. These results substantiate the future potential for Ag-NPs and ZnO-NPs to become established either as an anti-bacterial medication per se or as an adjunct to established anti-microbial therapies. It is suggested that future studies could evaluate the effects of NPs delivered alongside conventional anti-microbial agents. Such work could facilitate the implementation of NPs as an additional mode of treatment against infectious disease. In order to achieve this, additional investigations conducted both in vitro and on a molecular level are required to gain a greater understanding of the toxic effects of the released Ag and Zn metal ions. Additionally, longitudinal studies are merited to obtain a complete adverse event profile for these agents in the long term and to establish their potential for mutagenic or carcinogenic effects. This research is paramount in order to clarify that NPs could be implemented in the clinical domain without hazard. The way in which both Ag-NPs and ZnO-NPs interact with innate system immune cells could also be assessed by future research, as this may influence their anti-microbial potency and effect on established biofilms.

Supplementary Materials: The following supporting information can be downloaded at: https://www.mdpi.com/article/10.3390/ph17020255/s1, Figure S1: color change in the reaction mixture indicating formation of Ag-NPs and ZnO-NPs; Table S1: Biofilm forming ability of *P.acne*

Author Contributions: H.A.-M. was responsible for the study design and supervised M.A., D.A.B., L.I. and H.A.B. when performing the experiments. He analysed data, prepared figures, and co-wrote the manuscript. M.A., D.A.B., L.I. and H.A.B. are research assistants and were responsible for performing the experiments under the supervision of H.A.-M., B.A.A., I.A., S.H., S.A.H.M. and M.I.M. was responsible for the biosynthesis of Ag-NPs and ZnO-NPs and characterisation. All authors have read and agreed to the published version of the manuscript.

Funding: This research was funded by Department of scientific research at The Jordanian Hashemite University grant number [580].

Institutional Review Board Statement: The study was conducted in accordance with the Declaration of Helsinki and approved by the Institutional Review Board of The Hashemite University (NO.7/62022/2023).

Informed Consent Statement: Informed consent was obtained from all subjects involved in the study.

Data Availability Statement: The datasets used and/or analysed during the current study are available from the corresponding author on reasonable request.

Acknowledgments: The researchers wish to thank the Department of scientific research at The Jordanian Hashemite University for their financial support.

Conflicts of Interest: The authors declare no conflict of interest.

References

1. Schommer, N.N.; Gallo, R.L. Structure and function of the human skin microbiome. *Trends Microbiol.* **2013**, *21*, 660–668. [CrossRef]
2. Tuchayi, S.M.; Makrantonaki, E.; Ganceviciene, R.; Dessinioti, C.; Feldman, S.R.; Zouboulis, C.C. Acne vulgaris. *Nat. Rev. Dis. Primers.* **2015**, *1*, 15029. [CrossRef] [PubMed]
3. Sachdeva, M.; Tan, J.; Lim, J.; Kim, M.; Nadeem, I.; Bismil, R. The prevalence, risk factors, and psychosocial impacts of acne vulgaris in medical students: A literature review. *Int. J. Dermatol.* **2020**, *60*, 792–798. [CrossRef]
4. Prasad, S.B. Acne vulgaris: A review on pathophysiology and treatment. *Asian J. Pharm. Clin. Res.* **2016**, *9*, 54–59.
5. Taylor, M.; Gonzalez, M.; Porter, R. Pathways to inflammation: Acne pathophysiology. *Eur. J. Dermatol.* **2011**, *21*, 323–333. [CrossRef]
6. Dréno, B.; Pécastaings, S.; Corvec, S.; Veraldi, S.; Khammari, A.; Roques, C. Cutibacterium acnes (Propionibacterium acnes) and acne vulgaris: A brief look at the latest updates. *J. Eur. Acad. Dermatol. Venereol.* **2018**, *32* (Suppl. S2), 5–14. [CrossRef]
7. Liu, P.-F.; Hsieh, Y.-D.; Lin, Y.-C.; Two, A.; Shu, C.-W.; Huang, C.-M. Propionibacterium acnes in the Pathogenesis and Immunotherapy of Acne Vulgaris. *Curr. Drug Metab.* **2015**, *16*, 245–254. [CrossRef]
8. Ogé, L.K.; Broussard, A.; Marshall, M.D. Acne Vulgaris: Diagnosis and Treatment. *Am. Fam. Physician* **2019**, *100*, 475–484. [PubMed]
9. Eichenfield, D.Z.; Sprague, J.; Eichenfield, L.F. Management of Acne Vulgaris: A Review. *JAMA* **2021**, *326*, 2055–2067. [CrossRef]
10. Kayiran, M.A.; Karadag, A.S.; Al-Khuzaei, S.; Chen, W.; Parish, L.C. Antibiotic Resistance in Acne: Mechanisms, Complications and Management. *Am. J. Clin. Dermatol.* **2020**, *21*, 813–819. [CrossRef]

11. Zhu, T.; Zhu, W.; Wang, Q.; He, L.; Wu, W.; Liu, J.; Li, Y.; Sun, D. Antibiotic susceptibility of Propionibacterium Acnes isolated from patients with acne in a public hospital in Southwest China: Prospective cross-sectional study. *BMJ Open* **2019**, *9*, e022938. [CrossRef]
12. Nakase, K.; Aoki, S.; Sei, S.; Fukumoto, S.; Horiuchi, Y.; Yasuda, T.; Tanioka, M.; Sugai, J.; Huh, W.W.; Kakuta, M.; et al. Characterization of acne patients carrying clindamycin-resistant *Cutibacterium acnes*: A Japanese multicenter study. *J. Dermatol.* **2020**, *47*, 863–869. [CrossRef]
13. Platsidaki, E.; Dessinioti, C. Recent advances in understanding Propionibacterium acnes (*Cutibacterium acnes*) in acne. *F1000Research* **2018**, *7*, 1953. [CrossRef]
14. Yu, Y.; Champer, J.; Garbán, H.; Kim, J. Typing of *Propionibacterium acnes*: A review of methods and comparative analysis. *Br. J. Dermatol.* **2015**, *172*, 1204–1209. [CrossRef]
15. Burkhart, C.G.; Burkhart, C.N. Expanding the microcomedone theory and acne therapeutics: Propionibacterium acnes biofilm produces biological glue that holds corneocytes together to form plug. *J. Am. Acad. Dermatol.* **2007**, *57*, 722–724. [CrossRef]
16. Vestby, L.K.; Grønseth, T.; Simm, R.; Nesse, L.L. Bacterial Biofilm and its Role in the Pathogenesis of Disease. *Antibiotics* **2020**, *9*, 59. [CrossRef] [PubMed]
17. Bjarnsholt, T. The role of bacterial biofilms in chronic infections. *APMIS* **2013**, *121*, 1–58. [CrossRef] [PubMed]
18. Perni, S.; Caserta, S.; Pasquino, R.; Jones, S.A.; Prokopovich, P. Prolonged Antimicrobial Activity of PMMA Bone Cement with Embedded Gentamicin-Releasing Silica Nanocarriers. *ACS Appl. Bio Mater.* **2019**, *2*, 1850–1861. [CrossRef] [PubMed]
19. Artounian, K.; Bundogji, N.; Hoss, E.; Boen, M. Applications of Gold and Silver Nanoparticles in the Treatment of Acne Vulgaris: A Systematic Review. *J. Drugs Dermatol.* **2021**, *20*, 666–670. [CrossRef] [PubMed]
20. Chakraborty, N.; Narayanan, V.; Gautam, H.K. Nano-Therapeutics to Treat Acne Vulgaris. *Indian J. Microbiol.* **2022**, *62*, 167–174. [CrossRef] [PubMed]
21. Bruna, T.; Maldonado-Bravo, F.; Jara, P.; Caro, N. Silver Nanoparticles and Their Antibacterial Applications. *Int. J. Mol. Sci.* **2021**, *22*, 7202. [CrossRef]
22. Gold, K.; Slay, B.; Knackstedt, M.; Gaharwar, A.K. Antimicrobial Activity of Metal and Metal-Oxide Based Nanoparticles. *Adv. Ther.* **2018**, *1*, 1700033. [CrossRef]
23. Mba, I.E.; Nweze, E.I. Nanoparticles as therapeutic options for treating multidrug-resistant bacteria: Research progress, challenges, and prospects. *World J. Microbiol. Biotechnol.* **2021**, *37*, 108. [CrossRef] [PubMed]
24. Tekade, R.K.; Maheshwari, R.; Soni, N.; Tekade, M.; Chougule, M.B. Chapter 1—Nanotechnology for the Development of Nanomedicine. In *Nanotechnology-Based Approaches for Targeting and Delivery of Drugs and Genes*; Academic Press: Cambridge, MA, USA, 2017; pp. 3–61.
25. Dey, D.; Chowdhury, S.; Sen, R. Insight into recent advances on nanotechnology-mediated removal of antibiotic resistant bacteria and genes. *J. Water Process. Eng.* **2023**, *52*, 103535. [CrossRef]
26. Rieger, K.A.; Cho, H.J.; Yeung, H.F.; Fan, W.; Schiffman, J.D. Antimicrobial Activity of Silver Ions Released from Zeolites Immobilized on Cellulose Nanofiber Mats. *ACS Appl. Mater. Interfaces* **2016**, *8*, 3032–3040. [CrossRef] [PubMed]
27. Prakash, P.; Gnanaprakasam, P.; Emmanuel, R.; Arokiyaraj, S.; Saravanan, M. Green synthesis of silver nanoparticles from leaf extract of Mimusops elengi, Linn. for enhanced antibacterial activity against multi drug resistant clinical isolates. *Colloids Surf. B Biointerfaces* **2013**, *108*, 255–259. [CrossRef] [PubMed]
28. Kailasa, S.K.; Park, T.J.; Rohit, J.V.; Koduru, J.R. Chapter 14—Antimicrobial activity of silver nanoparticles. In *Nanoparticles in Pharmacotherapy*; William Andrew Publishing: Norwich, NY, USA, 2019; pp. 461–484.
29. Yusof, H.M.; Mohamad, R.; Zaidan, U.H.; Rahman, N.A.A. Microbial synthesis of zinc oxide nanoparticles and their potential application as an antimicrobial agent and a feed supplement in animal industry: A review. *J. Anim. Sci. Biotechnol.* **2019**, *10*, 57. [CrossRef]
30. Salem, W.; Leitner, D.R.; Zingl, F.G.; Schratter, G.; Prassl, R.; Goessler, W.; Reidl, J.; Schild, S. Antibacterial activity of silver and zinc nanoparticles against Vibrio cholerae and enterotoxic Escherichia coli. *Int. J. Med. Microbiol.* **2014**, *305*, 85–95. [CrossRef] [PubMed]
31. Al-Qubaisi, M.S.; El Zowalaty, M.E.; Rasedee, A.; Flaifel, M.H.; Ahmad, S.H.; Hussein-Al-Ali, S.H.; Hussein, M.Z.; Eid, E.E.E.; Zulkanain; Saeed, M.; et al. Cytotoxicity of nickel zinc ferrite nanoparticles on cancer cells of epithelial origin. *Int. J. Nanomed.* **2013**, *8*, 2497–2508. [CrossRef]
32. Premanathan, M.; Karthikeyan, K.; Jeyasubramanian, K.; Manivannan, G. Selective toxicity of ZnO nanoparticles toward Gram-positive bacteria and cancer cells by apoptosis through lipid peroxidation. *Nanomed. Nanotechnol. Biol. Med.* **2011**, *7*, 184–192. [CrossRef]
33. Shreyash, N.; Bajpai, S.; Khan, M.A.; Vijay, Y.; Tiwary, S.K.; Sonker, M. Green Synthesis of Nanoparticles and Their Biomedical Applications: A Review. *ACS Appl. Nano Mater.* **2021**, *4*, 11428–11457. [CrossRef]
34. Sharma, S.; Kumar, K.; Thakur, N.; Chauhan, S.; Chauhan, M.S. The effect of shape and size of ZnO nanoparticles on their antimicrobial and photocatalytic activities: A green approach. *Bull. Mater. Sci.* **2019**, *43*, 20. [CrossRef]
35. Marslin, G.; Siram, K.; Maqbool, Q.; Selvakesavan, R.K.; Kruszka, D.; Kachlicki, P.; Franklin, G. Secondary Metabolites in the Green Synthesis of Metallic Nanoparticles. *Materials* **2018**, *11*, 940. [CrossRef]

36. El-Seedi, H.R.; El-Shabasy, R.M.; Khalifa, S.A.M.; Saeed, A.; Shah, A.; Shah, R.; Iftikhar, F.J.; Abdel-Daim, M.M.; Omri, A.; Hajrahand, N.H.; et al. Metal nanoparticles fabricated by green chemistry using natural extracts: Biosynthesis, mechanisms, and applications. *RSC Adv.* **2019**, *9*, 24539–24559. [CrossRef] [PubMed]
37. Yadi, M.; Mostafavi, E.; Saleh, B.; Davaran, S.; Aliyeva, I.; Khalilov, R.; Nikzamir, M.; Nikzamir, N.; Akbarzadeh, A.; Panahi, Y.; et al. Current developments in green synthesis of metallic nanoparticles using plant extracts: A review. *Artif. Cells Nanomed. Biotechnol.* **2018**, *46*, 336–343. [CrossRef] [PubMed]
38. Ishak, N.A.I.M.; Kamarudin, S.K.; Timmiati, S.N. Green synthesis of metal and metal oxide nanoparticles via plant extracts: An overview. *Mater. Res. Express* **2019**, *6*, 112004. [CrossRef]
39. Nasrollahzadeh, M.; Sajjadi, M.; Sajadi, S.M.; Issaabadi, Z. Chapter 5—Green Nanotechnology. In *Interface Science and Technology*; Nasrollahzadeh, M., Sajadi, S.M., Sajjadi, M., Issaabadi, Z., Atarod, M., Eds.; Elsevier: Amsterdam, The Netherlands, 2019; Volume 28, pp. 145–198, ISBN 1573-4285.
40. Geraldes, A.N.; da Silva, A.A.; Leal, J.; Estrada-Villegas, G.M.; Lincopan, N.; Katti, K.V.; LugÃo, A.B. Green Nanotechnology from Plant Extracts: Synthesis and Characterization of Gold Nanoparticles. *Adv. Nanopart.* **2016**, *5*, 176–185. [CrossRef]
41. Marwat, S.K.; Rehman, F. Chapter 70—Medicinal and Pharmacological Potential of Harmala (*Peganum harmala* L.) Seeds. In *Nuts and Seeds in Health and Disease Prevention*; Preedy, V.R., Watson, R.R., Patel, V.B., Eds.; Academic Press: San Diego, CA, USA, 2011; pp. 585–599, ISBN 978-0-12-375688-6.
42. Moloudizargari, M.; Mikaili, P.; Aghajanshakeri, S.; Asghari, M.; Shayegh, J. Pharmacological and therapeutic effects of *Peganum harmala* and its main alkaloids. *Pharmacogn. Rev.* **2013**, *7*, 199–212. [CrossRef] [PubMed]
43. Asgarpanah, J.; Ramezanloo, F. Chemistry, pharmacology and medicinal properties of *Peganum harmala* L. *Afr. J. Pharm. Pharmacol.* **2012**, *6*, 1573–1580. [CrossRef]
44. Singleton, V.L.; Orthofer, R.; Lamuela-Raventós, R.M. Analysis of total phenols and other oxidation substrates and antioxidants by means of folin-ciocalteu reagent. *Methods Enzymol.* **1999**, *299*, 152–178. [CrossRef]
45. Vuolo, M.M.; Lima, V.S.; Junior, M.R.M. Phenolic compounds: Structure, classification, and antioxidant power. In *Bioactive Compounds*; Woodhead Publishing: Sawston, UK, 2019; pp. 33–50.
46. Singleton, V.L.; Rossi, J.A. Colorimetry of Total Phenolics with Phosphomolybdic-Phosphotungstic Acid Reagents. *Am. J. Enol. Vitic.* **1965**, *16*, 144–158. [CrossRef]
47. Pękal, A.; Pyrzynska, K. Evaluation of Aluminium Complexation Reaction for Flavonoid Content Assay. *Food Anal. Methods* **2014**, *7*, 1776–1782. [CrossRef]
48. Stepanović, S.; Vuković, D.; Hola, V.; Bonaventura, G.D.; Djukić, S.; Ćirković, I.; Ruzicka, F. Quantification of biofilm in microtiter plates: Overview of testing conditions and practical recommendations for assessment of biofilm production by staphylococci. *APMIS* **2007**, *115*, 891–899. [CrossRef]
49. Stockert, J.C.; Horobin, R.W.; Colombo, L.L.; Blázquez-Castro, A. Tetrazolium salts and formazan products in Cell Biology: Viability assessment, fluorescence imaging, and labeling perspectives. *Acta Histochem.* **2018**, *120*, 159–167. [CrossRef]
50. Grela, E.; Kozłowska, J.; Grabowiecka, A. Current methodology of MTT assay in bacteria—A review. *Acta Histochem.* **2018**, *120*, 303–311. [CrossRef]
51. Sabaeifard, P.; Abdi-Ali, A.; Soudi, M.R.; Dinarvand, R. Optimization of tetrazolium salt assay for *Pseudomonas aeruginosa* biofilm using microtiter plate method. *J. Microbiol. Methods* **2014**, *105*, 134–140. [CrossRef]
52. Motelica, L.; Vasile, B.-S.; Ficai, A.; Surdu, A.-V.; Ficai, D.; Oprea, O.-C.; Andronescu, E.; Mustățea, G.; Ungureanu, E.L.; Dobre, A.A. Antibacterial Activity of Zinc Oxide Nanoparticles Loaded with Essential Oils. *Pharmaceutics* **2023**, *15*, 2470. [CrossRef]
53. Dorofeev, G.A.; Streletskii, A.N.; Povstugar, I.V.; Protasov, A.V.; Elsukov, E.P. Determination of nanoparticle sizes by X-ray diffraction. *Colloid J.* **2012**, *74*, 675–685. [CrossRef]
54. Omer, H.; McDowell, A.; Alexeyev, O.A. Understanding the role of Propionibacterium acnes in acne vulgaris: The critical importance of skin sampling methodologies. *Clin. Dermatol.* **2017**, *35*, 118–129. [CrossRef] [PubMed]
55. Prabu, S.L.; Umamaheswari, A.; Rajakumar, S.; Bhuvaneswari, P.; Muthupetchi, S. Development and Evaluation of Gel Incorporated with Synthesized Silver Nanoparticle from Ocimum gratissimum for the Treatment of Acne Vulgaris. *Am. J. Adv. Drug Deliv.* **2017**, *5*, 303–311. [CrossRef]
56. Salem, S.S.; Fouda, A. Green Synthesis of Metallic Nanoparticles and Their Prospective Biotechnological Applications: An Overview. *Biol. Trace Elem. Res.* **2020**, *199*, 344–370. [CrossRef] [PubMed]
57. Dikshit, P.K.; Kumar, J.; Das, A.K.; Sadhu, S.; Sharma, S.; Singh, S.; Gupta, P.K.; Kim, B.S. Green Synthesis of Metallic Nanoparticles: Applications and Limitations. *Catalysts* **2021**, *11*, 902. [CrossRef]
58. Olszowy, M. What is responsible for antioxidant properties of polyphenolic compounds from plants? *Plant Physiol. Biochem.* **2019**, *144*, 135–143. [CrossRef] [PubMed]
59. Benbott, A.; Bahri, L.; Boubendir, A.; Yahia, A. Study of the chemical components of *Peganum harmala* and evaluation of acute toxicityof alkaloids extracted in the Wistar albino mice. *J. Mater. Environ. Sci.* **2013**, *4*, 558–565.
60. Miraj, S. A Review Study of Therapeutic Effects of *Peganum harmala*. Scholars Research Library. Available online: https://www.scholarsresearchlibrary.com/articles/a-review-study-of-therapeutic-effects-of-peganum-harmala.pdf (accessed on 10 November 2023).
61. Kutama, R.M.; Abdulkadir, S.; Kwalli, S.A.; Chiroma, G. Phytochemical Compositions in Some Nigerian Medicinal Plants and Their Pharmacological Properties: A Review. *J. Anesthesiol.* **2018**, *6*, 15. [CrossRef]

62. Senhaji, S.; Lamchouri, F.; Boulfia, M.; Lachkar, N.; Bouabid, K.; Toufik, H. Mineral composition, content of phenolic compounds and in vitro antioxidant and antibacterial activities of aqueous and organic extracts of the seeds of *Peganum harmala* L. *S. Afr. J. Bot.* **2022**, *147*, 697–712. [CrossRef]
63. Al-Momani, H.; Al Balawi, D.; Hamed, S.; Albiss, B.A.; Almasri, M.; AlGhawrie, H.; Ibrahim, L.; Al Balawi, H.; Mahmoud, S.A.H.; Pearson, J.; et al. The impact of biosynthesized ZnO nanoparticles from Olea europaea (Common Olive) on *Pseudomonas aeruginosa* growth and biofilm formation. *Sci. Rep.* **2023**, *13*, 5096. [CrossRef]
64. Al-Momani, H.; Almasri, M.; Al Balawi, D.; Hamed, S.; Albiss, B.A.; Aldabaibeh, N.; Ibrahim, L.; Albalawi, H.; Mahmoud, S.A.H.; Khasawneh, A.I.; et al. The efficacy of biosynthesized silver nanoparticles against *Pseudomonas aeruginosa* isolates from cystic fibrosis patients. *Sci. Rep.* **2023**, *13*, 8876. [CrossRef]
65. Desai, R.; Mankad, V.; Gupta, S.; Jha, P. Size Distribution of Silver Nanoparticles: UV-Visible Spectroscopic Assessment. *Nanosci. Nanotechnol. Lett.* **2012**, *4*, 30–34. [CrossRef]
66. Singh, P.; Kim, Y.J.; Singh, H.; Wang, C.; Hwang, K.H.; Farh, M.E.A.; Yang, D.C. Biosynthesis, characterization, and antimicrobial applications of silver nanoparticles. *Int. J. Nanomed.* **2015**, *10*, 2567–2577.
67. Pryshchepa, O.; Pomastowski, P.; Buszewski, B. Silver nanoparticles: Synthesis, investigation techniques, and properties. *Adv. Colloid Interface Sci.* **2020**, *284*, 102246. [CrossRef]
68. Kumar, A.; Dixit, C.K. Methods for characterization of nanoparticles. In *Advances in Nanomedicine for the Delivery of Therapeutic Nucleic Acids*; Nimesh, S., Chandra, R., Gupta, N., Eds.; Elsevier: Amsterdam, The Netherlands, 2017; pp. 43–55.
69. Tuan, T.Q.; Hao, P.V.; Quynh, L.M.; Luong, N.H.; Hai, N.H. Preparation and Properties of Silver Nanoparticles by Heat-combined Electrochemical Method. *VNU J. Sci. Math.-Phys.* **2015**, *31*, 36–44.
70. Bhattacharjee, S. DLS and zeta potential—What they are and what they are not? *J. Control. Release* **2016**, *235*, 337–351. [CrossRef] [PubMed]
71. Lee, J.-H.; Kim, Y.-G.; Cho, M.H.; Lee, J. ZnO nanoparticles inhibit *Pseudomonas aeruginosa* biofilm formation and virulence factor production. *Microbiol. Res.* **2014**, *169*, 888–896. [CrossRef]
72. Ali, S.G.; Ansari, M.A.; Alzohairy, M.A.; Alomary, M.N.; Jalal, M.; AlYahya, S.; Asiri, S.M.M.; Khan, H.M. Effect of Biosynthesized ZnO Nanoparticles on Multi-Drug Resistant *Pseudomonas Aeruginosa*. *Antibiotics* **2020**, *9*, 260. [CrossRef] [PubMed]
73. Tang, S.; Zheng, J. Antibacterial Activity of Silver Nanoparticles: Structural Effects. *Adv. Healthc. Mater.* **2018**, *7*, 1701503. [CrossRef] [PubMed]
74. Das, C.A.; Kumar, V.G.; Dhas, T.S.; Karthick, V.; Govindaraju, K.; Joselin, J.M.; Baalamurugan, J. Antibacterial activity of silver nanoparticles (biosynthesis): A short review on recent advances. *Biocatal. Agric. Biotechnol.* **2020**, *27*, 101593. [CrossRef]
75. Lv, H.; Cui, S.; Yang, Q.; Song, X.; Wang, D.; Hu, J.; Zhou, Y.; Liu, Y. AgNPs-incorporated nanofiber mats: Relationship between AgNPs size/content, silver release, cytotoxicity, and antibacterial activity. *Mater. Sci. Eng. C* **2020**, *118*, 111331. [CrossRef] [PubMed]
76. Munita Jose, M.; Arias Cesar, A. Mechanisms of Antibiotic Resistance. *Microbiol. Spectr.* **2016**, *4*, 464–473. [CrossRef]
77. Coenye, T.; Peeters, E.; Nelis, H.J. Biofilm formation by Propionibacterium acnes is associated with increased resistance to antimicrobial agents and increased production of putative virulence factors. *Res. Microbiol.* **2007**, *158*, 386–392. [CrossRef]
78. Gebreyohannes, G.; Nyerere, A.; Bii, C.; Sbhatu, D.B. Challenges of intervention, treatment, and antibiotic resistance of biofilm-forming microorganisms. *Heliyon* **2019**, *5*, e02192. [CrossRef]
79. Ansari, M.A.; Khan, H.M.; Khan, A.A.; Cameotra, S.S.; Pal, R. Antibiofilm efficacy of silver nanoparticles against biofilm of extended spectrum β-lactamase isolates of Escherichia coli and Klebsiella pneumoniae. *Appl. Nanosci.* **2013**, *4*, 859–868. [CrossRef]
80. LewisOscar, F.; Nithya, C.; Vismaya, S.; Arunkumar, M.; Pugazhendhi, A.; Nguyen-Tri, P.; Alharbi, S.A.; Alharbi, N.S.; Thajuddin, N. In vitro analysis of green fabricated silver nanoparticles (AgNPs) against *Pseudomonas aeruginosa* PA14 biofilm formation, their application on urinary catheter. *Prog. Org. Coat.* **2020**, *151*, 106058. [CrossRef]
81. Pompilio, A.; Geminiani, C.; Bosco, D.; Rana, R.; Aceto, A.; Bucciarelli, T.; Scotti, L.; Di Bonaventura, G. Electrochemically Synthesized Silver Nanoparticles Are Active Against Planktonic and Biofilm Cells of *Pseudomonas aeruginosa* and Other Cystic Fibrosis-Associated Bacterial Pathogens. *Front. Microbiol.* **2018**, *9*, 1349. [CrossRef] [PubMed]
82. Samanta, S.; Banerjee, J.; Das, B.; Mandal, J.; Chatterjee, S.; Ali, K.M.; Sinha, S.; Giri, B.; Ghosh, T.; Dash, S.K. Antibacterial potency of cytocompatible chitosan-decorated biogenic silver nanoparticles and molecular insights towards cell-particle interaction. *Int. J. Biol. Macromol.* **2022**, *219*, 919–939. [CrossRef]
83. Zhang, L.; Jiang, Y.; Ding, Y.; Daskalakis, N.; Jeuken, L.; Povey, M.; O'neill, A.J.; York, D.W. Mechanistic investigation into antibacterial behaviour of suspensions of ZnO nanoparticles against *E. coli*. *J. Nanopart. Res.* **2009**, *12*, 1625–1636. [CrossRef]
84. Xie, Y.; He, Y.; Irwin, P.L.; Jin, T.; Shi, X. Antibacterial Activity and Mechanism of Action of Zinc Oxide Nanoparticles against *Campylobacter jejuni*. *Appl. Environ. Microbiol.* **2011**, *77*, 2325–2331. [CrossRef]
85. Pati, R.; Mehta, R.K.; Mohanty, S.; Padhi, A.; Sengupta, M.; Vaseeharan, B.; Goswami, C.; Sonawane, A. Topical application of zinc oxide nanoparticles reduces bacterial skin infection in mice and exhibits antibacterial activity by inducing oxidative stress response and cell membrane disintegration in macrophages. *Nanomed. Nanotechnol. Biol. Med.* **2014**, *10*, 1195–1208. [CrossRef]
86. Siddiqi, K.S.; Rahman, A.U.; Tajuddin; Husen, A. Properties of Zinc Oxide Nanoparticles and Their Activity Against Microbes. *Nanoscale Res. Lett.* **2018**, *13*, 141. [CrossRef] [PubMed]
87. Xie, S.; Zhu, J.; Yang, D.; Xu, Y.; Zhu, J.; He, D. Low Concentrations of Zinc Oxide Nanoparticles Cause Severe Cytotoxicity Through Increased Intracellular Reactive Oxygen Species. *J. Biomed. Nanotechnol.* **2021**, *17*, 2420–2432. [CrossRef] [PubMed]

88. Ahmed, B.; Dwivedi, S.; Abdin, M.Z.; Azam, A.; Al-Shaeri, M.; Khan, M.S.; Saquib, Q.; Al-Khedhairy, A.A.; Musarrat, J. Mitochondrial and Chromosomal Damage Induced by Oxidative Stress in Zn2+ Ions, ZnO-Bulk and ZnO-NPs treated Allium cepa roots. *Sci. Rep.* **2017**, *7*, srep40685. [CrossRef] [PubMed]
89. Shi, L.-E.; Li, Z.-H.; Zheng, W.; Zhao, Y.-F.; Jin, Y.-F.; Tang, Z.-X. Synthesis, antibacterial activity, antibacterial mechanism and food applications of ZnO nanoparticles: A review. *Food Addit. Contam. Part A* **2014**, *31*, 173–186. [CrossRef] [PubMed]
90. Sirelkhatim, A.; Mahmud, S.; Seeni, A.; Kaus, N.H.M.; Ann, L.C.; Bakhori, S.K.M.; Hasan, H.; Mohamad, D. Review on Zinc Oxide Nanoparticles: Antibacterial Activity and Toxicity Mechanism. *Nano-Micro Lett.* **2015**, *7*, 219–242. [CrossRef] [PubMed]
91. Heinlaan, M.; Ivask, A.; Blinova, I.; Dubourguier, H.-C.; Kahru, A. Toxicity of nanosized and bulk ZnO, CuO and TiO2 to bacteria Vibrio fischeri and crustaceans Daphnia magna and Thamnocephalus platyurus. *Chemosphere* **2008**, *71*, 1308–1316. [CrossRef] [PubMed]
92. Motelica, L.; Oprea, O.-C.; Vasile, B.-S.; Ficai, A.; Ficai, D.; Andronescu, E.; Holban, A.M. Antibacterial Activity of Solvothermal Obtained ZnO Nanoparticles with Different Morphology and Photocatalytic Activity against a Dye Mixture: Methylene Blue, Rhodamine B and Methyl Orange. *Int. J. Mol. Sci.* **2023**, *24*, 5677. [CrossRef]
93. Motelica, L.; Vasile, B.-S.; Ficai, A.; Surdu, A.-V.; Ficai, D.; Oprea, O.-C.; Andronescu, E.; Jinga, D.C.; Holban, A.M. Influence of the Alcohols on the ZnO Synthesis and Its Properties: The Photocatalytic and Antimicrobial Activities. *Pharmaceutics* **2022**, *14*, 2842. [CrossRef]
94. Dayem, A.A.; Hossain, M.K.; Lee, S.B.; Kim, K.; Saha, S.K.; Yang, G.-M.; Choi, H.Y.; Cho, S.-G. The Role of Reactive Oxygen Species (ROS) in the Biological Activities of Metallic Nanoparticles. *Int. J. Mol. Sci.* **2017**, *18*, 120. [CrossRef]
95. Toscano, F.; Torres-Arias, M. Nanoparticles cellular uptake, trafficking, activation, toxicity and in vitro evaluation. *Curr. Res. Immunol.* **2023**, *4*, 100073. [CrossRef] [PubMed]
96. Akter, M.; Sikder, M.T.; Rahman, M.M.; Ullah, A.K.M.A.; Hossain, K.F.B.; Banik, S.; Hosokawa, T.; Saito, T.; Kurasaki, M. A systematic review on silver nanoparticles-induced cytotoxicity: Physicochemical properties and perspectives. *J. Adv. Res.* **2018**, *9*, 1–16. [CrossRef]
97. Siddique, M.H.; Aslam, B.; Imran, M.; Ashraf, A.; Nadeem, H.; Hayat, S.; Khurshid, M.; Afzal, M.; Malik, I.R.; Shahzad, M.; et al. Research article effect of silver nanoparticles on biofilm formation and EPS production of multidrug-resistant Klebsiella pneumonia. *Hindawi BioMed Res. Int.* **2020**, *2020*, 6398165. [CrossRef]
98. Marin, S.; Vlasceanu, G.M.; Tiplea, R.E.; Bucur, I.R.; Lemnaru, M.; Marin, M.M.; Grumezescu, A.M. Applications and Toxicity of Silver Nanoparticles: A Recent Review. *Curr. Top. Med. Chem.* **2015**, *15*, 1596–1604. [CrossRef] [PubMed]
99. Jaswal, T.; Gupta, J. A review on the toxicity of silver nanoparticles on human health. *Mater. Today Proc.* **2021**, *81*, 859–863. [CrossRef]
100. Salomoni, R.; Léo, P.; Montemor, A.; Rinaldi, B.; Rodrigues, M. Antibacterial effect of silver nanoparticles in *Pseudomonas aeruginosa*. *Nanotechnol. Sci. Appl.* **2017**, *10*, 115–121. [CrossRef] [PubMed]

pharmaceuticals

Article

Biosynthesis and Characterization of Silver Nanoparticles and Simvastatin Association in Titanium Biofilms

Sindy Magri Roque [1,2], Ana Carolina Furian [1], Marcela Kim Takemoto [2], Marta Cristina Teixeira Duarte [2,3], Rafaela Durrer Parolina [2], Adriano Luís Roque [4], Nelson Duran [5], Janaína de Cássia Orlandi Sardi [6], Renata Maria Teixeira Duarte [3] and Karina Cogo Muller [1,2,*]

1 Laboratório de Farmacologia de Antimicrobianos e Microbiologia, Faculdade de Ciências Farmacêuticas, Universidade Estadual de Campinas (UNICAMP), Campinas 13083-970, Brazil; s152591@dac.unicamp.br (S.M.R.); anafurian@hotmail.com (A.C.F.)

2 Departamento de Biociências, Faculdade de Odontologia de Piracicaba, Universidade Estadual de Campinas (UNICAMP), Piracicaba 13414-903, Brazil; takemotomarcela@gmail.com (M.K.T.); mduarte@cpqba.unicamp.br (M.C.T.D.); rafaelaparolina@gmail.com (R.D.P.)

3 Centro Pluridisciplinar de Pesquisas Químicas, Biológicas e Agrícolas—CPQBA, Universidade Estadual de Campinas (UNICAMP), Paulínia 13148-218, Brazil; duartemt@unicamp.br

4 Programa de Pós Graduação em Medicina (Cardiologia), Universidade Federal de São Paulo (UNIFESP), São Paulo 04021-001, Brazil; adriano.roque@unifesp.br

5 Laboratório de Carcinogenese Urogenital e Imunoterapia, Universidade Estadual de Campinas (UNICAMP), Campinas 13083-862, Brazil; nelsonduran1942@gmail.com

6 Divisão de Pesquisa em Odontologia, Universidade de Guarulhos (UNG), Guarulhos 07023-070, Brazil; janasardi@gmail.com

* Correspondence: karinacm@unicamp.br

Abstract: Introduction: Simvastatin is an antilipidemic drug that has already demonstrated antibacterial activities on oral and non-oral microorganisms. Silver nanoparticles also exhibit antimicrobial properties, particularly for coating implant surfaces. In this study, we evaluated the effects of combining simvastatin with silver nanoparticles on the formation and viability of biofilms consolidated on titanium discs. Methods: Silver nanoparticles were first biosynthesized using the fungus *Fusarium oxysporum* and then characterized using Dynamic Light Scattering, X-ray Diffraction, Transmission Electron Microscopy, and energy dispersive spectroscopy. Species of *Streptococcus oralis*, *Streptococcus mutans*, *Porphyromonas gingivalis*, Methicillin-sensitive *Staphylococcus aureus*, and Methicillin-resistant *Staphylococcus aureus* were used and tested using Minimum Inhibitory Concentration assays with concentrations of silver nanoparticles and simvastatin alone and in combination. Biofilm inhibition and viability tests were performed on titanium surfaces. Toxicity tests were also performed on *Galleria mellonella* moth larvae. Results: The silver nanoparticles had a spherical shape without the formation of aggregates as confirmed by Transmission Electron Microscopy. Dynamic Light Scattering revealed nanoparticles with an average diameter of 53.8 nm (±1.23 nm), a polydispersity index of 0.23 and a zeta potential of −25 mV (±2.19 mV). The silver nanoparticles inhibited the growth of the strains tested in the range of 0.001592 and 63.75, while simvastatin alone inhibited the growth of the same strains in the range of 3.125–62.5 µg/mL. The antibacterial activity test of the combination of the two substances showed a reduction in the Minimum Inhibitory Concentration of about two to eight times, showing synergistic effects on *Staphylococcus aureus* and additive effects on *Streptococcus oralis* and *Porphyromonas gingivalis*. As for biofilm, sub-inhibitory concentrations of the combination of substances showed better antibacterial activity in inhibiting the formation of *Streptococcus oralis* biofilm, and this combination also proved effective in eradicating already established biofilms compared to the substances alone. The combination of silver nanoparticles and simvastatin showed low toxicity to *Galleria mellonella* moth larvae. Conclusions: The results presented indicate that the combination of the two substances could be an alternative for the prevention and reduction of biofilms on implants. These findings open up new possibilities in the search for alternatives for the treatment of peri-implant infections, as well as the possibility of using lower doses compared to single drugs, achieving the same results and reducing potential toxic effects.

Keywords: simvastatin; anti-infective agents; dental implants; silver nanoparticles

1. Introduction

Currently, the use of metal implants to replace missing teeth has become a customary practice, but despite the high success rate and long-term survival, patients may develop infections and inflammations in the peri-implant region, leading to implant failure [1–3].

Among the diseases that can affect the peri-implant region, the most common is mucositis, which is characterized by the involvement of only the surrounding soft tissues, followed by peri-implantitis, which is caused by progressive inflammation of the alveolar bone crest that supports the implant, resulting in bone loss and surgical failure [4–7].

Peri-implantitis sites have been associated with bacterial diversity with the growth of pathogenic anaerobic bacteria, specifically members of the "red complex" group, *Porphyromonas gingivalis, Tannerella forsythia, Treponema denticola,* and also other species from the *Treponema* I to III and *Synergisteteso* groups [8,9]. In addition, *Staphylococcus aureus, Pseudomonas aeruginosa,* and *Candida* sp. have been detected in cases of implant inflammation and have been associated with early implant failure [4,10–12].

Some of the individual's pre-existing conditions, such as diabetes mellitus, smoking, and poor hygiene, may contribute to the development and progression of peri-implantitis [13]. However, the main etiology is the formation of biofilms, which are communities of microorganisms around implants that can trigger a host response resulting from the immunological interaction of toxins, antigens, and lipopolysaccharides with epithelial cells and granulocytes in the sulcus of the gingival mucosa [14].

It is important to emphasize that the different chemical composition of biomaterials used in implants is related to bacterial adhesion and succession during biofilm formation [15]. In particular, on titanium surfaces, the formation of an acquired film free of bacteria and rich in proteins such as proline, secretory IgA, α-amylase, and high molecular weight mucins provides an interface between the implant and initial colonizers such as *Streptococcus* sp. and *Actinomyces* sp. species that reach the film and titanium by fluid flow, Brownian motion, and chemotaxis [16].

Streptococci are highly prevalent during initial biofilm formation, and *Streptococcus oralis* in particular has been found to be an early colonizer of oral implants and associated with periodontitis [17]. Compared to other species such as *Acntinomyces naeslundi, Veillonela díspar* and *P. gingivalis,* it showed a higher potential for biomass formation [18]. Thus, the abundance of colonies of this species has been shown to favor the binding of pathogens to the biofilm through the expansion of signaling molecules and has been associated with greater tissue destruction during implant insertion [19,20].

The most common treatments are based on removal of the biofilm by mechanical debridement, which can be combined with chemical decontamination. However, the clinical outcomes of these treatments are lower than expected and there is no good evidence to support the usefulness of currently available chemical decontamination methods [21]. In addition, nonrational prophylaxis and treatment with antibiotics can cause adverse reactions and contribute to an increased risk of infection by resistant microorganisms such as *Enterobacter* sp., *Candida* sp., and *Staphylococcus* sp. [22–25]. In addition, inadequate doses may not reach poorly vascularized regions such as bone [25].

The development of new antibacterial compounds can be effective alternatives for both the control and prophylaxis of peri-implant infections. Among noble metal nanoparticles, silver nanoparticles (AgNP) have demonstrated biological activity and have therefore been used as highly effective, broad-spectrum agents for use in biomedical devices [26]. In addition, AgNP have exceptional physical properties, including high surface-to-volume ratio, high catalytic potential, and greater reactivity compared to their conventional form [27]. In dentistry, silver nanoparticles are used in the development of various antibacterial materials, such as orthodontic appliances, acrylic resins for prosthetics, composite resins for restorations, irrigation solutions, adhesives, and implant coatings [28].

The combination of AgNP with other antibiotics has shown a synergistic effect by increasing the antibacterial activity of already used antibiotics by redirecting them to specific targets and reducing antibacterial resistance [29,30].

AgNP are mainly synthesized by chemical and physical methods, which are generally more expensive and can be harmful to the environment due to the use of substances with specific biological risk potential [27]. Therefore, bio-based ecological approaches using bacteria, fungi, and plant extracts can be advantageous alternatives as they are economically viable, environmentally friendly, safe, and scalable [31]. Among the microorganisms used for the production of AgNP, fungi are considered true nanofactories due to the fact that they produce AgNP extracellularly and by biomimetic mineralization [32]. The production of silver nanoparticles by the fungus *Fusarium oxysporum* consists of the extracellular reduction of Ag^+ ions to Ag^0 in the presence of NADH-dependent reductases and electron-transporting quinones [31,32].

Another therapeutic approach that can be used to combat bacterial infections is the repurposing of drugs that have antibacterial activity as a side effect [33]. In this regard, statins are important lipid-lowering agents that reduce cholesterol synthesis by inhibiting the enzyme 3-hydroxy-3-methylglutaryl coenzyme A reductase-HMG-CoA, and have pleiotropic effects, i.e., effects that go beyond cholesterol reduction, such as antioxidant, anticarcinogenic, anticoagulant, anti-inflammatory, immunomodulatory, and antibacterial effects [34–36].

The antibacterial activity of isolated simvastatin has been demonstrated against *S. aureus* both in planktonic form and in biofilms [35] and in the inhibition of multi-species biofilms causing periodontal disease [37,38]. Similarly, AgNP have been tested for coating implants for antibacterial purposes [39–41].

The interaction between AgNP and simvastatin has previously been shown to be synergistic against standard strains of *S. aureus* [42], and the combination of these compounds showed antibacterial activity against biofilms of clinical strains of *S. aureus* and methicillin-resistant *S. aureus* (MRSA) [36]. Therefore, the aim of this study was to evaluate the antibacterial activity of the combination of simvastatin and AgNP on the formation and viability of mature biofilms on titanium discs against *Streptococcus oralis*.

2. Results and Discussion

2.1. Physical-Chemical Characterization of AgNP

The synthesis of silver nanoparticles (AgNP) was carried out by the biosynthetic method using the fungus *Fusarium oxysporum*. The filtrate initially had a yellowish color, and after the addition of $AgNO_3$, the solution turned yellowish-brown: the change in color of the solution is the first evidence of AgNP formation, was observed after 24 h and stabilized after 168 h, and was confirmed by UV-vis spectroscopy [43]. As shown in Figure 1A, there was a single peak with an absorbance value of 430 nm, which was attributed to the presence of surface plasmon resonance [44]. Thus, when metal nanoparticles are irradiated with light, the free electrons on their surfaces oscillate, causing some of the visible light to be absorbed, explaining the so-called plasmon resonance effect, which depends on the type of material, the size of the particle and its morphology [45,46]. The absorbance value found is in agreement with other studies using *Fusarium* sp. in AgNP biosynthesis, which found values between 415 and 440 nm [32,47,48].

The UV-vis analysis of the dispersion of AgNP was evaluated at pH 7.4, a temperature of 28 °C, and a fungal biomass concentration of 10%, using a concentration of 3 mM $AgNO_3$. The entire biosynthetic process was carried out in the dark.

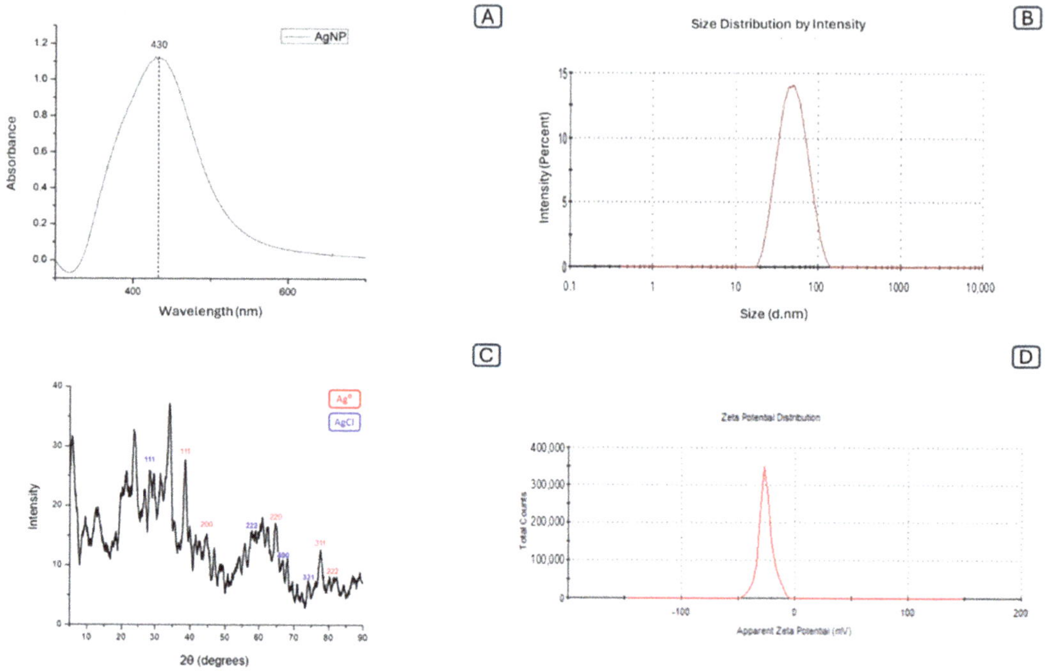

Figure 1. (**A**) UV-vis absorption spectrum of fungal filtrate after addition of $AgNO_3$. (**B**) AgNP size distribution versus intensity (Z-average 53.8). (**C**) X-ray diffraction pattern of AgNP (**D**) Zeta potential distribution (−25.66 mV).

As shown in Figure 1C, the evaluation of the crystalline nature of AgNP by X-ray diffraction (XRD) analysis showed Bragg reflections at $2\theta = 38.28°$, $44.53°$, $64.55°$, $77.64°$ and $81.33°$, which can be indexed as diffraction planes (111), (200), (220), (311) and (222), confirming the presence of AgNP with face-centered cubic crystalline structure [49]. Although to a lesser extent, other diffraction peaks were observed at $2\theta = 27.9°$, $57.6°$, $67.6°$, $74.6°$, representing facets of silver chloride nanoparticles (Ag/AgCl), a compound most commonly found in the final product of AgNP synthesized by biological routes [50], so they could be related to the partial oxidation of AgNP during synthesis due to the presence of chloride ions from the culture medium or metabolites from the fungal biomass. [51,52]. In addition, the AgNP produced showed a reflection at $2\theta = 33.9$, which refers to the plane (111) of Ag_2O. It is believed that the presence of oxide in the sample is due to the fact that the AgNP were not synthesized in an inert atmosphere [53].

Similar XRD patterns have been reported in studies using nanoparticles synthesized by *F. oxysporium* and in biogenic laccase nanoparticles produced by *Trametes versicolor* [54–56].

The EDS spectrum is an analytical technique used to determine the elemental composition and quantify specific elements [57]. The analyses presented in Figure 2D show a strong silver signal at 3 kev of oxygen ~0.5 kev, chlorine ~2.7 kev and carbon ~0.3 kev. In addition, the weight percentages of silver were 82.74%, oxygen 2.67%, chlorine 0.20% and carbon 12.37%, as shown in Table 1, confirming that the AgNP were the main products of biogenic synthesis. The presence of carbon as the second most contributing element may come from the proteins surrounding the nanoparticles. The average diameter of the nanoparticles was 53.8 nm (±1.23), as shown in Figure 1B, with 0.23 of polydispersity index (PDI), which indicates that the AgNP were monodisperse with a narrow size distribution [58]. In addition, the zeta potential was −25.66 ± (2.19 mV), a high zeta potential value, above ±30 mV, confers stability in colloidal systems so that the dispersion may resist aggregation, as shown in Figure 1D [59]. The spherical shape of the nanoparticles was confirmed by Transmission Electron Microscopy (TEM), and homogeneous and dispersed particles without aggregates were observed, as shown in Figure 2A,B.

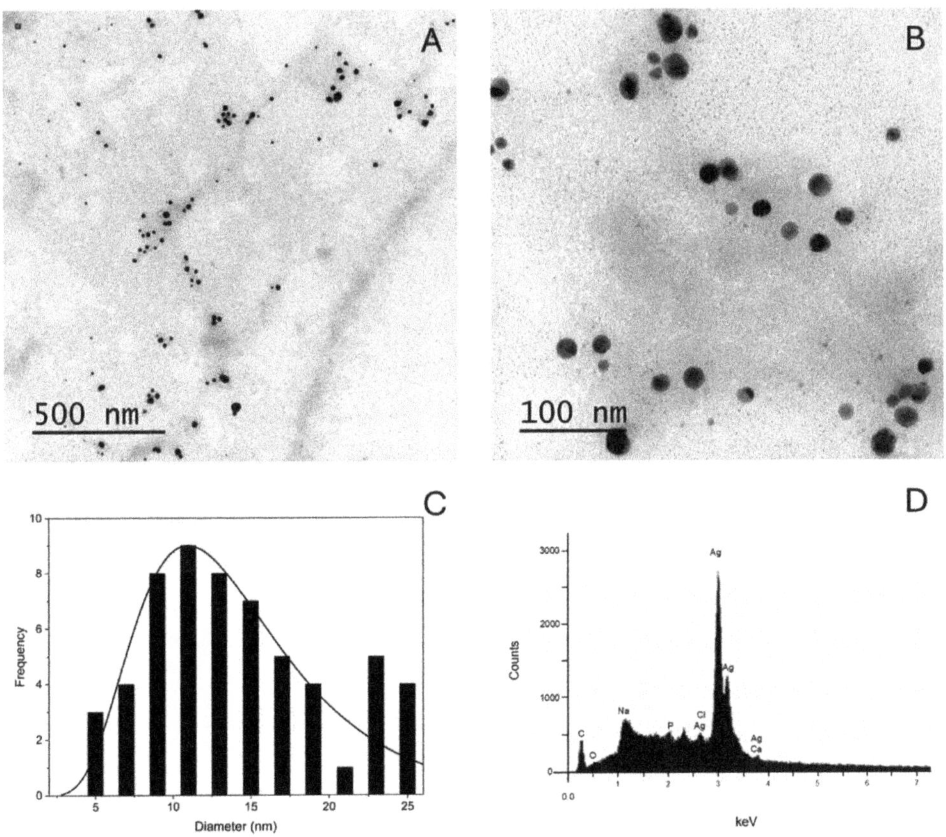

Figure 2. (**A**) Micrographs of biosynthesized AgNP obtained by TEM on scale of 500 nm. (**B**) AgNP on a scale of 100 nm. (**C**) Histogram of the size distribution of AgNP. (**D**) Energy dispersive X-ray (EDX) spectrum of AgNP.

Table 1. List of elements and their composition obtained in EDX analysis of AgNP.

Element	Weigth %	Atomic %
C	12.37	50.78
O	2.67	8.22
P	1.00	1.59
Cl	0.60	0.84
Ag	82.74	37.81
Ca	0.61	0.75

2.2. Minimum Inhibitory Concentration (MIC) Assay and Association of AgNP and SIM

AgNP showed MIC values between 0.0016 to 63.7 µg/mL against all tested strains. In addition, simvastatin presented MIC values between 3.125 and 62.5 µg/mL. Lower MIC values, such as those presented by AgNP, indicated better antibacterial efficacy on *P. gingivalis*, *S. mutans* and *S. oralis* species. All microorganisms were susceptible to the standard antibacterials, vancomycin (VAN), tested in a concentration range between 6.25 and

0.0031 μg/mL, ampicillin (AMP), 1.55 and 0.00076 μg/mL, and metronidazole (METRO), 3.12 and 0.0015 μg/mL, as shown in Table 2.

Table 2. Simvastatin MIC, AgNP and standard antibiotics: vancomycin (VAN), ampicillin (AMP), and metronidazole (METRO).

Microorganisms	MIC Simvastatin (μg/mL)	CIM—AgNP (μg/mL)	MIC—Antibiotics (μg/mL)
S. aureus MRSA 43300	62.5	63.75	VAN 1.56
S. aureus MRSA 33591	62.5	31.88	VAN 1.56
S. aureus ATCC 29213	31.25	31.88	VAN 1.56
S. aureus ATCC 6538	31.25	31.88	VAN 1.56
S. oralis ATCC 10557	15.62	15.94	AMP 0.024
S. mutans UA159	31.25	15.94	AMP 0.048
P. gingivalis ATCC W83	6.25	0.001592	METRO 0.195
P. gingivalis ATCC 33277	6.25	0.001592	METRO 0.390

These results are corroborated by studies evaluating the antibacterial activity of simvastatin against *S. aureus* strains, including methicillin-resistant *Staphylococcus aureus* (MRSA), which found MICs similar to the results of the present study [35,36]. They are also corroborated by studies that evaluated the effect of simvastatin alone and in combination with antibiotics on microorganisms present in oral infectious processes [38,56]. Finally, isolated AgNP concentrations that inhibited the growth of microbial strains were found in other studies evaluating AgNP against *S. aureus* and MRSA strains [36] and oral pathogens [60,61].

AgNP combined with simvastatin showed synergism in *S. aureus* ATCC 29213 but were not effective against other strains of *S. aureus* and *S. mutans*. For *S. oralis* and *P. gingivalis*, there was an additive effect with AgNP–SIM, as shown in Table 3. For *P. gingivalis*, *S. oralis* and *S. aureus*, the combination of SIM and AgNP reduced the MIC of the compounds by approximately two to eight times compared to the isolated compounds.

These results can be compared to previous studies that showed synergistic antibacterial activity of AgNP with tetracycline in reducing the inhibition range in *P. aeruginosa*, *E. coli* and *K. pneumoniae* [62], the combination of AgNP with amoxicillin in restorative material showed superior antibacterial effect compared to the isolated substances in *S. aureus* and *S. mutans* [63].

Other substances have shown synergistic effects in combination with AgNP, such as the interaction with tyrosol, an antibacterial molecule secreted by *Candida albicans*. The interaction of this molecule with AgNP inhibited the growth of *C. albicans* and *S. mutans* [64]. Another study evaluated the interaction between AgNP and oregano essential oil, and demonstrated a synergistic or additive effect against gram-positive and gram-negative bacterial species [65]. The interaction of AgNP and curcumin demonstrated a synergistic effect in *P. aeruginosa* and *E. coli* [66], and finally, the interaction between AgNP and simvastatin was effective against Methicillin-sensitive *Staphylococcus aureus* (MSSA), Methicillin-resistant *Staphylococcus aureus* (MRSA), and multidrug-resistant *Escherichia coli* [36,42].

Table 3. Comparison of simvastatin MIC, AgNP, standard antibiotics alone or in combination, FICI values and pharmacological interaction of the drug combination against oral bacteria.

Microorganisms	MIC SIM (μg/mL)	MIC AgNP (μg/mL)	MIC Antibiotic (μg/mL)	MIC SIM/AgNP (μ/mL)	FICI	Interaction
S. aureus MRSA 43300	62.5	63.75	VAN 1.56	62.5–63.75	2	----
S. aureus MRSA 33591	62.5	31.88	VAN 1.56	62.5–31.88	2	----
S. aureus ATCC 6538	31.25	31.88	VAN 1.56	31.25–31.88	2	----
S. aureus ATCC 29213	31.25	31.88	VAN 1.56	7.8–15.94	0.32	Synergistic
S. mutans UA159	31.25	15.94	AMP 0.048	31.25–15.94	2	----
S. oralis ATCC 10557	15.62	15.94	AMP 0.024	7.81–7.97	0.73	Additive
P. gingivalis ATCC W83	6.25	0.001592	METRO 0.195	0.781–0.00079	0.75	Additive
P. gingivalis ATCC 33277	6.25	0.001592	METRO 0.390	3.125–0.00079	1	Additive

2.3. *Inhibition of Biofilm Formation and Viability Assay of S. oralis*

Since the AgNP–SIM combination had positive effects against *S. oralis* 10,557 and due to the ability of this species to form biofilms [67], they were used for inhibition and viability tests in biofilm on titanium discs. Both simvastatin and AgNP, when isolated, similarly inhibited the formation of *S. oralis* biofilm. However, the combination of AgNP–SIM had a greater effect on inhibiting biofilm formation, which could be compared to ampicillin, as shown in Figure 3) ($p > 0.05$, ANOVA, Tukey's post-test).

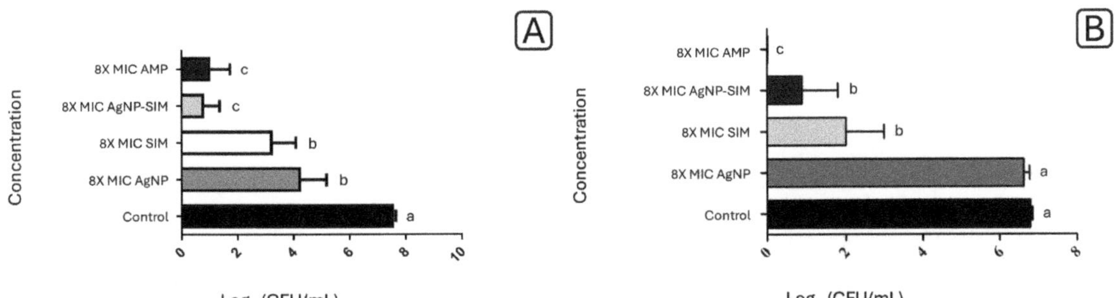

Figure 3. (**A**) *S. oralis* adhesion inhibition assay under exposure to AgNP, SIM, AgNP–SIM and AMP. (**B**) *S. oralis* biofilm viability assay under exposure to AgNP, SIM, AgNP–SIM and AMP for 24 h. The amount of biofilm formed is represented by means and standard deviations of log CFU/mL ($p < 0.05$, ANOVA, Tukey's post-test). Letters indicate statistical differences between the experimental groups compared to the control group, represent by the letter a.

Regarding the reduction of biofilm formed on titanium discs, AMP showed the best result, followed by the combination of AgNP–SIM and SIM alone. However, the discs treated with AgNP alone did not show any reduction in the number of viable cells. As observed in Figure 4. Scanning electron microscope (SEM) images confirmed these results, with a significant reduction in biofilm mass for the combination of AMP and AgNP–SIM, but no reduction for AgNP–SIM.

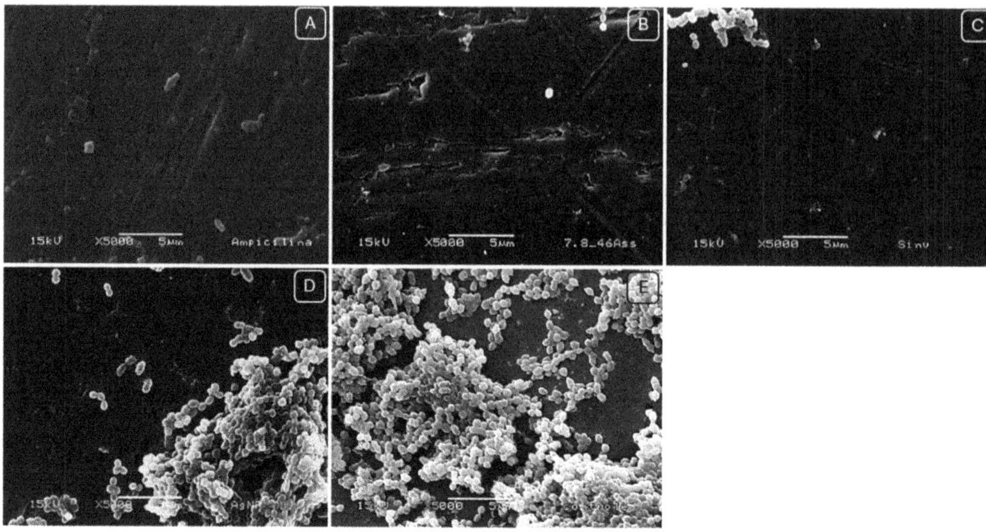

Figure 4. *S. oralis* biofilm on titanium disk treated with: (**A**) 8 × MIC of the combination of AgNP and SIM. (**B**) 8 × MIC of SIM. (**C**) 8 × MIC of AgNP. (**D**) 8 × MIC of Ampicillin. (**E**) No treatment, after 48 h of biofilm formation.

A study using AgNP between 10 and 20 nm coated with citrate enhanced the effect of tobramycin against biofilms of clinical strains of *P. aeruginosa* [30]. Another study testing the interaction of AgNP and chlorhexidine reported greater efficacy against multi-species biofilms compared to the isolated substances [48]. Finally, a previous study from our research group showed a synergistic effect of AgNP and simvastatin against a standard strain of *S. aureus* biofilm [36].

Due to its pleiotropic effects, simvastatin has demonstrated antibacterial activity against opportunistic bacteria and oral pathogens [35,36,38,42,68]. Previous studies have shown that simvastatin inhibits *S. aureus* biofilm at a concentration of 4 × MIC (62.5 µg/mL) and affects the production of insoluble extracellular polysaccharide [54]. Another study demonstrated that simvastatin inhibits *P. gingivalis* biofilm, which is commonly found in peri-implantitis [8], and a 79% reduction in metabolic activity was observed in multispecies biofilm of periodontal pathogens [38].

Similarly, AgNP reduced biofilm formation and can be compared with previous studies that showed an inhibitory effect of AgNP on oral biofilms clinically isolated from patients with and without periodontal disease [69], as well as a formulation containing AgNP that prevented biofilm formation of several species of *Streptococcus* and *E. faecalis* in vitro [70]. In addition, AgNP inhibited the formation of multidrug-resistant biofilms of *P. aeruginosa* [71].

Isolated AgNP had no effect on consolidated biofilms, but not because they developed resistance. Compared to other antibacterials, AgNP has multiple antibacterial mechanisms, including reduced ATP production by Ag^+ ions, generation of reactive oxygen species, and damage to the DNA and bacterial cell membrane [28,72]. Particularly against biofilms, AgNP interact with lipids and lipopolysaccharides (LPS), causing structural disruption. The penetration of nanoparticles into the biofilm depends on many factors, such as biofilm maturity, composition and chemistry of its surface, nanoparticle size, concentration, charge and surface chemistry [73].

Titanium discs were in contact with AgNP treatment for 48 h, which may not be sufficient time for biofilm eradication. Previous studies have shown a reduced antibacterial capacity of AgNP used as reticular canal irrigators, which was attributed to the short period of interaction as well as the low concentration (94 ppm) [74]. Another study demonstrated a potential effect of AgNP in the eradication of biofilm formed in root dentin when used as a treatment for 7 days, but the effect was limited as an irrigating solution, showing that the bactericidal treatment of biofilm is dependent on a longer period of exposure [75].

Another possible reason may be related to the possible interaction of these nanoparticles with the stabilizing proteins from the fungal filtrate. It has been reported that prior washing of AgNP resulted in improved antibacterial activity and was associated with a lower concentration of these proteins [76]. It is important to remember that the antibacterial activity of AgNP depends on the complexes they form with proteins present in biofluids that are responsible for coating the nanoparticle, the so-called protein corona, which determines the physical, chemical and biological properties of the nanoparticles [77,78]. These complexes can interfere with antibacterial activity, so it is the proteins in the corona that interact with cells, not the nanoparticles themselves [79,80].

Gnanadhas et al. [81] observed that unencapsulated AgNP showed no antibacterial activity in the presence of serum proteins due to interaction with bovine serum albumin (BSA). However, AgNP encapsulated with citrate or polyvinylpyrrolidone exhibited antibacterial properties due to minimized interactions with serum proteins. In the present study, the titanium discs were soaked in human saliva to form the acquired pellicle, which allowed bacterial adhesion. In addition, the culture medium for biofilm growth contained mucin, a glycoprotein present in saliva. Thus, proteins present in these substrates could interact with AgNP. However, these interactions need to be further investigated.

2.4. *Simvastatin and AgNP Toxicity In Vivo*

After 12 h exposure to 2 × MIC and 4 × MIC concentrations of the AgNP–SIM combination, the viability of *G. mellonella* larvae was reduced to 80%. After 24 h of evaluation, the 1 × MIC concentration of AgNP–SIM reduced viability to 90%. There was no reduction in viability at the 8 × MIC concentration or in the DMSO group used as a control. The AgNP group showed a reduction in larval viability to 90% at the 4 × MIC and 8 × MIC concentrations after 12 h exposure, and a reduction to 80% and 60% at these concentrations after 24 h exposure, $p = 0.029$. The simvastatin group showed a reduction in larval viability to 90% at the MIC concentration after 24 h and a reduction to 80% at the MIC concentration after 48 h ($p = 0.091$). Table 4 shows the doses of each compound injected into *G. mellonella*, as shown in Figure 5.

Table 4. Doses of compounds injected into *G. mellonella*.

Acute Toxicity Assessment—*G. mellonella*				
Compound (mg/Kg)	**1 × MIC**	**2 × MIC**	**4 × MIC**	**8 × MIC**
AgNP—SIM	26–53.1	52–103.3	104–212.5	208–423
AgNP	106.3	212.5	426	850
SIM	104.2	208.4	416.7	833

The toxicity assay of the AgNP–SIM combination was performed on *Galleria mellonella*, as shown in Figure 6, a model that replaces the use of mammals due to the similarity of its immune system, in addition to being widely accepted in the scientific literature [82]. The use of this model has been described in the activity of biogenic AgNP in larvae infected with *P. aeruginosa* [83]. It also has been tested for screening potential drugs against *Staphylococcus* strains, such as daptomycin and vancomycin [84]. At the highest concentrations (8 × MIC) of AgNP–SIM to test the biofilm viability, the larvae did not reduce the viability, however, at lower concentrations, viability was reduced by up to 80%, which can be explained by the higher levels of DMSO solvent used to solubilize SIM. AgNP showed greater toxicity only at the highest concentration (8 × MIC), where viability was reduced to 50%. In a similar study, the doses of isolated AgNP tested did not show a reduction in larval viability over the periods evaluated, but the highest dose tested was 5 mg/kg [85]. Since the concentrations of each substance are lower in the AgNP–SIM combination, this may explain the reduced toxicity of this combination. Thus, we can conclude that the AgNP–SIM combination is less toxic than AgNP alone in terms of MIC values. Our results showed that the AgNP–SIM combination may be an alternative for controlling infection on implants, which provides opportunities for further testing in preclinical studies.

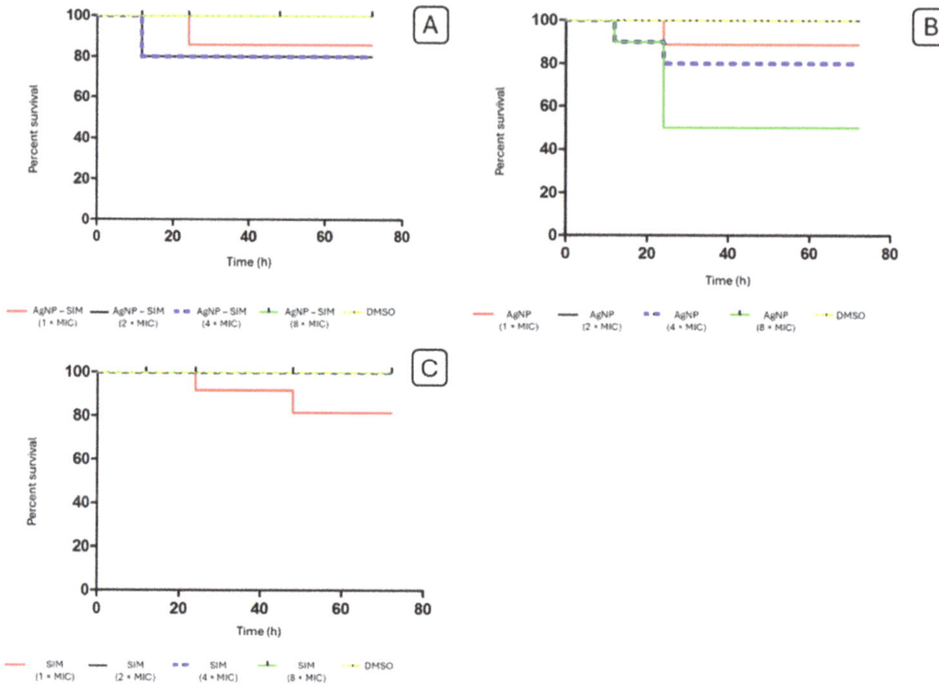

Figure 5. Survival curve of *G. mellonella* after treatment with different concentrations of (**A**) AgNP–SIM, (**B**) AgNP, and (**C**) SIM.

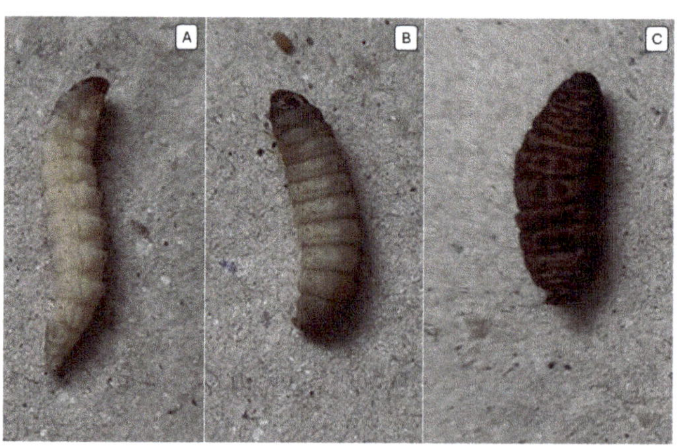

Figure 6. *Galleria mellonella* larvae. (**A**) Healthy larva without treatment; (**B**) Partially melanized larvae not counted as alive; (**C**) Melanized larvae not counted as alive.

3. Materials and Methods

3.1. Chemicals and Experimental Groups

Simvastatin (SIM), donated by EMS Pharma (Hortolândia, Sao Paulo, Brazil). Amoxicillin (AMOX, Sigma-Aldrich, St. Louis, MO, USA), metronidazole (METRO, Sigma-Aldrich, St. Louis, MO, USA), vancomycin (VAN, TEUTO Anápolis, Brazil) and ampicillin (AMP, Sigma-Aldrich, St. Louis, MO, USA) were used as standard antibacterials. SIM, and METRO were diluted in dimethyl sulfoxide (DMSO) to final concentrations of 2–2.5%, while AMOX, VAN, and AMP were dissolved in sterile distilled water.

The formulations were distributed in microplate wells as follows: (a) experimental groups (culture medium + bacteria + statin or antibacterial standard); (b) positive control (culture medium + bacteria); (c) vehicle control (culture medium + bacteria + DMSO); (d) negative control (culture medium + statin or standard antibacterial); (e) negative control of the medium (culture medium). All tests were performed with six replicates on at least two separate occasions.

3.2. Biosynthesis of Silver Nanoparticles

Silver nanoparticles (AgNP) were biosynthesized by fungi, according to the method previously described [32]. The strain 551 of the fungus *Fusarum oxysporum* used was obtained from the culture collection of molecular genetics laboratory of ESALQ-USP, Piracicaba-SP, Brazil. The fungus was grown on malt agar (Difco®) containing 0.5% yeast extract, 2% malt extract, 2% agar and distilled water for 7 days at 28 °C. Then, 10 g of fungal biomass (previously washed) from the culture medium were added to 100 mL of sterile distilled water and incubated for 72 h at 28 °C. After that, the supernatant was separated from the fungal biomass by vacuum filtration and $AgNO_3$ (Sigma-Aldrich®) was added for a final concentration of 3 mM. The system solution was incubated at 28 °C in the absence of light until AgNP were formed. The observation of AgNP formation was performed visually and by colorimetric analysis using a spectrophotometer (UV-vis) until the formation of nanoparticles at 430 nm. After purification, the AgNP were characterized on filters with 0.22 mm membranes (Orion Cientific, Rio de Janeiro, Brazil).

3.3. Characterization of Silver Nanoparticles

The hydrodynamic size, polydispersity index (PDI) and zeta potential of AgNP were determined by Dynamic Light Scattering—DLS (ZetaSizer NanoZS—Malvern Panalytical, Malvern, UK). Transmission Electron Microscopy—TEM (Jeol JEM-1400, Peabody, MA, USA) was performed to confirm AgNP morphology and size. X-ray diffraction (XRD) spectroscopy technique, XDR 7000 (Shimadzu, Kyoto, Japan) was used to determine and confirm the crystalline structure of AgNP and energy dispersive X-ray spectroscopy (EDS) (Vantage V.1.4 Rev. B, Noran Instruments, Middleton, WI, USA) was used to detect the elements on the surface of AgNP.

3.4. Bacterial Strains and Cultivation Conditions

Strains of *S. aureus* ATCC 29213 (MSSA), *S. aureus* ATCC 6538, *S. aureus* ATCC 43300 (MRSA; mecA gene present), *S. aureus* MRSA 33591, *Streptococcus oralis* ATCC 10557, *Streptococcus mutans* UA 159, and *Porphyromonas gingivalis* W83 and ATCC 33277 were used.

Stock cultures of *S. aureus* were grown in Mueller Hinton Broth (MHB, Difco Co., Detroit, MI, USA) medium for 24 h under aerobic conditions in an incubator (Solab, Piracicaba, Sao Paulo, Brazil) at 37 °C. Facultative anaerobic microorganisms *S. mutans* and *S. oralis* were cultured in Brain Heart Infusion Broth, (BHI, Difco Co., Detroit, MI, USA) medium for 24 h in an incubator (Sanyo Electric Co., Osaka, Japan, MCO-19AIC) at 37 °C with 5% CO_2 and *Porphyromonas gingivalis* were cultured in Tryptic Soy Agar (TSA, Difco Co, Detroit, MI, USA), supplemented with 7% sheep blood, 0.2% Yeast Extract (YE—Difco Co., Detroit, MI, USA), 5 μg/mL Hemin (Sigma Aldrich.—St. Louis, MO, USA, H5533), and 1 μg/mL Menadione (Sigma Aldrich.—St. Louis, MO, USA, M5625), incubated under anaerobic conditions for 48 h (80% N_2, 10% CO_2, 10% H_2 (MiniMacs Anaerobic Workstation;

Don Whitley Scientific, Shipley, UK) at 37 °C. The cultures were stored in Tryptic Soy Broth (TSB, Difco Co., Detroit, MI, USA) with 20% glycerol, at −80 °C.

The bacterial inoculum was adjusted for MIC and Checkerboard Microdilution Assay for an optical density of 0.08–0.1 (660 nm) grown in MHB in aerobiosis for 24 h for *S. aureus*. For the assays with *P. gingivalis*, an optical density of 0.5 (660 nm) was used, and after that, a 10-fold dilution was performed in 1.55% Tryptic Soy Broth added with 1.48% BHI, 0.2% YE, 5 μg/mL Hemin and 1 μg/mL Menadione, [86]. For *streptococcal* inoculum, cultures were grown for 24 h and suspensions were adjusted to an absorbance range of 0.08–0.1 (625 nm) in MHB [86].

3.5. *Minimum Inhibitory Concentration (MIC) Assay*

The minimum inhibitory concentration (MIC) was determined by microdilution assay in culture medium in 96-well microplates according to the guidance of the Clinical and Laboratory Standards Institute—CLSI [86]. Briefly, different concentrations of simvastatin (250 to 0.12 μg/mL) and AgNP (127.5 to 0.06 μg/mL) and standard antibiotics (10–0.001 μg/mL) were added by 2-fold dilution. Then, 100 μL of bacterial suspension prepared according to item 3.4 were inoculated and the 96-well plates were incubated under aerobic conditions for 24 h (*S. aureus*), under anaerobic conditions for 48 h (*P. gingivalis*) or in 5% CO_2 for 24 h (*streptococci*). The bacterial suspensions were adjusted according to the turbidity equivalent to the Mc Farland standard, resulting in a concentration of 1×10^8 CFU/mL. Then, 100 μL of the suspensions were diluted in 9.9 mL of MHB to obtain a suspension of 1×10^6 CFU/mL. Finally, 100 μL of the suspension was added to the plate obtaining a final concentration of 1×10^5 CFU/mL. The lowest concentration with any visible bacterial growth was taken as MIC. In addition, bacterial growth was assessed by optical density measurement and through the addition of 30 μL resazurin solution 0.01% [87]. This experiment was performed in triplicate of at least two independent assays.

3.6. *Antibacterial Combination Assay (Checkerboard Assay)*

The Checkerboard Microdilution Assay was used to verify the synergistic activity between simvastatin and AgNP, combining different concentrations of the compounds as previously described [35,88]. Different concentrations of SIM and AgNP combinations were diluted in MHB medium in 96-well plates. The concentrations of each substance used were the same as the MIC. After that, a 100 μL aliquot of bacterial suspension was added, at a final concentration of 1×10^5 CFU/mL. The plates were incubated according to the culture conditions of each strain. The plates were visually analyzed for turbidity and the absorbance was evaluated in a spectrophotometer (θ = 660 nm). Finally, 30 μL of 0.01% resazurin dye was added to each well, which were incubated for two hours and read.

To qualify the interaction between the two compounds, the fractional inhibitory concentration index (FICI) was calculated using combined MIC of both compounds (CIMAB) and MIC of each compound alone (CIMA), using the following equation:

$$\Sigma = \text{FICIA} + \text{FICIB} = \text{MICAB}/\text{MICA} + \text{MICBA}/\text{MICB}.$$

The FICI was interpreted according to the following index: ≤0.5, synergistic interaction effect; >0.5 and ≤1.0, additive interaction effect; >1 and <4, indifferent; and ≥4, antagonistic interaction effect [89].

3.7. *Inhibition Assay of S. oralis Adhesion on Titanium Discs*

Biofilm assays were performed in 24-well polystyrene plates coupled with sterilized titanium discs measuring 4.2 mm thick by 8 mm in diameter—Porous ® surface (Conexão prosthesis systems, Arujá, Sao Paulo, Brazil) secured by a metal apparatus. Because we used human saliva from donors, this study was previously approved by the research ethics committee (CEP) #2.805.995.

3.7.1. Saliva Preparation

Saliva was obtained from healthy volunteers in 10 mL aliquots. The sample was treated with 2.5 mmol L−1 of phenylmethylsulfonyl fluoride (Sigma Aldrich, St. Louis, MO, USA) to reduce salivary protein aggregation. After treatment, saliva was centrifuged at 10 min, 4 °C, 3800× *g* and the supernatant obtained was diluted (1:1) with AB solution (KCl—0.93 g, $CaCl_2$—0.02 g, $KHPO_4$—0.034 g, $MgCl_2$—0.005 g). The sample was then filtered and sterilized using a 0.22 µm Millex GV filter (Millipore, Millipore Corporation, Bedford, MA, USA). The saliva suspension was added to a 24-well plate and the titanium discs were positioned vertically, held by a metal wire, and then incubated in an orbital shaker (211DS Shaking Incubator, Labnet International, Inc., Edison, NJ, USA) at 37 °C, 60 rpm, for 2 h, for the formation of saliva biofilm.

3.7.2. Inhibition of Biofilm Formation and Biofilm Viability Assay of *S. oralis*

For biofilm formation, cultures of *S. oralis* ATCC 10,557 were grown in BHI medium supplemented with 2.5 g/L mucin, 1.0 g/L yeast extract, 0.1 g/L cysteine, 2.0 g/L sodium bicarbonate, 5.0 mg/mL hemin, and 1.0 mg/mL menadione [90].

After coating the discs with saliva film, they were placed in 24-well plates in a vertical position. For the biofilm formation inhibition assay, the treatments were added at time 0 h, before biofilm formation. In each well, 3 mL of culture medium with 8 × MIC concentrations of SIM, AgNP, AgNP–SIM and 0.3 mL of *S. oralis* culture at 1.0×10^8 CFU/mL were added to the wells containing the titanium discs. The plates were incubated for 48 h, in 5% of CO_2, at 37 °C. After this period, the discs were removed from the wells and washed in sterile saline solution to remove non-adhered cells and placed in tubes containing 5 mL of sterile 0.9% NaCl. The tubes were vortexed for one minute, after which they were sonicated at 5% amplitude, 6 pulses of 9.9 s with 5 s intervals for another minute (Vibra Cell 400 W, Sonics & Materials Inc., Newtown, CT, USA). The bacterial suspension was then diluted (10–100,000 times) and 0.01 mL of each dilution was plated on BHI agar medium. The plates were incubated in 5% CO_2 at 37 °C for 48 h. After this period, the colonies were quantified and the colony forming units per mL (CFU/mL) were calculated.

For the mature biofilm viability test, concentrations of each compound were added 24 h after biofilm formation. After adding the treatments, the discs were incubated for an additional 24 h in 5% CO_2 at 37 °C. After 48 h of contact with the substances, the discs were removed from the wells, washed with 0.9% NaCl solution and placed in tubes containing 5 mL of sterile 0.9% NaCl. The tubes were vortexed for one minute and then sonicated as previously described. Finally, the bacterial suspension was diluted and plated on BHI agar medium, and the plates were incubated for 48 h. After this period, the CFU/mL of each sample was calculated.

3.7.3. Scanning Electron Microscopy (SEM)

Scanning Electron Microscopy analyses were performed on *S. oralis* biofilms formed for 24 h and treated for 48 h with 8 × MIC concentrations of SIM, AgNP, AgNP–SIM. After growth and treatment of the biofilms on titanium discs, they were washed in 0.9% NaCl solution and after washing, the discs were fixed in 10% glutaraldehyde solution in Phosphate buffered saline solution (PBS) for 30 min. Then, the biofilms were immersed in 90% and 99% ethanol solutions for one minute, respectively. Finally, the discs were dried at room temperature for 12 h and the samples were fixed on a brass stub, and then metallized with gold. The discs were then evaluated in a Scanning Electron Microscope (JEOL, JSM5600LV, Tokyo, Japan) and images were taken at 15 KV.

3.7.4. Acute Toxicity Assay In Vivo in the *Galleria mellonella* Model

This assay was performed to evaluate possible acute toxic effects of the combination of AgNP–SIM, SIM and isolated AgNP. A total of 10 larvae weighing between 0.2 and 0.3 g were selected for each group. The larvae remained in the refrigerator for 30 min to facilitate the administration of the treatment solutions: 2.5% DMSO solution (diluent control) and

1 × MIC AgNP–SIM, 2 × MIC AgNP–SIM, 4 × MIC AgNP–SIM and 8 × MIC AgNP–SIM, 1 × MIC of SIM, 2 × MIC of SIM, 4 × MIC of SIM and 8 × MIC of SIM and 1 × MIC of AgNP, 2 × MIC of AgNP, 4 × MIC of AgNP and 8 × MIC of AgNP. The substances were injected into the hemocoel of each larva at the last progeny left using a 25 μL Hamilton syringe (Hamilton, Reno, NV, USA). The larvae were incubated at 30 °C and their survival was recorded at 12 h, 24 h, 48 h and 72 h intervals. Larvae that did not move after touching and showed myelination were counted as dead [91].

3.8. Statistics

The data were compared with the control group by analysis of variance (ANOVA) and Tukey's post-test. The analyses were performed with Bioestat 5.0 (Mamirauá, Belém, Brazil) and GraphPad Prism 8.0 (San Diego, CA, USA). For all comparisons, a "p" value of <0.05 was selected as the criterion for statistical significance. Survival assays were analyzed using Kaplan–Meier curves and Mantel–Cox tests.

4. Conclusions

Here, AgNP were biologically produced and their association with simvastatin showed an additive and synergistic effect against species of oral biofilm. Also, this association was able to inhibit and reduce the protection of the *S. oralis* biofilm in the titanium discs, with low in vivo toxicity tested in *Galleria mellonella*.

The association could be used as a potential drug in titanium implant coatings, contributing to the success of osteointegration. In this way, it would be guaranteed that concentrations close to or even above the MIC would not reach local infection or prevent microbial colonization. In addition, to date, there are no reports of antibacterial resistance to these drugs, which overcome the use of standard antibacterials. The synergistic effects provide a reduction in the concentration of both, which could reduce possible toxic effects.

Author Contributions: Conceptualization, S.M.R., N.D., J.d.C.O.S. and K.C.M.; Methodology, S.M.R., A.C.F., M.K.T., M.C.T.D., R.D.P., N.D., J.d.C.O.S., R.M.T.D. and K.C.M.; Validation, S.M.R. and K.C.M.; Formal analysis, S.M.R., A.L.R. and K.C.M.; Investigation, S.M.R., M.K.T. and K.C.M.; Resources, K.C.M.; Data curation, S.M.R., M.K.T., N.D., R.M.T.D. and K.C.M.; Writing—original draft, S.M.R., A.L.R. and K.C.M.; Writing—review & editing, S.M.R., A.L.R. and K.C.M.; Visualization, S.M.R., A.L.R., J.d.C.O.S. and K.C.M.; Supervision, K.C.M.; Project administration, K.C.M.; Funding acquisition, K.C.M. All authors have read and agreed to the published version of the manuscript.

Funding: This research was funded by Fundação de Amparo à Pesquisa do Estado de São Paulo—FAPESP, grant #2018/20593-0 and 2022/16461-6. Sindy Magri Roque acknowledges a scholarship provided by Conselho Nacional de Desenvolvimento Científico e Tecnológico—CNPq, grant #132811/2018-9.

Institutional Review Board Statement: The study was conducted in accordance with the Declaration of Helsinki, and approved by the Ethics Committee of Faculdade de Odontologia de Piracicaba, Universidade Estadual de Campinas (protocol code #2.805.995 and date of approval: 8 August 2018).

Informed Consent Statement: Informed consent was obtained from all subjects involved in the study.

Data Availability Statement: Data are contained within the article.

Conflicts of Interest: The authors declare no conflict of interest.

References

1. Ghensi, P.; Manghi, P.; Zolfo, M.; Armanini, F.; Pasolli, E.; Bolzan, M.; Bertelle, A.; Dell'Acqua, F.; Dellasega, E.; Waldner, R.; et al. Strong Oral Plaque Microbiome Signatures for Dental Implant Diseases Identified by Strain-Resolution Metagenomics. *NPJ Biofilms Microbiomes* **2020**, *6*, 47. [CrossRef] [PubMed]
2. Herrera, D.; Berglundh, T.; Schwarz, F.; Chapple, I.; Jepsen, S.; Sculean, A.; Kebschull, M.; Papapanou, P.N.; Tonetti, M.S.; Sanz, M. Prevention and Treatment of Peri-Implant Diseases-The EFP S3 Level Clinical Practice Guideline. *J. Clin. Periodontol.* **2023**, *50*, 4–76. [CrossRef] [PubMed]

3. Rodrigues, F.; Rodrigues da Silva, M.; Silva, F.S.; Madeira, S.; Carvalho, Ó. Electric Current Application on Dental Implant Biofilms: Review. *J. Funct. Biomater.* **2024**, *15*, 197. [CrossRef]
4. Charalampakis, G.; Belibasakis, G.N. Microbiome of Peri-Implant Infections: Lessons from Conventional, Molecular and Metagenomic Analyses. *Virulence* **2015**, *6*, 183–187. [CrossRef]
5. Dreyer, H.; Grischke, J.; Tiede, C.; Eberhard, J.; Schweitzer, A.; Toikkanen, S.E.; Glöckner, S.; Krause, G.; Stiesch, M. Epidemiology and Risk Factors of Peri-implantitis: A Systematic Review. *J. Periodontal Res.* **2018**, *53*, 657–681. [CrossRef] [PubMed]
6. Hussain, R.A.; Miloro, M.; Cohen, J.B. An Update on the Treatment of Periimplantitis. *Dent. Clin. N. Am.* **2021**, *65*, 43–56. [CrossRef]
7. Greenstein, G.; Eskow, R. High Prevalence Rates of Peri-Implant Mucositis and Peri-Implantitis Post Dental Implantations Dictate Need for Continuous Peri-Implant Maintenance. *Compend. Contin. Educ. Dent.* **2022**, *43*, 206–213; quiz 214.
8. Belibasakis, G.N.; Manoil, D. Microbial Community-Driven Etiopathogenesis of Peri-Implantitis. *J. Dent. Res.* **2021**, *100*, 21–28. [CrossRef]
9. Mulla, M.; Mulla, M.; Hegde, S.; Koshy, A.V. In Vitro Assessment of the Effect of Probiotic Lactobacillus Reuteri on Peri-Implantitis Microflora. *BMC Oral Health* **2021**, *21*, 408. [CrossRef]
10. Mombelli, A.; Décaillet, F. The Characteristics of Biofilms in Peri-Implant Disease. *J. Clin. Periodontol.* **2011**, *38* (Suppl. 11), 203–213. [CrossRef]
11. Persson, G.R.; Renvert, S. Cluster of Bacteria Associated with Peri-Implantitis. *Clin. Implant. Dent. Relat. Res.* **2014**, *16*, 783–793. [CrossRef] [PubMed]
12. do Nascimento, C.; Pita, M.S.; Fernandes, F.H.N.C.; Pedrazzi, V.; de Albuquerque Junior, R.F.; Ribeiro, R.F. Bacterial Adhesion on the Titanium and Zirconia Abutment Surfaces. *Clin. Oral Implant. Res.* **2014**, *25*, 337–343. [CrossRef] [PubMed]
13. Nibali, L.; Gkranias, N.; Mainas, G.; Di Pino, A. Periodontitis and Implant Complications in Diabetes. *Periodontol. 2000* **2022**, *90*, 88–105. [CrossRef] [PubMed]
14. Berglundh, T.; Jepsen, S.; Stadlinger, B.; Terheyden, H. Peri-Implantitis and Its Prevention. *Clin. Oral Implant. Res.* **2019**, *30*, 150–155. [CrossRef]
15. Song, X.; Li, L.; Gou, H.; Xu, Y. Impact of Implant Location on the Prevalence of Peri-Implantitis: A Systematic Review and Meta-Analysis. *J. Dent.* **2020**, *103*, 103490. [CrossRef]
16. Luke Yeo, I.-S. Dental Implants. *Dent. Clin. N. Am.* **2022**, *66*, 627–642. [CrossRef]
17. Chahal, G.; Quintana-Hayashi, M.P.; Gaytán, M.O.; Benktander, J.; Padra, M.; King, S.J.; Linden, S.K. *Streptococcus oralis* Employs Multiple Mechanisms of Salivary Mucin Binding That Differ Between Strains. *Front. Cell Infect. Microbiol.* **2022**, *12*, 889711. [CrossRef] [PubMed]
18. Kommerein, N.; Doll, K.; Stumpp, N.S.; Stiesch, M. Development and Characterization of an Oral Multispecies Biofilm Implant Flow Chamber Model. *PLoS ONE* **2018**, *13*, e0196967. [CrossRef]
19. Kolenbrander, P.E.; Palmer, R.J.; Periasamy, S.; Jakubovics, N.S. Oral Multispecies Biofilm Development and the Key Role of Cell–Cell Distance. *Nat. Rev. Microbiol.* **2010**, *8*, 471–480. [CrossRef]
20. Ingendoh-Tsakmakidis, A.; Mikolai, C.; Winkel, A.; Szafrański, S.P.; Falk, C.S.; Rossi, A.; Walles, H.; Stiesch, M. Commensal and Pathogenic Biofilms Differently Modulate Peri-implant Oral Mucosa in an Organotypic Model. *Cell Microbiol.* **2019**, *21*, e13078. [CrossRef]
21. de Waal, Y.C.M.; Winning, L.; Stavropoulos, A.; Polyzois, I. Efficacy of Chemical Approaches for Implant Surface Decontamination in Conjunction with Sub-marginal Instrumentation, in the Non-surgical Treatment of Peri-implantitis: A Systematic Review. *J. Clin. Periodontol.* **2023**, *50*, 212–223. [CrossRef] [PubMed]
22. Helovuo, H.; Hakkarainen, K.; Paunio, K. Changes in the Prevalence of Subgingival Enteric Rods, Staphylococci and Yeasts after Treatment with Penicillin and Erythromycin. *Oral Microbiol. Immunol.* **1993**, *8*, 75–79. [CrossRef] [PubMed]
23. Verdugo, F.; Laksmana, T.; Uribarri, A. Systemic Antibiotics and the Risk of Superinfection in Peri-Implantitis. *Arch. Oral Biol.* **2016**, *64*, 39–50. [CrossRef]
24. Berglundh, T.; Armitage, G.; Araujo, M.G.; Avila-Ortiz, G.; Blanco, J.; Camargo, P.M.; Chen, S.; Cochran, D.; Derks, J.; Figuero, E.; et al. Peri-implant Diseases and Conditions: Consensus Report of Workgroup 4 of the 2017 World Workshop on the Classification of Periodontal and Peri-Implant Diseases and Conditions. *J. Clin. Periodontol.* **2018**, *45*, S286–S291. [CrossRef]
25. ter Boo, G.A.; Grijpma, D.W.; Richards, R.G.; Moriarty, T.F.; Eglin, D. Preparation of Gentamicin Dioctyl Sulfosuccinate Loaded Poly(Trimethylene Carbonate) Matrices Intended for the Treatment of Orthopaedic Infections. *Clin. Hemorheol. Microcirc.* **2015**, *60*, 89–98. [CrossRef] [PubMed]
26. Zhu, Y.; Cao, H.; Qiao, S.; Gu, Y.; Luo, H.; Liu, X.; Lai, H.; Wang, M.; Meng, F. Hierarchical Micro/Nanostructured Titanium with Balanced Actions to Bacterial and Mammalian Cells for Dental Implants. *Int. J. Nanomed.* **2015**, *10*, 6659–6674. [CrossRef]
27. Ilahi, N.; Haleem, A.; Iqbal, S.; Fatima, N.; Sajjad, W.; Sideeq, A.; Ahmed, S. Biosynthesis of Silver Nanoparticles Using Endophytic *Fusarium oxysporum* Strain NFW16 and Their in Vitro Antibacterial Potential. *Microsc. Res. Tech.* **2022**, *85*, 1568–1579. [CrossRef]
28. Noronha, V.T.; Paula, A.J.; Durán, G.; Galembeck, A.; Cogo-Müller, K.; Franz-Montan, M.; Durán, N. Silver Nanoparticles in Dentistry. *Dent. Mater.* **2017**, *33*, 1110–1126. [CrossRef] [PubMed]
29. Franci, G.; Falanga, A.; Galdiero, S.; Palomba, L.; Rai, M.; Morelli, G.; Galdiero, M. Silver Nanoparticles as Potential Antibacterial Agents. *Molecules* **2015**, *20*, 8856–8874. [CrossRef]

30. Habash, M.B.; Goodyear, M.C.; Park, A.J.; Surette, M.D.; Vis, E.C.; Harris, R.J.; Khursigara, C.M. Potentiation of Tobramycin by Silver Nanoparticles against *Pseudomonas aeruginosa* Biofilms. *Antimicrob. Agents Chemother.* **2017**, *61*, e00415-17. [CrossRef]
31. Siddiqi, K.S.; Husen, A.; Rao, R.A.K. A Review on Biosynthesis of Silver Nanoparticles and Their Biocidal Properties. *J. Nanobiotechnol.* **2018**, *16*, 14. [CrossRef]
32. Durán, N.; Marcato, P.D.; Alves, O.L.; De Souza, G.I.; Esposito, E. Mechanistic Aspects of Biosynthesis of Silver Nanoparticles by Several *Fusarium oxysporum* Strains. *J. Nanobiotechnol.* **2005**, *3*, 8. [CrossRef]
33. Foletto, V.S.; da Rosa, T.F.; Serafin, M.B.; Bottega, A.; Hörner, R. Repositioning of Non-Antibiotic Drugs as an Alternative to Microbial Resistance: A Systematic Review. *Int. J. Antimicrob. Agents* **2021**, *58*, 106380. [CrossRef] [PubMed]
34. Jerwood, S.; Cohen, J. Unexpected Antimicrobial Effect of Statins. *J. Antimicrob. Chemother.* **2007**, *61*, 362–364. [CrossRef] [PubMed]
35. Graziano, T.S.; Cuzzullin, M.C.; Franco, G.C.; Schwartz-Filho, H.O.; de Andrade, E.D.; Groppo, F.C.; Cogo-Müller, K. Statins and Antimicrobial Effects: Simvastatin as a Potential Drug against *Staphylococcus aureus* Biofilm. *PLoS ONE* **2015**, *10*, e0128098. [CrossRef]
36. da Silva, A.C.F.; Roque, S.M.; Duarte, M.C.T.; Nakazato, G.; Durán, N.; Cogo-Müller, K. Modulation of *Staphylococcus aureus* Biofilm Formation through Subinhibitory Concentrations of Biogenic Silver Nanoparticles and Simvastatin. *Future Pharmacol.* **2024**, *4*, 3–16. [CrossRef]
37. de Carvalho, R.D.P.; Casarin, R.C.V.; de Lima, P.O.; Cogo-Müller, K. Statins with Potential to Control Periodontitis: From Biological Mechanisms to Clinical Studies. *J. Oral Biosci.* **2021**, *63*, 232–244. [CrossRef]
38. Parolina de Carvalho, R.D.; de Andrade Moreno, J.; Roque, S.M.; Chan, D.C.H.; Torrez, W.B.; Stipp, R.N.; Bueno-Silva, B.; de Lima, P.O.; Cogo-Müller, K. Statins and Oral Biofilm: Simvastatin as a Promising Drug to Control Periodontal Dysbiosis. *Oral Dis.* **2024**, *30*, 669–680. [CrossRef]
39. Huang, R.; Li, M.; Gregory, R.L. Bacterial Interactions in Dental Biofilm. *Virulence* **2011**, *2*, 435–444. [CrossRef]
40. De Giglio, E.; Cafagna, D.; Cometa, S.; Allegretta, A.; Pedico, A.; Giannossa, L.C.; Sabbatini, L.; Mattioli-Belmonte, M.; Iatta, R. An Innovative, Easily Fabricated, Silver Nanoparticle-Based Titanium Implant Coating: Development and Analytical Characterization. *Anal. Bioanal. Chem.* **2013**, *405*, 805–816. [CrossRef]
41. Massa, M.A.; Covarrubias, C.; Bittner, M.; Fuentevilla, I.A.; Capetillo, P.; Von Marttens, A.; Carvajal, J.C. Synthesis of New Antibacterial Composite Coating for Titanium Based on Highly Ordered Nanoporous Silica and Silver Nanoparticles. *Mater. Sci. Eng. C* **2014**, *45*, 146–153. [CrossRef] [PubMed]
42. Figueiredo, E.; Ribeiro, J.; Nishio, E.; Scandorieiro, S.; Costa, A.; Cardozo, V.; de Oliveira, A.; Durán, N.; Panagio, L.; Kobayashi, R.; et al. New Approach For Simvastatin As An Antibacterial: Synergistic Effect With Bio-Synthesized Silver Nanoparticles Against Multidrug-Resistant Bacteria. *Int. J. Nanomed.* **2019**, *14*, 7975–7985. [CrossRef] [PubMed]
43. Durán, N.; Marcato, P.D.; De Souza, G.I.H.; Alves, O.L.; Esposito, E. Antibacterial Effect of Silver Nanoparticles Produced by Fungal Process on Textile Fabrics and Their Effluent Treatment. *J. Biomed. Nanotechnol.* **2007**, *3*, 203–208. [CrossRef]
44. Zhou, H.; Zhu, X.-D.; Ge, P.; Hang, T.; Li, S.; Guo, F.; Wu, Y.; Li, C. Synergistic Coupling of Surface Plasmon Resonance with Metal-Organic Frameworks Based Biomimetic Z-Scheme Catalyst for Enhanced Photoelectrochemical Water Splitting. *Appl. Surf. Sci.* **2022**, *605*, 154693. [CrossRef]
45. Haes, A.J.; Haynes, C.L.; McFarland, A.D.; Schatz, G.C.; Van Duyne, R.P.; Zou, S. Plasmonic Materials for Surface-Enhanced Sensing and Spectroscopy. *MRS Bull.* **2005**, *30*, 368–375. [CrossRef]
46. Philip, A.; Kumar, A.R. The Performance Enhancement of Surface Plasmon Resonance Optical Sensors Using Nanomaterials: A Review. *Coord. Chem. Rev.* **2022**, *458*, 214424. [CrossRef]
47. Birla, S.S.; Gaikwad, S.C.; Gade, A.K.; Rai, M.K. Rapid Synthesis of Silver Nanoparticles from *Fusarium oxysporum* by Optimizing Physicocultural Conditions. *Sci. World J.* **2013**, *2013*, 796018. [CrossRef]
48. Pineda, M.; Barón, M.; Pérez-Bueno, M.L. Diverse Projected Climate Change Scenarios Affect the Physiology of Broccoli Plants to Different Extents. *Physiol. Plant* **2024**, *176*, e14269. [CrossRef]
49. Erenler, R.; Gecer, E.N.; Hosaflioglu, I.; Behcet, L. Green Synthesis of Silver Nanoparticles Using Stachys Spectabilis: Identification, Catalytic Degradation, and Antioxidant Activity. *Biochem. Biophys. Res. Commun.* **2023**, *659*, 91–95. [CrossRef]
50. Durán, N.; Nakazato, G.; Seabra, A.B. Antimicrobial Activity of Biogenic Silver Nanoparticles, and Silver Chloride Nanoparticles: An Overview and Comments. *Appl. Microbiol. Biotechnol.* **2016**, *100*, 6555–6570. [CrossRef]
51. Liu, J.; Hurt, R.H. Ion Release Kinetics and Particle Persistence in Aqueous Nano-Silver Colloids. *Environ. Sci. Technol.* **2010**, *44*, 2169–2175. [CrossRef]
52. Li, G.; He, D.; Qian, Y.; Guan, B.; Gao, S.; Cui, Y.; Yokoyama, K.; Wang, L. Fungus-Mediated Green Synthesis of Silver Nanoparticles Using *Aspergillus terreus*. *Int. J. Mol. Sci.* **2012**, *13*, 466–476. [CrossRef]
53. Gao, X.; Feng, H.-L.; Zhang, Z.-Y.; Ma, J.-M. Study on the Crystalline Structure and Thermal Stability of Silver Oxide Films Deposited by Direct-Current Reactive Magnetron Sputtering Methods. *J. Korean Phys. Soc.* **2010**, *56*, 1176–1179. [CrossRef]
54. Bocate, K.P.; Reis, G.F.; de Souza, P.C.; Oliveira Junior, A.G.; Durán, N.; Nakazato, G.; Furlaneto, M.C.; de Almeida, R.S.; Panagio, L.A. Antifungal Activity of Silver Nanoparticles and Simvastatin against Toxigenic Species of *Aspergillus*. *Int. J. Food Microbiol.* **2019**, *291*, 79–86. [CrossRef]
55. Durán, N.; Cuevas, R.; Cordi, L.; Rubilar, O.; Diez, M.C. Biogenic Silver Nanoparticles Associated with Silver Chloride Nanoparticles (Ag@AgCl) Produced by Laccase from *Trametes versicolor*. *Springerplus* **2014**, *3*, 645. [CrossRef]

56. Emani, S.; Gunjiganur, G.; Mehta, D. Determination of the Antibacterial Activity of Simvastatin against Periodontal Pathogens, *Porphyromonas gingivalis* and *Aggregatibacter actinomycetemcomitans*: An in Vitro Study. *Contemp. Clin. Dent.* **2014**, *5*, 377. [CrossRef]
57. Almulaiky, Y.Q.; Alkabli, J.; El-Shishtawy, R.M. Sustainable Immobilization of β-Glucosidase onto Silver Ions and AgNPs-Loaded Acrylic Fabric with Enhanced Stability and Reusability. *Polymer* **2023**, *15*, 4361. [CrossRef]
58. Hamedi, M.M.; Ainla, A.; Güder, F.; Christodouleas, D.C.; Fernández-Abedul, M.T.; Whitesides, G.M. Integrating Electronics and Microfluidics on Paper. *Adv. Mater.* **2016**, *28*, 5054–5063. [CrossRef]
59. Șuică-Bunghez, I.R.; Senin, R.M.; Sorescu, A.A.; Ganciarov, M.; Răut, I.; Firincă, C.; Constantin, M.; Gifu, I.C.; Stoica, R.; Fierăscu, I.; et al. Application of Lavandula Angustifolia Mill. Extracts for the Phytosynthesis of Silver Nanoparticles: Characterization and Biomedical Potential. *Plants* **2024**, *13*, 333. [CrossRef] [PubMed]
60. Panpaliya, N.P.; Dahake, P.T.; Kale, Y.J.; Dadpe, M.V.; Kendre, S.B.; Siddiqi, A.G.; Maggavi, U.R. In Vitro Evaluation of Antimicrobial Property of Silver Nanoparticles and Chlorhexidine against Five Different Oral Pathogenic Bacteria. *Saudi Dent. J.* **2019**, *31*, 76–83. [CrossRef] [PubMed]
61. Ahmed, O.; Sibuyi, N.R.S.; Fadaka, A.O.; Madiehe, A.M.; Maboza, E.; Olivier, A.; Meyer, M.; Geerts, G. Antimicrobial Effects of Gum Arabic-Silver Nanoparticles against Oral Pathogens. *Bioinorg. Chem. Appl.* **2022**, *2022*, 9602325. [CrossRef]
62. Rogowska, A.; Rafińska, K.; Pomastowski, P.; Walczak, J.; Railean-Plugaru, V.; Buszewska-Forajta, M.; Buszewski, B. Silver Nanoparticles Functionalized with Ampicillin. *Electrophoresis* **2017**, *38*, 2757–2764. [CrossRef]
63. Enan, E.T.; Ashour, A.A.; Basha, S.; Felemban, N.H.; Gad El-Rab, S.M.F. Antimicrobial Activity of Biosynthesized Silver Nanoparticles, Amoxicillin, and Glass-Ionomer Cement against *Streptococcus mutans* and *Staphylococcus aureus*. *Nanotechnology* **2021**, *32*, 215101. [CrossRef]
64. Souza, J.A.S.; do Amaral, J.G.; Monteiro, D.R.; Fernandes, R.A.; Fernandes, G.L.; Gorup, L.F.; de Souza Neto, F.N.; de Camargo, E.R.; Agostinho, A.M.; Barbosa, D.B.; et al. 'Green' Silver Nanoparticles Combined with Tyrosol as Potential Oral Antimicrobial Therapy. *J. Dent.* **2024**, *143*, 104867. [CrossRef]
65. Scandorieiro, S.; de Camargo, L.C.; Lancheros, C.A.C.; Yamada-Ogatta, S.F.; Nakamura, C.V.; de Oliveira, A.G.; Andrade, C.G.T.J.; Duran, N.; Nakazato, G.; Kobayashi, R.K.T. Synergistic and Additive Effect of Oregano Essential Oil and Biological Silver Nanoparticles against Multidrug-Resistant Bacterial Strains. *Front. Microbiol.* **2016**, *7*, 760. [CrossRef]
66. Alves, T.F.; Chaud, M.V.; Grotto, D.; Jozala, A.F.; Pandit, R.; Rai, M.; dos Santos, C.A. Association of Silver Nanoparticles and Curcumin Solid Dispersion: Antimicrobial and Antioxidant Properties. *AAPS PharmSciTech* **2018**, *19*, 225–231. [CrossRef]
67. Xu, H.; Sobue, T.; Bertolini, M.; Thompson, A.; Vickerman, M.; Nobile, C.J.; Dongari-Bagtzoglou, A.S. Oralis Activates the Efg1 Filamentation Pathway in C. Albicans to Promote Cross-Kingdom Interactions and Mucosal Biofilms. *Virulence* **2017**, *8*, 1602–1617. [CrossRef]
68. Liao, J.K.; Laufs, U. Pleiotropic Effects of Statins. *Annu. Rev. Pharmacol. Toxicol.* **2005**, *45*, 89–118. [CrossRef]
69. Hernández-Venegas, P.A.; Martínez-Martínez, R.E.; Zaragoza-Contreras, E.A.; Domínguez-Pérez, R.A.; Reyes-López, S.Y.; Donohue-Cornejo, A.; Cuevas-González, J.C.; Molina-Frechero, N.; Espinosa-Cristóbal, L.F. Bactericidal Activity of Silver Nanoparticles on Oral Biofilms Related to Patients with and without Periodontal Disease. *J. Funct. Biomater.* **2023**, *14*, 311. [CrossRef]
70. Schwass, D.R.; Lyons, K.M.; Love, R.; Tompkins, G.R.; Meledandri, C.J. Antimicrobial Activity of a Colloidal AgNP Suspension Demonstrated In Vitro against Monoculture Biofilms: Toward a Novel Tooth Disinfectant for Treating Dental Caries. *Adv. Dent. Res.* **2018**, *29*, 117–123. [CrossRef]
71. El-Telbany, M.; El-Sharaki, A. Antibacterial and Anti-Biofilm Activity of Silver Nanoparticles on Multi-Drug Resistance *Pseudomonas aeruginosa* Isolated from Dental-Implant. *J. Oral Biol. Craniofac. Res.* **2022**, *12*, 199–203. [CrossRef]
72. Durán, N.; Marcato, P.D.; De Conti, R.; Alves, O.L.; Costa, F.T.M.; Brocchi, M. Potential Use of Silver Nanoparticles on Pathogenic Bacteria, Their Toxicity and Possible Mechanisms of Action. *J. Braz. Chem. Soc.* **2010**, *21*, 949–959. [CrossRef]
73. Ikuma, K.; Decho, A.W.; Lau, B.L.T. When Nanoparticles Meet Biofilms-interactions Guiding the Environmental Fate and Accumulation of Nanoparticles. *Front. Microbiol.* **2015**, *6*, 591. [CrossRef]
74. Rodrigues, C.T.; de Andrade, F.B.; de Vasconcelos, L.R.S.M.; Midena, R.Z.; Pereira, T.C.; Kuga, M.C.; Duarte, M.A.H.; Bernardineli, N. Antibacterial Properties of Silver Nanoparticles as a Root Canal Irrigant against *Enterococcus faecalis* Biofilm and Infected Dentinal Tubules. *Int. Endod. J.* **2018**, *51*, 901–911. [CrossRef]
75. Wu, D.; Fan, W.; Kishen, A.; Gutmann, J.L.; Fan, B. Evaluation of the Antibacterial Efficacy of Silver Nanoparticles against *Enterococcus faecalis* Biofilm. *J. Endod.* **2014**, *40*, 285–290. [CrossRef] [PubMed]
76. Ballottin, D.; Fulaz, S.; Souza, M.L.; Corio, P.; Rodrigues, A.G.; Souza, A.O.; Gaspari, P.M.; Gomes, A.F.; Gozzo, F.; Tasic, L. Elucidating Protein Involvement in the Stabilization of the Biogenic Silver Nanoparticles. *Nanoscale Res. Lett.* **2016**, *11*, 313. [CrossRef]
77. Miclăuş, T.; Bochenkov, V.E.; Ogaki, R.; Howard, K.A.; Sutherland, D.S. Spatial Mapping and Quantification of Soft and Hard Protein Coronas at Silver Nanocubes. *Nano Lett.* **2014**, *14*, 2086–2093. [CrossRef] [PubMed]
78. Sarker, P.; Sajib, M.S.J.; Tao, X.; Wei, T. Multiscale Simulation of Protein Corona Formation on Silver Nanoparticles: Study of Ovispirin-1 Peptide Adsorption. *J. Phys. Chem. B* **2022**, *126*, 601–608. [CrossRef] [PubMed]
79. Monopoli, M.P.; Åberg, C.; Salvati, A.; Dawson, K.A. Biomolecular Coronas Provide the Biological Identity of Nanosized Materials. *Nat. Nanotechnol.* **2012**, *7*, 779–786. [CrossRef]

80. Durán, N.; Silveira, C.P.; Durán, M.; Martinez, D.S.T. Silver Nanoparticle Protein Corona and Toxicity: A Mini-Review. *J. Nanobiotechnol.* **2015**, *13*, 55. [CrossRef]
81. Gnanadhas, D.P.; Ben Thomas, M.; Thomas, R.; Raichur, A.M.; Chakravortty, D. Interaction of Silver Nanoparticles with Serum Proteins Affects Their Antimicrobial Activity In Vivo. *Antimicrob. Agents Chemother.* **2013**, *57*, 4945–4955. [CrossRef]
82. Allegra, E.; Titball, R.W.; Carter, J.; Champion, O.L. *Galleria mellonella* Larvae Allow the Discrimination of Toxic and Non-Toxic Chemicals. *Chemosphere* **2018**, *198*, 469–472. [CrossRef]
83. Thomaz, L.; Gustavo de Almeida, L.; Silva, F.R.O.; Cortez, M.; Taborda, C.P.; Spira, B. In Vivo Activity of Silver Nanoparticles Against *Pseudomonas aeruginosa* Infection in *Galleria mellonella*. *Front. Microbiol.* **2020**, *11*, 582107. [CrossRef]
84. Desbois, A.P.; Coote, P.J. Wax Moth Larva (*Galleria mellonella*): An in Vivo Model for Assessing the Efficacy of Antistaphylococcal Agents. *J. Antimicrob. Chemother.* **2011**, *66*, 1785–1790. [CrossRef]
85. Rigotto Caruso, G.; Tonani, L.; Marcato, P.D.; von Zeska Kress, M.R. Phenothiazinium Photosensitizers Associated with Silver Nanoparticles in Enhancement of Antimicrobial Photodynamic Therapy. *Antibiotics* **2021**, *10*, 569. [CrossRef]
86. Cockerill, F.R.; Wikler, M.A.; Alder, J.; Dudley, M.N.; Eliopoulos, G.M.; Ferraro, M.J.; Hardy, D.J.; Hecht, D.W.; Hindler, J.A.; Patel, J.B.; et al. *Methods for Dilution Antimicrobial Susceptibility Tests for Bacteria That Grow Aerobically*; Clinical and Laboratory Standards Institute: Wayne, PA, USA, 2012; Volume 32.
87. Palomino, J.-C.; Martin, A.; Camacho, M.; Guerra, H.; Swings, J.; Portaels, F. Resazurin Microtiter Assay Plate: Simple and Inexpensive Method for Detection of Drug Resistance in *Mycobacterium tuberculosis*. *Antimicrob. Agents Chemother.* **2002**, *46*, 2720–2722. [CrossRef]
88. Odds, F.C. Synergy, Antagonism, and What the Chequerboard Puts between Them. *J. Antimicrob. Chemother.* **2003**, *52*, 1. [CrossRef]
89. Doern, C.D. When Does 2 Plus 2 Equal 5? A Review of Antimicrobial Synergy Testing. *J. Clin. Microbiol.* **2014**, *52*, 4124–4128. [CrossRef]
90. Sánchez, M.C.; Llama-Palacios, A.; Fernández, E.; Figuero, E.; Marín, M.J.; León, R.; Blanc, V.; Herrera, D.; Sanz, M. An in Vitro Biofilm Model Associated to Dental Implants: Structural and Quantitative Analysis of in Vitro Biofilm Formation on Different Dental Implant Surfaces. *Dent. Mater.* **2014**, *30*, 1161–1171. [CrossRef]
91. Sardi, J.d.C.O.; Polaquini, C.R.; Freires, I.A.; Galvão, L.C.d.C.; Lazarini, J.G.; Torrezan, G.S.; Regasini, L.O.; Rosalen, P.L. Antibacterial Activity of Diacetylcurcumin against *Staphylococcus aureus* Results in Decreased Biofilm and Cellular Adhesion. *J. Med. Microbiol.* **2017**, *66*, 816–824. [CrossRef]

pharmaceuticals

MDPI

Article

Immobilization of Silver Nanoparticles with Defensive Gum of *Moringa oleifera* for Antibacterial Efficacy Against Resistant Bacterial Species from Human Infections

Liaqat Ali [1], Nisar Ahmad [1,*], Muhammad Nazir Uddin [1], Mostafa A. Abdel-Maksoud [2], Hina Fazal [3], Sabiha Fatima [4], Mohamed A. El-Tayeb [4], Bushra Hafeez Kiani [5], Wajid Khan [1], Murad Ali Rahat [1], Mohammad Ali [1], Yaqub Khan [1], Kamran Rauf [6], Salman Khan [1], Sami Ullah [1], Tanveer Ahmad [1], Afshan Salam [1] and Sajjad Ahmad [1]

1 Centre for Biotechnology and Microbiology, University of Swat, Swat 19120, Pakistan; liaqatbiotech23@gmail.com (L.A.); nazir@uswat.edu.pk (M.N.U.); w.khan@uswat.edu.pk (W.K.); muradrahat@uswat.edu.pk (M.A.R.); alimoh@uswat.edu.pk (M.A.); shaazkhan068@gmail.com (Y.K.); salmanbiotech6168@gmail.com (S.K.); samibiotech22@gmail.com (S.U.); tanveerbiotech88@gmail.com (T.A.); awaisnaveed085@gmail.com (A.S.); sajjad.std.mus@gmail.com (S.A.)

2 Botany and Microbiology Department, College of Science, King Saud University, P.O. Box 2455, Riyadh 11451, Saudi Arabia; mabdmaksoud@ksu.edu.sa

3 Pakistan Council for Scientific and Industrial Research (PCSIR) Laboratories Complex, Peshawar 25120, Pakistan; hina_fazalso@yahoo.com or hina_fazalso@pcsir-pesh.gov.pk

4 Department of Clinical Laboratory Science, College of Applied Medical Sciences, King Saud University, P.O. Box 10219, Riyadh 12371, Saudi Arabia; sabmehdi@ksu.edu.sa (S.F.); mali5@ksu.edu.sa (M.A.E.-T.)

5 Department of Biology and Biotechnology, Worcester Polytechnic Institute, Worcester, MA 01609, USA; bushra.hafeez@iiu.edu.pk

6 Department of Horticulture, The University of Agriculture Peshawar, Peshawar 25120, Pakistan; raufkamran317@gmail.com

* Correspondence: ahmadn@uswat.edu.pk

Abstract: Background: The worldwide misuse of antibiotics is one of the main factors in microbial resistance that is a serious threat worldwide. Alternative strategies are needed to overcome this issue. **Objectives**: In this study, a novel strategy was adopted to suppress the growth of resistant pathogens through immobilization of silver nanoparticles (AgNPs) in gum of *Moringa oleifera*. **Methods**: The AgNPs were prepared from the leaves of *Moringa oleifera* and subsequently characterized through UV-spectrophotometry, FTIR, SEM, and XRD. The differential ratios of characterized AgNPs were immobilized with gum of *M. oleifera* and investigated for antimicrobial potential against highly resistant pathogens. **Results**: The immobilized AgNPs displayed promising activities against highly resistant *B. subtilis* (23.6 mm; 50 µL:200 µL), *E. coli* (19.3 mm; 75 µL:200 µL), *K. pneumoniae* (22 mm; 200 µL:200 µL), *P. mirabilis* (16.3 mm; 100 µL:200 µL), *P. aeruginosa* (22 mm; 175 µL:200 µL), and *S. typhi* (19.3; 25 µL:200 µL) than either AgNPs alone or gum. The immobilized AgNPs released positive sliver ions that easily attached to negatively charged bacterial cells. After attachment and permeation to bacterial cells, the immobilized NPs alter the cell membrane permeability, protein/enzymes denaturation, oxidative stress (ROS), damage DNA, and change the gene expression level. It has been mechanistically considered that the immobilized AgNPs can kill bacteria by damaging their cell membranes, dephosphorylating tyrosine residues during their signal transduction pathways, inducing cell apoptosis, rupturing organelles, and inhibiting cell division, which finally leads to cell death. **Conclusions**: This study proposes a potential alternative drug for curing various infections.

Keywords: *Moringa oleifera*; organic synthesis of silver nanoparticles; defensive gum; immobilization of AgNPs; antibiotic resistance; antibacterial activity; alternative antimicrobials

1. Introduction

Moringa oleifera (*M. oleifera*), the "Miracle tree", thrives globally in almost all tropical and subtropical regions, but it is believed to be native to India, Bangladesh, Pakistan and Afghanistan [1]. The *Moringa* genus, belonging to the *Moringaceae* family, is also known as the drumstick tree, horseradish tree and benzoyl tree and can grow in a wide range of environmental conditions [2–7]. Moreover, *M. oleifera* is a rich source of different phytochemicals [8–11]. *M. oleifera* is a highly nutritional plant, and its various anatomical structures have been used for centuries to treat a variety of health conditions and possess widespread biological properties [12–17].

M. oleifera has been shown to have antimicrobial and antifungal activity. The plant contains compounds that can inhibit the growth of bacteria such as *Pseudomonas aeruginosa, Salmonella typhi, Vibrio cholera, Escherichia coli, Staphylococcus aureus, Klebsiella pneumoniae* and *Candida albicans* [18,19], and fungi such as *Rhizopus stolonifera, Neurospora crassa, Aspergillus niger,* and *Microsporum gypseum* [20], including pterygospermin and ethanolic extracts of the leaves, and alkaloids, flavonoids, and steroids in the fruits [19], *M. oleifera* has been shown to have antioxidant properties. The plant contains compounds that can scavenge free radicals [21], such as kaempferol [22], myricetin, isoquercetin, astragalin, and crypto-chlorogenic acid [23]. This antioxidant potential can help to protect cells from damage and reduce the risk of chronic diseases.

M. oleifera bark extract has anti-inflammatory activity similar to diclofenac and is thought to work by regulating the c-Jun N-terminal kinase and neutrophil pathways [24,25] due to the presence of flavonoids, alkaloids, vanillin, moringin, phenols, tannins, carotenoids, hydroxymellein, Beta-sitosterol, and ß-sitostenol [26]. *M. oleifera* has been shown to have both fertility and anti-fertility properties. The aqueous extract of the plant has been found to increase abortifacient and anti-fertility at doses of 200 and 400 mg/kg [15]. A recent study suggested that the ingestion of *M. oleifera* before, after and during pregnancy may lead to adverse fetal developmental outcomes [27].

The seed extract was able to reduce histamine release and suppress anaphylaxis induced by anti-immunoglobulin G. The mechanism underlying this effect is thought to be the membrane-stabilizing potential of the extract on mast cells [28]. The leaf extract can prevent gastric ulcers by reducing free radicals, neutralizing stomach acid, and increasing capillary resistance [29,30]. Some active constituents such as niazirmin A, niazirmin B, and niazimicin play a key role in lowering cholesterol levels, and avenasterol, stigmasterol, campesterol, and beta-sistosterol have diuretic activity [28,31,32]. The presence of quercetin, kaempferol, flavonoids, and benzylglucosinolate can protect the liver from damage [33,34]. The leaves, seeds, and dried pulp have shown health-inducing properties [28,35,36]. It is a nutrient-rich plant with a high protein content, as well as significant amounts of vitamins, minerals, fat carbohydrates, and dietary fibers [37–39].

Plant exudates are a diverse group of compounds that can be released from all parts of the plant [40]. Gums are complex carbohydrates that can absorb water and form gels [41]. Plant gums are bioavailable and have been used for centuries in a variety of applications, including food, medicine, and industry [41,42]. In pharmaceutical formulations, plant-based gums and mucilages are the key ingredients due to their bootability, widespread availability, non-toxicity, and affordability [43]. Scientists and pharmaceutical companies are interested in using plant-based gums and mucilages as drug delivery systems, gene therapy vectors, and biosynthetic materials. By modifying these natural substances, researchers have developed a new class of innovative drug products with potential applications in a variety of advanced fields [41]. Plant-based gums are non-toxic and biodegradable [41,44]. They have shown antimicrobial activity against a variety of microorganisms, including bacteria, fungi, and viruses [45]. Potential mechanisms of action include the inhibition of the bacterial cell membrane, chelation of essential metal ions, production of reactive oxygen species, and modulation of the host immune response [46,47]. Plant-based gums could be used to develop a variety of antimicrobial products, such as food additives, pharmaceutical products, and agricultural products [47].

Nanomaterials are at the forefront of nanotechnology, a rapidly developing field with the potential to revolutionize many areas of human activity [48]. Nanoparticles are particles with a maximum size of 100 nanometers (nm), which is about 1/100,000th the width of a human hair [49]. Nanoparticles exhibit unique properties that make them superior and indispensable in many applications, including combating microbes, drug delivery, catalysis, water purification, the treatment of environmental waste, in the food industry, in the textile industry, biolabeling, and cancer treatment [50]. Silver nanoparticles (AgNPs) are a promising antimicrobial agent because they are effective against a wide range of microorganisms, including bacteria, fungi, and viruses [51,52]. They are also stable and reduce the likelihood of bacteria developing antibiotic resistance. AgNPs are being investigated for use in a variety of applications, such as medicine, medical devices, and food packaging [53,54].

Immobilization is a powerful technique that allows for reuse and recovery [55], improved stability [56], controlled reactivity, and easier separation of molecules [57]. It is used in a wide range of applications, including bio-catalysis [58], sensors [59], diagnostics [60], and environmental remediation [61]. The immobilization of AgNPs is a versatile technique that can be used to improve their stability, control their reactivity, and make them easier to use in a variety of applications: AgNPs have strong antimicrobial properties and can be used to create coatings that can kill bacteria and other microorganisms [62], AgNPs can be used to create sensors that are sensitive to specific chemicals or biological signals, AgNPs can be used as catalysts for a variety of chemical reactions, and AgNPs can be used to degrade pollutants in water and soil [63].

AgNPs alone have proven antimicrobial potential, while the gum is released in response to pathogen attacks in plants. Here, the dual and synergistic potential of AgNPs along with the gum was investigated for the growth inhibition of infectious strains. Immobilized AgNPs have potential to kill infectious strains by disrupting the membranes by inducing pores and causing cytoplasmic leakage and bacterial cell death. It is possible that immobilized AgNPs can stimulate the defense system of bacterial cells more rapidly than either NPs alone or using gum alone. The immobilization strategy most probably releases huge quantities of reactive oxygen species or other radicals that directly react and inhibit major functions such as metabolism, replication, translation, and denaturation and cause DNA damage.

The gum of this miracle plant possesses strong antimicrobial potential against various pathogens. Similarly, silver nanoparticles are widely used in the medical sector due to their high inhibiting efficacy against microorganisms. Therefore, the main objective of the current study was to investigate the synergistic and high efficacy of immobilized silver nanoparticles encapsulated in *M. oleifera* gum against highly resistant microbes and to develop a possible antimicrobial mechanism for the immobilized AgNPs.

2. Results

2.1. Biogenic Synthesis of Nanoparticles and Its Characterization

M. Oleifera leaves were mixed with different volumes of salt solution, keeping the reactant volume constant. The change in color representing the formation of NPs was observed in two different ways. Upon exposing the reactants to sunlight or incubation for 24 h, the observation showed that a 4 mg/mL:4 mM ratio displayed the darkest color and characteristic peak between 300 and 600 nm. The other differential ratios were less effective in the formation of NPs.

2.1.1. UV–Visible Spectrophotometry of Leaf-Derived AgNPs

The initial step in identifying the formation of silver nanoparticles from leaf extracts involved using an Elite Double-beam UV spectrophotometer to measure the absorbance at 300–600 nm for 24 h. The reactants (4 mg/mL:4 mM) showed the greatest absorbance in the 400–450 nm range, with a peak at 430 nm. Furthermore, the solution's color changed from light brown to dark brown, possibly indicating the formation of nanoparticles as shown in Figure 1.

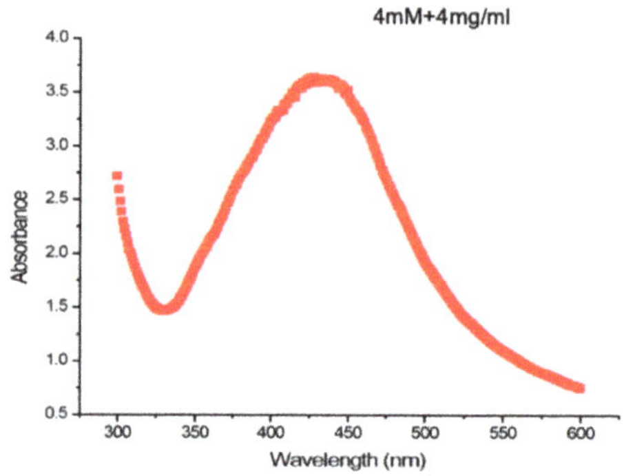

Figure 1. UV–visible spectroscopy of Moringa leaf-derived silver nanoparticles.

2.1.2. Fourier Transform Infrared Spectroscopy (FTIR) ML-Derived AgNPs

FTIR was used to analyze the chemicals in the silver nanoparticles. The FTIR spectra displayed different plant substances (phenolics functional group), like proteins and alcohols/carbonyl rings/groups, and aromatic amines and this all helped the nanoparticles. X-rays showed that the nanoparticles were round-shaped and about 25 to 40 nanometers in size (Figure 2). The broad peak was observed at 2000, corresponding to carboxylic acids with an OH group with alcohol stretching. The peak at 3000 to 2900 represents the major intramolecular bonds with OH groups. The C-H of Aldehydic amines was represented by the spectra with a peak area of 2800 with C-H stretching, while after the sp3 hybridized groups, the O=C=O displayed a peak area ranging from 2400 to 2100. Below the 1700 peak area, double carbon bonding was observed, showing the presence of alkenes. N alone or O alone or in various groups either in nitro compounds in FTIR spectra was observed at the peak area below 1500, while the OH of the amine and phenolic compounds was observed from 1300 to 1450. Peaks below 650 cm^{-1} were attributed to the AgNPs (Figure 2).

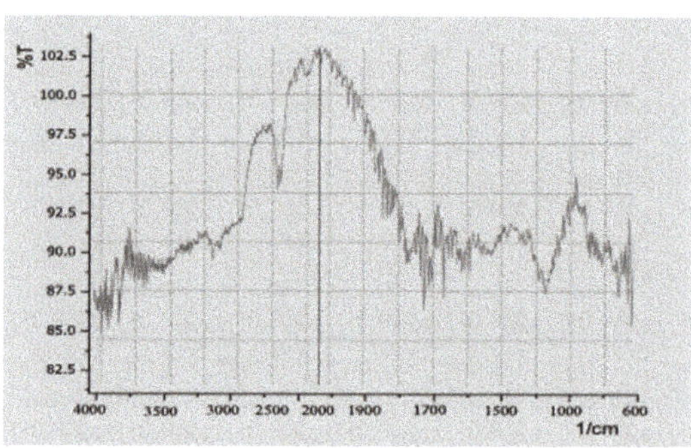

Figure 2. FTIR spectra of Moringa leaf (ML)-derived silver nanoparticles.

2.1.3. X-Ray Diffraction Spectrum (XRD) Analysis of Biogenic AgNPs

X-ray diffraction (XRD) analysis of the biogenic silver nanoparticles synthesized from *M. oleifera* leaf extract revealed a mostly round/cubic crystalline structure with three strong Bragg reflections at 32.201, 37.27, and 45.6, corresponding to the (42), (40), and (120) planes, respectively. The interplanar distances were calculated as 2.15 Å, 2.11 Å, and 1.38 Å, respectively. The particle size, determined by the Debye–Scherrer formula, was 25 nm (Figure 3). These findings confirm the characteristics of silver nanoparticles derived from

Moringa oleifera. The XRD analysis was conducted using a diffractometer with Cu K-alpha radiation at 40 kV and 30 mA. The scanning range was from 0 to 80 degrees 2θ with a scan rate of 10 degrees/min. The XRD analysis was performed using a Goniometer PW3050/60 and analyzed with Xpert-PRO software (https://www.xpert-pro.com/home.php, (accessed on 29 October 2024)).

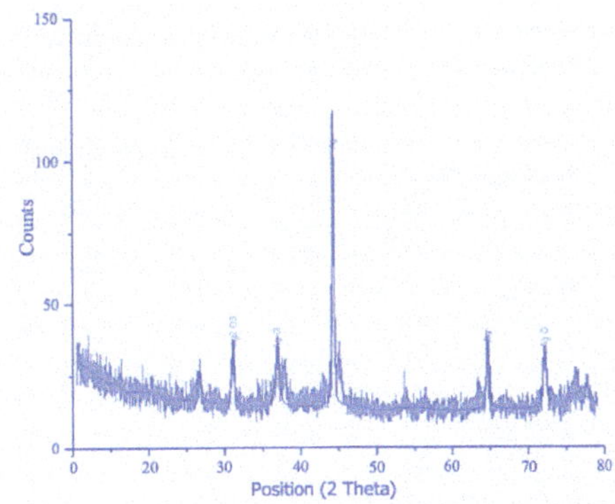

Figure 3. XRD spectra of ML-derived silver nanoparticles.

2.1.4. Transmission Electron Microscopy of ML-Derived AgNPs

The ML-derived AgNPs were analyzed by Transmission Electron Microscopy (TEM) to determine their size, shape, and morphology. The TEM images displayed that most of the ML-derived AgNPs were spherical in shape, and they may be individual or in aggregated morphologies (Figure 4). The presence of bioactive phytochemicals in the leaves of medicinally important *M. oleifera* extract was the main characteristic responsible for the formation of spherical-shape nanoparticles. The scale on the TEM images indicates that the size varies from 25 nm to 40 nm to 120 nm, as shown in Figure 4.

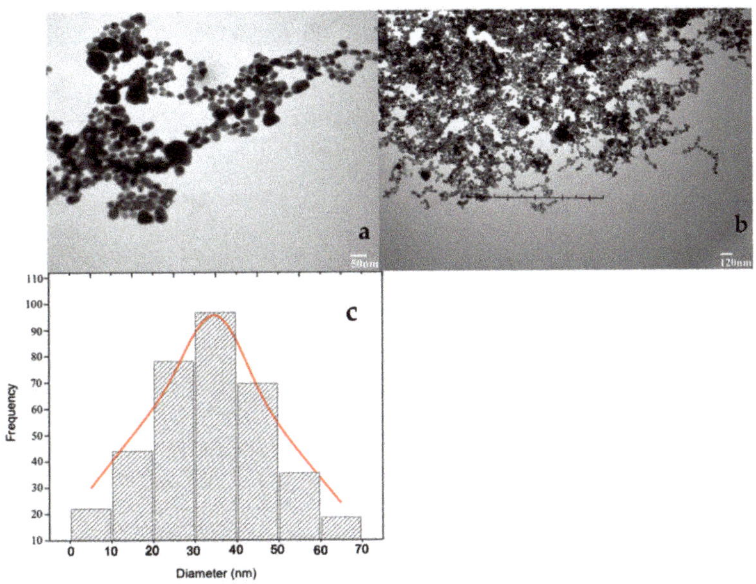

Figure 4. TEM images of ML-derived silver nanoparticles: (**a**) 50 nm, (**b**) 120 nm, and (**c**) histogram.

2.2. Morphological Identification of Bacterial Isolates

To identify bacterial species, morphological identification was carried out. *E. coli* on MAC agar has a bright, smooth, pink-colored elevated colony that is transparent; *K. pneumoniae* on MAC agar revealed the development of small to large-sized mucoid colonies with a creamy pink and yellow appearance, as shown in Figure 5b; *P. aeruginosa* on CLED agar showed green colonies with a typical matte surface and rough periphery—its scent was "sweet" and it was colored blue-green, as shown in Figure 5c. *S. typhi* on MAC agar appeared pale, colorless, smooth, and transparent, with raised colonies, as shown in Figure 5d.

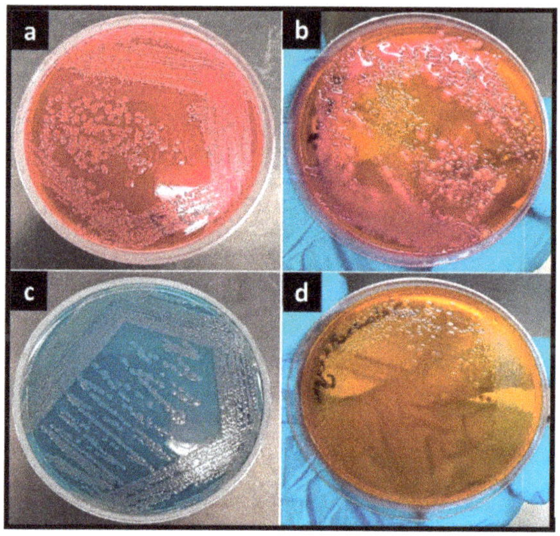

Figure 5. Morphological representation of different bacterial strains on MAC agar and CLED agar plates. (**a**) *E. coli*, (**b**) *K. pneumoniae* (**c**) *P. aeruginosa*, and (**d**) *S. typhi*.

2.3. Identification Through Microscopy

Morphology and staining characteristics of *E. coli*, *K. pneumoniae*, *P. aeruginosa*, and *S. typhi* were observed under microscope. *E. coli* was observed as Gram-negative, rod-shaped, pink, and grouped in single or paired/short, as shown in Figure 6a. *K. pneumoniae*, was bacilli in shape and Gram-negative, as shown in Figure 6b. *P. aeruginosa* was rod-shaped, Gram-negative bacteria, typically 0.5–1.0 µm in width and 1–4 µm in length, as shown in Figure 6c, and *S. typhi* was short, singly arranged, Gram-negative rod-shaped bacteria, as shown in Figure 6d.

2.4. Antibiotic Susceptibility Pattern

The sensitivity patterns of *B. subtilis*, *E. coli*, *K. pneumoniae*, *P. aeruginosa*, *P. mirabilis, and S. typhi* isolates were investigated using the disk diffusion technique. Doxycycline (DO), Ceftriaxone (CRO), Cefotaxime (CTX), Sulbactam/cefoperazone (SCF), Erythromycin (E), Trimethoprim/sulfamethoxazole (SXT), Imipenem (IPM), and Azithromycin (AZM) were applied on each bacterial strain for a susceptibility test, as shown in Table 1 and Figure 7. *B. subtilis* was totally resistant to E, SXT, and AZM. *E. coli* displayed resistance to SCF, E, and AZM. *K. pneumoniae* showed resistance to CRO, E, and SXT. *P. aeruginosa* exhibited resistance to CRO, CTX, SCF, E, and SXT. *P. mirabilis* was resistant to CRO, SXT, and AZM. *S. typhi* was resistant to CRO, SXT, and AZM.

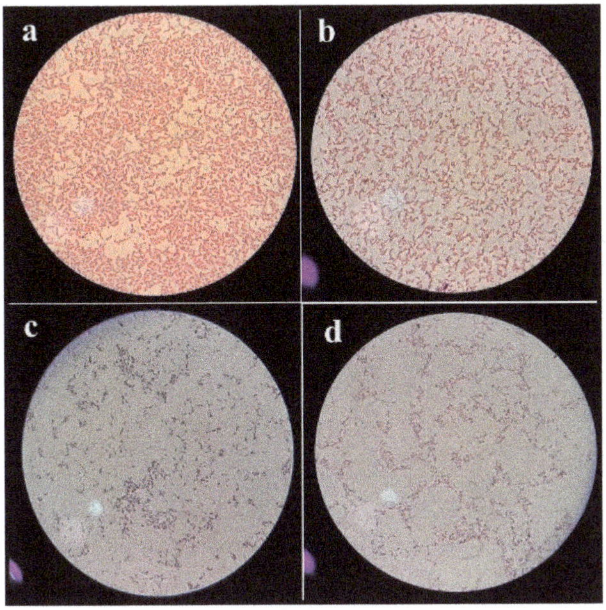

Figure 6. Microscopic representation of different bacterial strains. (**a**) *E. coli*, (**b**) *K. pneumoniae*, (**c**) *P. aeruginosa*, and (**d**) *S. typhi*.

Table 1. Antibiotic sensitivity status and zone of inhibition in mm of different drugs.

Pathogenic Species	Zones of Inhibition (mm) of Different Antibiotics							
	Do	CRO	CTX	SCF	E	SXT	IPM	AZM
B. subtilis	10.1 ± 0.1	12.2 ± 0.4	15.3 ± 0.3	17.3 ± 0.3	**R**	**R**	---	**R**
E. coli	8.3 ± 0.1	10.2 ± 0.1	13.5 ± 0.4	**R**	**R**	14.6 ± 0.5	15.1 ± 0.3	**R**
K. pneumoniae	10.5 ± 0.2	**R**	10.6 ± 0.6	17.3 ± 0.3	**R**	**R**	15.4 ± 0.7	10.2 ± 0.4
P. aeruginosa	8.9 ± 0.2	**R**	**R**	**R**	**R**	**R**	10.2 ± 0.8	**R**
P. mirabilis	18.2 ± 0.4	**R**	10.3 ± 0.1	18.4 ± 0.6	---	**R**	12.4 ± 0.2	**R**
S. typhi	14.3 ± 0.1	**R**	10.2 ± 0.3	15.2 ± 0.5	---	**R**	12.3 ± 0.5	**R**

2.5. Antibacterial Potential of Immobilized AgNPs

Many microorganisms that cause human diseases are becoming resistant to antibiotics due to the misuse of antibiotics. This means that there is a need to find novel antibacterial substances derived from plants and other natural sources. To find traditionally utilized therapeutic herbs that are very effective against both Gram-positive and Gram-negative bacteria, different concentrations of *M. oleifera* gums (gums alone, gums + AgNPs, and AgNPs alone) were applied to investigate antibacterial activities. The synergistic combination boosted the antibacterial efficacy against resistant bacteria. Furthermore, several secondary metabolites, including alkaloids, flavonoids, glycosides, phenols, saponins, and sterols, are some of the active phytochemicals that give medicinal plants their therapeutic qualities. Various plant extracts, such as of the root, stem, bark, and seeds, have been shown to contain these metabolites. Therefore, preliminary screening tests are useful for finding bioactive compounds that could result in their finding to launch novel pharmaceuticals. Additionally, these tests can help to quantify and qualitatively separate chemicals with pharmacological action [64]. Both the AgNPs and gum of *M. oleifera* have high antimicrobial potential, and their immobilization further enhances the antibacterial capability by inhibiting the growth of resistant bacterial strains. The immobilization of AgNPs and gum is presented in the following Figure 8.

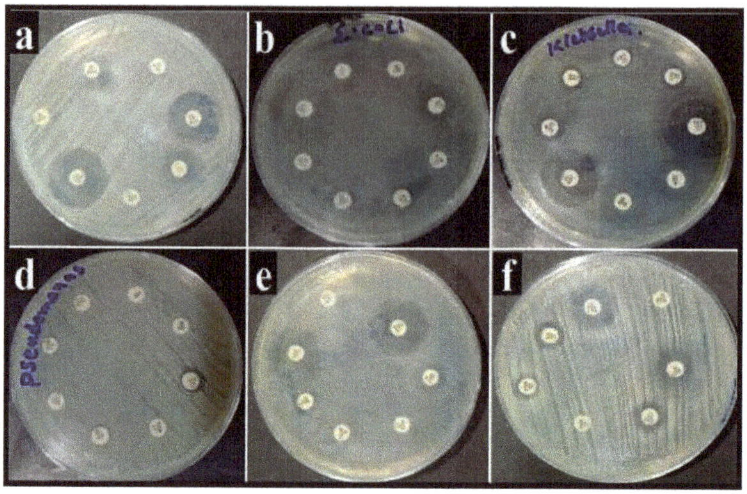

Figure 7. Pictorial representation of zones of inhibition of various drugs against different bacterial strains (**a**) *B. subtilis*, (**b**) *E. coli*, (**c**) *K. pneumoniae*, (**d**) *P. aeruginosa*, (**e**) *P. mirabilis*, and (**f**) *S. typhi*.

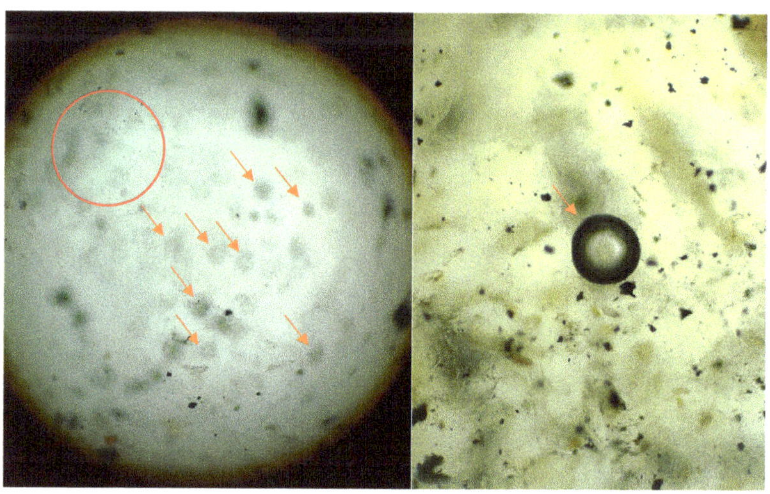

Figure 8. Micrographs of immobilization of silver nanoparticles and gum of *M. oleifera*. The red circle indicates the encapsulation of NPs in gum, while red arrows refers to strong binding of gum with maximum AgNPs, and the black circle (indicated by red arrow) represent the accumulation of NPs that appear in circular shape after zooming.

2.6. Immobilized AgNP-Induced Growth Inhibition of Highly Resistant B. subtilis

The zone of inhibition of the synergistic combination of *M. oleifera* gum and AgNPs against highly resistant *B. subtilis* displayed variable activities: T1 (25 μL AgNPs:200 μL gums) showed a 19.3 mm zone inhibition; T2 (50 μL AgNPs:200 μL gums), 23.6 mm; T3 (75 μL AgNPs:200 μL gums), 20.6 mm; T4 (100 μL AgNPs:200 μL gums), 17 mm; T5 (125 μL AgNPs:200 μL gums), 15.6 mm; T6 (150 μL AgNPs:200 μL gums), 14.6 mm; T7 (175 μL AgNPs:200 μL gums), 16 mm; T8 (200 μL AgNPs:200 μL gums), 21.3 mm; T9 (225 μL AgNPs:200 μL gums), 19.3 mm; and T10 (250 μL AgNPs:200 μL gums), 11.6 mm. This mean that these combinations of immobilized AgNPs were able to kill bacteria within a radius of 11.6 to 23.6 mm. AgNPs alone as C1 (100 μL AgNPs) and gums alone as

200 μL gums showed zones of inhibition of 16.3 mm and 19 mm, respectively. These results suggest that the immobilized AgNPs were more effective at killing highly resistant *B. subtilis* than either AgNPs or gums alone, as shown in Figure 9a. The zones of inhibition of each treatment are shown in Figure 10.

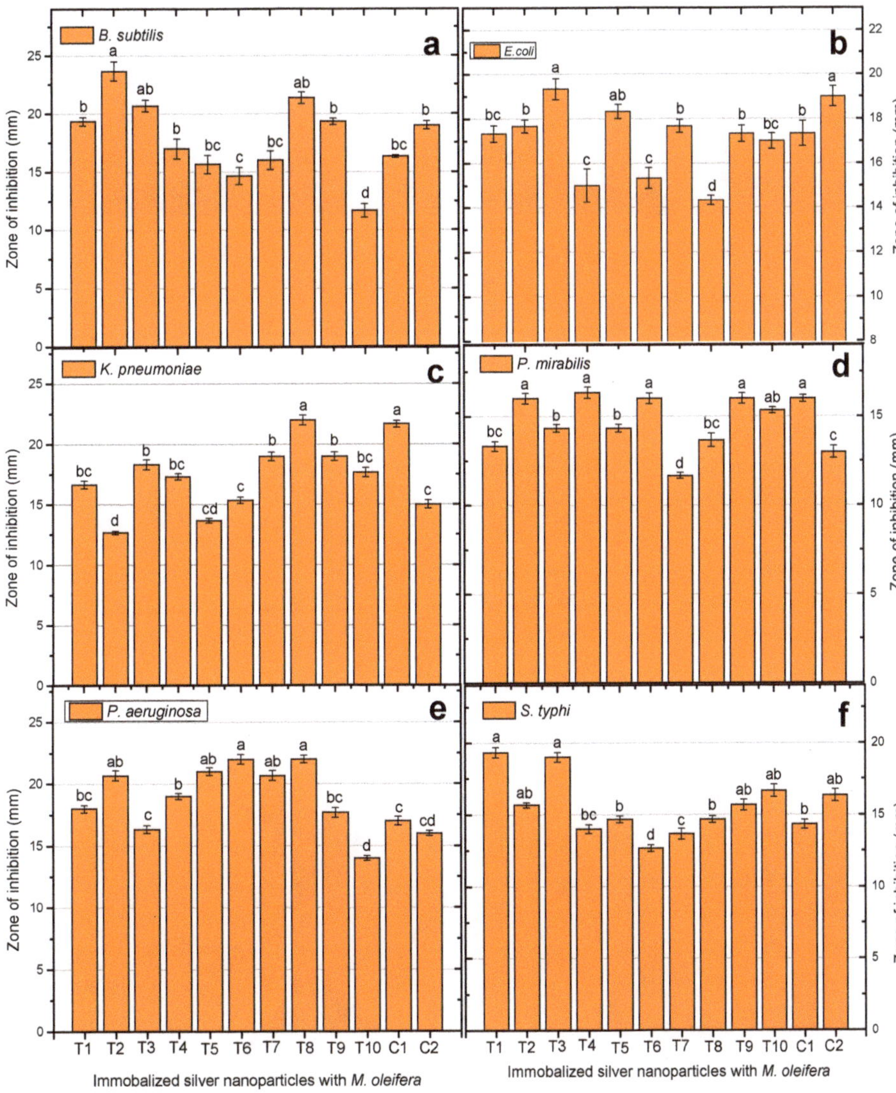

Figure 9. Antibacterial potential of different treatments of immobilized AgNPs (T1: 25 μL AgNPs + 200 μL gums; T2: 50 μL AgNPs + 200 μL gums; T3: 75 μL AgNPs + 200 μL gums; T4: 100 μL AgNPs + 200 μL gums; T5: 125 μL + 200 μL gums; T6: 150 μL AgNPs + 200 μL gums; T7: 175 μL AgNPs + 200 μL gums; T8: 200 μL AgNPs + 200 μL gums; T9: 225 μL AgNPs + 200 μL gums; T10: 250 μL AgNPs + 200 μL gums; AgNPs alone and gums alone against (**a**) *B. subtilis*, (**b**) *E. coli*, (**c**) *K. pneumoniae*, (**d**) *P. mirabilis*, (**e**) *P. aeruginosa*, and (**f**) *S. typhi*). Bars with alphabets and standard errors represents least significant differences among mean values from triplicates.

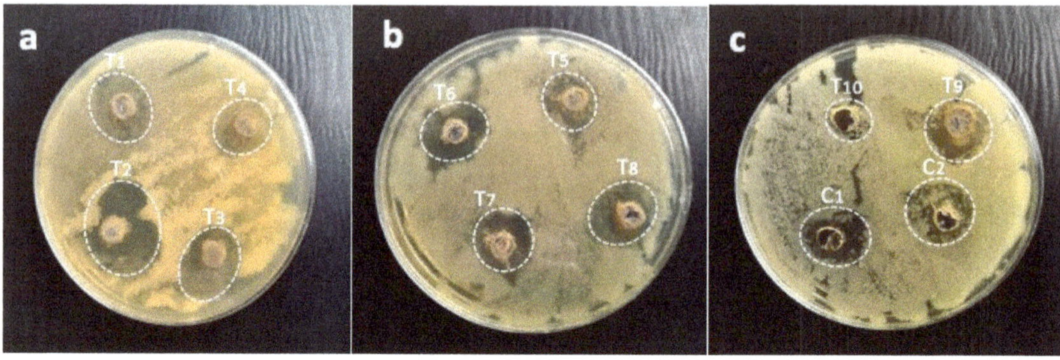

Figure 10. Pictorial presentation of zones of inhibitions of immobilized AgNPs against *B. subtilis* as (**a**) T1 (25 µL AgNPs + 200 µL gums), T2 (50 µL AgNPs + 200 µL gums), T3 (75 µL AgNPs + 200 µL gums), and T4 (100 µL AgNPs + 200 µL gums); (**b**) T5 (125 µL + 200 µL gums), T6 (150 µL AgNPs + 200 µL gums), T7 (175 µL AgNPs + 200 µL gums), and T8 (200 µL AgNPs + 200 µL gums); and (**c**) T9 (225 µL AgNPs + 200 µL gums), T10 (250 µL AgNPs + 200 µL gums), C1 (100 µL AgNPs alone), and C2 (200 µL gums alone).

2.7. Immobilized AgNP-Induced Growth Inhibition of Highly Resistant *E. coli*

The immobilized AgNPs also exhibited excellent inhibiting potential against highly resistant *E. coli* and displayed a 17.3 mm zone using T1 (25 µL AgNPs:200 µL gums), while, the other treatments, such as T2 (50 µL AgNPs:200 µL gums), showed a 17.6 mm zone; T3 (75 µL AgNPs:200 µL gums), 19.3 mm; T4 (100 µL AgNPs:200 µL gums), 15 mm; T5 (125 µL AgNPs:200 µL gums), 18.3 mm; T6 (150 µL AgNPs:200 µL gums), 15.3 mm; T7 (175 µL AgNPs:200 µL gums), 17.6 mm; T8 (200 µL AgNPs:200 µL gums), 14.3 mm; T9 (225 µL AgNPs:200 µL gums), 17.3 mm; and T10 (250 µL AgNPs:200 µL gums), 17 mm. By comparison, this was more than C1 and C2. This means that the immobilized AgNPs were found to be dominant in killing resistant *E. coli* compared to other treatments (Figure 9b), and the zones of inhibitions are given in Figure 11.

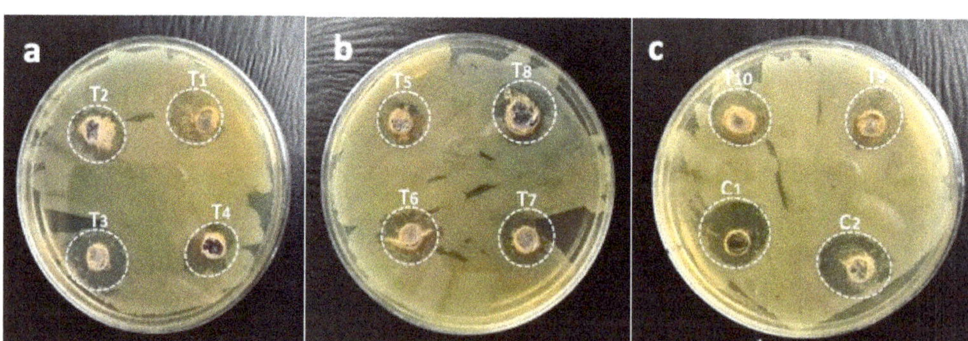

Figure 11. Pictorial presentation of zones of inhibitions of immobilized AgNPs against *E. coli* as (**a**) T1 (25 µL AgNPs + 200 µL gums), T2 (50 µL AgNPs + 200 µL gums), T3 (75 µL AgNPs + 200 µL gums), and T4 (100 µL AgNPs + 200 µL gums); (**b**) T5 (125 µL + 200 µL gums), T6 (150 µL AgNPs + 200 µL gums), T7 (175 µL AgNPs + 200 µL gums), and T8 (200 µL AgNPs + 200 µL gums); and (**c**) T9 (225 µL AgNPs + 200 µL gums), T10 (250 µL AgNPs + 200 µL gums), C1 (100 µL AgNPs alone), and C2 (200 µL gums alone).

2.8. Immobilized AgNP-Induced Inhibition of Highly Resistant K. pneumoniae

In this study, the immobilized AgNPs presented potent activities against resistant *K. pneumoniae* as T1 (25 µL AgNPs:200 µL gums), 16.6 mm; T2 (25 µL AgNPs:200 µL gums), 12.6 mm; T3 (75 µL AgNPs:200 µL gums), 18.3 mm; T4 (100 µL AgNPs:200 µL gums), 17.3 mm; T5 (125 µL AgNPs:200 µL gums), 13.6 mm; T6 (150 µL AgNPs:200 µL gums), 15.3 mm; T7 (175 µL AgNPs:200 µL gums), 19 mm; T8 (200 µL AgNPs:200 µL gums), 22 mm; T9 (225 µL AgNPs:200 µL gums), 19 mm; and T10 (250 µL AgNPs:200 µL gums), 17.6 mm. The C1 and C2 displayed lower activities than the immobilized AgNPs. The inhibiting efficacy against highly resistant *K. pneumoniae* is shown in Figures 9c and 12.

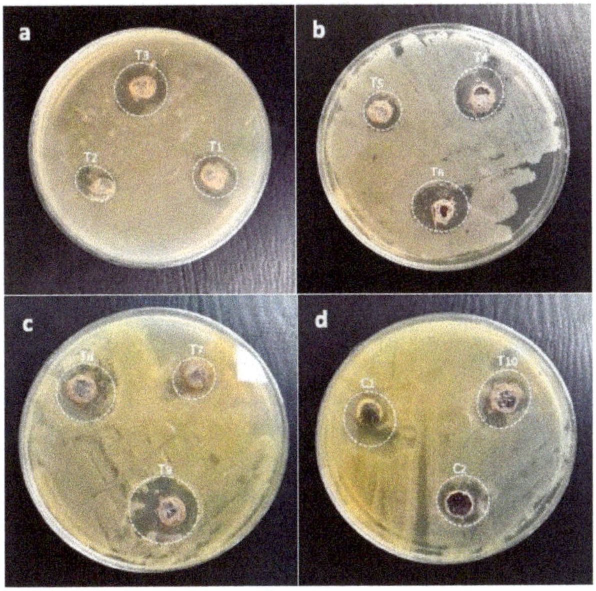

Figure 12. Pictorial presentation of zones of inhibitions of immobilized AgNPs against *K. pneumoniae* as (**a**) T1 (25 µL AgNPs + 200 µL gums), T2 (50 µL AgNPs + 200 µL gums), and T3 (75 µL AgNPs + 200 µL gums); (**b**) T4 (100 µL AgNPs + 200 µL gums), T5 (125 µL + 200 µL gums), and T6 (150 µL AgNPs + 200 µL gums); (**c**) T7 (175 µL AgNPs + 200 µL gums), T8 (200 µL AgNPs + 200 µL gums), and T9 (225 µL AgNPs + 200 µL gums); and (**d**) T10 (250 µL AgNPs + 200 µL gums), C1 (100 µL AgNPs alone), and C2 (200 µL gums alone).

2.9. Immobilized AgNP-Induced Growth Inhibition of Highly Resistant P. mirabilis and the Zones of Inhibition of the Synergistic Combination of M. oleifera Gums

AgNPs (immobilized) against highly resistant *P. mirabilis* were recorded as follows: T1 (25 µL AgNPs:200 µL gums) displayed 13.3 mm; T2 (50 µL AgNPs:200 µL gums), 16 mm; T3 (75 µL AgNPs:200 µL gums), 14.3 mm; T4 (100 µL AgNPs:200 µL gums), 16.3 mm; T5 (125 µL AgNPs:200 µL gums), 14.3 mm; T6 (150 µL AgNPs:200 µL gums), 16 mm; T7 (175 µL AgNPs:200 µL gums), 11.6 mm; T8 (200 µL AgNPs:200 µL gums), 13.6 mm; T9 (225 µL AgNPs:200 µL gums), 16 mm; and T10 (250 µL AgNPs:200 µL gums) 15 mm. However, the C1 (100 µL AgNPs) and gums alone as C2 (200 µL gums) have shown 16 mm and 13 mm zones of inhibition, respectively. These results confirm that the immobilized nanoparticles were superior in efficacy compared to the AgNPs or gum of medicinal plants used alone against highly resistant *P. mirabilis*, as shown in Figures 9d and 13.

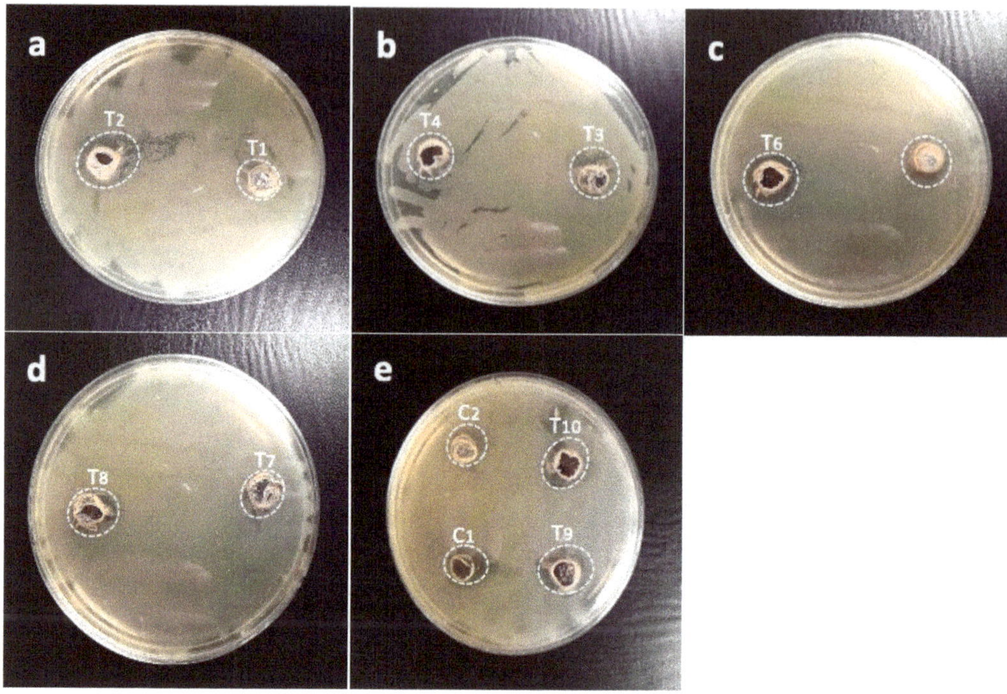

Figure 13. Pictorial presentation of zones of inhibitions of immobilized AgNPs against *P. mirabilis* as (**a**) T1 (25 µL AgNPs + 200 µL gums) and T2 (50 µL AgNPs + 200 µL gums); (**b**) T3 (75 µL AgNPs + 200 µL gums) and T4 (100 µL AgNPs + 200 µL gums); (**c**) T5 (125 µL + 200 µL gums) and T6 (150 µL AgNPs + 200 µL gums); (**d**) T7 (175 µL AgNPs + 200 µL gums) and T8 (200 µL AgNPs + 200 µL gums; and (**e**) T9 (225 µL AgNPs + 200 µL gums), T10 (250 µL AgNPs + 200 µL gums), C1 (100 µL AgNPs alone), and C2 (200 µL gums alone).

2.10. Immobilized AgNP-Induced Inhibition of Highly Resistant P. aeruginosa

The immobilized AgNPs exhibited optimal activities against the highly resistant *P. aeruginosa*. The coating of NPs with gum enhanced the antibacterial effectiveness, as shown in Figures 9e and 14. The differential treatments of immobilized AgNPs exhibited differential activities against *P. aeruginosa* and the activities in terms of inhibition zones were T1 (25 µL AgNPs:200 µL gums), 18 mm; T2 (50 µL AgNPs:200 µL gums), 20.6 mm; T3 (75 µL AgNPs:200 µL gums), 16.3 mm; T4 (100 µL AgNPs:200 µL gums), 19 mm; T5 (125 µL AgNPs:200 µL gums), 21 mm; T6 (150 µL AgNPs:200 µL gums), 22 mm; T7 (175 µL AgNPs:200 µL gums), 20 mm; T8 (200 µL AgNPs:200 µL gums), 22 mm; T9 (225 µL AgNPs:200 µL gums), 17.6 mm; and T10 (250 µL AgNPs:200 µL gums), 14 mm. The AgNPs alone, C1 (100 µL AgNPs), and gums alone, C2 (200 µL gums), exhibited 17 mm and 16 mm zones of inhibition, which are comparatively less than immobilized AgNPs and more effective in killing the highly resistant *P. aeruginosa*, as shown in Figures 9e and 14.

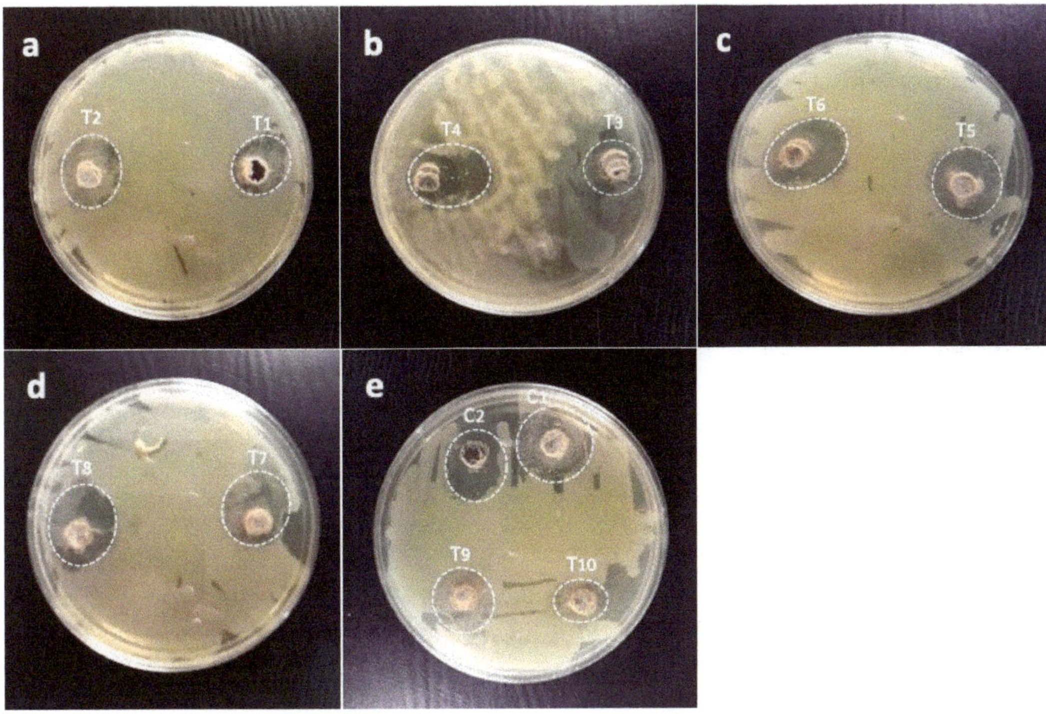

Figure 14. Pictorial presentation of zones of inhibitions of immobilized AgNPs against *P. aeruginosa* as (**a**) T1 (25 μL AgNPs + 200 μL gums) and T2 (50 μL AgNPs + 200 μL gums); (**b**) T3 (75 μL AgNPs + 200 μL gums) and T4 (100 μL AgNPs + 200 μL gums); (**c**) T5 (125 μL + 200 μL gums) and T6 (150 μL AgNPs + 200 μL gums); (**d**) T7 (175 μL AgNPs + 200 μL gums) and T8 (200 μL AgNPs + 200 μL gums); and (**e**) T9 (225 μL AgNPs + 200 μL gums), T10 (250 μL AgNPs + 200 μL gums), C1 (100 μL AgNPs alone), and C2 (200 μL gums alone).

2.11. Immobilized AgNP-Induced Growth Inhibition of S. typhi

Herewith, the zones of inhibition of the immobilized AgNPs against highly resistant *S. typhi* were recorded as T1 (25 μL AgNPs:200 μL gums), 19.3 mm; T2 (50 μL AgNPs:200 μL gums), 15.6 mm; T3 (75 μL AgNPs:200 μL gums), 19 mm; T4 (100 μL AgNPs:200 μL gums), 14 mm; T5 (125 μL AgNPs:200 μL gums), 14.6 mm; T6 (150 μL AgNPs:200 μL gums), 12.6 mm; T7 (175 μL AgNPs:200 μL gums), 13.6 mm; T8 (200 μL AgNPs:200 μL gums), 14.6 mm; T9 (225 μL AgNPs:200 μL gums), 15.6 mm; and T10 (250 μL AgNPs:200 μL gums), 16.6 mm. The differential ratios of immobilized AgNPs displayed antibacterial potential within the range of 12.6 to 19.3 mm, which was significantly slightly higher than that of C1 (100 μL AgNPs) and C2 (200 μL gums), which exhibited 14.3 mm and 16.3 mm zones of inhibition, respectively. This means that the immobilized AgNPs were also more effective than NPs or gum alone against resistant *S. typhi*, as shown in Figures 9f and 15.

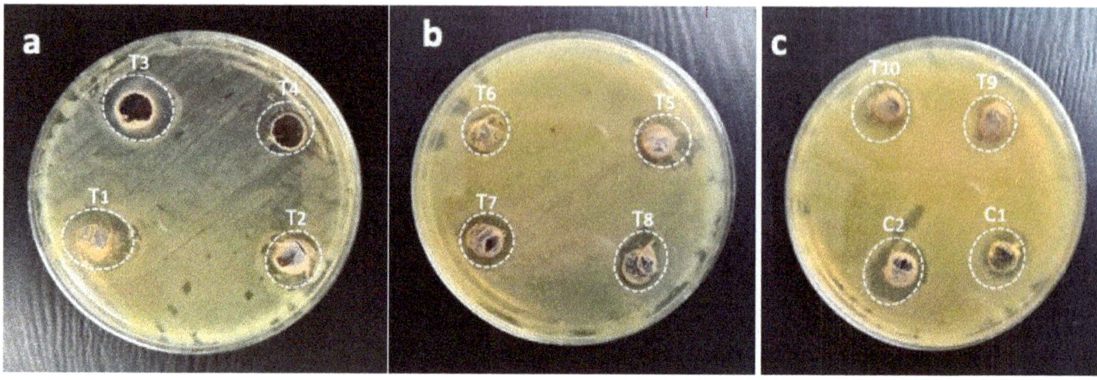

Figure 15. Pictorial presentation of zones of inhibitions of immobilized AgNPs against *S. typhi* as (**a**) T1 (25 μL AgNPs + 200 μL gums), T2 (50 μL AgNPs + 200 μL gums), T3 (75 μL AgNPs + 200 μL gums), and T4 (100 μL AgNPs + 200 μL gums); (**b**) T5 (125 μL + 200 μL gums), T6 (150 μL AgNPs + 200 μL gums), T7 (175 μL AgNPs + 200 μL gums), and T8 (200 μL AgNPs + 200 μL gums); and (**c**) T9 (225 μL AgNPs + 200 μL gums), T10 (250 μL AgNPs + 200 μL gums), C1 (100 μL AgNPs alone), and C2 (200 μL gums alone).

3. Discussion

Plant gums are natural substances that are not harmful to humans or to the environment. They are also sustainable, meaning that they can be produced and used without depleting natural resources. Additionally, they are recyclable, cost-effective, and biodegradable. These properties make them ideal for use in a variety of industries, including pharmaceuticals, nanoparticle synthesis, and food. *M. oleifera* is a highly important medicinal plant that is found in both tropical and subtropical regions around the globe. Numerous significant phenols, amino acids, proteins, vitamins, and betacarotenes may be found in all anatomical structures of the plant. Antiulcer, antidiuretic, anticancer, antipyretic, anti-inflammatory, antidiabetic, antihypertensive, antidiabetic, cholesterol-lowering, and antioxidant qualities are found in all parts of this plant. Traditional medical systems have traditionally used this herb since ancient times, particularly in south Asia [65].

Multidrug-resistant (MDR) bacteria are extremely dangerous and pose a serious threat to global health systems because they can survive antibiotic treatments. These bacteria are able to adapt to antibiotics by changing their genetic makeup to become resistant to known antibiotics and their combinations [66]. Nanoparticles are a new type of antimicrobial agent that are being researched as a way to combat these MDR bacteria; they target the bacterial cells in multiple ways, making it difficult for the bacteria to escape [67]. The emergence of antibiotic-resistant bacteria has made it difficult to treat bacterial infections. There is an urgent need for new and powerful antibacterial agents. AgNPs have shown excellent antibacterial activity. AgNPs can target bacterial cells in multiple ways, such as by altering cell membrane permeability and protein denaturation, causing oxidative stress, deactivating enzymes, generating ROS, damaging DNA, and changing gene expression. These unique properties make it difficult for bacteria to develop resistance to AgNPs.

In this study, immobilized AgNPs were effective against both Gram-positive and Gram-negative MDR bacteria. These synergistic combinations showed exceptional activity against *B. subtilis* in T2 (50 μL AgNPs:200 μL gums) with a zone of inhibition of 23.66 mm. They also showed excellent activity against *K. pneumoniae* in T8 (200 μL:200 μL) with a zone of inhibition of 22 mm and good activity against *P. aeruginosa* in T6 (150 μL:200 μL) with a zone of inhibition of 22 mm. Against *E. coli*, T3 (75 μL:200 μL) displayed a zone of inhibition of 19.33 mm, and 19.33 mm against *S. typhi* as T1. Additionally, they showed activity against *P. mirabilis* in T4 (100 μL:200 μL) with zone of inhibition of 16.33 mm. The authors of [68] reported that the antimicrobial activity of AgNPs against *K. pneumonia* was

14.33 mm, 15.66 mm against *P. aeruginosa*, 15.33 mm against *E. coli*, and 13.33 mm against *P. mirabilis*, and further reported that the antimicrobial activity of streptomycin against *K. pneumoniae* was 16.33 mm, 16.0 mm against *P. aeruginosa*, 16.0 mm against *E. coli*, and 15.33 mm against *P. mirabilis*. They further investigated the antimicrobial activity of the combination of AgNPs and streptomycin against *K. pneumoniae* (19.66 mm), *P. aeruginosa* (20.0 mm), *E. coli* (20.3 mm), and *P. mirabilis* (17.66 mm). The authors of [69] reported that the antimicrobial activity of levofloxacin against *S. typhi* was 15.0 mm and the combination of levofloxacin and AgNPs possesses antimicrobial activity against *S. typhi* with a 20 mm zone of inhibition.

M. oleifera has been shown to have antifungal, antibacterial, and water-purification properties. The compound pterygospermin found in the roots and flowers of the plant has antifungal activity against *Neurospora crassa*, *Rhizopus stolonifera*, *Microsporum gypseum*, and *Aspergillus niger* [20]. A range of microbes, including *P. aeruginosa*, *Vibrio cholera*, and *S. typhi*, are resistant to the ethanolic extract of the leaves [18]. The seed extracts of the plants have been demonstrated to inhibit the growth of bacteria in both liquid and on solid media, suggesting that they could be used in water purification [70]. Methanol extracts of the leaves have also been shown to repress microbes such as *K. pneumoniae* and *Staphylococcus aureus* of the urinary tract infections. Alkaloids, flavonoids, and steroids found in *M. oleifera* fruits have an inhibiting impact on Candida albicans cultures either through protein denaturation or by residing in the spore's germination through their steroid ring [19].

In this study, the immobilized AgNPs mechanistically cause the cell death of resistant bacterial strains by disrupting the cell membrane, leading to the leakage of cellular contents and then cell death. The immobilized AgNPs generated reactive oxygen species (ROS), which damage cellular components, such as proteins, DNA, and lipids. In addition, immobilized AgNPs denature bacterial proteins, disrupting important cellular processes such as metabolism, DNA replication, and protein synthesis. The immobilized AgNPs kill bacterial cells through a combination of mechanisms, including membrane disruption, oxidative stress, protein denaturation, and DNA damage, as shown in Figure 16.

However, the exact mechanism through which immobilized AgNPs kill bacteria is still not fully understood. However, it is thought that immobilized AgNPs may release silver ions (Ag+); this is likely one of the ways that AgNPs kill bacteria [71]. The silver ions (Ag+) are essential for the antibacterial and toxicity activities of silver (Ag). To maintain these activities, silver must be in its ionized state (Ag+) [72]. Ag+ can bind to nucleic acids, and they prefer to bind to nucleosides (the sugar-base units) rather than the phosphate groups [73]. This is why all silver-based materials that have antibacterial activity ultimately release silver ions [74]. Some studies have shown that positively charged nanoparticles (NPs) are attracted to negatively charged bacterial cells [75]. These NPs have been proposed to be very effective at killing bacteria [76]. Ag+ ions are attracted to sulfur-containing proteins in the cytoplasm and cell wall of bacteria. This attraction causes the Ag+ ions to attach to the bacteria and make their cell walls more permeable. This allows the Ag+ ions to enter the bacteria and kill them [77]. Once Ag+ enter bacteria, they deactivate the enzymes such as respiratory enzymes. This causes the bacteria to produce reactive oxygen species (ROS), which are toxic agents that damage the bacteria's DNA and other important molecules. The Ag+ ions also prevent the bacteria from producing energy such as in interrupting adenosine triphosphate (ATP) release [78]. ROS can play a major role in damaging the cell membrane and deoxyribonucleic acid (DNA); the DNA is mainly made up of phosphorus and sulfur, and when it interacts with Ag+ ions, a number of difficulties can be caused, including the prevention of DNA replication and cell division. In addition, the Ag+ ions can also efficiently stop protein synthesis by denaturing cytoplasmic ribosomal components [79].

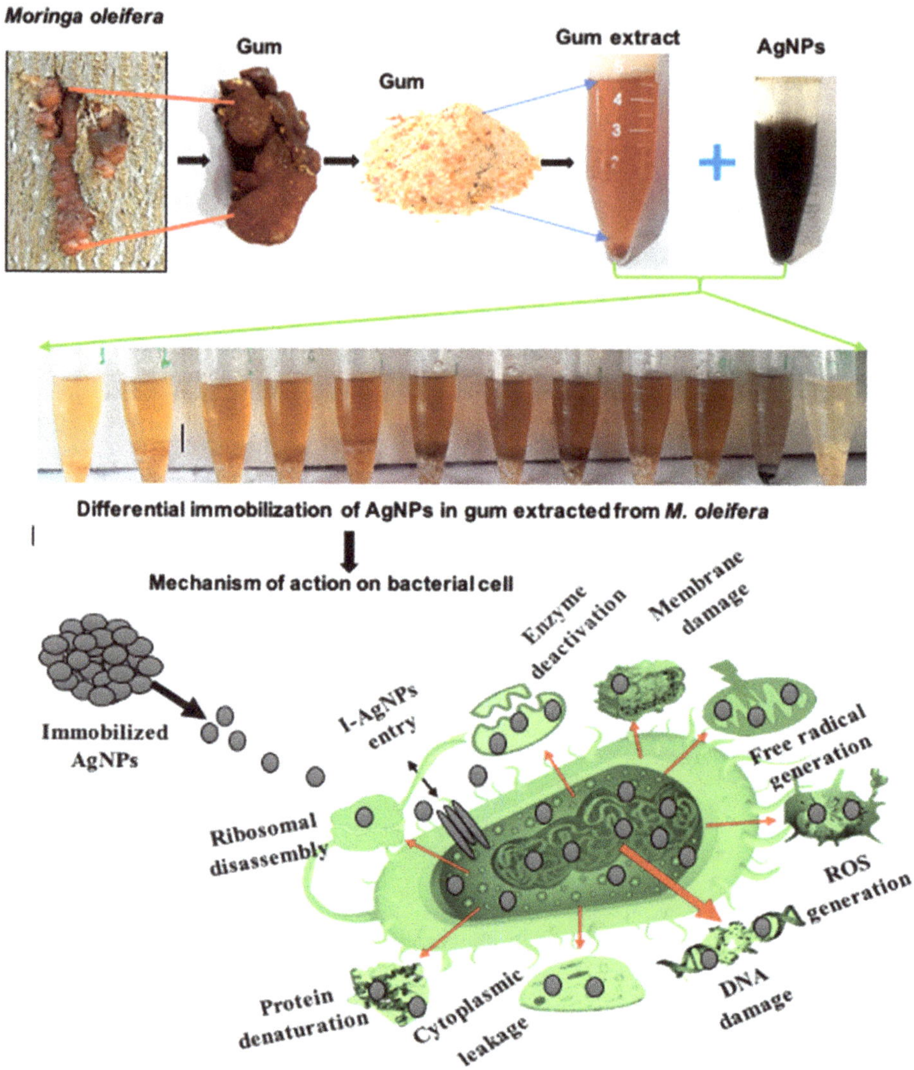

Figure 16. Mechanism of bacterial cell death through the application of immobilized AgNPs.

Furthermore, AgNPs can kill bacteria even if they are not Ag+ ions, which can damage the cell membranes of bacteria, and due to the nanoscale size, they can also enter bacteria and change the way the cell membrane works [79]. Therefore, immobilized AgNPs can kill bacteria by damaging their cell membranes and disrupting their signal transduction pathways, causing the organelles inside bacteria to rupture, which can lead to cell death. AgNPs can also dephosphorylate tyrosine residues on protein substrates, which can interfere with the bacteria's signal transduction pathways. This disruption of signal transduction can lead to cell apoptosis (programmed cell death) and the inhibition of cell division [80].

4. Materials and Methods

4.1. Collection of Plant Materials

The gum of *M. oleifera* was gathered from healthy and fresh plants from the Medicinal Botanic Garden (MBG), Medicinal Botanic Center (MBC), Pakistan Council of Scientific and Industrial Research (PCSIR), Laboratories Complex, Peshawar, Pakistan. Furthermore, all methods were carried out according to institutional and national guidelines, which comply with international standards.

4.2. Authentication of Plant Materials

Samples were collected from three-year-old *M. oleifera* trees in March 2024 (Spring season), grown in clay soil with a suitable soil pH (5.8) and temperature range, from 28 to 32 ± 2 °C (a Moring tree picture is in the Supplementary File). These plant materials (gum and *M. oleifera*) were recognized and verified by Dr. Hina Fazal (a specialist in plant taxonomy), and the herbarium specimen with Voucher No. MBC-PES-10811 was deposited in the herbarium of the Medicinal Botanic Center (MBC), Pakistan Council of Scientific and Industrial Research (PCSIR), Laboratories Complex, Peshawar, Pakistan.

4.3. Extract Preparation

For antimicrobial activity, active parts (gum) of the plants were powdered; 1.0, 2.5, and 5.0 g of powdered gum was dissolved in HPLC-grade water (Sigma; Aldrich; Darmstadt, Germany) to obtain a final volume of 10 mL. The colloidal solution was stored at 4 °C in airtight small bottles after accurate weighing before activities and its immobilization with silver nanoparticles.

4.4. Biogenic Synthesis of Silver Nanoparticles

Leaves of *M. oleifera* plant were collected from the Medicinal Botanic Garden (MBG), PCSIR Labs Complex, Peshawar, Pakistan. The leaves were oven-dried at 50 °C for 24 h and subsequently grinded with the help of a grinder. Distilled water (1000 mL) and powdered leaves (5 g) was boiled for 5 min, filtered twice, and then cooled at 4 °C for further usage. A silver nitrate ($AgNO_3$) solution of 8.0 mM was prepared upon dissolving the appropriate amount of silver nitrate in deionized water. The solution was mixed using a vortex machine, and further dilutions of 6.0 mM, 4.0 mM, and 2.00 mM were made from the stock solution, following the equation $C_1V_1 = C_2V_2$. Plant extracts were combined with silver nitrate solutions in order to produce silver nanoparticles using the protocol in [81]. In a series of reactions including equal volumes of a twofold dilution of plant extract (8.0 mg/mL to 2.0 mg/mL) and $AgNO_3$ (8.0 mg/mL to 2.0 mg/mL), various concentrations of plant extract and $AgNO_3$ were mixed to select the most efficient concentration for the synthesis of AgNPs. Here, 5 mL of reactant in 15 mL tube was kept at room temperature for 24 h, and any change in color indicated the development of AgNPs. The best biosynthesized nanoparticle was selected based on the surface plasmon resonance and peak area. The biogenic nanoparticles were collected as pellets after centrifugation at 13,000 rpm for 15 min at room temperature. The supernatant was discarded, and the pellet was dissolved in deionized water and centrifuged again using the same protocol. This process was repeated thrice. The final supernatant was discarded, and the pellets were dried and stored in a refrigerator as biogenic nanoparticles.

4.5. Characterization of Silver Nanoparticles

4.5.1. UV–Spectrophotometry

A UV–visible spectrophotometer was used to measure the formation of silver nanoparticles using light absorption between 300 and 600 nanometers [82].

4.5.2. Fourier Transform Infrared Spectroscopy (FTIR)

FTIR analysis was performed to investigate the functional groups on the nanoparticles according to the protocol in [83]. Free biomass residues and non-capping ligand impurities were eliminated. The remaining solution was centrifuged at 10,000 rpm for 10 min, and the final suspension was reconstituted in 2 mL of distilled water. This centrifugation and redispersion process were repeated three times, after which the purified suspension was freeze-dried. The resulting powder was then used for FTIR analysis.

4.5.3. X-Ray Diffraction

X-ray diffraction (XRD) analysis was employed to study the overall oxidation state and crystalline structure of silver nanoparticles [84]. Through the centrifugation and redispersion of the pellets into deionized water, prepared nanoparticles were purified and freeze-dried and analyzed through XRD.

4.5.4. TEM Analysis

Transmission Electron Microscopy (TEM) was performed to investigate the size, morphology, and distribution of the silver nanoparticles. A drop of a sample was loaded on copper grids coated with carbon and placed on the grid. Further, the film on the grid was left to dry at room temperature and analyzed through a Transmission Electron Microscope. An elemental analysis of the biosynthesized silver nanoparticles conducted calibrated using an energy-dispersive X-ray (EDX) detector [83].

4.6. Selection of Nanoparticles

The silver nanoparticles (AgNPs) were selected for the growth inhibition of resistant microorganisms including both Gram-positive and Gram-negative; however, some reports suggested that these AgNPs can also inhibit the growth of fungi and viruses by disrupting the cell membrane and generating ROS [85].

4.7. Selection of Pathogens

In this study, M. oleifera gums and AgNPs were applied against *Bacillus subtilis* (*B. subtilis*), *Escherichia coli* (*E. coli*), *Klebsiella pneumoniae* (*K. pneumoniae*), *Proteus mirabilis* (*P. mirabilis*) *Pseudomonas aeruginosa* (*P. aeruginosa*), and *Salmonella typhi* (*S. typhi*), which cause various infections in humans [86–90]. These infectious microbes (Table 2) were received from different hospitals through the Pakistan Council of Scientific and Industrial Research (PCSIR) Laboratories Complex, Peshawar, Pakistan. These microorganisms were kept at 4 °C before antimicrobial activities.

Table 2. Collected bacterial strains, voucher specimen numbers, strain types, and sources. The strains were Gram-positive (G+ve) and Gram-negative (G-ve).

Voucher Specimen Numbers	Bacterial Strain	Types	Source
MBC-MIC-208	*B. subtilis*	G + ve	PCSIR Peshawar
MBC-MIC-003	*E. coli*	G − ve	PCSIR Peshawar
MBC-MIC-459	*K. pneumoniae*	G − ve	PCSIR Peshawar
MBC-MIC-405	*P. mirabilis*	G − ve	PCSIR Peshawar
MBC-MIC-051	*P. aeruginosa*	G − ve	PCSIR Peshawar
MBC-MIC-104	*S. typhi*	G − ve	PCSIR Peshawar

4.8. Nutrient Agar Preparation

To make nutrient agar media, 900 mL of distilled water and 28 g of nutrient agar (15 g/L agar, 5 g/L gelatin component, 5 g/L NaCl, 1 g/L beef extract, and 2 g/L yeast extract) (Sigma, Aldrich, Darmstadt, Germany) were added to a 1 L screw-capped container. The solution was heated while being thoroughly agitated, the volume was increased to 1 L, and the bottle was sealed. The nutritional agar media bottle and the tools (Wire loops, Flasks, Glass tubes, Eppendorf tubes, swabs, cell spreaders, micropipette tips, and disks) that were used in the next tests were autoclaved at 121 °C for 20 min at 1.5 pounds per square inch (PSI) to sanitize them. The nutritional agar medium and sterilized equipment were added to the laminar flow unit (LFU) once it had cooled to 55 °C. Under sterile circumstances, the medium was transferred onto Petri dishes with approximately 35 milliliters of media applied to each plate. After being left for half an hour to form, the Petri dishes were covered with lids. The Petri dishes were turned upside down and incubated for 24 h at 37 °C to check for contamination. After that, these plates were put through testing for antibacterial activity [91]. Gram staining was performed for all isolated colonies according to the standard procedure in [92].

4.9. Antibiotic Susceptibility Test

The disk diffusion method and the Kirby–Bauer method of antibiotics was performed for the microbial sensitivity. Nutrient broth (1.3 g/100 mL) and nutrient agar (2.8 g/100 mL) were combined with hot distilled water to prepare the cultures for testing. The mixture was then transferred into test tubes (6–7 mL), Petri dishes (20 mL), and flasks (18–23 mL). To check for undesirable microbial development, the medium was sterilized at 121 °C for 20 min at 15 pressure and then incubated overnight at 37 °C. The microorganisms were streaked onto solid medium plates from the stock cultures, and cultured containers were placed for 24 h at 37 °C.

After being moved to liquid medium on the second day, the bacterial cultures were incubated for 10 h at 100 rpm in a GLSC-SBR-04-28 water bath at 32 °C. The optical density (OD) of the growing culture was maintained between 0.1 and 0.2, and the turbidity of the microbial growth in the test tubes was standardized by comparing it to the 0.5 McFarland standard. After that, solid media plates were covered with 0.1 mL of the standardized cultures, and they were refrigerated for 15 min to allow for absorption. Each cultivated plate's surface was meticulously coated in three copies of a standard disk containing each antibiotic. A negative control disk was utilized, which lacked antibiotics. In order to determine if the bacterium is sensitive or resistant to antibiotics, the cultured plates were incubated for 24 h at 37 °C. The antimicrobial efficiency was then assessed using the millimeter diameter of the zones of inhibition surrounding the disks [93].

4.10. Antimicrobial Assay of Immobilized AgNPs

The physical mixing method was applied for the immobilization of AgNPs in gum of *M. oleifera*. In preliminary experiments, 10% to 80% gum solution was less effective for the encapsulation of AgNPs. Here, 85% was the best candidate for the immobilization process, while more than 85% was unable to move/flow in suspension. The different concentrations of AgNPs suspension were maintained using a magnetic stirrer/ultrasonicator, and 85% gum solution (slightly heated) was added to the suspension drop-wise, followed by cooling to form round shaped bodies for easy attachment to the bacterial cell. After the successful uniform and homogenous polymerization of NPs with gum, differential AgNPs were allowed for immobilization with gum (85%).

In this study, six different bacterial strains were used for antimicrobial assay. These bacterial strains included *B. subtilis*, *E coli*, *K pneumoniae*, *P. mirabilis*, *P. aeruginosa*, and *S. typhi*. The well diffusion method was utilized for the antibacterial activity of nanoparticles and gums, and the procedure was repeated for synergistic combinations/differential ratios of nanoparticles + gums (Table 3) [94]. The zone of inhibition was measured in mm as the diameter around the well. The bacterial strains were streaked in plates, and the wells were bored in each plate.

The following treatments contained immobilized AgNPs with gum of *M. oleifera*: T1 (25 µL AgNPs + 200 µL gums), T2 (50 µL AgNPs + 200 µL gums), T3 (75 µL AgNPs + 200 µL gums), T4 (100 µL AgNPs + 200 µL gums), T5 (125 µL + 200 µL gums), T6 (150 µL AgNPs + 200 µL gums), T7 (175 µL AgNPs + 200 µL gums), T8 (200 µL AgNPs + 200 µL gums), T9 (225 µL AgNPs + 200 µL gums), T10 (250 µL AgNPs + 200 µL gums), C1 (100 µL AgNPs alone), and C2 (200 µL gums alone). These combinations were applied for the determination of antimicrobial activities. All the plates (containing bacteria and a combination of AgNPs + gum) were kept at 37 °C in an incubator for one day. After that, the zones of inhibition were recorded in millimeters (mm).

Table 3. Differential treatments/concentrations of AgNPs and gum of *M. oleifera* for immobilization.

Treatments	Applied Combinations
T1	25 µL AgNPs + 200 µL gums
T2	50 µL AgNPs + 200 µL gums
T3	75 µL AgNPs + 200 µL gums
T4	100 µL AgNPs + 200 µL gums
T5	125 µL AgNPs + 200 µL gums
T6	150 µL AgNPs + 200 µL gums
T7	175 µL AgNPs + 200 µL gums
T8	200 µL AgNPs + 200 µL gums
T9	225 µL AgNPs + 200 µL gums
T10	250 µL AgNPs + 200 µL gums
C1	100 µL AgNPs alone
C2	200 µL gums alone

4.11. Statistical Analysis

The antimicrobial activity of different treatments was measured three times. Excel was used to calculate descriptive statistics (mean values ± standard error). One-way analysis of variance (ANOVA) was conducted through Statistics software (Version 8.1; Tallahassee, FL, USA) (V. 8.1; USA) and for determining significance and least significant differences. Origin Lab software (Version 8.5; Northampton, MA, USA) was used to create graphical representations of the data.

5. Conclusions

The immobilized AgNPs displayed promising potential by inhibiting the growth of highly resistant *B. subtilis, E. coli, K. pneumoniae, P. mirabilis, P. aeruginosa,* and *S. typhi*. These results conclude that the immobilized AgNPs have proven antimicrobial activities; however, the gum of *M. oleifera* may serve as a stabilizing or immobilizing agent for silver nanoparticles, enhancing their antibacterial effects. Silver nanoparticles are known to exhibit antimicrobial properties by interfering with bacterial cell membranes and other cellular structures, leading to the inhibition of bacterial growth. The immobilization strategy enhanced the antimicrobial efficacy that may be attributed to the natural polymerization of gum and their stability and controlled release of silver ions. Further research and validation are needed to confirm the effectiveness, understand the underlying mechanisms, and assess the safety of such formulations for practical applications, especially in medical or environmental contexts. This study shows the nanoparticles' potential to be adopted by pharmaceutical industries as highly effective antibacterial alternatives to synthetic drugs.

Supplementary Materials: The following supporting information can be downloaded at https://www.mdpi.com/article/10.3390/ph17111546/s1.

Author Contributions: Conceptualization, L.A., N.A. and M.N.U.; methodology, N.A., L.A., Y.K. and H.F.; software, M.A.R.; validation, M.A.; formal analysis, K.R.; investigation, N.A., L.A., Y.K., S.K. and S.U.; resources, N.A. and H.F.; data curation, T.A. and S.A.; writing—original draft preparation, N.A. and L.A.; writing—review and editing, N.A., H.F. and L.A.; visualization, L.A., Y.K. and N.A.; supervision, N.A., M.N.U. and W.K.; project administration, N.A. and M.N.U.; funding acquisition, M.A.A.-M., S.F., M.A.E.-T. and B.H.K.; revision, A.S. All authors have read and agreed to the published version of the manuscript.

Funding: The authors extend their appreciation to the Researchers Supporting Project (number RSPD2024R966), King Saud University, Riyadh, Saudi Arabia.

Institutional Review Board Statement: All experimental protocols were approved by the Bioethical committee of the Center for Biotechnology and Microbiology, University of Swat, with approved certificate "BC-IBC- Reference N. 0023-UoS; Date: 30 December 2023". We confirm that all the protocols and methods used in this experiment were conducted according to the approved guidelines of the institution. We confirm that the gum collected from *Moringa oleifera* was in accordance with the guidelines/regulations/of PCSIR and UoS without harming the plants.

Informed Consent Statement: Not applicable.

Data Availability Statement: The presented data in the current manuscript will be provided upon request to the corresponding author.

Conflicts of Interest: The authors declare no conflicts of interest.

References

1. Fuglie, L.J. *Producing Food Without Pesticides, Local Solutions to Crop Pest Control in West Africa*; Church World Service, West Africa Office: Accra, Ghana, 1998.
2. Abd Rani, N.Z.; Husain, K.; Kumolosasi, E. *Moringa* genus: A review of phytochemistry and pharmacology. *Front. Pharmacol.* **2018**, *9*, 108. [CrossRef]
3. Edward, E. Survival, growth and biomass production of *Moringa oleifera* provenances at Gairo inland plateau and Ruvu Coastal Region in Tanzania. *Afr. J. Plant Sci.* **2014**, *8*, 54–64. [CrossRef]
4. Jikah, A.N.; Edo, G.I. *Moringa oleifera*: A valuable insight into recent advances in medicinal uses and pharmacological activities. *J. Sci. Food Agric.* **2023**, *103*, 7343–7361. [CrossRef]
5. Yerima, B.P.K.; Ayuk, G.M.; Enang, R.K.; Guehjung, N.; Tiamgne, Y.A. Germination and early seedling growth of *Moringa oleifera* Lam with different seeds soaking time and substrates at the Yongka Western Highlands Research Garden Park (YWHRGP) Nkwen-Bamenda, North-West Cameroon. *Am. J. Plant Sci.* **2016**, *7*, 2173–2185. [CrossRef]
6. Kome, G.K.; Enang, R.K.; Tabi, F.O.; Yerima, B.P.K. Influence of clay minerals on some soil fertility attributes: A review. *Open J. Soil. Sci.* **2019**, *9*, 155–188. [CrossRef]
7. Abd El-Hack, M.E.; Alagawany, M.; Elrys, A.S.; Desoky, E.S.M.; Tolba, H.M.; Elnahal, A.S.; Elnesr, S.S.; Swelum, A.A. Effect of forage *Moringa oleifera* L. (moringa) on animal health and nutrition and its beneficial applications in soil, plants and water purification. *Agriculture* **2018**, *8*, 145. [CrossRef]
8. Mahmood, K.T.; Mugal, T.; Haq, I.U. *Moringa oleifera*: A natural gift-A review. *J. Pharm. Sci. Res.* **2010**, *2*, 775.
9. Bhattacharya, A.; Ghosh, G.; Agrawal, D.; Sahu, P.K.; Kumar, S.; Mishra, S.S. GC-MS profiling of ethanolic extract of *Moringa oleifera* leaf. *Int. J. Pharm. Bio Sci.* **2014**, *5*, 263275.
10. Faizi, S.; Siddiqui, B.S.; Saleem, R.; Siddiqui, S.; Aftab, K.; Gilani, A.U.H. Isolation and structure elucidation of new nitrile and mustard oil glycosides from *Moringa oleifera* and their effect on blood pressure. *J. Nat. Prod.* **1994**, *57*, 1256–1261. [CrossRef]
11. Saini, R.K.; Shetty, N.P.; Giridhar, P. Carotenoid content in vegetative and reproductive parts of commercially grown *Moringa oleifera* Lam. cultivars from India by LC–APCI–MS. *Eur. Food Res. Technol.* **2014**, *238*, 971978. [CrossRef]
12. Patel, S.; Thakur, A.S.; Chandy, A.; Manigauha, A. *Moringa oleifera*: A review of their medicinal and economical importance to the health and nation. *Drug Invent. Today* **2010**, *2*, 339–342.
13. Guevara, A.P.; Vargas, C.; Sakurai, H.; Fujiwara, Y.; Hashimoto, K.; Maoka, T.; Kozuka, M.; Ito, Y.; Tokuda, H.; Nishino, H. An antitumor promoter from *Moringa oleifera* Lam. *Mutat. Res./Genet. Toxicol. Environ. Mutagen.* **1999**, *440*, 181–188. [CrossRef] [PubMed]
14. Mohd Fisall, U.F.; Ismail, N.Z.; Adebayo, I.A.; Arsad, H. Dichloromethane fraction of *Moringa oleifera* leaf methanolic extract selectively inhibits breast cancer cells (MCF7) by induction of apoptosis via upregulation of Bax, p53 and caspase 8 expressions. *Mol. Biol. Rep.* **2021**, *48*, 4465–4475. [CrossRef]
15. Upadhyay, P.; Yadav, M.K.; Mishra, S.; Sharma, P.; Purohit, S. *Moringa oleifera*: A review of the medical evidence for its nutritional and pharmacological properties. *Int. J. Res. Pharm. Sci.* **2015**, *5*, 12–16.
16. Balogun, T.A.; Buliaminu, K.D.; Chukwudozie, O.S.; Tiamiyu, Z.A.; Idowu, T.J. Anticancer potential of *Moringa oleifera* on BRCA-1 gene: Systems biology. *Bioinform. Biol. Insights* **2021**, *15*, 11779322211010703. [CrossRef] [PubMed]
17. Villarruel-López, A.; López-De La Mora, D.A.; Vázquez-Paulino, O.D.; Puebla-Mora, A.G.; Torres-Vitela, M.R.; Guerrero-Quiroz, L.A.; Nuño, K. Effect of *Moringa oleifera* consumption on diabetic rats. *BMC Complement. Altern. Med.* **2018**, *18*, 1–10. [CrossRef]
18. Valle Jr, D.L.; Cabrera, E.C.; Puzon, J.J.M.; Rivera, W.L. Antimicrobial activities of methanol, ethanol and supercritical CO_2 extracts of Philippine *Piper betle L.* on clinical isolates of gram positive and gram-negative bacteria with transferable multiple drug resistance. *PLoS ONE* **2016**, *11*, e0146349. [CrossRef]
19. Moodley, J.S.; Krishna, S.B.N.; Pillay, K.; Sershen, F.; Govender, P. Green synthesis of silver nanoparticles from *Moringa oleifera* leaf extracts and its antimicrobial potential. *Adv. Nat. Sci. Nanosci. Nanotechnol.* **2018**, *9*, 015011. [CrossRef]
20. Dalhoumi, W.; Guesmi, F.; Bouzidi, A.; Akermi, S.; Hfaiedh, N.; Saidi, I. Therapeutic strategies of *Moringa oleifera* Lam. (*Moringaceae*) for stomach and forestomach ulceration induced by HCl/EtOH in rat model. *Saudi J. Biol. Sci.* **2022**, *29*, 103284. [CrossRef]
21. Singh, A.; Navneet, X. Ethnomedicinal, pharmacological and antimicrobial aspects of *Moringa oleifera* Lam. A review. *J. Phytopharm.* **2018**, *7*, 45–50. [CrossRef]
22. Mishra, G.; Singh, P.; Verma, R.; Kumar, S.; Srivastav, S.; Jha, K.K.; Khosa, R.L. Traditional uses, phytochemistry and pharmacological properties of *Moringa oleifera* plant: An overview. *Der Pharm. Lett.* **2011**, *3*, 141–164.

23. Vongsak, B.; Mangmool, S.; Gritsanapan, W. Antioxidant activity and induction of mRNA expressions of antioxidant enzymes in HEK-293 cells of *Moringa oleifera* leaf extract. *Planta Medica* **2015**, *81*, 1084–1089. [CrossRef] [PubMed]
24. Okaiyeto, K.; Oguntibeju, O.O. African herbal medicines: Adverse effects and cytotoxic potentials with different therapeutic applications. *Int. J. Environ. Res. Public Health* **2021**, *18*, 5988. [CrossRef]
25. Akinyede, K.A.; Ekpo, O.E.; Oguntibeju, O.O. Ethnopharmacology, therapeutic properties and nutritional potentials of *Carpobrotus edulis*: A comprehensive review. *Sci. Pharm.* **2020**, *88*, 39. [CrossRef]
26. Adeyanju, A.A.; Oyenihi, O.R.; Oguntibeju, O.O. Antioxidant-Rich Vegetables: Impact on Human Health. In *Vegetable CropsHealth Benefits and Cultivation*; IntechOpen: London, UK, 2021.
27. Attah, A.F.; Moody, J.O.; Sonibare, M.A.; Salahdeen, H.H.; Akindele, O.O.; Nnamani, P.O.; Diyaolu, O.A.; Raji, Y. Aqueous extract of *Moringa oleifera* leaf used in Nigerian ethnomedicine alters conception and some pregnancy outcomes in Wistar rat. *S. Afr. J. Bot.* **2020**, *129*, 255–262. [CrossRef]
28. Bhattacharya, A.; Tiwari, P.; Sahu, P.K.; Kumar, S. A review of the phytochemical and pharmacological characteristics of *Moringa oleifera*. *J. Pharm. Bioallied Sci.* **2018**, *10*, 181.
29. Ijioma, S.N.; Nwaogazi, E.N.; Nwankwo, A.A.; Oshilonya, H.; Ekeleme, C.M.; Oshilonya, L.U. Histological exhibition of the gastroprotective effect of *Moringa oleifera* leaf extract. *Comp. Clin. Pathol.* **2018**, *27*, 327–332. [CrossRef]
30. Amrutia, J.N.; Lala, M.; Srinivasa, U.; Shabaraya, A.R.; Semuel, M.R. Anticonvulsant activity of *Moringa oleifera* leaf. *Int. Res. J. Pharm.* **2011**, *2*, 160–162.
31. Panda, S.; Kar, A.; Sharma, P.; Sharma, A. Cardioprotective potential of *N*, *α-l*-rhamnopyranosyl vincosamide, an indole alkaloid, isolated from the leaves of *Moringa oleifera* in isoproterenol induced cardiotoxic rats: In vivo and in vitro studies. *Bioorganic Med. Chem. Lett.* **2013**, *23*, 959–962. [CrossRef]
32. Salehi, B.; Quispe, C.; Sharifi-Rad, J.; Cruz-Martins, N.; Nigam, M.; Mishra, A.P.; Konovalov, D.A.; Orobinskaya, V.; Abu-Reidah, I.M.; Zam, W.; et al. Phytosterols: From preclinical evidence to potential clinical applications. *Front. Pharmacol.* **2021**, *11*, 1819. [CrossRef]
33. Mbikay, M. Therapeutic potential of *Moringa oleifera* leaves in chronic hyperglycemia and dyslipidemia: A review. *Front. Pharmacol.* **2012**, *3*, 24. [CrossRef] [PubMed]
34. Almatrafi, M.M.; Vergara-Jimenez, M.; Murillo, A.G.; Norris, G.H.; Blesso, C.N.; Fernandez, M.L. *Moringa* leaves prevent hepatic lipid accumulation and inflammation in *guinea* pigs by reducing the expression of genes involved in lipid metabolism. *Int. J. Mol. Sci.* **2017**, *18*, 1330. [CrossRef]
35. Muhammad, A.A.; Arulselvan, P.; Cheah, P.S.; Abas, F.; Fakurazi, S. Evaluation of wound healing properties of bioactive aqueous fraction from *Moringa oleifera* Lam on experimentally induced diabetic animal model. *Drug Des. Dev. Ther.* **2016**, *10*, 1715–1730. [CrossRef] [PubMed]
36. Awodele, O.; Oreagba, I.A.; Odoma, S.; da Silva, J.A.T.; Osunkalu, V.O. Toxicological evaluation of the aqueous leaf extract of *Moringa oleifera* Lam. (Moringaceae). *J. Ethnopharmacol.* **2012**, *139*, 330–336. [CrossRef]
37. Anwar, F.; Latif, S.; Ashraf, M.; Gilani, A.H. *Moringa oleifera*: A food plant with multiple medicinal uses. *Phytother. Res. An Int. J. Devoted Pharmacol. Toxicol. Eval. Nat. Product Deriv.* **2007**, *21*, 17–25. [CrossRef] [PubMed]
38. Sultana, B.; Anwar, E. Flavonols (kaempeferol, quercetin, myricetin) contents of selected fruits, vegetables and medicinal plants. *Food Chem.* **2008**, *108*, 879–884. [CrossRef] [PubMed]
39. Islam, Z.; Islam, S.R.; Hossen, F.; Mahtab-ul-Islam, K.; Hasan, M.R.; Karim, R. *Moringa oleifera* is a prominent source of nutrients with potential health benefits. *Int. J. Food Sci.* **2021**, *2021*, 6627265. [CrossRef] [PubMed]
40. Avachat, A.M.; Dash, R.R.; Shrotriya, S.N. Recent investigations of plant based natural gums, mucilages and resins in novel drug delivery systems. *Ind. J. Pharm. Edu. Res.* **2011**, *45*, 86–99.
41. Amiri, M.S.; Mohammadzadeh, V.; Yazdi, M.E.T.; Barani, M.; Rahdar, A.; Kyzas, G.Z. Plant-based gums and mucilages applications in pharmacology and nanomedicine: A review. *Molecules* **2021**, *26*, 1770. [CrossRef]
42. Amiri, M.S.; Yazdi, M.E.T.; Rahnama, M. Medicinal plants and phytotherapy in Iran: Glorious history, current status and future prospects. *Plant Sci. Today* **2021**, *8*, 95–111. [CrossRef]
43. Nair, L.S.; Laurencin, C.T. Biodegradable polymers as biomaterials. *Progr. Polym. Sci.* **2007**, *32*, 762–798. [CrossRef]
44. Zare, E.N.; Makvandi, P.; Borzacchiello, A.; Tay, F.R.; Ashtari, B.; Padil, V.V. Antimicrobial gum bio-based nanocomposites and their industrial and biomedical applications. *Chem. Commun.* **2019**, *55*, 14871–14885. [CrossRef]
45. Mohammadzadeh, V.; Barani, M.; Amiri, M.S.; Yazdi, M.E.T.; Hassanisaadi, M.; Rahdar, A.; Varma, R.S. Applications of plant-based nanoparticles in nanomedicine: A review. *Sustain. Chem. Pharm.* **2022**, *25*, 100606. [CrossRef]
46. Shukla, A.; Desai, K.; Modi, N. In vitro antioxidant and antimicrobial potential of Sterculia urens Roxb. root extract and its bioactive phytoconstituents evaluation. *Future J. Pharm. Sci.* **2020**, *6*, 1–11. [CrossRef]
47. Yuan, L.; Wu, Y.; Qin, Y.; Yong, H.; Liu, J. Recent advances in the preparation, characterization and applications of locust bean gum-based films. *J. Renew. Mater.* **2020**, *8*, 1565–1579. [CrossRef]
48. Rastogi, P.K.; Ganesan, V.; Krishnamoorthi, S. Microwave assisted polymer stabilized synthesis of silver nanoparticles and its application in the degradation of environmental pollutants. *Mater. Sci. Eng. B* **2012**, *177*, 456–461. [CrossRef]
49. Costa, C.O.N.T.E.; Conte, A.; Buonocore, G.G.; Del Nobile, M.A. Antimicrobial silver-montmorillonite nanoparticles to prolong the shelf life of fresh fruit salad. *Int. J. Food Microbiol.* **2011**, *148*, 164–167. [CrossRef] [PubMed]

50. De Moura, M.R.; Mattoso, L.H.; Zucolotto, V. Development of cellulose-based bactericidal nanocomposites containing silver nanoparticles and their use as active food packaging. *J. Food Eng.* **2012**, *109*, 520–524. [CrossRef]
51. Haroon, M.; Zaidi, A.; Ahmed, B.; Rizvi, A.; Khan, M.S.; Musarrat, J. Effective inhibition of phytopathogenic microbes by eco-friendly leaf extract mediated silver nanoparticles (AgNPs). *Indian J. Microbiol.* **2019**, *59*, 273–287. [CrossRef]
52. Jo, Y.K.; Seo, J.H.; Choi, B.H.; Kim, B.J.; Shin, H.H.; Hwang, B.H.; Cha, H.J. Surface-independent antibacterial coating using silver nanoparticle-generating engineered mussel glue. *ACS Appl. Mater. Interfaces* **2014**, *6*, 20242–20253. [CrossRef]
53. Zhao, L.; Chu, P.K.; Zhang, Y.; Wu, Z. Antibacterial coatings on titanium implants. *J. Biomed. Mater. Res. Part B Appl. Biomater.* **2009**, *91*, 470–480. [CrossRef] [PubMed]
54. Rai, M.; Yadav, A.; Gade, A. Silver nanoparticles as a new generation of antimicrobials. *Biotechnol. Adv.* **2009**, *27*, 76–83. [CrossRef] [PubMed]
55. Arakawa, Y.; Wiesner, M.; Wennemers, H. Efficient recovery and reuse of an immobilized peptidic organocatalyst. *Adv. Synth. Catal.* **2011**, *353*, 1201–1206. [CrossRef]
56. Mateo, C.; Palomo, J.M.; Fernandez-Lorente, G.; Guisan, J.M.; Fernandez-Lafuente, R. Improvement of enzyme activity, stability and selectivity via immobilization techniques. *Enzym. Microb. Technol.* **2007**, *40*, 1451–1463. [CrossRef]
57. Tischer, W.; Wedekind, F. Immobilized enzymes: Methods and applications. In *Biocatalysis-from Discovery to Application*; Springer: Berlin/Heidelberg, Germany, 1999; pp. 95–126.
58. Miletić, N.; Nastasović, A.; Loos, K. Immobilization of biocatalysts for enzymatic polymerizations: Possibilities, advantages, applications. *Bioresour. Technol.* **2012**, *115*, 126–135. [CrossRef]
59. Yang, Z.; Castrignanò, E.; Estrela, P.; Frost, C.G.; Kasprzyk-Hordern, B. Community sewage sensors towards evaluation of drug use trends: Detection of cocaine in wastewater with DNA-directed immobilization aptamer sensors. *Sci. Rep.* **2016**, *6*, 21024. [CrossRef] [PubMed]
60. Balamurugan, S.; Obubuafo, A.; Soper, S.A.; Spivak, D.A. Surface immobilization methods for aptamer diagnostic applications. *Anal. Bioanal. Chem.* **2008**, *390*, 1009–1021. [CrossRef]
61. Wu, C.; Zhi, D.; Yao, B.; Zhou, Y.; Yang, Y.; Zhou, Y. Immobilization of microbes on biochar for water and soil remediation: A review. *Environ. Res.* **2022**, *212*, 113226. [CrossRef]
62. Huang, L.; Zhao, S.; Wang, Z.; Wu, J.; Wang, J.; Wang, S. In situ immobilization of silver nanoparticles for improving permeability, antifouling and anti-bacterial properties of ultrafiltration membrane. *J. Membr. Sci.* **2016**, *499*, 269–281. [CrossRef]
63. GhavamiNejad, A.; Aguilar, L.E.; Ambade, R.B.; Lee, S.H.; Park, C.H.; Kim, C.S. Immobilization of silver nanoparticles on electropolymerized polydopamine films for metal implant applications. *Colloids Interface Sci. Commun.* **2015**, *6*, 5–8. [CrossRef]
64. Mallikharjuna, P.B.; Rajanna, L.N.; Seetharam, Y.N.; Sharanabasappa, G.K. Phytochemical studies of *Strychnos potatorum* Lf-A medicinal plant. *J. Chem.* **2007**, *4*, 510–518. [CrossRef]
65. Carnachan, S.M.; Bell, T.J.; Hinkley, S.F.; Sims, I.M. Polysaccharides from New Zealand native plants: A review of their structure, properties, and potential applications. *Plants* **2019**, *8*, 163. [CrossRef]
66. Medina, E.; Pieper, D.H. Tackling threats and future problems of multidrug-resistant bacteria. In *How to Overcome the Antibiotic Crisis: Facts, Challenges, Technologies and Future Perspectives*; Springer: Cham, Switzerland, 2016; pp. 3–33.
67. Baptista, P.V.; McCusker, M.P.; Carvalho, A.; Ferreira, D.A.; Mohan, N.M.; Martins, M.; Fernandes, A.R. Nano-strategies to fight multidrug resistant bacteria—"*A Battle of the Titans*". *Front. Microbiol.* **2018**, *9*, 1441. [CrossRef] [PubMed]
68. Maniraj, A.; Kannan, M.; Rajarathinam, K.; Vivekanandhan, S.; Muthuramkumar, S. Green synthesis of silver nanoparticles and their effective utilization in fabricating functional surface for antibacterial activity against multi-drug resistant Proteus mirabilis. *J. Clust. Sci.* **2019**, *30*, 1403–1414. [CrossRef]
69. Thomas, R.; Nair, A.P.; Kr, S.; Mathew, J.; Ek, R. Antibacterial activity and synergistic effect of biosynthesized AgNPs with antibiotics against multidrugresistant biofilm-forming coagulase-negative *staphylococci* isolated from clinical samples. *Appl. Biochem. Biotechnol.* **2014**, *173*, 449–460. [CrossRef]
70. Chandrashekar, S.; Vijayakumar, R.; Chelliah, R.; Oh, D.H. Identification and purification of potential bioactive peptide of *Moringa oleifera* seed extracts. *Plants* **2020**, *9*, 1445. [CrossRef] [PubMed]
71. Bapat, R.A.; Chaubal, T.V.; Joshi, C.P.; Bapat, P.R.; Choudhury, H.; Pandey, M.; Gorain, B.; Kesharwani, P. An overview of application of silver nanoparticles for biomaterials in dentistry. *Mater. Sci. Eng. C* **2018**, *91*, 881–898. [CrossRef]
72. Klueh, U.; Wagner, V.; Kelly, S.; Johnson, A.; Bryers, J.D. Efficacy of silver coated fabric to prevent bacterial colonization and subsequent device based biofilm formation. *J. Biomed. Mater. Res. Off. J. Soc. Biomater. Jpn. Soc. Biomater. Aust. Soc. Biomater. Korean Soc. Biomater.* **2000**, *53*, 621–631. [CrossRef]
73. Yakabe, Y.; Sano, T.; Ushio, H.; Yasunaga, T. Kinetic studies of the interaction between silver ion and deoxyribonucleic acid. *Chem. Lett.* **1980**, *9*, 373–376. [CrossRef]
74. Chouhan, S.; Guleria, S. Green synthesis of AgNPs using *Cannabis sativa* leaf extract: Characterization, antibacterial, antiyeast and α-amylase inhibitory activity. *Mater. Sci. Energy Technol.* **2020**, *3*, 536–544. [CrossRef]
75. Cao, R.J.; Mirkin, C.A. DNA-modified core− shell Ag/Au nanoparticles. *J. Am. Chem. Soc.* **2001**, *123*, 7961–7962. [CrossRef] [PubMed]
76. Wright, J.B.; Lam, K.; Hansen, D.; Burrell, R.E. Efficacy of topical silver against fungal burn wound pathogens. *Am. J. Infect. Control* **1999**, *27*, 344–350. [CrossRef] [PubMed]

77. Khorrami, S.; Zarrabi, A.; Khaleghi, M.; Danaei, M.; Mozafari, M.R. Selective cytotoxicity of green synthesized silver nanoparticles against the MCF-7 tumor cell line and their enhanced antioxidant and antimicrobial properties. *Int. J. Nanomed.* **2018**, *13*, 8013–8024. [CrossRef]
78. Das, S.S.; Alkahtani, S.; Bharadwaj, P.; Ansari, M.T.; ALKahtani, M.D.; Pang, Z.; Hasnain, M.S.; Nayak, A.K.; Aminabhavi, T.M. Molecular insights and novel approaches for targeting tumor metastasis. *Int. J. Pharm.* **2020**, *585*, 119556. [CrossRef] [PubMed]
79. Pareek, V.; Gupta, R.; Panwar, J. Do physico-chemical properties of silver nanoparticles decide their interaction with biological media and bactericidal action? A review. *Mater. Sci. Eng. C* **2018**, *90*, 739–749. [CrossRef]
80. Ahmad, S.A.; Das, S.S.; Khatoon, A.; Ansari, M.T.; Afzal, M.; Hasnain, M.S.; Nayak, A.K. Bactericidal activity of silver nanoparticles: A mechanistic review. *Mater. Sci. Energy Technol.* **2020**, *3*, 756–769. [CrossRef]
81. Khan, A.; Ahmad, N.; Fazal, H.; Ali, M.; Akbar, F.; Khan, I.; Tayyab, M.; Uddin, M.N.; Ahmad, N.; Abdel-Maksoud, M.A.; et al. Biogenic synthesis of silver nanoparticles using Rubus fruticosus extract and their antibacterial efficacy against Erwinia caratovora and Ralstonia solanacearum phytopathogens. *RSC Adv.* **2024**, *14*, 5754–5763. [CrossRef]
82. Ali, M.; Kim, B.; Belfield, K.D.; Norman, D.; Brennan, M.; Ali, G.S. Green synthesis and characterization of silver nanoparticles using *Artemisia absinthium* aqueous extract—A comprehensive study. *Mater. Sci. Eng. C* **2016**, *58*, 359–365. [CrossRef]
83. Li, X.; Wang, Y.; Huang, D.; Jiang, Z.; He, Z.; Luo, M.; Lei, J.; Xiao, Y. Nanomaterials Modulating the Fate of Dental-Derived Mesenchymal Stem Cells Involved in Oral Tissue Reconstruction: A Systematic Review. *Int. J. Nanomed.* **2023**, *18*, 5377–5406. [CrossRef]
84. Singh, A.; Agrawal, M.; Marshall, F.M. The role of organic vs. inorganic fertilizers in reducing phytoavailability of heavy metals in a wastewater-irrigated area. *Ecol. Eng.* **2010**, *36*, 1733–1740. [CrossRef]
85. Kato, A.; Yoshifuji, A.; Komori, K.; Aoki, K.; Taniyama, D.; Komatsu, M.; Fujii, K.; Yamada, K.; Ishii, Y.; Kikuchi, T.; et al. A case of *Bacillus subtilis* var. natto *bacteremia* caused by ingestion of natto during COVID-19 treatment in a maintenance hemodialysis patient with multiple myeloma. *J. Infect. Chemother.* **2022**, *28*, 1212–1215. [CrossRef] [PubMed]
86. Cabrera-Sosa, L.; Ochoa, T.J. Escherichia coli diarrhea. In *Hunter's Tropical Medicine and Emerging Infectious Diseases*; Elsevier: Amsterdam, The Netherlands, 2020; pp. 481–485. [CrossRef]
87. Gupta, A. Hospital-acquired infections in the neonatal intensive care unit-*Klebsiella pneumoniae*. In *Seminars in Perinatology*; Elsevier: Amsterdam, The Netherlands, 2002. [CrossRef]
88. Jacobsen, S.M.; Stickler, D.J.; Mobley, H.L.; Shirtliff, M.E. Complicated catheter-associated urinary tract infections due to *Escherichia coli* and *Proteus mirabilis*. *Clin. Microbiol. Rev.* **2008**, *21*, 26–59. [CrossRef] [PubMed]
89. Arancibia, F.; Bauer, T.T.; Ewig, S.; Mensa, J.; Gonzalez, J.; Niederman, M.S.; Torres, A. Community-acquired pneumonia due to gram-negative bacteria and *Pseudomonas aeruginosa*: Incidence, risk, and prognosis. *Arch. Intern. Med.* **2002**, *162*, 1849–1858. [CrossRef]
90. Raffatellu, M.; Wilson, R.P.; Winter, S.E.; Baumler, A.J. Clinical pathogenesis of typhoid fever. *J. Infect. Dev. Ctries* **2008**, *2*, 260–266. [CrossRef] [PubMed]
91. Fazal, H.I.N.A.; Ahmad, N.; Ullah, I.; Inayat, H.; Khan, L.; Abbasi, B.H. Antibacterial potential in *Parthenium hysterophorus*, *Stevia rebaudiana* and *Ginkgo biloba*. *Pak. J. Bot.* **2011**, *43*, 1307–1313.
92. Merchant, I.A. *Veterinary Bacteriology and Virology*, 4th ed.; Iowa State College Press, the University of California: Ames, IA, USA, 1950.
93. Ahmad, N.; Ali, S.; Abbas, M.; Fazal, H.; Saqib, S.; Ali, A.; Ullah, Z.; Zaman, S.; Sawati, L.; Zada, A. Sohail, Antimicrobial efficacy of *Mentha piperata*-derived biogenic zinc oxide nanoparticles against UTI-resistant pathogens. *Sci. Rep.* **2023**, *13*, 14972. [CrossRef]
94. Ahmad, N.; Muhammad, J.; Khan, K.; Ali, W.; Fazal, H.; Ali, M.; Rahman, L.U.; Khan, H.; Uddin, M.N.; Abbasi, B.H.; et al. Silver and gold nanoparticles induced differential antimicrobial potential in calli cultures of Prunella vulgaris. *BMC Chem.* **2022**, *16*, 20. [CrossRef]

pharmaceuticals

MDPI

Article

Therapeutic Potential of Novel Silver Carbonate Nanostructures in Wound Healing and Antibacterial Activity Against *Pseudomonas chengduensis* and *Staphylococcus aureus*

Tehmina Khan [1], Ali Umar [1], Zakia Subhan [2,3], Muhammad Saleem Khan [1,*], Hafeeza Zafar Ali [3], Hayat Ullah [4,*], Sabeen Sabri [5], Muhammad Wajid [1], Rashid Iqbal [6,7], Mashooq Ahmad Bhat [8] and Hamid Ali [9]

1 Department of Zoology, Faculty of Life Sciences, University of Okara, Okara 56130, Pakistan; aumar2102@gmail.com (A.U.)
2 Department of Pharmacology, Institute of Medical Science (KMU-IMS), Khyber Medical University, Kohat 26000, Pakistan
3 Institute of Pharmaceutical Sciences, Khyber Medical University, Peshawar 25000, Pakistan
4 Department of Chemistry, University of Okara, Okara 56130, Pakistan
5 Department of Microbiology and Molecular Genetics, Faculty of Life Sciences, University of Okara, Okara 56130, Pakistan
6 Department of Agronomy, Faculty of Agriculture and Environment, The Islamia University of Bahawalpur, Bahawalpur 63100, Pakistan; rashid.iqbal@iub.edu.pk
7 Department of Life Sciences, Western Caspian University, Baku AZ1001, Azerbaijan
8 Department of Pharmaceutical Chemistry, College of Pharmacy, King Saud University, Riyadh 11451, Saudi Arabia; mabhat@ksu.edu.sa
9 School of Material Science and Engineering, Tiangong University, Tianjin 300387, China
* Correspondence: samiikhan@uo.edu.pk (M.S.K.); ayaanwazir366@gmail.com (H.U.)

Abstract: Background/Objectives: Metallic NPs have been explored for various therapeutic uses owing to utilitarian physicochemical characteristics such as antibacterial, anti-inflammatory, and healing properties. The objective of this study is to evaluate the therapeutic potential of novel silver carbonate nanostructures in promoting wound healing and their antibacterial activity against *Pseudomonas chengduensis* and *Staphylococcus aureus*. **Methods**: In this work, we prepared Ag_2CO_3 nanoparticles through a two-step methodology that was expected to improve the material's biomedical performance and biocompatibility. The characterization and assessment of synthesized NPs biocompatibility were conducted using hemolysis assays on the blood of a healthy male human. Further, we performed molecular docking analysis to confirm interactions of silver NPs with biological molecules. **Results**: In detail, the synthesized NPs showed <5% hemolysis activity at various concentrations, confirming their therapeutic applicability. Additionally, the NPs had good metabolic activities; they raised the T3/T4 hormone content and acted effectively on Insulin-like Growth Factor 1 (IGF-1) in diabetic models. They also facilitated the rate of repair by having the diabetic wounds reach 100% re-epithelialization by day 13, unlike the control group, which reached the same level only by day 16. The synthesized Ag_2CO_3 NPs exhibited high antimicrobial potential against both *Pseudomonas chengduensis* and *Staphylococcus aureus*, hence being a potential material that can be used for infection control in biomedical tissue engineering applications. **Conclusions**: These findings concluded that novel synthesis methods lead to the formation of NPs with higher therapeutic prospects; however, studies of their metaphysical and endocrinological effects are necessary.

Keywords: Ag_2CO_3 nanoparticles; biocompatibility; metabolic effects; insulin; molecular docking

1. Introduction

Among all metallic nanostructures, silver has been widely investigated in recent years primarily because of its attractive physicochemical characteristics, which have been identified as ideal for various applications, particularly in the purification of water and air, as well as in the biomedical field. These nanostructures have a high surface area and, therefore, increased reactivity, which enhances their catalytic and antimicrobial properties. Among the synthesis approaches, chemical reduction methods can be considered effective for forming silver nanostructures with pre-set nano shapes and sizes [1]. This method offers good control over the synthesis, thereby producing nanostructures that demonstrate high performance in various applications [2].

Silver nanostructures also have tremendous applications in the biomedical sector, including wound healing, metabolic regulation, and antimicrobial activity. The antibacterial characteristics of AgNPs are well known, as they are effective against Gram-positive and Gram-negative bacterial and fungal pathogens, as well as viruses. This makes silver nanostructures irreplaceable in preventing infections and treating injuries [3]. These nanostructures have enlarged surfaces, allowing for a more effective interface with microbial cells, thus enhancing their antimicrobial properties [4]. Furthermore, they are biocompatible, stimulate cell growth, and facilitate tissue formation, which shortens healing time [5].

The wound healing potential of silver nanostructures is thought to stem from their ability to decrease inflammation and increase collagen synthesis. This is due to the release of silver ions, which are believed to have antibacterial and anti-inflammatory effects, especially when used in hydrogels or other wound dressings [6]. This slow release is particularly desirable when treating chronic wounds, and materials containing silver nanoparticles have been designed to release medication gradually over a long period. Research has shown that incorporating silver nanoparticles into wound dressings improves their effectiveness, especially in treating diabetic ulcers and burns [7].

Another potential application of silver nanostructures in biomedicine is metabolic activity regulation. These nanostructures can positively affect cellular metabolism, which is beneficial for therapeutic applications. For instance, silver nanoparticles have been shown to alter oxidative stress and inflammatory activity levels in cells, making them useful for treating wound infections and other related biomedical issues [8]. Modulating cellular metabolic processes through silver nanostructures creates the foundation for personalized treatments and better patient outcomes [9]. Moreover, chemical reduction methods for preparing silver nanostructures improve their environmental and biomedical prospects while also supporting sustainable development goals [10]. These methods utilize appropriate chemicals to reduce Ag ions to Ag NPs, producing higher-quality nanostructures with uniform characteristics [11]. Due to their improved activity and biocompatibility, chemically synthesized silver nanostructures have potential applications across many sectors [12].

Despite the many opportunities, there are some challenges concerning the application of silver nanostructures in environmental and biomedical fields. For example, there is a possibility of bioaccumulation and toxicity to nontarget organisms, along with concerns about nanoparticle durability in different environments and the need for long-term studies [13]. Addressing these issues will require collaboration across materials science, toxicology, and environmental science, as well as advancements in the synthesis of safe and promising silver nanostructures [14].

The increasing need for solutions to environmental pollution and the ongoing search for better biomedical treatments underscores the importance of this work. The objective of the current research is to prepare silver nanostructures using a chemical reduction process and assess their catalytic efficiencies in degrading methylene orange dye and agricultural pesticides, as well as their wound healing, metabolic, and antimicrobial properties. This research is relevant because it could lead to the development of environmentally friendly methods for pollution treatment and effective therapeutic approaches for wound and infection treatment. Enhancing the knowledge of chemically synthesized silver nanostructures through this study promotes technological growth, which will benefit society as a whole.

2. Results

2.1. Synthesis and Characterization

The Ag_2CO_3 nanoparticles were synthesized via a chemical reduction method. The characterization of these NPs was performed through SEM, FTIR, and XRD analysis. SEM analysis showed that Ag_2CO_3 nanoparticles have an irregular and aggregated shape with a rough and jack-surfaced morphology. These particles seem to be irregular in size and can be seen coalescing to form clusters with an impression of agglomeration. Yet, the most apparent change is related to surface texture; it is rather rough, which may affect the reactivity of the material or its uses. For such morphology, we can encounter a nonuniform synthesis process, which is characteristic of many nanoparticle fabrication techniques (Figure 1). The size of synthesized NPs was 10.29 nm (Figure 2).

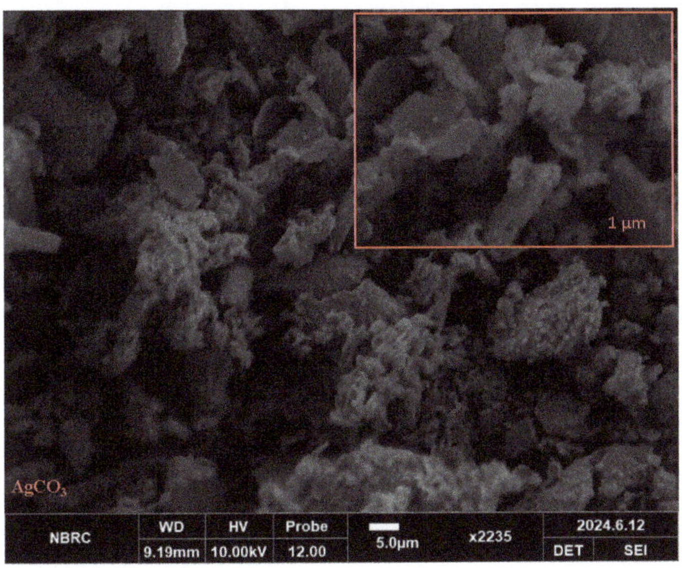

Figure 1. SEM analysis of Ag_2CO_3 nanoparticles.

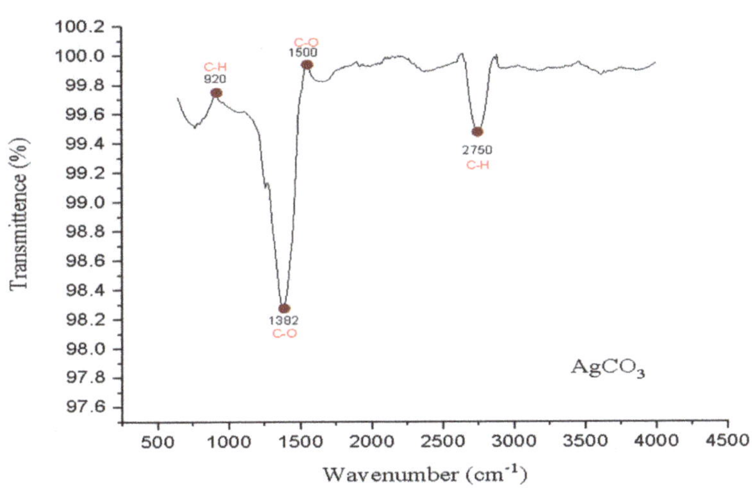

Figure 2. FTIR analysis of Ag_2CO_3 nanoparticles.

In the present study, the FTIR spectrum of Ag_2CO_3 nanoparticles has been observed to have peaks that characterize certain functional groups. The intense characteristic peaks at 1382 cm^{-1} and 1500 cm^{-1} may be assigned to C-O for the carbonate group. The peak at 920 cm^{-1} is assigned to C-H bending, while the peak at 2750 cm^{-1} corresponds to the stretching of C-H, indicating the presence of some forms of organic residues or surface changes. These peaks further illustrate the existence of carbonate groups and other functional groups in the Ag_2CO_3 nanoparticles and prove the chemical composition and structure of the nanoparticles. Functional groups are indicated in red on the specified peaks identifying the functional group associated with each peak. (Figure 2).

The X-ray diffraction pattern of Ag_2CO_3 nanoparticles shows a number of intense and sharp peaks, which confirm the crystalline behavior of the compound. The diffraction peaks at some 2θ values, evident as high-intensity peaks, belong to the characteristic crystal planes of Ag_2CO_3. These peaks are more intense and sharper, which indicates high crystallinity; they provide the essence of the material depending on its properties and uses (Figure 3).

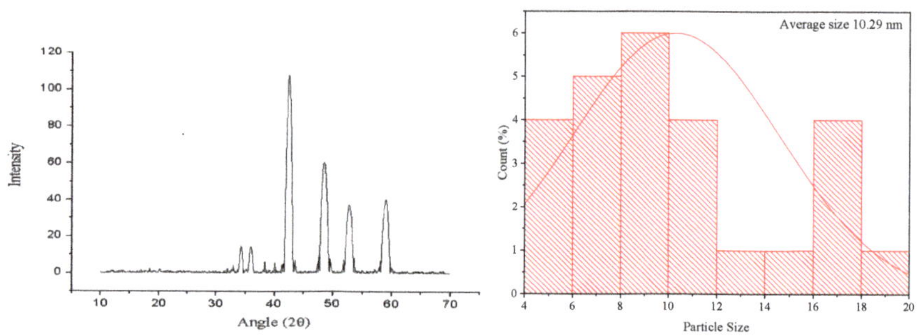

Figure 3. XRD analysis (**left** side) and histogram for NPs size (**right** side) of Ag_2CO_3 nanoparticles.

2.2. Biocompatibility

Biocompatibility assessment in terms of hemolytic analysis showed dose-dependent hemolysis of RBCs treated with Ag_2CO_3 nanoparticles. At a concentration of 75 µg/mL, the level of hemolysis was observed at 3.37%. In this case, rates of hemolysis lower than 5% are generally believed to point to good biocompatibility [15]. Therefore, it is possible to conclude that the Ag_2CO_3 NPs could be considered biocompatible by means of red blood cells' integrity at different concentrations. This low level of hemolysis favors the possibility of using these nanoparticles in biomedical applications and suggests that they might not pose a high degree of hemolytic toxicity in biological systems. This finding is relevant for the safe incorporation of Ag_2CO_3 NPs in therapeutic or diagnostic applications (Table 1).

Table 1. Hemolytic activity of different concentrations of Ag_2CO_3 NPs.

Sr No	Concentration (µg/mL)	Hemolysis %	F Value	*p* Value
1	25	2.55 ± 0.041	408.8	<0.0001 ***
2	50	2.98 ± 0.033		
3	75	3.37 ± 0.035		

*** = Highly significant.

2.3. Metabolic Effects

Results of metabolic investigations showed that Ag_2CO_3 nanoparticles can alter the metabolic pattern of diabetic albino mice in a dose-dependent manner. The high dose of NPs (50 mg/kg) significantly increased the levels of T3, T4, TSH, and insulin, which may suggest a Ag_2CO_3-induced stimulatory effect on thyroid hormone production that was not observed at the low dose. Thus, this study brings to light the multifaceted relationship between Ag_2CO_3 NPs and endocrinal functions, which suggests the need to understand the nature of any therapeutic or deleterious impact of these NPs in diabetes (Figure 4).

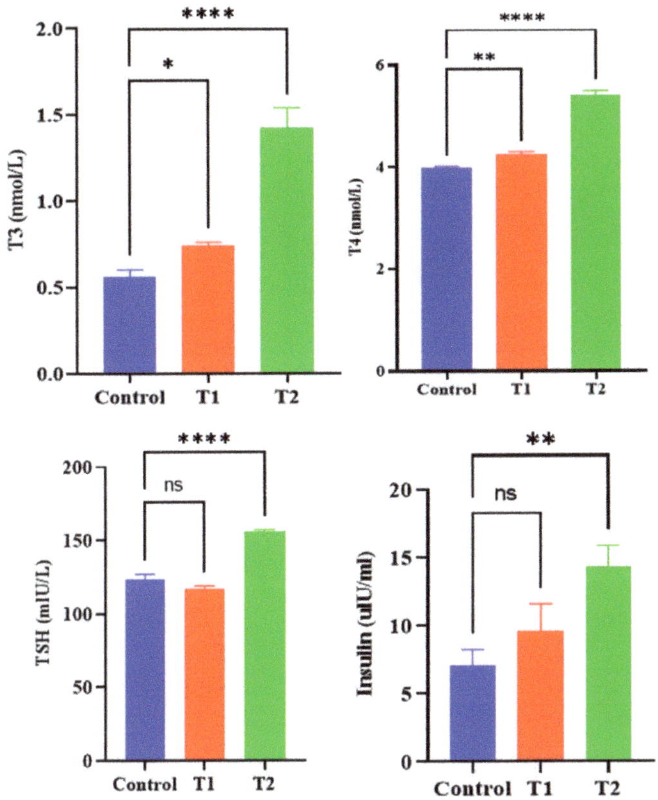

Figure 4. Effect of Ag_2CO_3 nanoparticles on metabolic profile of diabetic albino mice. *: $p < 0.05$—indicates a significant difference. **: $p < 0.01$—indicates a very significant difference. ****: $p < 0.0001$—indicates an extremely significant difference. ns: $p > 0.05$—indicates non-significant difference.

2.4. Wound Healing

The data indicate that wounds treated with Ag_2CO_3 nanoparticles exhibit a significantly faster healing rate compared to the control group. Starting from day 2, the treated wounds show a more rapid reduction in wound size, with the healing process accelerating notably from day 5 onwards. By day 12, the treated wounds are nearly healed and, by day 13, complete healing is achieved. In contrast, the control group continues to show gradual wound closure, with complete healing not occurring until day 16. These results suggest that Ag_2CO_3 nanoparticles effectively enhance the wound healing process in diabetic conditions, potentially due to their antimicrobial properties and ability to promote tissue regeneration. This accelerated healing in the treated group highlights the potential therapeutic benefits of Ag_2CO_3 NPs in managing diabetic wounds, which are typically challenging to treat due to impaired healing mechanisms in diabetic patients (Figures 5 and 6).

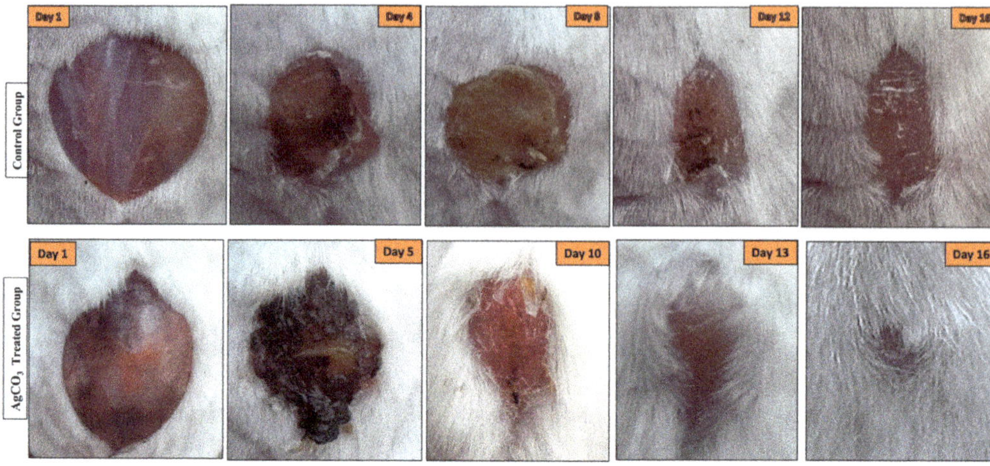

Figure 5. Comparison of wound healing progress between control and Ag_2CO_3-nanoparticle-treated diabetic wounds.

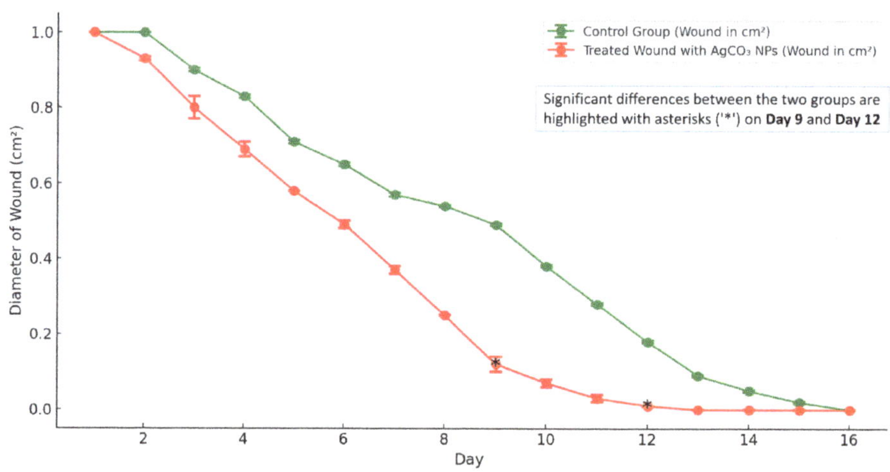

Day	Control Mean	Control STD	Treated Mean	Treated STD	Day	Control Mean	Control STD	Treated Mean	Treated STD
1	1.000	0.000	1.000	0.000	9	0.492	0.002	0.130	0.014
2	1.000	0.000	0.935	0.007	10	0.382	0.002	0.065	0.007
3	0.903	0.004	0.815	0.021	11	0.282	0.002	0.025	0.007
4	0.833	0.004	0.700	0.014	12	0.182	0.002	0.010	0.000
5	0.712	0.004	0.580	0.000	13	0.092	0.002		
6	0.653	0.004	0.500	0.014	14	0.052	0.002	Healed	Healed
7	0.573	0.004	0.375	0.007	15	0.022	0.002		
8	0.542	0.002	0.250	0.000	16	Healed	Healed		

Figure 6. Graphical representation of wound healing progress between control and Ag_2CO_3-nanoparticle-treated diabetic wounds.

2.5. Antimicrobial Activity

According to the data, 1 mg/mL Ag_2CO_3 solution has a bacteriostatic effect on both *P. chengduensis* and *S. aureus*, with the zone of inhibition growing with the increase in volume of the tested solution. *Pseudomonas chengduensis* is more sensitive to Ag_2CO_3 at lower concentrations (25 µL and 50 µL), as there were larger zones of inhibition at lower concentrations. Nevertheless, the inhibition seen at 75 µL and 100 µL is comparable and, in this case, it can be postulated that increasing the volume leads to increased inhibition of both bacteria by Ag_2CO_3 because of the accelerated antimicrobial effect of the compound. These results indicate that Ag_2CO_3 has pronounced broad-spectrum antimicrobial activity, with a slight tendency towards higher effectiveness than *Pseudomonas chengduensis* at high concentrations (Table 2; Figure 7).

Table 2. Antimicrobial activity (zone of inhibition) of Ag NPs.

Concentration of Ag_2CO_3 (1 mg/mL)	Zone of Inhibition (mm)		T Value	*p* Value
	Pseudomonas chengduensis	*Staphylococcus aureus*		
25 µL	6.52 ± 0.49	4.375 ± 0.38	18.65	0.0341 *
50 µL	7.255 ± 0.19	5.865 ± 0.27	3.022	0.2035
75 µL	7.86 ± 0.26	7.76 ± 0.26	21.0	0.0303 *
100 µL	8.405 ± 0.29	8.175 ± 0.275	23.0	0.0277 *

*: $p < 0.05$—indicates a significant difference.

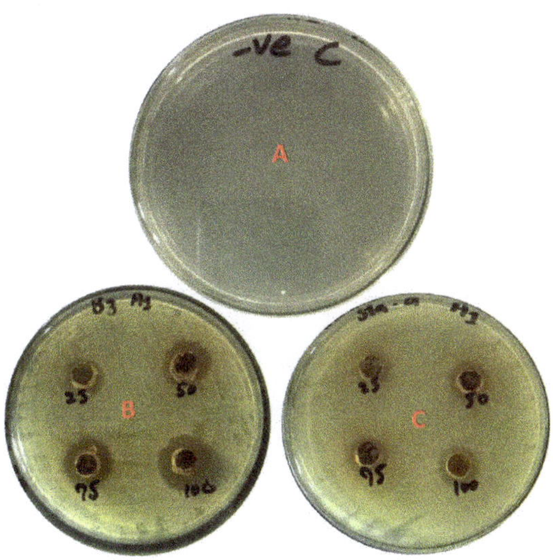

Figure 7. Antimicrobial activity of Ag_2CO_3 nanoparticle against different bacterial strains: (**A**) Control; (**B**) *Pseudomonas chengduensis;* (**C**) Staphylococcus *aureus*.

2.6. Conformation of Interaction Between Ag_2CO_3 and Biological Proteins Involved in Metabolism Regulation and Antimicrobial Activity Through Molecular Docking Analysis

2.6.1. Molecular Interaction Between Ag_2CO_3 and Thyroxine (T4) (PDB: 2CEO)

The molecular docking analysis presented highlights the interactions between Ag_2CO_3 and the thyroxine-binding protein (PDB). Records from this study portrayed the gene as 2CEO, which is known to have an important function in metabolism. The schemes at the left represent 2D depictions of the interaction between Ag_2CO_3 and the key amino acid residues for binding to thyroxine. Green-shaded residues, such as ALA256, ILE198, LEU261,

PHE258, and TYR262, represent good van der Waals interactions that are crucial for the stabilization of the ligand in the active site and, thus, they adopted potential modulation of metabolic rate. Nonetheless, the residues colored in red (ARG260, GLU259, and PHE165) define steric or spatial hindrances expressed as "bad contacts" or "unfavorable bumps" that, potentially, lower the binding ability of Ag_2CO_3.

From the 3D diagram on the right, the spatial position of Ag_2CO_3 within the binding site is described in more detail. The red dotted lines show that the interactions are unfavorable with Arg260, Glu 259, and Phe165 residues in particular. Such clashes may imply that, in order to obtain a better binding fit for Ag_2CO_3, changes may need to be made structurally so that the compound may be able to occupy a more relevant position in its interaction with the protein more effectively. This means that the observed Glide XP GScore of −3.52 indicates that there is moderate binding affinity; it shows that, while forming a stable complex with thyroxine-binding protein, there is still an area of opportunity for improvement in the binding of Ag_2CO_3. Since thyroxine controls metabolic processes and Ag_2CO_3 is involved in binding pocket, it might disturb protein conformation or flexibility and therefore disturb its role in the management of metabolic rates. Ag_2CO_3 could either augment or suppress all or some of the metabolic regulatory functions of thyroxine depending on the change in the overall conformation and activity of the protein induced by the ligand binding (Figure 8).

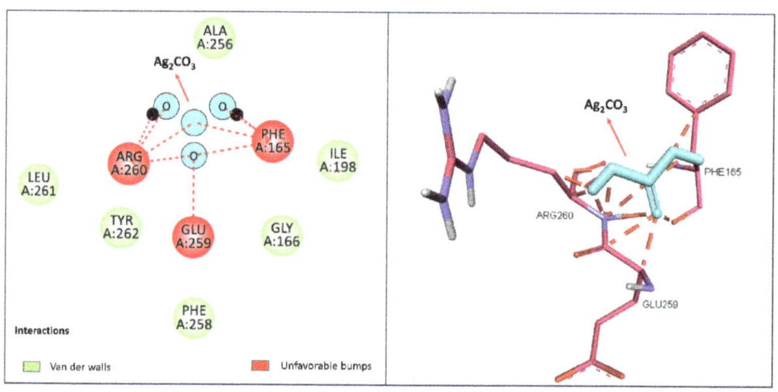

Figure 8. Molecular docking analysis of Ag_2CO_3 with thyroxine-binding protein (PDB: 2CEO): left-side figure shows 2D interactions, while right panel displays 3D binding pose.

Figure 9 shows an iMODS validation chart related to the docking analysis, where the major interest is on the protein–ligand complex motion. Normal mode analysis used in the work is proved by the arrows in the top-left diagram, where the location of protein motion is described. This facilitates visualizing flexibility in the protein structure during the interaction process. The deformability graph, in the bottom left of the figure, represents areas of protein that are capable of changing their structures, as identified by peaks. The B-factor plot (middle left) is a graph of NMA-predicted flexibility (red line) against the flexibility as obtained from the PDB (grey bar plot), and alignment of the peaks on the two graphs indicates that the flexibility calculated by the NMA simulation was correct.

Based on the eigenvalue plot (top right), it is low (1.06×10^{-6}), representing flexibility of the system and the ability to undergo conformational changes upon ligand binding. The variance graph (bottom right) indicates that flexibility and lower modes account for much of the motion, and higher modes have less influence in the system. The covariance matrix in the middle right shows red for correlated motions and blue for anti-correlated motions between residues. Lastly, there is the elastic network model (bottom right) that relates the forces between atoms, where the black areas indicate strong interactions diagonally along the protein structure. In summary, to the validation of the iMODS results, there is flexibility of the protein–ligand complex, implying that the protein changes its conformation in order to interact with Ag_2CO_3; this is a key means through which the protein is able to maintain the kinetic control of the metabolic system.

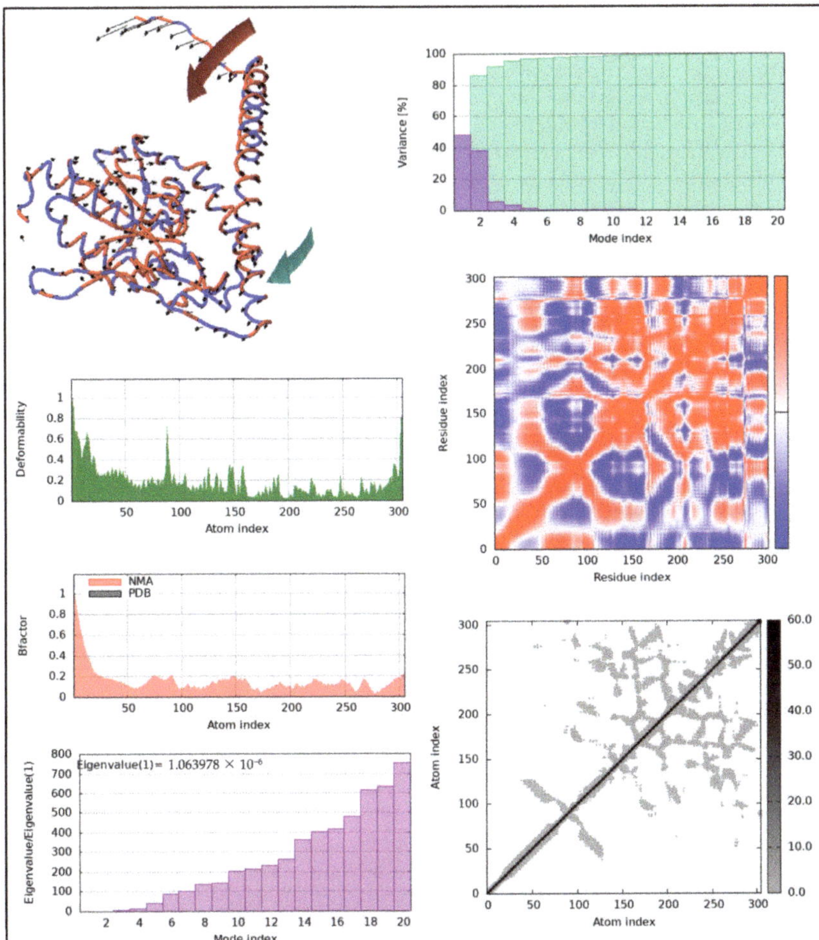

Figure 9. iMODS validation of thyroxine–Ag_2CO_3 complex: analysis of protein flexibility, deformability, and motion through normal mode analysis (NMA), highlighting dynamic conformational changes and stable interactions in the docked structure.

2.6.2. Molecular Interaction Between Ag_2CO_3 and Thymidylate Kinase (PDB ID: 4GQQ)

The molecular docking analysis between Ag_2CO_3 and thymidylate kinase (PDB: Protein P4GQQ) has functional domains that suggest interactions critical to understanding its function in the antimicrobial property. The 2D interaction diagram (left) also depicts no covalent link between the enzyme and the inhibitor; however, Ag_2CO_3 has a conventional hydrogen bond with GLU161 with a green dashed line, meaning that there is a stabilizing contribution from this source to the inhibition of the enzyme. Nevertheless, residues GLU165, ILE164, and VAL163 exhibited steric clashes, and the introduction of red dashed lines indicates that this is actually a detrimental factor that may weaken Ag_2CO_3 binding because there may be spatial hindrance.

In the case of the 3D diagram (right), spatial positioning of Ag_2CO_3 is shown, especially its hydrogen bonding interaction with the GLU161 residue. However, several favorable interactions with nearby residues include the induction of six hydrogen bonds with CDR-H loop residues; however, steric clashes were also observed with nearby residues such as ILE 164 and GLU 165, which could have been minimized perfectly. At an XP GScore of −3.55, it can be argued that the binding affinity of Ag_2CO_3 is moderate to thymidylate kinase, and better ligand optimization can be performed to minimize steric hindrance.

Thymidylate kinase is involved in DNA replication as well as the DNA repair process in microorganisms; hence, it is highly probable that Ag_2CO_3 acting as an inhibitor binds on the active site of the enzyme and prevents its proper working. This may inhibit microbial DNA replication, which could also account for the compound's antibacterial properties. Thus, the analysis of docking suggests that Ag_2CO_3 can be used as an antimicrobial agent through interaction with the important enzyme of microbial reproduction, though further enhancement in binding energy could be conducted by structural modification (Figure 10).

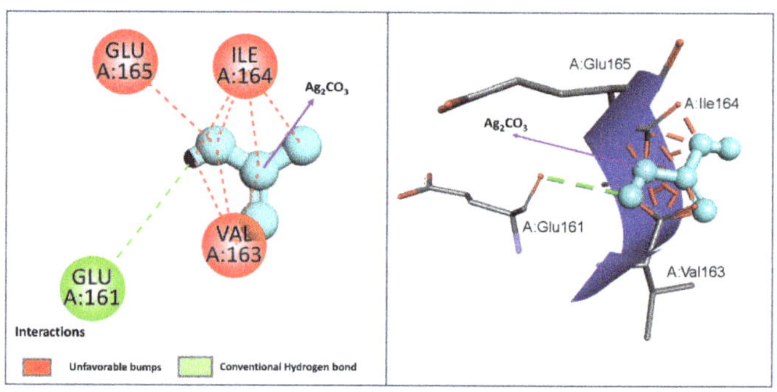

Figure 10. Molecular docking analysis of Ag_2CO_3 with thymidylate kinase (PDB ID: 4GQQ): left-side figure shows 2D interactions, while right panel displays 3D binding pose.

This presents the iMODS validation of the thymidylate kinase–Ag_2CO_3, including the protein's flexibility, deformability, and dynamic movement derived from normal mode analysis (NMA). The various figures provide a clear description of the stability of the complex and its interactivity behavior. The top left structure shows the whole conformation change of the protein using arrows to represent the direction of the flexibility for each region of the structure to illustrate the collective motions of the protein in the NMA. The deformability plot (bottom left) shows peaks that are in line with the regions where higher flexibility is confirmed, along with specific residues that indicate areas more sensitive to conformational changes.

The B-factor plot (middle left) overlays the experimental B-factor derived from the PDB with the corresponding predicted values in NMA, and the closeness of the graphs about the same axis reflects the correlation between the experimental and computational data, further affirming the docking outcomes. The variance and eigenvalue plots at the top right and bottom left prove the contribution of each mode to the overall movement, and lower modes are highly significant in overall conformational changes.

The heatmaps (right side) also give the residue–residue contact analysis, which shows how various regions of the protein change position relative to another. The colored correlation matrix in the middle right shows an overall co-operation in motion, while the grayscale in the bottom right shows a detailed interaction of the protein. Collectively, these analyses verify the stability of the thymidylate kinase–Ag_2CO_3 structure and provide the cinematographic view of the protein-induced fit mechanism as to how specificity is maintained while the overall protein presents conformational flexibility (Figure 11).

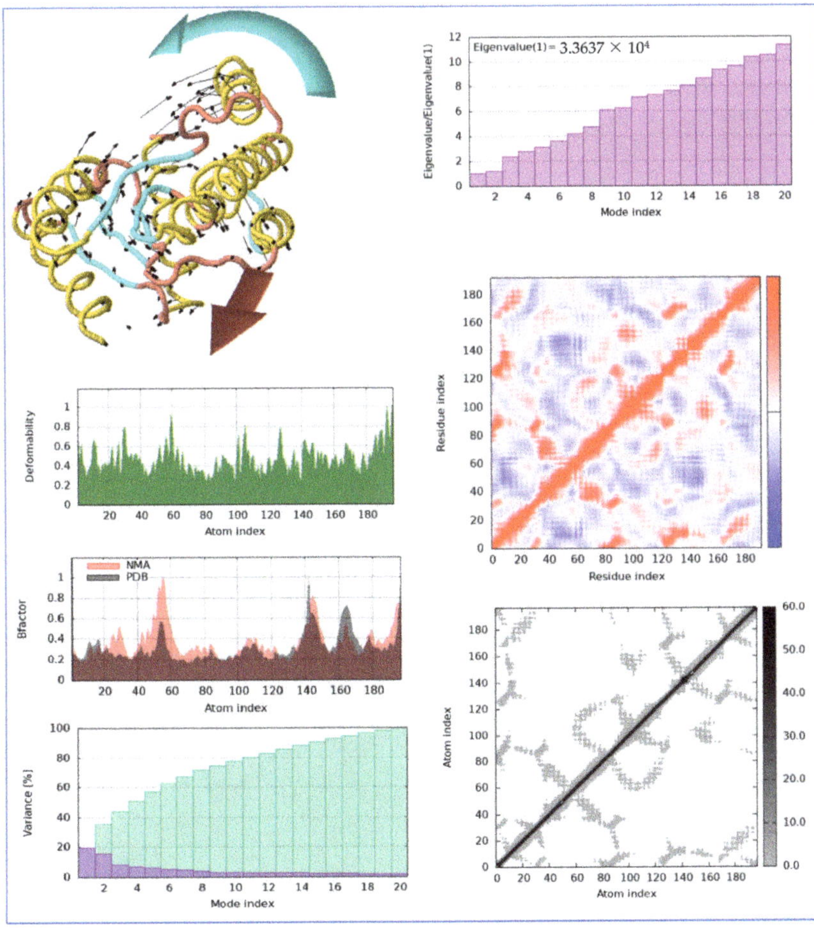

Figure 11. iMODS validation of thymidylate kinase–Ag_2CO_3 complex: analysis of protein flexibility, deformability, and motion through normal mode analysis (NMA), highlighting dynamic conformational changes and stable interactions in the docked structure.

3. Discussion

The FTIR spectrum of Ag_2CO_3 nanoparticles shows some intense peaks that clearly identify functional groups present in the nanoparticles. The two sharp peaks at 1382 cm^{-1} and 1500 cm^{-1} can be ascribed to C-O bonds present in the carbonate group, which is similar to findings by Pan et al. [16] in Ag_2CO_3 nanocomposites with photocatalytic applications. The 920 cm^{-1} peak is attributed to C-H bending and the 2750 cm^{-1} peak to C-H stretching, which implies the presence of organic residues or surface modifications, as pointed out by Rabchinskii et al. [17], where carbon–hydrogen peaks are attributed to surface changes. Furthermore, the appearance of these peaks is confirmed by Ebrahimi et al. [18], who identified Ag_2CO_3-based nanocomposites using FTIR, stressing the role of functional groups in the FTIR spectra of the nanoparticles. Altogether, these results confirm the presence of carbonate groups and possible surface changes in the Ag_2CO_3 nanoparticles.

The biocompatibility implications of Ag_2CO_3 nanoparticles (NPs) indicate the possibility and safety of the compound being used in biomedical applications. Hemolysis assays show the effect of concentration; the percentage of hemolysis is still below 5% at the tested range and even at the highest concentration of 75 µg/mL. Due to the low degree of hemolysis, it can be concluded that Ag_2CO_3 NPs provide stability to red blood cells, which is consistent with other works stating the biological compatibility of silver nanoparticles. For example, Burdușel et al. argue that, although silver nanoparticles have been shown to be toxic in high concentrations or when introduced into the human body, they are biocompatible when used in moderate quantities. This suggests that Ag_2CO_3 can be used in medicine, for instance, in wound dressing and infection control [5]. This is crucial, as biocompatibility must be achieved to reduce side effects, such as hemolytic toxicity, making the nanoparticles suitable for diagnosis and treatment [6].

One cannot overlook the metabolic impacts associated with Ag_2CO_3 NPs. The observed elevation of T3, T4, TSH, and insulin levels in experimental diabetic mice suggests that Ag_2CO_3 has the capability to stimulate thyroid hormone synthesis, which may directly affect global glucose homeostasis. These observations align with other studies that have shown silver nanoparticles affecting metabolic pathways. Jarak et al. further noted that the metabolic effects of silver nanoparticles include changes in various organs, indicating that the effects of Ag_2CO_3 on thyroid hormones are likely to have a general impact [19]. Moreover, these changes could lead to better glycemic control, which could be beneficial in managing diabetes, as seen in the study by Paul et al. [19] on the effects of silver nanoparticles on diabetes. However, the metabolic effects suggest interactive qualities, requiring further investigation to ensure that these nanoparticles do not negatively interfere with endocrine balance [20].

As to the general wound-healing abilities of Ag_2CO_3 NPs, the results highlight the positive impact of the developed conjugates on boosting wound closure rates, especially under diabetic conditions. The nanoparticles promoted faster wound healing, with complete closure by the 13th day, compared to the control group, which saw closure on the 16th day. These findings are consistent with previous research that highlights the positive effects of silver nanoparticles on wound healing due to their enhanced antibacterial properties and tissue remodeling function [7]. Similarly, studies by Adibhesami et al. and Bhagavathy & Kancharla indicate that silver nanoparticles significantly improve wound healing, particularly in open or diabetic wounds [21,22]. Ag_2CO_3 NPs are promising for wound healing applications due to their broad-spectrum antimicrobial activity and ability to promote cell proliferation in the affected area. In this study, the results obtained against *Pseudomonas chengduensis* and *Staphylococcus aureus* confirm their bacteriostatic activity, enhancing their therapeutic value in wound healing [12].

Regarding molecular interactions, data from docking studies show that Ag_2CO_3 NPs can affect the conformational structure of thyroxine, potentially altering thyroid hormone levels in the body. These changes could impact glucose homeostasis and insulin signaling since thyroid hormone modifications affect many metabolic processes [22]. Surprisingly, this study did not establish a direct interaction between Ag_2CO_3 and insulin but, given the observed effects on thyroid hormone secretion, it can be inferred that Ag_2CO_3 may indirectly influence insulin. This is consistent with the existing literature on thyroid dysfunction's effects on insulin sensitivity and glucose metabolism, as reported by Sulaiman et al. [23].

The molecular docking and interaction analysis of Ag_2CO_3 with thymidylate kinase (PDB ID: 4GQQ) further suggest that this compound may inhibit bacterial thymidylate kinase activity. The docking results indicate that Ag_2CO_3 engages in both positive and negative interactions with critical amino acids essential for the enzyme's function, particularly Glu161, Glu165, and Ile164. This interaction profile corresponds with the assertion of Jayanthi and Azam that thymidylate kinase is a prime target for new antibacterial agents [24]. Additionally, normal mode analysis (NMA) by iMODS confirmed the stability and dynamic conformational flexibility of the thymidylate kinase–Ag_2CO_3 complex, predicting its potential as a strong inhibitor. Khan et al. [25] also validated the effectiveness of structure-based design in identifying inhibitors targeting viral kinases, while Patel et al. [26] affirmed that computational modeling and molecular dynamics are useful in evaluating the efficacy of phytochemical inhibitors [25,26]. Altogether, these works underscore the importance of computationally guided approaches in identifying and optimizing effective thymidylate kinase inhibitors for antibacterial and antiviral applications.

4. Materials and Methods

4.1. Research Design

The research design of this study was systematically planned based on synthesizing silver carbonate nanostructures (Ag_2CO_3-NS) using controlled chemical reduction and characterizing them by XRD, SEM, and FTIR to confirm their structure composition, morphology, and properties, respectively. The bacterial properties of Ag_2CO_3-NS were evaluated by in vitro tests using different types of pathogenic bacteria. After that, the in vivo part of the study was carried out with albino mice in order to assess the metabolic performance of the nanostructures, paying attention to glucose level, lipid profile, and the general metabolic situation of the animal models.

4.2. Synthesis and Characterization

Silver nanostructures were synthesized using a chemical reduction method adopted from Umar et al. [27]. Silver nitrate (Sigma Aldrich; Lot# SZBF1070V; Darmstadt, Germany) was used as the precursor, while sodium borohydride (Sigma Aldrich; Darmstadt, Germany) was used as the reducing agent. There are two reaction conditions preparing two kinds of nanostructures. These synthesized nanoparticles were then confirmed using X-ray diffraction pattern (D8 advanced Burker; Karlsruhe, Germany), and scanning electron micrograph. These techniques are valuable to measure the size, shape, crystalline nature, and surface morphology of the nanostructures.

4.2.1. Synthesis

The synthesis of 20 mM Ag_2CO_3 NPs was conducted via a two-step process adopted from Umar et al. [27]. Firstly, 15 mL of 20 mM $AgNO_3$ solution was mixed with high-purity $AgNO_3$ powder in about 15 mL deionized water, stirring continuously until glimmer transparent. After this, 10 mL of 20 mM Na_2CO_3 (Sigma Aldrich; Darmstadt, Germany) solution was dropped slowly into the above solution to form a silver carbonate precipitate. Such a dropwise addition also enabled the slow and controlled formation of silver carbonate so as to facilitate homogeneous nucleation of nanoparticles.

Once the addition of Na_2CO_3 was completed, there was use of an anionic reducing agent called $NaBH_4$ (Sigma Aldrich; Darmstadt, Germany). This step formed the reduction process, which produced the silver carbonate nanoparticles within 10 min. However, to maintain stability in the nanoparticles, an additional 20 min of stirring were needed. During this period, the particles that had begun to grow in size acquired a fixed size and shape so that there was no agglomeration.

After nanoparticle synthesis was fully attained, the colloidal solution was centrifuged at 10,000 rpm for 15 min in order to precipitate nanoparticles from the reaction mixture. The liquid part of the suspension was removed and the collected solid nanoparticle pellet was washed with deionized water several times to eliminate residual amounts of the precursors or other products formed during the process. After washing, the nanoparticles were dried to obtain the final powdery form of silver carbonate nanoparticles, which were then used for characterizations.

4.2.2. Characterization

Following the synthesis of silver carbonate nanoparticles (Ag_2CO_3 NPs), various characterization techniques were employed to thoroughly analyze their physical, chemical, and structural properties.

Fourier transform infrared spectroscopy (FT-IR; Cary630, Agilent Technologies, Santa Clara, CA, USA): The functional groups and chemical bonds of the nanoparticles synthesized were further identified with the help of FT-IR spectroscopy. The spectra were obtained and scanned from 4000 cm^{-1} to 400 cm^{-1} to determine the presence of the carbonate functional group, $CO^{3}-$, and to confirm that of Ag_2CO_3. The characteristic diffraction peaks for carbonate ions were evidenced, and these allowed for understanding of the binding environment and chemistry of the nanoparticles.

X-ray diffraction (XRD): Structural analysis was conducted by XRD to establish the crystallite structure, phase composition, and size of the synthesized Ag_2CO_3 NPs. The analysis was made with an X-ray source Cu-Kα radiation Fizeau (λ = 1.5406 Å) in a range of 2θ = 10–80. The diffraction patterns were compared with standard reference patterns to ensure the obtained silver carbonate phase. The broadening of the peaks was used in conjunction with Scherrer's equation to determine the average crystallite size of the nanoparticles produced.

Scanning electron microscopy (SEM): The studies of surface morphology and spatial distribution of nanoparticles were carried out using SEM (JSM-IT100; JEOL Ltd., Tokyo, Japan). High protocols of SEM gave details of particles that included shape, surface morphology, and aspects of agglomeration. The SEM analysis supported the earlier observation and conclusion that the nanoparticles synthesized were uniformly distributed, with almost equal particle size, which were usually spherical or irregular.

4.3. *Research Animals*

Albino mice were used as experimental animals. Healthy adult albino mice (n = 18–20) with an average age of 8 $\pm$ 1 week and a weight of 30 $\pm$ 5 g were purchased from Animal House University of Punjab, Lahore, Pakistan. Mice were kept in a controlled environment, both in terms of temperature and humidity, in plastic cages (temperature: 25.2 °C, humidity: 55%, and light/dark cycles: 12 h). A regular chow meal with 21% protein, 48.8% carbohydrate, and 3% fat were fed to the animals. The mice were acclimatized for a week before the trial. This experimental study was conducted in the Animal House, Department of Zoology, University of Okara.

4.3.1. Diabetes Induction

Diabetes was induced in albino mice using alloxan, a compound known to selectively destroy pancreatic beta cells. The mice were administered a single intraperitoneal dose of 150 mg/kg of alloxan, which generated reactive oxygen species, leading to oxidative stress and the destruction of beta cells. This resulted in a significant decrease in insulin production, causing hyperglycemia and mimicking type 1 diabetes. The induced diabetic state allowed for further study of diabetes-related mechanisms and potential treatments.

4.3.2. Blood Sampling and Euthanasia Procedure

The blood samples of albino mice were collected through a noninvasive technique to ensure the well-being of albino mice. Blood can be collected from several sites of albino mice [28], i.e., the lateral tail vein [29], the saphenous vein [30], the retroorbital sinus, and the cardiac puncher. In the current study, blood samples were collected from the lateral tail vein due to its accessibility and relatively low stress induced in albino mice. The vein was warmed to dilate the veins just before collecting the blood in the required amount [28]. To prevent blood clotting and contamination, blood was collected for metabolic profiling. At the end of the experiment, no death was observed.

Metabolic Evaluation

The concentration of circulating T3, T4, TSH, and insulin was estimated using Enzyme-linked Immunosorbent Assay (ELISA) kits (Sigma-Aldrich (Merck) Darmstadt, Germany). These hormone levels were then compared between the treated groups and the control in order to compare the metabolic loading of the treatment. The hormone scores were compared between the groups to assess if there was a significant difference.

4.3.3. Hemolysis

The hemolysis assay was performed using blood collected from a 27-year-old male with a B-positive blood group. The blood was drawn into EDTA-coated tubes to prevent clotting. Red blood cells (RBCs) were isolated by washing the blood three times with phosphate-buffered saline (PBS) and centrifuging at 1500 rpm for 5 min after each wash. The washed RBCs were then resuspended in PBS to create a 2% erythrocyte suspension. To assess hemolysis, 100 μL of the RBC suspension was added to test tubes containing 100 μL of either the test compound, distilled water (positive control), or PBS (negative control). The samples were incubated at 37 °C for 1 h. After incubation, the tubes were centrifuged again to pellet any remaining intact RBCs, and the supernatant was collected. The degree of hemolysis was quantified by measuring the absorbance of the supernatant at 540 nm using a spectrophotometer. Percent hemolysis was calculated by comparing the absorbance of the experimental samples to the positive and negative controls. This procedure allowed for the assessment of the hemolytic potential of the compounds tested on human RBCs.

$$\text{Percent Hemolysis} = \left(\frac{Absorbance\ of\ sample - Absorbance\ of\ negative\ control}{\text{Absorbance of positive control} - \text{Absorbance of negative control}}\right) \times 100$$

4.4. Wound Healing

To determine the ability of the NPs in wound healing, two full-thickness standardized punched excisions (1 cm^2) were made on the back of each albino mouse. The mice were divided into two groups, which included a control group injected with saline and an experimental group receiving silver nanostructures. The nanostructures were used locally on the wound areas once daily. The wound healing procedure was followed and assayed from digital photographic records. To find the rate of wound closure, the wound size was determined at different time points [31].

4.5. Antimicrobial Activity

An investigation of the synthesized silver nanostructures against pathogenic bacteria such as *Staphylococcus aureus* and Escherichia coli was also evaluated. The well diffusion method was followed, in which bacterial cultures were streaked on agar plates and wells were made to inoculate the nanostructures. The plates were incubated at 37 °C for 24 h, after which the zone of inhibition around each well was checked to determine probabilities of the antimicrobial activities.

4.6. Docking Study

For the docking analysis, two proteins were selected: thyroxine-binding protein (PDB ID: 2CEO), which plays a role in metabolism regulation, and thymidylate kinase (PDB ID: 4GQQ), with antimicrobial activity. Both proteins were prepared using the Protein Preparation Wizard in Maestro 12.5 software. This comprised of reading in the PDB structures, appraisal of the bonds, inclusion of hydrogen atoms, and addressing of missing side chains and loops that were missing through the PMV Prime module. In addition, hydrogen bonds were adjusted, and the structures' geometry was fully optimized with the help of the OPLS3e force field. Additional water molecules that do not play a role with ligand interactions were clipped off from the protein structure.

Ligands were first built with the help of the LigPrep module of Maestro. This was aided by geometry optimization and energy minimization apart from tautomeric and ionization states at a pH of 7.0 ± 2.0. The structures of the ligands used in the analysis were chosen from the conformations exhibiting the least energy in their configurational space. Receptor grids were created for each protein using the Receptor Grid Generation option in the Maestro suite. This specific grid establishes the docking area and, therefore, ligands bind within the defined active site. The grid for 2CEO was constructed based on the thyroxine-binding pocket and the thymidylate kinase active site for 4GQQ. Certain modifications were made to the Van der Waals radii of all nonpolar atoms in order to achieve better flexibility within the docking space.

The ligands were then placed into their respective receptor grids using the Glide docking tool of the Maestro application. There, depending on the level of accuracy demanded, either the single-part precision docking (SP) or the double-part extra-precision docking (XP) technique was used. What was found was that the docking process provided flexible ligand sampling, which means that various conformations of the ligand can be sampled. Evaluation was conducted using the Glide Score function that takes into consideration hydrogen bonding, hydrophobic contacts, and shape complementarity. The most-ranked ligand–receptor complexes were solely considered for further analysis.

Subsequently, the protein–ligand interactions were analyzed; although, docking the protein, the interacting energies were analyzed, which include hydrogen bonds, π-π stacking, and hydrophobic interactions. Following each identified ligand, multiple poses were scrutinized to set the correct position of the ligand for binding. Finally, the docked complexes were summarized and viewed in Discovery Studio (BIOVIA Discovery Studio Client 2024). With Discovery Studio tools, detailed 2D and 3D diagrams were prepared that illustrated the interactions with and between ligands and protein residues, such as hydrogen bonds, hydrophobic pockets, and π-pi stacks. The visualization aided in the continuation of the docking results and their validation [32].

4.7. Statistical Analysis

All experimental data were analyzed using the statistical software (GraphPad prism v 10). The data were summarized and presented using mean $\pm$ standard deviation (SD) on the value of the variables. One-way analysis of variance (ANOVA) was used to compare the results of the control and the treatment groups. The p-value is desirable and significant, with a level usually below 0.05 being viewed as statistically meaningful.

5. Conclusions

In conclusion, this study explores that, by employing silver carbonate (Ag_2CO_3) NPs, there are tremendous opportunities to use them in various biomedical applications. The new morphology of the synthesized Ag_2CO_3 NPs with irregular and aggregated shapes provides better activity on the catalyst support. This was further supported by biocompatibility data showing their low hemolytic potential for safe use in therapeutic systems. There was further proof that Ag_2CO_3 NPs could exert metabolic effects and therefore may have endocrine-related potential benefits or risks. Moreover, the wound healing experience revealed enhanced diabetic healing involving the use of Ag_2CO_3 NPs effectively enhancing tissue repair. Our results indicate that they have a wide spectrum of antibacterial action against *Pseudomonas chengduensis* and *Staphylococcus aureus* and, hence, could be used as potent inhibitors against microbial infections via influencing microbial enzymes such as thymidylate kinase. Molecular docking and iMODS reaffirmed the solidity in structure and functionality of Ag_2CO_3 on metabolic and antimicrobial interfaces. Taken together, these works reveal that Ag_2CO_3 NPs have numerous potential uses in the therapeutic domain, ranging from the management of wounds to antimicrobial treatments and metabolic conditions

Author Contributions: Conceptualization, M.S.K. and M.W.; methodology, A.U. and T.K.; software, A.U.; validation, H.U., Z.S. and S.S.; formal analysis, M.S.K. and H.U.; investigation, M.S.K.; resources, M.W. and S.S.; data curation, Z.S. and H.Z.A.; writing—original draft preparation, T.K.; writing—review and editing, M.A.B. and H.A.; visualization, R.I., M.A.B., H.Z.A. and H.A.; supervision, M.S.K. All authors have read and agreed to the published version of the manuscript.

Funding: Researchers Supporting Project number (RSPD2024R740), King Saud University, Riyadh, Saudi Arabia.

Institutional Review Board Statement: Ethical Committee University of Okara approved the current research work (Reference no. UO/ETH/2024/TK1).

Informed Consent Statement: Informed consent was obtained from all subjects involved in the study.

Data Availability Statement: All the data are available in the manuscript.

Acknowledgments: We are thankful to the Researchers Supporting Project number (RSPD2024R740), King Saud University, Riyadh, Saudi Arabia.

Conflicts of Interest: The authors declare no conflicts of interest.

References

1. Suriyakala, S.; Kumar, R.; Singh, N. Silver nanostructures: Recent trends in environmental and biomedical applications. *J. Nanomater.* **2021**, *8*, 142–153.
2. Rani, S.; Sharma, P.; Verma, D. Chemical reduction synthesis of silver nanoparticles for diverse applications. *J. Chem.* **2022**, *10*, 108–115.
3. Almatroudi, A. Silver nanoparticles: Antimicrobial properties and applications in wound healing. *J. Pathog.* **2020**, *9*, 77–89.
4. Zahoor, M.; Rashid, S.; Asim, A. Biocompatibility and antimicrobial activity of silver nanoparticles. *J. Biomed. Nanotechnol.* **2021**, *17*, 95–106.
5. Burdușel, A.C.; Grumezescu, A.M.; Mogoanta, L.; Ficai, A.; Andronescu, E. Biocompatibility and cytotoxicity of silver nanoparticles: A comprehensive review. *Front. Pharmacol.* **2018**, *9*, 622.
6. Paladini, F.; Pollini, M. Silver nanoparticles and wound healing: A critical review. *Mater. Sci. Eng. C* **2019**, *104*, 109873.
7. Nam, S.; Yong, T.; Fang, X.; Kim, M.J.; Hwang, B. Silver nanoparticles in wound healing applications. *J. Nanotechnol.* **2015**, *8*, 95–107.
8. Mao, B.; Zhang, X.; Liu, Y.; Chen, Y. Silver nanoparticles affect oxidative stress and inflammatory pathways in cells. *J. Biomed. Mater. Res.* **2017**, *105*, 1938–1947.
9. Nicolae-Maranciuc, S.; Petrescu, I.; Popescu, T. Modulation of metabolic processes through silver nanostructures for therapeutic purposes. *Nanomed. Nanotechnol. Biol. Med.* **2022**, *42*, 102435.
10. Naganthran, N.; Tan, Y.N.; Chew, K.W. Advances in the chemical reduction synthesis of silver nanoparticles. *J. Colloid Interface Sci.* **2022**, *612*, 567–577.
11. da Silva, S.L.; Andrade, F.K.; Pereira, M.M. Enhanced biocompatibility and catalytic activity of silver nanoparticles in environmental applications. *J. Environ. Manag.* **2021**, *292*, 113340.
12. Vidhu, V.K.; Philip, D. Silver and silver-based nanoparticles for environmental and biomedical applications. *Environ. Chem. Lett.* **2014**, *12*, 493–517.
13. Babu, P.J.; Mohan, R.; Selvaraj, K. Toxicology and environmental science of silver nanostructures. *J. Nanopart. Res.* **2018**, *20*, 123.
14. Jarak, M.; Kovacevic, T.; Kravic, D. Metabolic effects of silver nanoparticles in various organs. *Nanomedicine* **2017**, *13*, 987–995.
15. Malehmir, S.; Esmaili, M.A.; Khaksary Mahabady, M.; Sobhani-Nasab, A.; Atapour, A.; Ganjali, M.R.; Ghasemi, A.; Moradi Hasan-Abad, A. A review: Hemocompatibility of magnetic nanoparticles and their regenerative medicine, cancer therapy, drug delivery, and bioimaging applications. *Front. Chem.* **2023**, *11*, 1249134. [CrossRef] [PubMed]
16. Pan, S.; Jia, B.; Fu, Y. Ag_2CO_3 nanoparticles decorated g-C_3N_4 as a high-efficiency catalyst for photocatalytic degradation of organic contaminants. *J. Mater. Sci. Mater. Electron.* **2021**, *32*, 14464–14476. [CrossRef]
17. Rabchinskii, M.K.; Ryzhkov, S.A.; Besedina, N.A.; Brzhezinskaya, M.; Malkov, M.N.; Stolyarova, D.Y.; Arutyunyan, A.F.; Struchkov, N.S.; Saveliev, S.D.; Diankin, I.D. Guiding graphene derivatization for covalent immobilization of aptamers. *Carbon* **2022**, *196*, 264–279. [CrossRef]
18. Ebrahimi, S.; Rezvani Jalal, M.; Hosseini, S.F. Optical, Structural and Mechanical Properties of Ag_2O_2/Ag_2CO_3 Nanocomposite Synthesized by Air-Plasma Electrolysis. *Iran. J. Sci.* **2024**, *11*, 1249134. [CrossRef]
19. Paul, T.; Smith, J.; Gupta, R. Silver nanoparticles and glycemic control in diabetes. *Diabetes Res. Ther.* **2024**, *6*, 311–321.
20. Adibhesami, M.; Hasani, M.; Taher, A. Silver nanoparticles and wound healing: Therapeutic perspectives. *J. Nanobiotechnol.* **2017**, *15*, 20.
21. Bhagavathy, S.; Kancharla, R. The influence of silver nanoparticles on wound closure. *J. Nanosci. Nanotechnol.* **2016**, *16*, 2147–2153.
22. Foretz, M.; Viollet, B.; Vaulont, S. The role of thyroid hormones in glucose homeostasis. *Endocrinology* **2019**, *160*, 1042–1051.
23. Sulaiman, M.; Iqbal, J.; Hussain, A. Thyroid dysfunction and its effects on insulin sensitivity and glucose metabolism. *J. Clin. Endocrinol. Metab.* **2018**, *103*, 2678–2685.
24. Jayanthi, R.; Azam, M.A. Targeting thymidylate kinase for antibacterial agents: A structure-based approach. *J. Mol. Biol.* **2024**, *441*, 156–169.
25. Khan, Z.; Ahmad, S.; Farooq, M. Structure-based design of viral kinase inhibitors. *Virol. J.* **2023**, *20*, 1–12.
26. Patel, R.; Kumar, A.; Desai, P. Computational modeling and molecular dynamics in assessing phytochemical inhibitors. *J. Mol. Model.* **2023**, *29*, 82–97.
27. Umar, A.; Khan, M.S.; Wajid, M.; Khan, M.U. Dose-Dependent Effects of Cobalt Nanoparticles on Antioxidant Systems, Hematological Parameters, and Organ Morphology in Albino Mice. *BioNanoScience* **2024**, *14*, 3078–3098. [CrossRef]
28. Hoff, J. Features-Technique-Methods of Blood Collection in the Mouse. *Lab Anim.* **2000**, *29*, 47–54.

29. Parasuraman, S.; Raveendran, R.; Kesavan, R. Blood sample collection in small laboratory animals. *J. Pharmacol. Pharmacother.* **2010**, *1*, 87–93.
30. Hem, A.; Smith, A.J.; Solberg, P. Saphenous vein puncture for blood sampling of the mouse, rat, hamster, gerbil, guinea pig, ferret and mink. *Lab. Anim.* **1998**, *32*, 364–368. [CrossRef]
31. Umar, A.; Khan, M.S.; Wajid, M.; Ullah, H. Biocompatibility, antimicrobial efficacy, and therapeutic potential of cobalt carbonate nanoparticles in wound healing, sex hormones, and metabolic regulation in diabetic albino mice. *Biochem. Biophys. Res. Commun.* **2024**, *734*, 150773. [CrossRef] [PubMed]
32. Eliseev, A.; Yashina, M.L. Brzhezinskaya, M. Chernysheva, M. Kharlamova, N. Verbitsky, A. Lukashin, N. Kiselev, A. Kumskov, and R. Zakalyuhin, Structure and electronic properties of AgX (X = Cl, Br, I)-intercalated single-walled carbon nanotubes. *Carbon* **2010**, *48*, 2708–2721. [CrossRef]

pharmaceuticals

MDPI

Article

Green-Synthesized Characterization, Antioxidant and Antibacterial Applications of CtAC/MNPs-Ag Nanocomposites

Ayşe Baran [1], Erdal Ertaş [2], Mehmet Fırat Baran [2], Aziz Eftekhari [3,4,*], Zübeyir Gunes [5], Cumali Keskin [6], Sergey A. Usanov [7] and Rovshan Khalilov [8,9]

1 Department of Biology, Graduate Education Institute, Mardin Artuklu University, Mardin 47200, Turkey; ayse.gorgec43@gmail.com
2 Department of Food Technology, Vocational School of Technical Sciences, Batman University, Batman 72000, Turkey; erdalertas21@gmail.com (E.E.); mfiratbaran@gmail.com (M.F.B.)
3 Department of Biochemistry, Faculty of Science, Ege University, Izmir 35040, Turkey
4 Department of Life Sciences, Western Caspian University, Baku AZ1072, Azerbaijan
5 Department of Crops and Animal Production, Mardin Artuklu University, Mardin 47200, Turkey; zubeyirgunes@artuklu.edu.tr
6 Department of Medical Services, Vocational School of Health Services, Mardin Artuklu University, Mardin 47200, Turkey; ckeskinoo@gmail.com
7 Institute of Bioorganic Chemistry, National Academy of Sciences of Belarus, 220141 Minsk, Belarus
8 Department of Biophysics and Biochemistry, Baku State University, Baku AZ1148, Azerbaijan
9 Institute of Radiation Problems, Ministry of Science and Education Republic of Azerbaijan, Baku AZ1143, Azerbaijan
* Correspondence: eftekhari.aziz@gmail.com

Abstract: The emergence of antibiotic resistance, caused by the improper use of antibiotics, is a significant challenge in combating infectious diseases, leading to millions of annual fatalities. The occurrence of antimicrobial side effects catalyzes the investigation of novel antimicrobial compounds and sources of drugs. Consequently, the research on biological activity that is conducted on plants, plant extracts, and compounds that are produced from plant components is of utmost significance. In this study, CtAC/MNPs were obtained by the reaction of activated carbon (AC) obtained from the fruits of the *Celtis tournefortii* (Ct) plant and magnetic nanoparticles (MNPs), and a CtAC/MNPs-Ag nanocomposite was synthesized by the reduction in silver ions added to the reaction. The synthesized CtAC/MNPs and CtAC/MNPs-Ag nanocomposites were analyzed spectroscopically (FTIR, XRD), microscopically (SEM, EDX), optically (DLS), electrochemically (zeta potential) and magnetically (VSM). The antibacterial activities of CtAC/MNPs and CtAC/MNPs-Ag nanocomposites against *S. aureus* and *E. coli* were investigated by microdilution method using minimal inhibitory concentration (MIC) and disk diffusion methods. Antioxidant activity study, including total phenolic content and DPPH and cuprac assays, revealed the remarkable effect of the CtAC/MNPs-Ag nanocomposite. This study has the advantages of obtaining CtAC/MNPs and CtAC/MNPs-Ag nanocomposites in a short time without requiring energy, and most importantly, the reaction takes place without using any toxic substances. In addition, according to the data obtained in the study, the CtAC/MNPs-Ag nanocomposite is thought to shed light on biomedical research.

Keywords: *Celtis tournefortii*; biological activity; CtAC/MNPs-Ag nanocomposite

1. Introduction

Nowadays, new technologies are being researched to reduce the size of materials and lighten them. This has occurred as a consequence of the application of nanotechnology, which enhances the properties of materials [1]. Nanotechnology is responsible for the development and production of the required nanoparticles [2,3]. Nanoparticles are materials that range in size from one to one hundred nanometers. These small particles have been utilized in numerous applications [4,5]

To comprehend and utilize nanoparticles, it is necessary to categorize them based on their size, shape, and content [6–8]. Nanoparticles are commonly classified based on their size. Nanoparticles are categorized based on their size into three groups: ultra-fine (1–100 nm), fine (100–2500 nm), and coarse (>2500 nm) [9]. The size classification of nanoparticles determines their surface area, reactivity, and toxicity [10]. Morphology is another method of nanoparticle classification. Nanoparticles can exhibit several morphologies, including spherical, rod-like, tubular, or wire-like structures [11,12]. The shape of the nanoparticle influences its optical, electrical, and mechanical characteristics. Furthermore, it can be classified according to the nanoparticle composition. The chemical stability, biocompatibility, and magnetic properties of nanoparticles vary depending on the component [13].

Due to their unique properties, the potential applications of metal or metallic nanoparticles in various fields such as medicine, electronics, and environmental science have been the subject of intense research and interest in recent years. These nanoparticles consist of metal atoms typically less than 100 nm, giving them a large surface area to volume ratio and distinctive physicochemical properties. Metal nanoparticles have become one of the most important components of nanotechnology, which has attracted great attention in many fields in recent years. These nanoparticles are generally obtained from metals such as gold, copper, silver, titanium, palladium, and platinum [14,15].

Silver nanoparticles are an important nanotechnology product that has been widely used in many industrial and medical fields in recent years. Silver nanoparticles are preferred in many applications due to their small size and unique properties [16,17]. Due to their small size, silver nanoparticles can be easily applied to the surface of many materials and positively affect the properties of the material. Additionally, silver nanoparticles have become one the popular study subjects due to their wide range of applications such as environmental friendliness, pollution reduction, energy saving, electrical and thermal conductivity, anti-cancer, anti-inflammatory, drug transport, wound healing, biosensor, antimicrobial, antioxidant and biocatalysts [18,19].

Activated carbon, also known as activated charcoal, is a highly porous material widely used for water purification, air filtration, and removal of impurities in various substances. One of the sources of activated carbon is plants. The process of obtaining activated carbon from plant sources involves heating the raw material at high temperatures in the presence of steam. This creates small pores and cracks in the carbon structure, increasing its surface area and resulting in an increase in surface capacity. Activated carbon can then be processed into various forms such as powder, granules, or pellets, depending on the intended application. Production of activated carbon using the fruit part of plants is a sustainable and environmentally friendly method of obtaining this valuable material [20–22].

Support materials are used to increase the activity and selectivity of silver nanoparticles, but activated carbon has proven to be one of the most effective options for this purpose [23]. The success of activated carbon in supporting nanoparticles increases the thermal and mechanical stability of the material and maximizes catalytic efficiency by increasing the effective surface area thanks to its high surface area [24]. However, since activated carbon is biologically compatible with microorganisms and can increase the proliferation of bacteria, it would be advantageous to use silver to give activated carbon antibacterial properties to eliminate this disadvantage that may occur during its use in different applications [25]. In addition, by binding silver ions to a support material to produce silver-bonded (doped) nanocomposites, agglomeration of nanocomposites can be prevented, and recycling and reuse of silver nanoparticles supported on activated carbon in various industrial applications can be achieved [26]. Moreover, activated carbon stands out as an ideal support material for silver nanoparticles due to its high surface area and pore volume [27].

MNP nanoparticles are important materials widely used in many industrial and medical fields today. The modification of these nanoparticles is especially important for biomedical applications because the control of surface properties is important for effectively directing the nanoparticles to targeted cells. Activated carbon obtained from Dardagan fruit is a potential material for surface modification of nanoparticles. The effect of activated carbon on MNPs may offer advantages such as increasing the biocompatibility of nanoparticles, improving their target orientation, and enabling their more effective use in environmental applications. The use of activated carbon obtained from daffodil fruit for the modification of MNPS may offer significant advantages to enable the more effective use of these nanoparticles in biological and environmental applications [28–30].

Dardagan, also known by its scientific name *Celtis tournefortii*, is a species of flowering plant belonging to the Cannabaceae family. Native to the Middle East, particularly Iran and Iraq, the Dardagan is a small to medium-sized species that can reach heights of up to 15 m. It is known for its distinctive appearance, with dark green, oval leaves and small, round fruits that turn purplish-black when ripe [31,32].

One of the most striking features of Dardagan is its adaptability to various climates and soil types. It can grow in both arid and semi-arid regions and is also a plant species that is resistant to drought and requires low maintenance.

In this study, for the first time, the antimicrobial activity effects of CtAC/MNPs and CtAC/MNPs-Ag nanocomposites obtained by using the Ct plant on *E. coli* and *S. aureus* bacteria and the determination of the antioxidant activity effects and total phenolic content of the CtAC/MNPs-Ag nanocomposite are comprehensively explained.

2. Result and Discussion

2.1. FT-IR Analysis

Celtis tournefortii fruits were used as biological sources in the synthesis of both AC-MNPs and Ag nanoparticles. The only source of phenolic compounds in the synthesized CtAC/MNPs-Ag nanocomposite was the extract obtained from *Celtis tournefortii* fruits. Spectrum shifts detected in the FTIR spectrum indicate the presence of functional groups of the compounds in the extract. FTIR spectroscopy was used to evaluate the synthesis of CtAC composite, CtAC/MNPs, and CtAC/MNPs-Ag nanocomposites. The results are presented in Figure 1. The CtAC composite's FT-IR spectrum has a peak at 2113 cm^{-1}, which corresponds to the C=C stretching vibration of alkyne [33,34]. In addition, the peaks observed at 1423 and 1023 cm^{-1} were attributed to the stretching vibrations of -CH_2 and C−OH [35] while the peaks at 875 and 711 cm^{-1} are probably attributable to out-of-plane deformation of C=C and C-H bonds in the benzene ring [35,36].

The 3369 cm^{-1} peak of the CtAC/MNPs nanocomposite can be assigned to the O-H bond due to the hydroxyl on the surface of the structure. hydroxyl groups (OH), possibly attributable to the presence of water molecules that do not fully dry on the surface of the nanocomposite for analysis after synthesis, the formation of long-chain acid and hydroxy compounds, or the decomposition or recombination of oxygen-containing rings [37–39]. The analysis of the spectra of CtAC/MNPs and CtAC/MNPs-Ag nanocomposites reveals the existence of alkyne and C-H groups, as evidenced by the absorbance peaks observed at 2109, 2113, 2011, 1994, and 1990 cm^{-1}. The observed peaks at 1636 and 1580 cm^{-1}, which correspond to the carbonyl C=O group. The increase in the peak intensity of C=O groups, which was not visible in the FTIR analysis of CtAC, indicates that the functional groups on the surface of the activated carbon structure improve the peak intensity as a result of surface modification of the activated carbon with MNPs [40]. Furthermore, the absorption peak observed at 1386 cm^{-1} in CtAC/MNPs and CtAC/MNPs-Ag nanocomposites signifies the bending vibration of –OH and C-H bonds, whereas the peak at 1069 cm^{-1} indicates the existence of C-O and C-N functional groups [41]. The strong peak observed at 536 cm^{-1} in Figure 1 is related to the presence of the Fe-O-Fe stretching vibration component in the core of CtAC/MNPs and CtAC/MNPs-Ag nanocomposites [42]. FT-IR results show that Fe_3O_4 is indeed dispersed with various functional bonds (such as hydroxyl, carbonyl, and amine groups) abundantly attached to the porous surfaces of activated carbon [35].

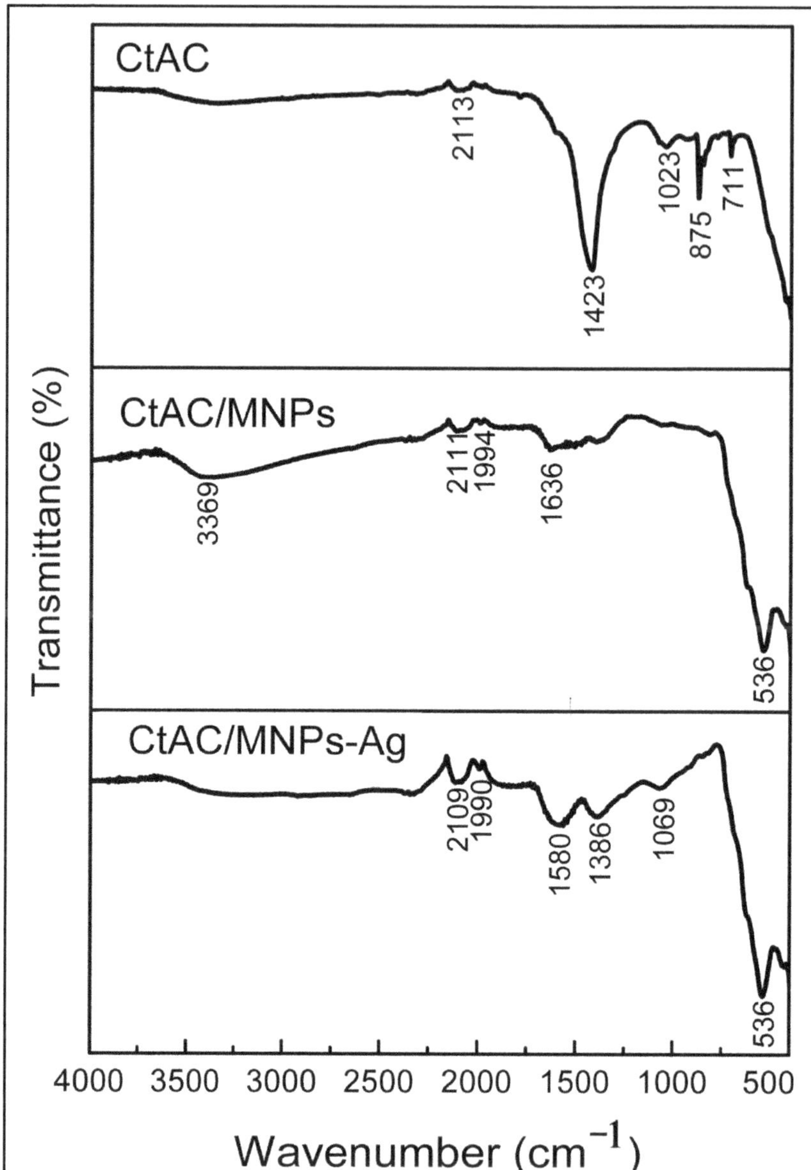

Figure 1. FTIR spectrum comparison of CtAC, CtAC/MNPs, and CtAC/MNPs-Ag.

2.2. SEM and EDX Analysis

The surface morphologies of CtAC/MNPs and CtAC/MNPs-Ag nanocomposites were examined using scanning electron microscopy (SEM). The elemental composition of these nanocomposites was determined by EDX analysis. This study presents scanning electron microscopy (SEM) images of CtAC/MNPs and CtAC/MNPs-Ag nanocomposites in Figure 2a,b, while EDX spectra are depicted in Figure 3a,b.

The nanocomposite of CtAC/MNPs exhibits a granular surface with diverse pore sizes. The surface form and pore structures of the CtAC/MNPs-Ag nanocomposite undergo modifications after its acquisition. The presence of heterogeneity and irregular distribution on the surface of the CtAC/MNPs composite leads to the attachment and subsequent smoothing of Ag ions [43,44].

The EDX analysis of the CtAC/MNPs nanocomposite indicates the presence of carbon (C), oxygen (O), zinc (Zn), and iron (Fe), which are important components of the nanocomposite. In the process of analyzing the CtAC/MNPs-Ag nanocomposite using EDX, it was observed that the element silver (Ag) was also detected. The relative amounts of Fe and Ag in CtAC/MNPs-Ag were measured as 53% and 2%, respectively. Iron and silver components have been verified in CtAC/MNPs and CtAC/MNPs-Ag nanocomposites using EDX analysis, as depicted in Figure 3a,b [45–47].

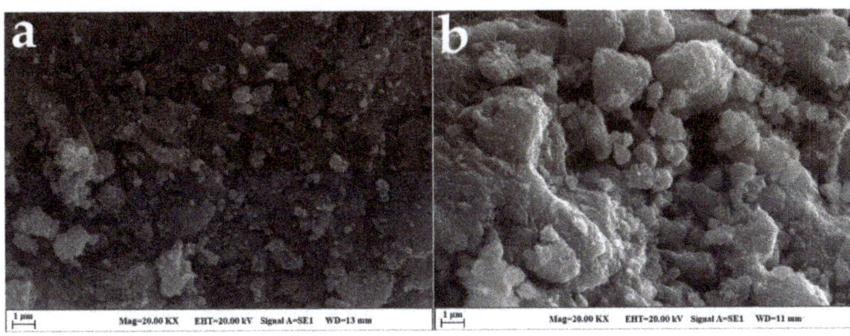

Figure 2. SEM images (**a**) CtAC/MNPs; (**b**) CtAC/MNPs-Ag.

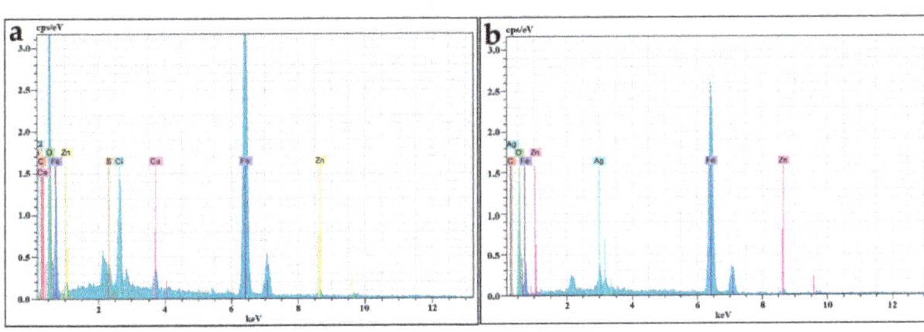

Figure 3. EDX images (**a**) CtAC/MNPs; (**b**) CtAC/MNPs-Ag.

2.3. Particle Size and Zeta Potential Analysis

In Figure 4, the results of the DLS analysis are presented following the dispersion of 10 mg of CtAC/MNPs and CtAC/MNPs-Ag nanocomposites in 100 mL of purified water using an ultrasonic bath. The particle size distribution inside a solid–liquid mixture can be determined through the utilization of DLS analysis. As an illustration, upon examination of the outcomes derived from the DLS analysis, it is evident that the mean size distribution of CtAC/MNPs is 91 nm, while the mean size distribution of CtAC/MNPs-Ag is 122 nm [48].

The zeta potential study of CtAC/MNPs and CtAC/MNPs-Ag nanocomposites is shown in Figure 5. The zeta potential on any material gives its surface electric charge. To prevent agglomeration and clustering of CtAC/MNPs and CtAC/MNPs-Ag nanocomposites and assure stability, high positive or negative zeta potential findings are needed. Under optimal conditions, CtAC/MNPs and CtAC/MNPs-Ag nanocomposites had potential values of −17.0 and −16.6 mV. In line with this, CtAC/MNPs and CtAC/MNPs-Ag nanocomposites had little agglomeration and stable suspensions for months [49–51].

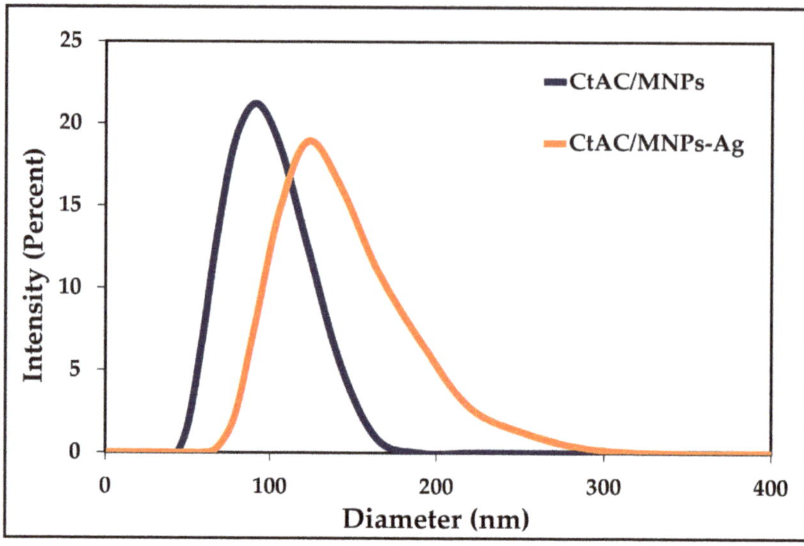

Figure 4. DLS analysis of CtAC/MNPs and CtAC/MNPs-Ag.

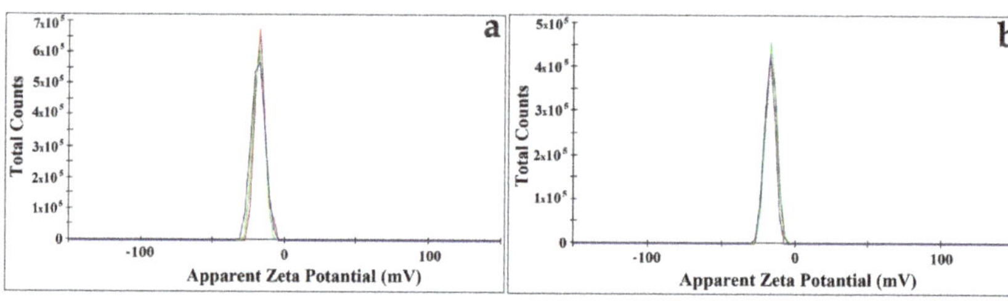

Figure 5. Zeta potential for (**a**) CtAC/MNPs (**b**) CtAC/MNPs-Ag nanocomposite.

2.4. VSM Analysis

Figure 6 shows the MNPs's and CtAC/MNPs nanocomposite's magnetic behavior. The magnetic saturation value for MNPs was 73.7 emu/g, and for the CtAC/MNPs nanocomposite, it was 67.72 emu/g. The magnetic saturation parameter of the CtAC/MNPs nanocomposite might vary depending on particle size, concentration, and oxygen absorption [36].

2.5. XRD Analysis CtAC/MNPs and CtAC/MNPs-Ag Nanocomposites

Figure 7 displays the X-ray diffraction pattern of CtAC/MNPs and CtAC/MNPs-Ag nanocomposites' crystal phases. The CtAC/MNPs nanocomposite exhibits crystal reflection patterns of (111) and (200), whereas the CtAC/MNPs-Ag nanocomposite displays crystal reflection patterns of (111), (200) and (311) [52]. In this work, the Joint Committee on Powder Diffraction Standards (JCPDS) value of the CtAC/MNPs nanocomposite was 28-0491, and for CtAC/MNPs-Ag nanocomposites, it was 65-2871 [53]. According to the Scherrer equation, the greatest peak values of 35.440 and 38.021 determined the crystal size of CtAC/MNPs and CtAC/MNPs-Ag nanocomposites as 24.67 and 28.59 nm. XRD shows that CtAC/MNPs and CtAC/MNPs-Ag nanocomposites were synthesized.

The Ct-ACMnNPs and Ct-ACMnNPs crystal dimensions were determined using the $D = K\lambda/(\beta \cos\theta)$ formula. D is the particle size, K is the constant value (1.504), λ is the X-ray wavelength value (0.90), β is half of the FWHM value of the peak with the maximum height, and θ is the high peak's Bragg angle (Ct-ACMNPs = 0.591 Ct-ACMNPs-Ag = 0.513) in the formula.

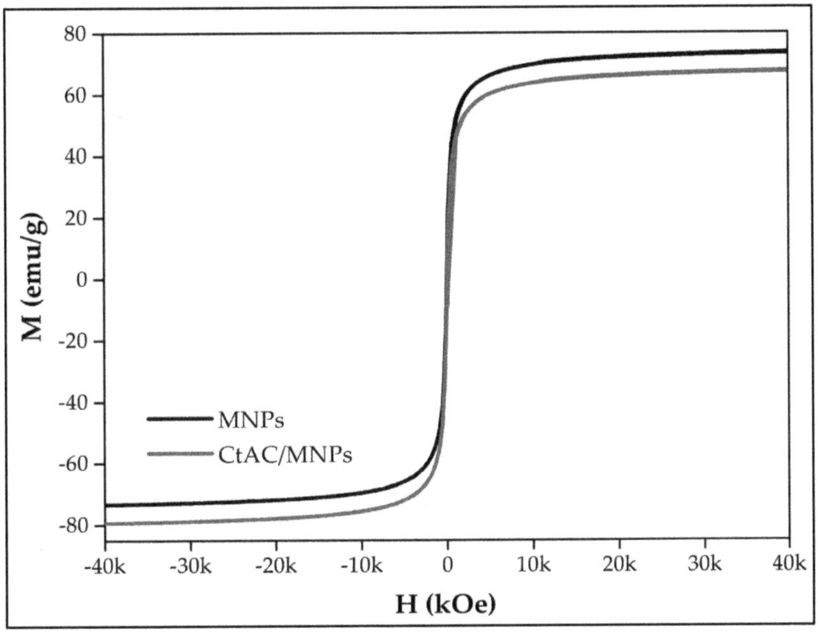

Figure 6. VSM analysis of MNPs and CtAC/MNPs nanocomposite.

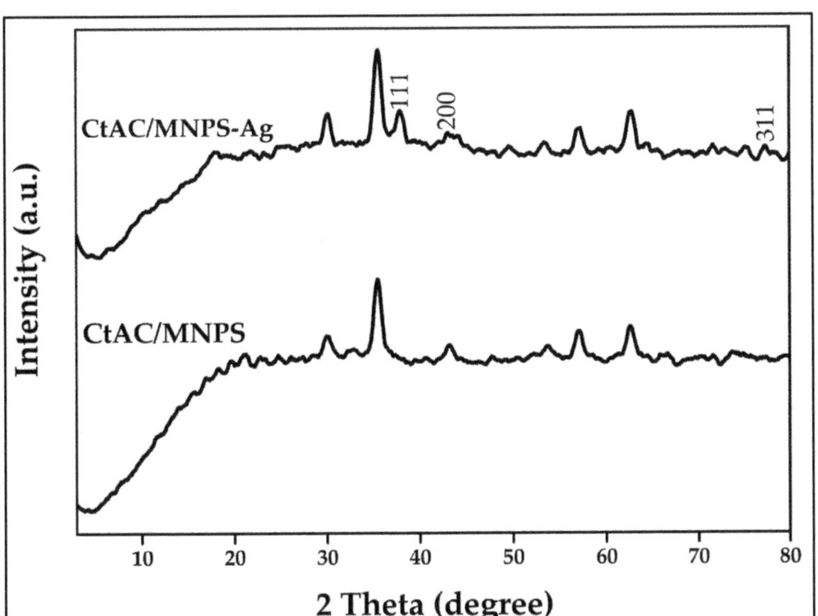

Figure 7. XRD patterns of CtAC/MNPs and CtAC/MNPs-Ag.

2.6. CtAC/MNPs and CtAC/MNPs-Ag Nanocomposites Antibacterial Effect

Disc diffusion and microdilution methods were employed to study the antibacterial properties of the CtAC/MNPs-Ag and CtAC/MNPs nanocomposite. The data from Table 1 show that the CtAC/MNPs-Ag nanocomposite had a substantial impact on two different bacterial species: Gram-positive and Gram-negative. The CtAC/MNPs-Ag nanocomposite demonstrated greater efficacy against Gram-positive *S. aureus* in the microdilution test, requiring a lower dosage than the antibiotic. This result is additionally corroborated by the disc diffusion approach (Table 1). The CtAC/MNPs-Ag nanocomposite exhibited higher efficacy against *S. aureus* bacteria compared to *E. coli*. Gram-positive bacteria possess a more substantial peptidoglycan coating compared to Gram-negative bacteria. Within this stratum, linear polysaccharide chains are connected by cross-links containing short peptides. Conversely, the wall architectures of Gram-negative bacteria are intricate. Gram-negative bacteria possess lipopolysaccharide plates, a feature absent in Gram-positive bacteria. The variation in wall architectures significantly influences how nano-sized objects impact two distinct species at varying concentrations [54–56].

Table 1. Gram (−) *E. coli* and gram (+) *S. aureus* bacteria were treated with colistin and vancomycin antibiotics, respectively, for comparative analysis. DW: Distilled water.

MICROORGANISM	MICRODILUTION METHOD (μg/mL)			DISC DIFFUSION METHOD Inhibition Zone (mm)				
				Control Disc			Image	
	Antibiotic	CtAC/MNPs	CtAC/MNPs-Ag	DW	CtAC/MNPs	CtAC/MNPs-Ag	CtAC/MNPs	CtAC/MNPs-Ag
S. aureus	1.00	32	1.17	1.00	0.00	12.00	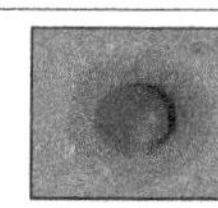	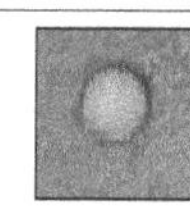
E. coli	2.00	128	2.34	2.00	0.00	11.00	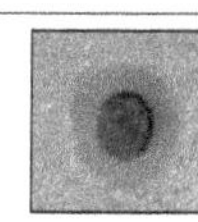	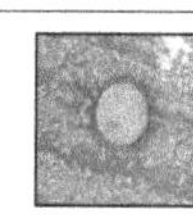

Metallic nanoparticles are valuable products that are constantly being developed due to their multiple antimicrobial effects as opposed to the specific effect of the antibiotic [57–59]. The antibacterial properties of silver ions have long been recognized. Silver ions that are ionized or diffuse exhibit high reactivity. Through the electrostatic force of attraction, they come together and interact with other microbes in the same environment. The effects that are shown in Figure 8 are assumed to be the mechanism that is responsible for the inactivation of bacteria by CtAC/MNPs-Ag. Several reports have suggested that this inactivation is related to the production of reactive oxygen species (ROS), depletion of antioxidants, and protein dysfunction (Figure 8) [60–63]. Considering the aforementioned works and the discoveries of the current investigation, we have put up a credible and comprehensive procedure. The antimicrobial action may occur in two different aspects. Ag depletion may lead to the creation of irregularly shaped pits in the outer bacterial membrane and alter its permeability, resulting in the leaking of cellular substances. Alternatively, we hypothesized that the antibacterial action of CtAC/MNPs-Ag was linked to the generation of free radicals, which in turn led to membrane degradation. Then, because of the rise in reactive oxygen species (ROS), they result in flaws in the membrane structure of microorganisms. Due to its strong affinity for reactive oxygen species (ROS), RNA disrupts the structure and activities of essential biomolecules like DNA and essential enzymes. Microorganisms perish all of these factors that obstruct essential functions (Figure 8) [56,60–66].

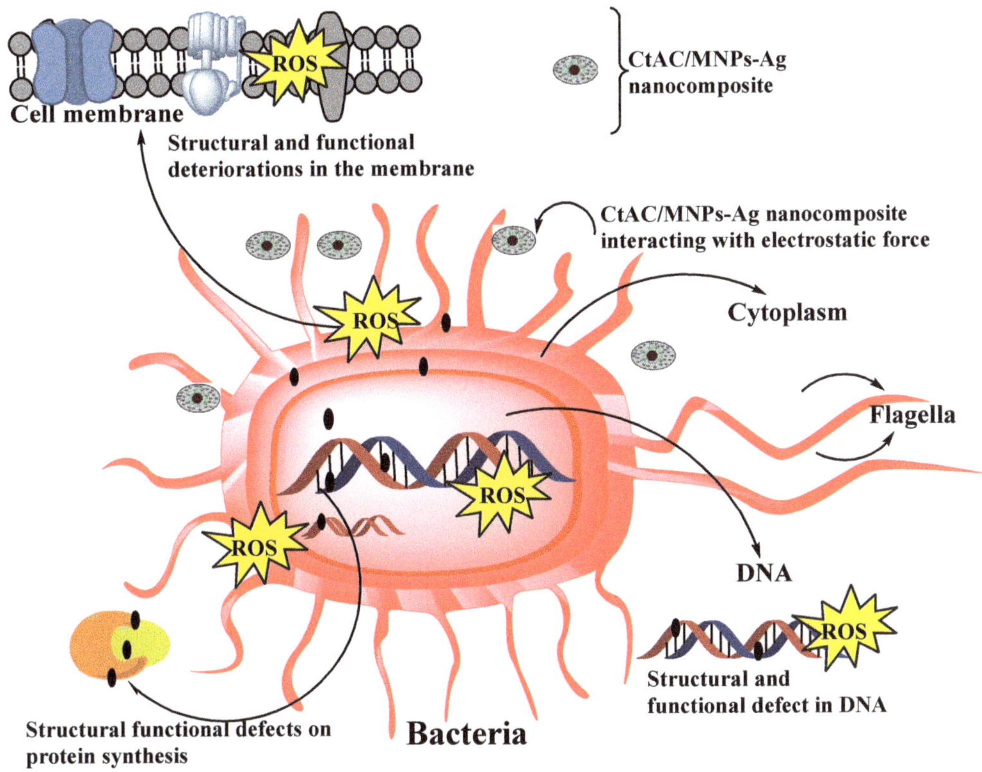

Figure 8. Mechanism of antimicrobial activity.

2.7. The Total Phenolic Content

The total phenolic content was evaluated by creating a calibration curve using five different amounts of gallic acid. The plant extract gallic acid equivalents (mg GAE/g) were calculated based on this curve. The total phenolic content of 1 mg/mL aqueous extracts of nanoparticles derived from plant extracts is presented in Table 2. The morphology of the CtAC/MNPs-Ag nanocomposite remains unchanged; however, the phenolic content of the plant extract has a substantial impact on the phenolic content of the nanoparticles. The overall phenolic content of the CtAC/MNPs-Ag nanocomposite was found to be 10.68 ± 0.435 mg GAE/g, as reported in reference [67].

Table 2. Total phenolic content and antioxidant capacity (DPPH and CUPRAC) of CtAC/MNPs-Ag nanocomposite.

Samples	Total Phenolic Content (mg GAE/g)	DPPH (%)	CUPRAC (μM TE/100 mL)
CtAC/MNPs-Ag	10.68 ± 0.435	70.37 ± 0.64	32.70 ± 1.035

2.8. Antioxidant Capacity

DPPH free radical scavenging experiments compared the CtAC/MNPs-Ag nanocomposite to crude extracts for antioxidant activity. Hydrogen ions and antioxidant compound free electrons neutralize the nitrogen atom's unpaired electron in the DPPH assay. This turns purple DPPH into yellow hydrazine. The CtAC/MNPs-Ag nanocomposite was evaluated for antioxidant activity by the DPPH radical scavenging method (Table 2). The CtAC/MNPs-Ag nanocomposite at the highest concentration showed an inhibition percentage of 70.37 ± 0.64. The spherical CtAC/MNPs-Ag nanocomposite may have better antioxidant capabilities than the extract due to bioactive component adsorption. Polyphenols' antioxidant properties and the CtAC/MNPs-Ag nanocomposite's catalytic actions may also help [68]. The CtAC/MNPs-Ag nanocomposite, produced using nanoparticles, showed a Copper Ion Reducing Antioxidant Capacity (CUPRAC) of 32.70 ± 1.035 (Table 2).

2.9. Comparison of Antimicrobial Effect of Various Silver Nanoparticles

The diameter of the inhibition zones (in millimeters) of silver nanoparticles synthesized from different structures against *S. aureus* and *E. coli* using the disc diffusion method is shown in Table 3.

Table 3. A comparison of antimicrobial effect of different silver nanoparticles for *S. aureus* and *E. coli*.

Samples	*S.aureus*	*E. coli*	References
AgNP (*Ferocactus echidne*)	2.10	1.80	[69]
AgNP (*Ziziphus spina-christi*)	5.20	4.40	[70]
AgNP (*Streptomyces enissocaesilis*)	16.60	16.30	[71]
AgNP (*Duchesnea indica*)	11.64	11.35	[72]
Ag/CNSAC	11.00	8.00	[73]
AgNP (*Linumusitatissimum* L.)	8.90	11.00	[74]
AgNP (*Zanthoxylum armatum*)	21.00	19.00	[75]
CtAC/MNPs-Ag	**12.00**	**11.00**	**This study**

3. Materials and Methods

3.1. Chemicals and Reagents

All chemicals were used without any further purification. Ferric chloride hexahydrate ($FeCl_3 \cdot 6H_2O$, ≥99% purity), ferrous chloride tetrahydrate ($FeCl_2 \cdot 4H_2O$, 98% purity), silver nitrate ($AgNO_3 \geq 99.0\%$ purity), sodium borohydride ($NaBH_4$, 99% purity), hydrochloric acid (HCl, 37% purity), sodium hydroxide ($NaOH \geq 97.0\%$ purity), ammonium hydroxide (NH_3, 28.0–30.0% purity), and zinc chloride ($ZnCl_2$, ≥98% purity) purchased from Sigma-Aldrich (St. Louis, MO, USA). All chemicals were used without any further purification. In this study, deionized (DI) water was used in the synthesis phase, during solution preparation, and for other purposes.

3.2. Synthesis of CtAC

In the process of synthesizing activated carbon, the fruit parts of the Ct plant were subjected to initial washing and drying steps to eliminate foreign contaminants. The fruits were pulverized to increase the activation surface area. A quantity of 10 g of powdered plant material was measured and placed into a 500 mL conical flask. Then, a solution of zinc chloride with a concentration of 1 M (during the activation process, the use of activating agents such as $ZnCl_2$ tends to promote dehydration of activated carbon and can lead to charring and aromatization with the formation of pores) [35] was added and mixed. The mixture was then subjected to stirring in a water bath set at a temperature of 90 °C for one hour.

Following cooling to ambient temperature, the mixed precipitate was homogeneously put in a big container and dried in an oven at 110 °C for 24 h. Then, the dried mixture was transferred to porcelain crucibles under room conditions and carbonized in a muffle furnace at 550 °C for 4 h, and thus, activated carbon was synthesized (Ct-AC) using *Celtis tournefourtii* fruits (Dardagan). Carbonization increases the surface area by creating pores in the carbon structure. The HCl solution was washed several times with 0.1 N to remove the remaining ions that did not react on the surface of CtAC. After washing the HCl solution, the composite was washed with distilled water and left to dry in an oven set at 75 °C [35,76].

3.3. Synthesis of CtAC/MNPs Nanocomposite

CtAC/MNPs were synthesized by the co-precipitation method, which is a simple and useful approach, with some modifications as stated in the literature [77]. After 6.0 g of iron (III) hexahydrate was dissolved in 100 mL of distilled water, a few drops of concentrated HCl solution were added to the solution to avoid hydrolysis of iron (III) ions in the solution environment. In the next step, 4 g of iron (II) tetrahydrate was added to the solution and the temperature of the solution mixture was slowly increased to 90 °C this process continued for 30 min and the solution was mixed. At the end of 30 min, 10 mL of 28% ammonia solution was added to the mixture and stirring was continued for another 30 min at this temperature until the solution turned black. In the next step, the prepared solution of 0.50 g of CtAC in 50 mL of water was added to the mixture. One hour after the addition of CtAC, the system was turned off in a shaking water bath and the CtAC/MNPs obtained were allowed to cool at room temperature. The synthesized CtAC/MNPs nanocomposite was separated from the mixture with an external magnet, washed, and dried in a desiccator at room temperature [43,78]. To remove the substances that did not react with CtAC/MNPs and remained in the environment, the CtAC/MNPs nanocomposite was washed 4–5 times with distilled water and then left to dry in the oven (set at 75 °C). The CtAC/MNPs nanocomposite was stored in a dark environment for use in other studies.

3.4. Synthesis of CtAC/MNPs-Ag Nanocomposite

For the synthesis of the CtAC/MNPs-Ag nanocomposite, 50 mL of deionized water was added to 1 g of the CtAC/MNPs nanocomposite and dispersed in the ultrasonic bath. After 25 mL of 5 mM $AgNO_3$ solution was slowly added to the mixture, mixing was continued for 1 h at 70 °C in the magnetic stirrer. In the next stage, to reduce the silver ions in the mixture to Ag-containing nanoparticles, 0.5 g of $NaBH_4$ was quickly added to the mixed solution, and the solution at 75 °C was shaken vigorously in the mixer for 3 h. The synthesized CtAC/MNPs-Ag nanocomposite was removed from the solution environment by an external magnet [44,79,80]. The synthesis mechanism of the CtAC/MNPS-Ag nanocomposite is shown in Figure 9.

3.5. Characterization

The FTIR spectra of CtAC, CtAC/MNPs, and CtAC/MNPs-Ag nanocomposites were determined with an Agilent Cary 630 FTIR-ATR spectrometer at a wavelength range of 400–4000 cm^{-1}. XRD patterns for the CtAC/MNPs and CtAC/MNPs-Ag nanocomposites were performed using a Rigaku RadB- Dmax II at $2\theta = 3°–80°$ with a scan rate of 1°/min. Surface images of CtAC/MNPs and CtAC/MNPs-Ag nanocomposites were taken using a LEO-EVO 40/Cambridge electron microscope at an accelerating voltage of 20 kV, and a 125 eV Bruker detector EDX system mounted on this system was used. The magnetic properties of CtAC/MNPs and CtAC/MNPs-Ag nanocomposites were observed at 25 °C using a VSM (Quantum Design PPMS-9T). Particle size and zeta potential of CtAC/MNP and CtAC/MNPs-Ag nanocomposites were measured using Zetasizer Nano ZS90 (Malvern Co., Malvern, UK). Before measurements were taken, the samples were used from the stock solution by making the necessary dilutions with pure water.

3.6. CtAC/MNPs-Ag and CtAC/MNPs Nanocomposites Antibacterial Effect

The antibacterial properties of CtAC/MNPs-Ag and CtAC/MNPs nanocomposites on the pathogens *E. coli* ATCC 25922 and *S. aureus* ATCC 25923 were investigated by the Disc

Diffusion (1) and Micro Dilution (2) methods. The bacteria were cultured in the suitable media under optimal conditions in an incubator set at 37 °C. Merck's Mueller-Hinton agar and broth were utilized to assess the antibacterial impact. Microorganism strains were produced with a concentration of 1.5×10^8 CFU/mL using the McFarland 0.5 turbidity standard [81,82].

After loading sterile discs with CtAC/MNPs-Ag and CtAC/MNPs nanocomposites, as well as a control with sterile distilled water, each microbe was grown on a Muller–Hinton agar medium. The discs were placed in Petri dishes and incubated at 37 °C for 24 h to allow the active components to interact with the dish. After the period ended, observations were conducted, and the inhibition zones were measured in millimeters.

Various concentrations of CtAC/MNPs-Ag and CtAC/MNP nanocomposites were diluted using a micropipette and added to the wells of a microplate serially. The antibiotics underwent the same microdilution processes for comparison. Bacterial suspensions made using the McFarland 0.5 turbidity standard were added to each well, and the microplates were incubated at 37 degrees Celsius for 24 h. After the experiment, a growth control was conducted to establish the Minimum Inhibitory Concentrations (MIC) at which growth was inhibited.

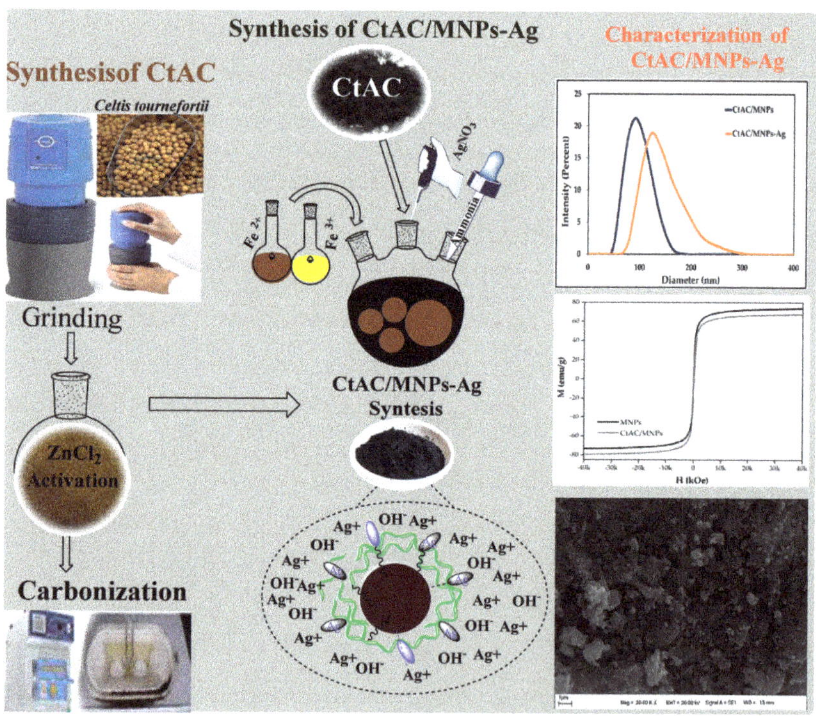

Figure 9. Synthesis mechanism of the CtAC/MNPS-Ag nanocomposite.

3.7. *Determination of Total Phenol Content*

The phenolic substance of the CtAC/MNPs-Ag nanocomposite was selected using a Folin–Ciocalteu reagent, which may consist of phosphotungstate phosphomolybdate, and gallic acid (as a standard). The phenolic compounds were observed to undergo complexation with the Folin–Ciocalteu reagent under standard circumstances, leading to the formation of a predominantly pure purple-violet color. Following a 2 h incubation period, the maximum absorbance of these compounds was obtained at a wavelength of 760 nm. The analysis results were computed in terms of gallic acid equivalent (mg GAE/g) [83].

3.8. Determination of the Efficacy of CtAC/MNPs-Ag Nanocomposite to Scavenge DPPH Radicals

The DPPH (1,1-diphenyl-2-picrylhydrazyl) assay was employed to assess the antioxidant potential of the CtAC/MNPs-Ag nanocomposite in scavenging free radicals. Initially, a solution of DPPH reagent at a concentration of 0.1 mM was produced using methanol. Next, a mixture was prepared by combining 0.4 mL of a 1000 µg/mL CtAC/MNPs-Ag nanocomposite with 0.4 mL of a 0.1 mM DPPH reagent solution, along with 3.2 mL of methanol. As the standard reference, ascorbic acid was employed, and the DPPH scavenging activity was assessed at various particle concentrations (50, 100, and 200 µg/mL). After a comprehensive mixing process, the mixtures were allowed to incubate in a light-free environment at ambient temperature for a duration of 30 min [84]. Subsequently, absorbance measurements were conducted at a wavelength of 517 nm, and the percentage of DPPH radical scavenging was determined utilizing the specified mathematical procedure.

$$\text{Scavenging effect } (\%) = \frac{(A_{\text{control}} - A_{\text{sample}})}{A_{\text{control}}} \times 100$$

In this context, A_{control} denotes the absorbance of the reaction mixture in the absence of samples, while A_{sample} signifies the absorbance of the reaction mixture when samples are present. The DPPH radical percentage scavenging was determined using the average values obtained from three replicates [85].

3.9. Determination of Reduction Force According to the Cuprac Method

The CUPRAC assay for the produced CtAC/MNPs-Ag nanocomposite was modified by Apak et al. (2008) [86]. Test tubes included 1 mL of a CMAC/MNPs-Ag bio nanocomposite and standard antioxidant solutions at 100–1000 µg/mL level. After that, 1 mL of 10 mM Copper (II) Chloride), 7.5 mM neocuprin in ethanol, and 1 mL of 1 M NH_4Ac buffer solution (pH: 7) were added to the test tubes, followed by distilled water and the final solution. After vortexing, the 8 mL mixture was incubated at room temperature for 30 min. The combination absorbed 450 nm.

4. Conclusions

Activated carbon material with a high surface area was synthesized from the fruit of the Ct plant by chemical activation of $ZnCl_2$. The CtAC/MNPs nanocomposite was formed by combining activated carbon derived from the Ct plant with magnetic nanoparticles produced through co-precipitation. Then, silver ions were effectively doped into ACs by chemical means, using sodium borohydride as the reducing agent. Nanocomposites characterized by SEM, XRD, FTIR, VSM, DLS, and zeta potential techniques show the formation of activated carbon and silver nanoparticles. In the XRD analysis, the crystal structure of CtAC/MNPs and CtAC/MNPs-Ag nanocomposites were examined and their dimensions were measured as 24.80 and 28.59 nm, respectively. It was determined that the zeta potentials of CtAC/MNPs and CtAC/MNPs-Ag nanocomposites had values of −17.0 and −16.6 mV. Moreover, the PDI average values of CtAC/MNPs and CtAC/MNPs-Ag nanocomposites were found to be 0.701 ± 0.186 and 0.546 ± 0.112, respectively. The total phenolic substance content of the CtAC-MNPs-Ag nanocomposite was determined as 10.68 ± 0.435 mg GAE/g, the DPPH radical scavenging activity was determined as %70.37 ± 0.64, and the CUPRAC reducing power activity was determined as 32.70 ± 1.035 µM TE/100 mL. The antibacterial activity of CtAC/MNPs and CtAC/MNPs-Ag nanocomposites against *E. coli* and *S. aureus* is shown in Table 1. CMAC-MNPs nanocomposites shows higher antibacterial activity than the CtAC/MNPs-Ag nanocomposite. CtAC/MNPs and CtAC/MNPs-Ag nanocomposites can potentially be used as antibacterial agents in various products.

Author Contributions: Conceptualization, A.B. and E.E.; methodology, M.F.B.; software, A.E.; validation, A.E. and E.E.; formal analysis, A.B., M.F.B. and E.E.; investigation, A.B. resources, C.K.; data curation, A.B., M.F.B., E.E. and Z.G. writing—original draft preparation, A.B., S.A.U., R.K. and

E.E.; writing—review and editing, A.E., S.A.U., R.K. and Z.G. visualization, C.K. supervision, A.B. and A.E. project administration, S.A.U., R.K. and C.K. funding acquisition, M.F.B. All authors have read and agreed to the published version of the manuscript.

Funding: This research received no external funding.

Institutional Review Board Statement: Not applicable.

Informed Consent Statement: Not applicable.

Data Availability Statement: All data and materials are available.

Conflicts of Interest: The authors declare no conflicts of interest.

References

1. Khalilov, R.; Bakishzade, A.; Nasibova, A. Future prospects of biomaterials in nanomedicine. *Adv. Biol. Earth Sci.* **2024**, *9*, 5–10. [CrossRef]
2. Erdil, N. Cardiovascular disease, signaling, gene/cell therapy and advanced nanobiomaterials. *Adv. Biol. Earth Sci.* **2024**, *9*, 58–80. [CrossRef]
3. Salahshour, P.; Abdolmaleki, S.; Monemizadeh, S.; Gholizadeh, S.; Khaksar, S. Nanobiomaterials/bioinks based scaffolds in 3d bioprinting for tissue engineering and artificial human organs. *Adv. Biol. Earth Sci.* **2024**, *9*, 97–104. [CrossRef]
4. Babanli, S.; Ahmadov, I.; Khalilov, R. Effect of nano zinc oxide on the chlorophyll content of bean plants under drought stress. *Adv. Biol. Earth Sci.* **2024**, *9*, 40–52. [CrossRef]
5. Li, B.; Wang, W.; Zhao, L.; Li, M.; Yan, D.; Li, X.; Zhang, J.; Gao, Q.; Feng, Y.; Zheng, J.; et al. Aggregation-Induced Emission-Based Macrophage-Like Nanoparticles for Targeted Photothermal Therapy and Virus Transmission Blockage in Monkeypox. *Adv. Mater.* **2023**, *36*, e2305378. [CrossRef]
6. Jiang, Z.; Shi, H.; Tang, X.; Qin, J. Recent advances in droplet microfluidics for single-cell analysis. *TrAC Trends Anal. Chem.* **2023**, *159*, 116932. [CrossRef]
7. Harish, V.; Ansari, M.; Tewari, D.; Yadav, A.B.; Sharma, N.; Bawarig, S.; García-Betancourt, M.-L.; Karatutlu, A.; Bechelany, M.; Barhoum, A. Cutting-edge advances in tailoring size, shape, and functionality of nanoparticles and nanostructures: A review. *J. Taiwan Inst. Chem. Eng.* **2023**, *149*, 105010. [CrossRef]
8. Prasad, R.B.; Prasad, S.R.; Singha, S.B.; Sinha, P.; Saxena, S.; Vaidya, A.K.; Teli, S.B.B.; Saxena, U.R.; Harale, A.; Deshmukh, M.B.; et al. A Review on Modern Characterization Techniques for Analysis of Nanomaterials and Biomaterials. *ES Energy Environ.* **2024**, *23*, 1087. [CrossRef]
9. Gawai, A.A.; Sarode, R.J.; Biyani, K.R. A Review on nanoparticles, their preparation and applications. *Int. J. Pharma Sci.* **2020**, *11*, 6540.
10. Salem, S.S.; Hammad, E.N.; Mohamed, A.A.; El-Dougdoug, W. A comprehensive review of nanomaterials: Types, synthesis, characterization, and applications. Biointerface Res. *Appl. Chem.* **2022**, *13*, 41.
11. Tadic, M.; Kopanja, L.; Panjan, M.; Lazovic, J.; Tadic, B.V.; Stanojevic, B.; Motte, L. Rhombohedron and plate-like hematite (α-Fe_2O_3) nanoparticles: Synthesis, structure, morphology, magnetic properties and potential biomedical applications for MRI. *Mater. Res. Bull.* **2021**, *133*, 111055. [CrossRef]
12. Zhang, W.; Taheri-Ledari, R.; Ganjali, F.; Mirmohammadi, S.S.; Qazi, F.S.; Saeidirad, M.; KashtiAray, A.; Zarei-Shokat, S.; Tian, Y.; Maleki, A. Effects of morphology and size of nanoscale drug carriers on cellular uptake and internalization process: A review. *RSC Adv.* **2022**, *13*, 80–114. [CrossRef] [PubMed]
13. Nair, G.M.; Sajini, T.; Mathew, B. Advanced green approaches for metal and metal oxide nanoparticles synthesis and their environmental applications. *Talanta Open* **2022**, *5*, 100080. [CrossRef]
14. Yaqoob, A.A.; Ahmad, H.; Parveen, T.; Ahmad, A.; Oves, M.; Ismail, I.M.I.; Qari, H.A.; Umar, K.; Ibrahim, M.N.M. Recent Advances in Metal Decorated Nanomaterials and Their Various Biological Applications: A Review. *Front. Chem.* **2020**, *8*, 341. [CrossRef] [PubMed]
15. Altammar, K.A. A review on nanoparticles: Characteristics, synthesis, applications, and challenges. *Front. Microbiol.* **2023**, *14*, 1155622. [CrossRef] [PubMed]
16. Almatroudi, A. Silver nanoparticles: Synthesis, characterisation and biomedical applications. *Open Life Sci.* **2020**, *15*, 819–839. [CrossRef] [PubMed]
17. Dawadi, S.; Katuwal, S.; Gupta, A.; Lamichhane, U.; Thapa, R.; Jaisi, S.; Lamichhane, G.; Bhattarai, D.P.; Parajuli, N. Current Research on Silver Nanoparticles: Synthesis, Characterization, and Applications. *J. Nanomater.* **2021**, *2021*, 1–23. [CrossRef]
18. Zahoor, M.; Nazir, N.; Iftikhar, M.; Naz, S.; Zekker, I.; Burlakovs, J.; Uddin, F.; Kamran, A.W.; Kallistova, A.; Pimenov, N.; et al. A Review on Silver Nanoparticles: Classification, Various Methods of Synthesis, and Their Potential Roles in Biomedical Applications and Water Treatment. *Water* **2021**, *13*, 2216. [CrossRef]
19. Rosic, G.; Selakovic, D.; Omarova, S. Cancer signaling, cell/gene therapy, diagnosis and role of nanobiomaterials. *Adv. Biol. Earth Sci.* **2024**, *9*, 11–34. [CrossRef]

20. Chew, T.W.; H'ng, P.S.; Abdullah, B.C.T.G.L.C.; Chin, K.L.; Lee, C.L.; Hafizuddin, B.M.S.M.N.; TaungMai, L. A Review of Bio-Based Activated Carbon Properties Produced from Different Activating Chemicals during Chemicals Activation Process on Biomass and Its Potential for Malaysia. *Materials* **2023**, *16*, 7365. [CrossRef]
21. Jjagwe, J.; Olupot, P.W.; Menya, E.; Kalibbala, H.M. Synthesis and Application of Granular Activated Carbon from Biomass Waste Materials for Water Treatment: A Review. *J. Bioresour. Bioprod.* **2021**, *6*, 292–322. [CrossRef]
22. Ahmadpour, A. Using of activated carbon adsorption in wastewater industries. *J. Chem. Lett.* **2022**, *3*, 2–9.
23. Luceri, A.; Francese, R.; Lembo, D.; Ferraris, M.; Balagna, C. Silver Nanoparticles: Review of Antiviral Properties, Mechanism of Action and Applications. *Microorganisms* **2023**, *11*, 629. [CrossRef] [PubMed]
24. He, X.; Jiang, Z.; Akakuru, O.U.; Li, J.; Wu, A. Nanoscale covalent organic frameworks: From controlled synthesis to cancer therapy. *Chem. Commun.* **2021**, *57*, 12417–12435. [CrossRef] [PubMed]
25. Zhang, F.; Tao, Y.; Chen, S.; Lu, Y. Preparation and properties of the silver loaded activated carbon fibers. *Fibers Polym.* **2015**, *16*, 2003–2010. [CrossRef]
26. Kazmi, S.J.; Shehzad, M.; Mehmood, S.; Yasar, M.; Naeem, A.; Bhatti, A. Effect of varied Ag nanoparticles functionalized CNTs on its anti-bacterial activity against *E. coli*. *Sens. Actuators A Phys.* **2014**, *216*, 287–294. [CrossRef]
27. Chingombe, P.; Saha, B.; Wakeman, R.J. Sorption of atrazine on conventional and surface modified activated carbons. *J. Colloid Interface Sci.* **2006**, *302*, 408–416. [CrossRef] [PubMed]
28. Yi, J.; Li, L.; Yin, Z.-J.; Quan, Y.-Y.; Tan, R.-R.; Chen, S.-L.; Lang, J.-R.; Li, J.; Zeng, J.; Li, Y.; et al. Polypeptide from Moschus Suppresses Lipopolysaccharide-Induced Inflammation by Inhibiting NF-κ B-ROS/NLRP3 Pathway. *Chin. J. Integr. Med.* **2023**, *29*, 895–904. [CrossRef] [PubMed]
29. Fatima, T.; Mushtaq, A. Efficacy and challenges of carbon-based nanomaterials in water treatment: A review. *Int. J. Chem. Biochem. Sci.* **2023**, *23*, 232–248.
30. Baabu, P.R.S.; Kumar, H.K.; Gumpu, M.B.; Babu, K.J.; Kulandaisamy, A.J.; Rayappan, J.B.B. Iron Oxide Nanoparticles: A Review on the Province of Its Compounds, Properties and Biological Applications. *Materials* **2022**, *16*, 59. [CrossRef]
31. Baran, A.; Keskin, C.; Kandemir, S.İ. Rapid biosynthesis of silver nanoparticles by *Celtis tournefortii* LAM. leaf extract; investigation of antimicrobial and anticancer activities. *KSÜ Tarım Doğa Derg.* **2022**, *25*, 72–84. [CrossRef]
32. Baran, A.; Keskin, C. Determination of Constituents of Extract of *Celtis tournefortii* Lam. by LC-MS/MS, Investigation of Enzyme Inhibition, Antimicrobial and Anticancer Effects. *Int. J. Pure Appl. Sci.* **2023**, *9*, 56–65. [CrossRef]
33. Hamat, N.A.B.A.C.; Phaik-Ching, A.; Ibrahim, M.N.M.; Abu Bakar, N.H.H.; Tan, T.-W.; Amin, N.F.B.M.; Garba, Z.N.; Perumal, V.; Raja, P.B. *Cocos Nucifera's* lignin mediated silver nanoparticle and their photocatalytic activity. *Inorg. Chem. Commun.* **2024**, *160*, 111845. [CrossRef]
34. Maniom, M.; Gunasegaran, Y.R. Performance of Waste Tire Activated Carbon on Methylene Blue. *Multidiscip. Appl. Res. Innov.* **2023**, *4*, 83–90.
35. Veerakumar, P.; Muthuselvam, I.P.; Hung, C.-T.; Lin, K.-C.; Chou, F.-C.; Liu, S.-B. Biomass-Derived Activated Carbon Supported Fe_3O_4 Nanoparticles as Recyclable Catalysts for Reduction of Nitroarenes. *ACS Sustain. Chem. Eng.* **2016**, *4*, 6772–6782. [CrossRef]
36. Islam, M.A.; Tan IA, W.; Benhouria, A.; Asif, M.; Hameed, B.H. Mesoporous and adsorptive properties of palm date seed activated carbon prepared via sequential hydrothermal carbonization and sodium hydroxide activation. *Chem. Eng. J.* **2015**, *270*, 187–195. [CrossRef]
37. Anyika, C.; Asri, N.A.M.; Majid, Z.A.; Yahya, A.; Jaafar, J. Synthesis and characterization of magnetic activated carbon developed from palm kernel shells. *Nanotechnol. Environ. Eng.* **2017**, *2*, 16. [CrossRef]
38. Zhang, Y.; Cheng, X.; Wang, Z.; Tahir, M.H.; Wang, Z.; Wang, X.; Wang, C. Full recycling of high-value resources from *cabbage* waste by multi-stage utilization. *Sci. Total Environ.* **2022**, *804*, 149951. [CrossRef] [PubMed]
39. Xiong, B.; Zhang, W.; Wu, Z.; Liu, R.; Yang, C.; Hui, A.; Huang, X.; Xian, Z. Preparation, characterization, antioxidant and anti-inflammatory activities of acid-soluble pectin from okra (*Abelmoschus esculentus* L.). *Int. J. Biol. Macromol.* **2021**, *181*, 824–834. [CrossRef]
40. Kristianto, H.; Arie, A.A.; Susanti, R.F.; Halim, M.; Lee, J.K. The effect of activated carbon support surface modification on characteristics of carbon nanospheres prepared by deposition precipitation of Fe-catalyst. *IOP Conf. Ser. Mater. Sci. Eng.* **2016**, *162*, 012034. [CrossRef]
41. Nguyen, D.T.; Tran, H.N.; Juang, R.-S.; Dat, N.D.; Tomul, F.; Ivanets, A.; Woo, S.H.; Hosseini-Bandegharaei, A.; Nguyen, V.P.; Chao, H.-P. Adsorption process and mechanism of acetaminophen onto commercial activated carbon. *J. Environ. Chem. Eng.* **2020**, *8*, 104408. [CrossRef]
42. Al-Musawi, T.J.; Mahvi, A.H.; Khatibi, A.D.; Balarak, D. Effective adsorption of ciprofloxacin antibiotic using powdered activated carbon magnetized by iron(III) oxide magnetic nanoparticles. *J. Porous Mater.* **2021**, *28*, 835–852. [CrossRef]
43. Kakavandi, B.; Jonidi, A.; Rezaei, R.; Nasseri, S.; Ameri, A.; Esrafily, A. Synthesis and properties of Fe_3O_4-activated carbon magnetic nanoparticles for removal of aniline from aqueous solution: Equilibrium, kinetic and thermodynamic studies. *Iran. J. Environ. Health Sci. Eng.* **2013**, *10*, 19. [CrossRef] [PubMed]
44. Chishti, A.N.; Guo, F.; Aftab, A.; Ma, Z.; Liu, Y.; Chen, M.; Diao, G. Synthesis of silver doped Fe_3O_4/C nanoparticles and its catalytic activities for the degradation and reduction of methylene blue and 4-nitrophenol. *Appl. Surf. Sci.* **2021**, *546*, 149070. [CrossRef]

45. Amiri, O.; Beshkar, F.; Ahmed, S.S.; Hamad, B.W.; Mahmood, P.H.; Dezaye, A.A. Magnetically-driven Ag/Fe_3O_4/graphene ternary nanocomposite as efficient photocatalyst for desulfurization of thiophene under visible-light irradiation. *Int. J. Hydrog. Energy* **2021**, *46*, 19913–19925. [CrossRef]
46. Huang, T.; AlSalem, H.S.; Binkadem, M.S.; Al-Goul, S.T.; El-Kott, A.F.; Alsayegh, A.A.; Majdou, G.J.; Batiha, G.E.-S.; Karmakar, B. Green synthesis of Ag/Fe_3O_4 nanoparticles using *Mentha* extract: Preparation, characterization and investigation of its anti-human lung cancer application. *J. Saudi Chem. Soc.* **2022**, *26*, 101505. [CrossRef]
47. Ravichandran, R.; Annamalai, K.; Annamalai, A.; Elumalai, S. Solid state–Green construction of starch- beaded Fe_3O_4@Ag nanocomposite as superior redox catalyst. *Colloids Surf. A Physicochem. Eng. Asp.* **2023**, *664*, 131117. [CrossRef]
48. Pop, D.; Buzatu, R.; Moacă, E.-A.; Watz, C.G.; Pînzaru, S.C.; Tudoran, L.B.; Nekvapil, F.; Avram, Ș.; Dehelean, C.A.; Crețu, M.O.; et al. Development and Characterization of Fe_3O_4@Carbon Nanoparticles and Their Biological Screening Related to Oral Administration. *Materials* **2021**, *14*, 3556. [CrossRef] [PubMed]
49. Lopes, K.L.; de Oliveira, H.L.; Serpa, J.A.S.; Torres, J.A.; Nogueira, F.G.E.; de Freitas, V.A.A.; Borges, K.B.; Silva, M.C. Nanomagnets based on activated carbon/magnetite nanocomposite for determination of endocrine disruptors in environmental water samples. *Microchem. J.* **2021**, *168*, 106366. [CrossRef]
50. Rodrigues, S.C.; Silva, M.C.; Torres, J.A.; Bianchi, M.L. Use of Magnetic Activated Carbon in a Solid Phase Extraction Procedure for Analysis of 2,4-dichlorophenol in Water Samples. *Water Air Soil Pollut.* **2020**, *231*, 294. [CrossRef]
51. Forest, V.; Pourchez, J. Preferential binding of positive nanoparticles on cell membranes is due to electrostatic interactions: A too simplistic explanation that does not take into account the nanoparticle protein corona. *Mater. Sci. Eng. C* **2017**, *70*, 889–896. [CrossRef] [PubMed]
52. Ma, Y.-Z.; Zheng, D.-F.; Mo, Z.-Y.; Dong, R.-J.; Qiu, X.-Q. Magnetic lignin-based carbon nanoparticles and the adsorption for removal of methyl orange. *Colloids Surf. A Physicochem. Eng. Asp.* **2018**, *559*, 226–234. [CrossRef]
53. Patil, M.P.; Singh, R.D.; Koli, P.B.; Patil, K.T.; Jagdale, B.S.; Tipare, A.R.; Kim, G.-D. Antibacterial potential of silver nanoparticles synthesized using *Madhuca longifolia* flower extract as a green resource. *Microb. Pathog.* **2018**, *121*, 184–189. [CrossRef] [PubMed]
54. Reith, J.; Mayer, C. Peptidoglycan turnover and recycling in Gram-positive bacteria. *Appl. Microbiol. Biotechnol.* **2011**, *92*, 1–11. [CrossRef] [PubMed]
55. Velmurugan, P.; Anbalagan, K.; Manosathyadevan, M.; Lee, K.-J.; Cho, M.; Lee, S.-M.; Park, J.-H.; Oh, S.-G.; Bang, K.-S.; Oh, B.-T. Green synthesis of silver and gold nanoparticles using *Zingiber officinale* root extract and antibacterial activity of silver nanoparticles against food pathogens. *Bioprocess Biosyst. Eng.* **2014**, *37*, 1935–1943. [CrossRef] [PubMed]
56. Ahmed, B.; Hashmi, A.; Khan, M.S.; Musarrat, J. ROS mediated destruction of cell membrane, growth and biofilms of human bacterial pathogens by stable metallic AgNPs functionalized from bell pepper extract and quercetin. *Adv. Powder Technol.* **2018**, *29*, 1601–1616. [CrossRef]
57. Hatipoğlu, A.; Baran, A.; Keskin, C.; Baran, M.F.; Eftekhari, A.; Omarova, S.; Janas, D.; Khalilov, R.; Adican, M.T.; Kandemir, S.I. Green synthesis of silver nanoparticles based on the *Raphanus sativus* leaf aqueous extract and their toxicological/microbiological activities. *Environ. Sci. Pollut. Res.* **2023**, 1–13. [CrossRef]
58. Susanti, D.; Haris, M.S.; Taher, M.; Khotib, J. Natural Products-Based Metallic Nanoparticles as Antimicrobial Agents. *Front. Pharmacol.* **2022**, *13*, 895616. [CrossRef]
59. Alsaiari, N.S.; Alzahrani, F.M.; Amari, A.; Osman, H.; Harharah, H.N.; Elboughdiri, N.; Tahoon, M.A. Plant and Microbial Approaches as Green Methods for the Synthesis of Nanomaterials: Synthesis, Applications, and Future Perspectives. *Molecules* **2023**, *28*, 463. [CrossRef]
60. Keskin, C.; Ölçekçi, A.; Baran, A.; Baran, M.F.; Eftekhari, A.; Omarova, S.; Khalilov, R.; Aliyev, E.; Sufianov, A.; Beilerli, A.; et al. Green synthesis of silver nanoparticles mediated *Diospyros kaki* L. (Persimmon): Determination of chemical composition and evaluation of their antimicrobials and anticancer activities. *Front. Chem.* **2023**, *11*, 1187808. [CrossRef]
61. Anand, K.K.H.; Mandal, B.K. Activity study of biogenic spherical silver nanoparticles towards microbes and oxidants. *Spectrochim. Acta Part A Mol. Biomol. Spectrosc.* **2015**, *135*, 639–645. [CrossRef] [PubMed]
62. Nagajyothi, P.; Sreekanth, T.; Lee, J.-I.; Lee, K.D. Mycosynthesis: Antibacterial, antioxidant and antiproliferative activities of silver nanoparticles synthesized from *Inonotus obliquus* (*Chaga mushroom*) extract. *J. Photochem. Photobiol. B Biol.* **2014**, *130*, 299–304. [CrossRef] [PubMed]
63. Stadtman, E.R.; Levine, R.L. Free radical-mediated oxidation of free amino acids and amino acid residues in proteins. *Amino Acids* **2003**, *25*, 207–218. [CrossRef] [PubMed]
64. Chen, T.; Geng, Y.; Wan, H.; Xu, Y.; Zhou, Y.; Kong, X.; Wang, J.; Qi, Y.; Yao, B.; Gao, Z. Facile preparation of Fe3O4/Ag/RGO reusable ternary nanocomposite and its versatile application as catalyst and antibacterial agent. *J. Alloys Compd.* **2021**, *876*, 160153. [CrossRef]
65. Furlan, P.Y.; Fisher, A.J.; Furlan, A.Y.; Melcer, M.E.; Shinn, D.W.; Warren, J.B. Magnetically Recoverable and Reusable Antimicrobial Nanocomposite Based on Activated Carbon, Magnetite Nanoparticles, and Silver Nanoparticles for Water Disinfection. *Inventions* **2017**, *2*, 10. [CrossRef]
66. Qamar, M.A.; Javed, M.; Shahid, S. Designing and investigation of enhanced photocatalytic and antibacterial properties of 3d (Fe, Co, Ni, Mn and Cr) metal-doped zinc oxide nanoparticles. *Opt. Mater.* **2022**, *126*, 112211. [CrossRef]

67. Elakremi, M.; Sillero, L.; Ayed, L.; Mannai, F.; BEN Salem, R.; Labidi, J.; Moussaoui, Y. Chemical composition and biological activity of *Pistacia vera* L. leaves: Beneficial effects of female leaves extract on food products. *Cellul. Chem. Technol.* **2022**, *56*, 309–319. [CrossRef]
68. Senthilkumar, S.R.; Sivakumar, T.; Arulmozhi, K.T.; Mythili, N. FT-IR analysis and correlation studies on the antioxidant activity, total phenolics and total flavonoids of Indian commercial teas (*Camellia sinensis* L.)-A novel approach. *Int. Res. J. Biol. Sci.* **2017**, *6*, 1–7.
69. Shah, A.T.; Din, M.I.; Bashir, S.; Qadir, M.A.; Rashid, F. Green Synthesis and Characterization of Silver Nanoparticles Using *Ferocactus echidne* Extract as a Reducing Agent. *Anal. Lett.* **2015**, *48*, 1180–1189. [CrossRef]
70. Abdelkader, H.; Alzahrani, H.; Al-Ayafi, A.; Al-Mulah, H.; Al-Zubaidi, S. Green synthesis, characterization and antimicrobial activity of biosynthesized silver nanoparticles using *Ziziphus spina-christi* leaf extracts. *Adv. Microbiol. Res.* **2019**, 3, 10. [CrossRef]
71. Shaaban, M.T.; Mohamed, B.S.; Zayed, M.; El-Sabbagh, S.M. Antibacterial, antibiofilm, and anticancer activity of silver-nanoparticles synthesized from the cell-filtrate of *Streptomyces enissocaesilis*. *BMC Biotechnol.* **2024**, *24*, 8. [CrossRef] [PubMed]
72. Kim, S.-M.; Choi, H.-J.; Lim, J.-A.; Woo, M.-A.; Chang, H.-J.; Lee, N.; Lim, M.-C. Biosynthesis of Silver Nanoparticles from *Duchesnea indica* Extracts Using Different Solvents and Their Antibacterial Activity. *Microorganisms* **2023**, *11*, 1539. [CrossRef] [PubMed]
73. Ramasundaram, S.; Manikandan, V.; Vijayalakshmi, P.; Devanesan, S.; Bin Salah, M.; Babu, A.R.; Priyadharsan, A.; Oh, T.H.; Ragupathy, S. Synthesis and investigation on synergetic effect of activated carbon loaded silver nanoparticles with enhanced photocatalytic and antibacterial activities. *Environ. Res.* **2023**, *233*, 116431. [CrossRef] [PubMed]
74. Alzubaidi, A.K.; Al-Kaabi, W.J.; Al Ali, A.; Albukhaty, S.; Al-Karagoly, H.; Sulaiman, G.M.; Asiri, M.; Khane, Y. Green Synthesis and Characterization of Silver Nanoparticles Using *Flaxseed* Extract and Evaluation of Their Antibacterial and Antioxidant Activities. *Appl. Sci.* **2023**, *13*, 2182. [CrossRef]
75. Habib, U.; Ahmad Khan, A.; Rahman, T.U.; Zeb, M.A.; Liaqat, W. Green synthesis, characterization, and antibacterial activity of silver nanoparticles using stem extract of *Zanthoxylum armatum*. *Microsc. Res. Tech.* **2022**, *85*, 3830–3837. [CrossRef] [PubMed]
76. Jamaludin, N.F.M.; Jamali, N.S.; Abdullah, L.C.; Idrus, S.; Engliman, N.S.; Abdul, P.M. Biohydrogen production with utilisation of magnetite nanoparticles embedded in granular activated carbon from coconut shell. *Int. J. Hydrog. Energy* **2023**, *48*, 11695–11708. [CrossRef]
77. Foroutan, R.; Peighambardoust, S.J.; Peighambardoust, S.H.; Pateiro, M.; Lorenzo, J.M. Adsorption of crystal violet dye using activated carbon of lemon wood and activated carbon/Fe_3O_4 magnetic nanocomposite from aqueous solutions: A kinetic, equilibrium and thermodynamic study. *Molecules* **2021**, *26*, 2241. [CrossRef] [PubMed]
78. Yadav, S.; Asthana, A.; Chakraborty, R.; Jain, B.; Singh, A.K.; Carabineiro, S.A.C.; Susan, A.B.H. Cationic Dye Removal Using Novel Magnetic/Activated Charcoal/β-Cyclodextrin/Alginate Polymer Nanocomposite. *Nanomaterials* **2020**, *10*, 170. [CrossRef] [PubMed]
79. Tomke, P.D.; Rathod, V.K. Facile fabrication of silver on magnetic nanocomposite (Fe_3O_4@ Chitosan–AgNP nanocomposite) for catalytic reduction of anthropogenic pollutant and agricultural pathogens. *Int. J. Biol. Macromol.* **2020**, *149*, 989–999. [CrossRef]
80. Wang, Y.; Gao, P.; Wei, Y.; Jin, Y.; Sun, S.; Wang, Z.; Jiang, Y. Silver nanoparticles decorated magnetic polymer composites (Fe_3O_4@PS@Ag) as highly efficient reusable catalyst for the degradation of 4-nitrophenol and organic dyes. *J. Environ. Manag.* **2021**, *278*, 111473. [CrossRef]
81. Acay, H.; Baran, M.F.; Eren, A. Investigating antimicrobial activity of silver nanoparticles produced through green synthesis using leaf extract of common grape (*Vitis vinifera*). *Appl. Ecol. Environ. Res.* **2019**, *17*, 4539–4546. [CrossRef]
82. Zapata, A.; Ramirez-Arcos, S. A Comparative Study of McFarland Turbidity Standards and the Densimat Photometer to Determine Bacterial Cell Density. *Curr. Microbiol.* **2015**, *70*, 907–909. [CrossRef] [PubMed]
83. Srećković, N.Z.; Nedić, Z.P.; Monti, D.M.; D'Elia, L.; Dimitrijević, S.B.; Mihailović, N.R.; Mihailović, V.B. Biosynthesis of silver nanoparticles using *Salvia pratensis* L. aerial part and root extracts: Bioactivity, biocompatibility, and catalytic potential. *Molecules* **2023**, *28*, 1387. [CrossRef] [PubMed]
84. Nagalingam, M.; Rajeshkumar, S.; Balu, S.K.; Tharani, M.; Arunachalam, K. Anticancer and Antioxidant Activity of *Morinda citrifolia* Leaf Mediated Selenium Nanoparticles. *J. Nanomater.* **2022**, *2022*, 1–7. [CrossRef]
85. Abdel-Aty, A.M.; Barakat, A.Z.; Bassuiny, R.I.; Mohamed, S.A. Statistical optimization, characterization, antioxidant and antibacterial properties of silver nanoparticle biosynthesized by saw palmetto seed phenolic extract. *Sci. Rep.* **2023**, *13*, 15605. [CrossRef]
86. Apak, R.; Güçlü, K.; Özyürek, M.; Çelik, S.E. Mechanism of antioxidant capacity assays and the CUPRAC (cupric ion reducing antioxidant capacity) assay. *Microchim. Acta* **2007**, *160*, 413–419. [CrossRef]

pharmaceuticals

Article

Exploring the Antimicrobial, Antioxidant, and Antiviral Potential of Eco-Friendly Synthesized Silver Nanoparticles Using Leaf Aqueous Extract of *Portulaca oleracea* L.

Mohammed Ali Abdel-Rahman [1], Khalid S. Alshallash [2,*], Ahmed M. Eid [1], Saad El-Din Hassan [1], Mutaz Salih [3], Mohammed F. Hamza [4,5] and Amr Fouda [1,*]

1 Botany and Microbiology Department, Faculty of Science, Al-Azhar University, Nasr City, Cairo 11884, Egypt; mohamedali@azhar.edu.eg (M.A.A.-R.); aeidmicrobiology@azhar.edu.eg (A.M.E.); saad_hassan@azhar.edu.eg (S.E.-D.H.)

2 Department of Biology, College of Science, Imam Mohammad Ibn Saud Islamic University (IMSIU), Riyadh 11623, Saudi Arabia

3 Department of Chemistry, College of Science, Imam Mohammad Ibn Saud Islamic University (IMSIU), Riyadh 11623, Saudi Arabia; meamin@imamu.edu.sa

4 School of Nuclear Science and Technology, University of South China, Hengyang 421001, China

5 Nuclear Materials Authority, P.O. Box 530, El-Maadi, Cairo 11728, Egypt

* Correspondence: ksalshallash@imamu.edu.sa (K.S.A.); amr_fh83@azhar.edu.eg (A.F.)

Abstract: Herein, the prospective applications of green fabricated silver nanoparticles (Ag-NPs) within the biomedical field were investigated. The leaf aqueous extract of *Portulaca oleracea* L., a safe, cheap, and green method, was used to fabricate Ag-NPs. The maximum plasmon resonance of synthesized NPs has appeared at 420 nm. The various biomolecules present in the plant extract to assemble spherical Ag-NPs with sizes of 5–40 nm were analyzed using Fourier transform infrared and transmission electron microscopy. The Ag was the major content of the formed Ag-NPs with an atomic percent of 54.95% and weight percent of 65.86%, as indicated by EDX. The crystallographic structure of synthesized NPs was confirmed by the diffraction of the X-ray. The dynamic light scattering exhibits the homogeneity and mono-dispersity nature with a polydispersity index of 0.37 in the colloidal fluid and a zeta potential value of –36 mV. The synthesized Ag-NPs exhibited promising antimicrobial efficacy toward various prokaryotic and eukaryotic pathogenic microorganisms with low MIC values of 12.5 $\mu g\ mL^{-1}$ and 6.25 $\mu g\ mL^{-1}$, respectively. Additionally, the *P. oleracea*-formed Ag-NPs showed optimistic antioxidant activity assessed by DPPH and H_2O_2 assay methods with the highest scavenging percentages of 88.5 ± 2.3% and 76.5 ± 1.7%, respectively, at a concentration of 200 $\mu g\ mL^{-1}$. Finally, the biosynthesized Ag-NPs showed high antiviral properties toward the hepatitis A virus and Cox-B4 with inhibition percentages of 79.16 ± 0.5% and 73.59 ± 0.8%, respectively. Overall, additional research is essential to explore the Ag-NP-based aqueous extract of *P. oleracea* for human health. In the current investigation the use of synthesized Ag-NPs as antimicrobial, antioxidant, and antiviral agents to protect against pathogenic microbes, degenerative diseases caused by various oxidative stresses, and deadly viruses is recommended.

Keywords: green synthesis; *Portulaca oleracea*; silver nanoparticles; biomedical applications; antimicrobial; antiviral activity

1. Introduction

Nanobiotechnology has appeared as an interesting study area for different researchers due to its wide applications in varied sectors such as agriculture, wastewater treatment, catalysis, cloth manufacture, optical and electrical sensors, cosmetics, drug delivery, and medications [1,2]. Nanoparticles (NPs) have unique features such as small sizes (1 nm to 100 nm), thermal conductivity, shapes, plasmonic and magnetic characteristics, and a high surface area to volume [3,4] as compared to counter-bulk materials. Generally, these new active substances are produced by varied methods including chemical, physical, and biological ones. Unfortunately, those synthesized using chemical and physical methods are non-ecofriendly, have a low yield, require harsh environmental conditions, produce toxic by-products, [5,6]. Due to all these drawbacks, the use of NPs formed using chemical and physical methods is not preferred to be applied in medical sectors. Thus, there is an immediate need for methods that are non-toxic, cheap, and environmentally benign for synthesizing NPs. The green synthesis or biosynthesis methods use of natural products from plants or microorganisms, such as yeast, fungi, actinomycetes, bacteria, and algae, to reduce the metal precursor to form nanoscale substances [7,8]. Therefore, environmental friendliness, reduced environmental effect, and the possibility of creating NPs with improved biocompatibility are the reasons for the growing interest in green synthesis processes [9,10].

In this regard, the huge amount of metabolites secreted by the plant are used as reducing agents to form a wide range of NPs such as Au (gold), Ag (silver), Se (selenium), palladium (Pd), ZnO (zinc oxide), CuO (copper oxide) Fe (iron oxide), etc. Plant metabolites, such as phenols, proteins, carbohydrates, alkaloids, flavonoids, terpenoids, and polysaccharides, have dual roles as reducing metal ions to assemble NPs and coating the final nanostructure substances to increase their stability [11]. *Portulaca oleracea*, also called Purslane or Regla in Egypt, belongs to the portulacaceae family. Several reasons distinguished *P. oleracea* from other plant extracts, which led to its selection for the form of silver nanoparticles (Ag-NPs). Among these reasons, *P. oleracea* is well-known for its abundant phytochemical makeup, which includes polysaccharides, omega-3, flavonoids, vitamins (A, B, and C), alkaloids, min erals (Mg, Ca, K, and Fe), and terpenoids [12,13]. These compounds are thought to have powerful reducing and capping capabilities that are ideal for synthesizing nanoparticles. Moreover, *P. oleracea* is extensively spread and readily available. In addition, this plant is characterized by its medicinal importance, suggesting that synthesized Ag-NPs using their aqueous extract will have a wide range of biomedical applications. Due to these reasons, the aqueous extract of *P. oleracea* leaves is used to assemble varied NPs with specific sizes and shapes. For instance, the *P. oleracea*-aqueous extract was used to produce CuO-NPs which revealed promising activities involving antimicrobial, wastewater treatment, and the removal of heavy metals [14]. Additionally, *P. oleracea* was used to synthesize Ag-NPs and ZnO-NPs with anticancer efficacy [15]. Although there have been several investigations to produce Ag-NPs using different plants, the use of *P. oleracea* leaf extract for this objective has received very little attention to fill the gap between the medicinal characteristic of this plant and their efficacy to green synthesis of Ag-NPs.

The Ag-NPs have attracted the researcher's attention due to significant input in various medical, scientific, and industrial fields because of their unique characteristics. Ag-NPs are recognized as non-toxic to humans and extremely toxic to microbes such as bacteria and fungi [16]. In addition to antimicrobial activity, Ag-NPs have a wide range of applications such as wound healing, catalysis, optical properties, coating and conductive ink, drug delivery, cancer therapy, water and air purification, food packaging, diabetic treatment, cloth industry, cosmetics, and photothermal therapy [16,17]. Various published investigations have recorded the efficacy of plant extract to assembly the Ag-NPs, for instance, *Phaseolus vulgaris* [18], *Eugenia roxburghii* [7], *Calophyllum tomentosum* [17], *Malephora lutea* [19], *Crossopteryx febrifuga* [20], *Erythrina suberosa* [21], *Atrocarpus altilis* [22], *Prosopis farcta* [11], and *Psidium guajava* [23]. The synthesized Ag-NPs using plant extracts showed higher activities than those formed using other biological entities due to the varied capping agents that coated NPs and originated from plant extract [24]. In addition to the advantages of green synthesized methods compared to conventional approaches, our study fills a gap in the literature through the development and utilization of *P. oleracea*-synthesized Ag-NPs in various applications, including antimicrobial, antioxidant, and antiviral activities, which have significant implications for healthcare and environmental protection.

The purpose of this study is to contribute to the expanding body of knowledge on green nanotechnology and its participation in the healthcare and environmental sustainability. Following this, the Ag-NPs were synthesized by water extract of the *P. oleracea* and characterized using several analytical tools, including transmission electron microscopy, energy-dispersive ray, X-ray pattern, zeta potential, and UV-vis spectroscopy. The activity of Ag-NPs as an antimicrobial agent toward prokaryotic and eukaryotic pathogenic microorganisms, antioxidant compounds (assessed by DPPH and H_2O_2 assay method), and their effectiveness against HAV and Cox-B4 viruses were investigated.

2. Results and Discussion

2.1. *Portulaca oleracea-Mediated Biosynthesis of Ag-NPs*

Recently, the plant has attracted a lot of attention in the nanotechnology field due to the unusual qualities that it possesses, particularly in the biosynthesis of Ag-NPs [25]. This green synthesis method involves the utilization of plant extracts to convert silver ions into nanostructures that are both stable and biocompatible. Herein, the *P. oleracea* water extract was used in the environmentally friendly manufacture of NPs, and offers several advantages over traditional chemical approaches. One of the most important advantages is that the method is low impact on the environment. In contrast to chemical processes, which frequently involve the use of dangerous chemicals and result in the production of deleterious by-products [14]. Phenolic compounds in addition to flavonoids, alkaloids, and terpenoids are only some of the bioactive chemicals that are abundant in *P. oleracea* [26]. These bioactive compounds facilitate the reduction of Ag ions into Ag-NPs. In addition, the phytochemicals perform the function of capping agents, which prevents the NPs from aggregating and ensures NP stability. Ag-NPs with improved biocompatibility are produced as a result of this green synthesis method, which is not only beneficial to the atmosphere but also environmentally benign. In a similar study, various NPs were fabricated through the reducing action of active metabolites that exist in the water extract of the plant leaves [27,28].

2.2. *Characterization*

2.2.1. Optical Properties Using UV-Vis Spectroscopy

The change from colorless to yellowish-brown visually confirms the successful formation of Ag-NPs using the *P. oleracea* water extract. The shifting of the color can be attributed to the excitation of surface plasmon vibrations in the Ag-NPs, which is responsible for this phenomenon. Surface plasmon resonance (SPR) is a phenomenon that is defined by the collective oscillation of free electrons on the surface of a metal when it is exposed to light [29]. In order to verify the synthesis of NPs and determine their optical characteristics, particularly the maximum SPR, UV-vis spectroscopy is a technique that is commonly utilized. In this investigation, the UV-vis spectrum of *P. oleracea*-mediated Ag-NPs exhibited a prominent absorption peak at 420 nm (Figure 1A). This wavelength corresponds to the maximum absorption of light by the Ag-NPs during the SPR. Similarly, the Ag-NPs produced by *P. oleracea* exhibited their highest specific photo-response (SPR) at a 423 nm wavelength [28]. Dong and coauthors reported that the greenly produced Ag-NPs have a localized SPR in the 400 to 460 nm range [30].

The particular wavelength is related to the electron oscillation frequency on the NPs' surface, which is affected by their size, shape, and environmental factors [31]. A stable colloidal solution and nanoparticles with consistent sizes and shapes are indicated by the sharp and clearly defined peak. According to Taha et al., spherical Ag-NPs often exhibit a maximum SPR peak in the 410–420 nm range [32].

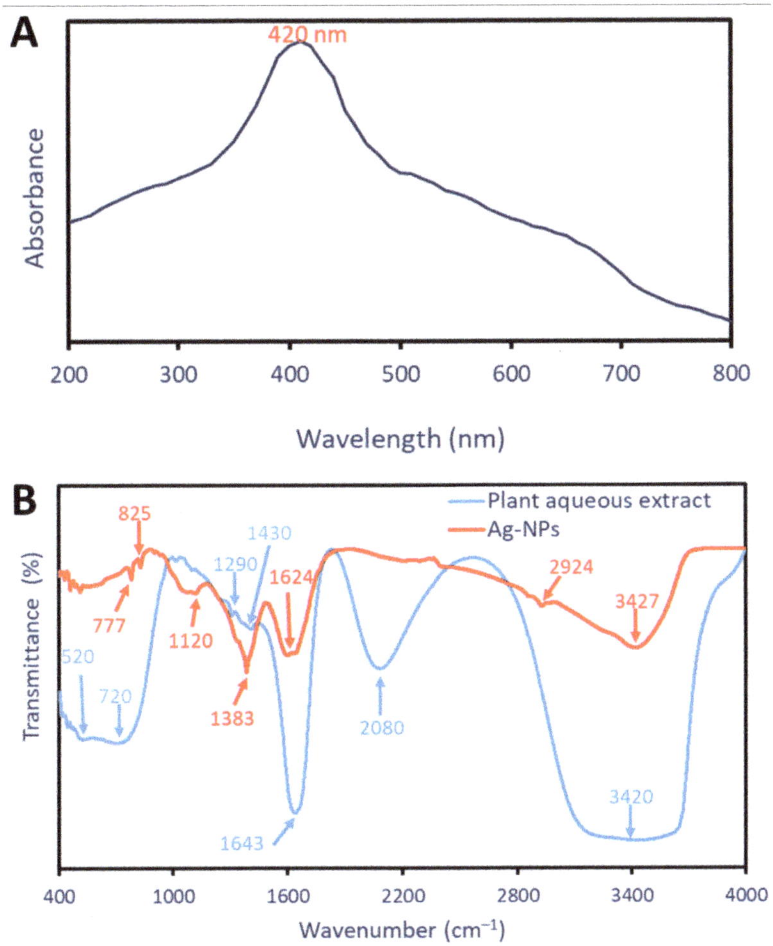

Figure 1. Green synthesized Ag-NPs exhibit maximal SPR at 420 nm in their optical characteristics (**A**), and a variety of functional groups in both the plant aqueous extract and the Ag-NPs (**B**) as shown by FT-IR.

2.2.2. Fourier Transform Infrared (FT-IR)

Fourier transform infrared spectroscopy (FT-IR) is a common method for identifying the functional groups in plant aqueous extracts and how they contribute to NP production. In addition, FT-IR was able to identify biosynthesized NPs with new functional groups or those with shifted presence groups. The *P. oleracea* water extract contains six peaks at 3420, 2080, 1643, 1430, 1290, 720, and 520 cm^{-1} (Figure 1B). These peaks were shifted or formed new peaks after the fabrication of Ag-NPs. The peak at 3420 cm^{-1} was signified by the O-H vibration stretching or N-H groups. These groups are associated with the different compounds such as sugars, phenolic compounds, or organic molecules present in plant aqueous extract [33]. The intensity of this peak decreased as well as their position was shifted at 3427 cm^{-1} after the Ag-NPs form. Moreover, the peak at 2080 cm^{-1} refers to the stretching C≡C due to the existence of alkynes or other compounds containing triple pond in plant aqueous extracts [34]. The peak localized at 1643 cm^{-1} is related to the C=O (carbonyl group) stretching of amides or ketones or refers to the N-H bending of secondary amines [35]. After the production of NPs, this peak was moved to a frequency of 1624 cm^{-1}. The peak at a frequency of 1430 cm^{-1} is linked to the bending C-H vibration of alkanes or methyl groups. These groups indicate the presence of organic compounds containing CH_3 such as certain types of carbohydrates or lipids [36]. The peak at 1290 cm^{-1} is related to the stretching of C-O that is associated with carbohydrates and polysaccharides [37]. The peaks at 720 and 520 cm^{-1} are associated with the out-of-plane bending of the aromatic ring in plant aqueous extract [38]. Because of the manufacturing of Ag-NPs, these peaks moved to the 825 and 777 cm^{-1} frequency range. The presence of new peaks due to Ag-NPs formation was observed at the wavenumbers of 2924, 1383, and 1120 cm^{-1}. The peaks at 2924 and 1383 cm^{-1} signify the stretching vibration of C-H in aliphatic compounds or organic molecules that act as a capping or stabilizing agent during Ag-NPs synthesis [39,40]. Finally, the peak at 1120 cm^{-1} is related to stretching C-O associated with molecules containing oxygen that have a role in the reduction and stabilization of as-formed Ag-NPs [41]. The FTIR spectra, in general, revealed functional groups that are indicative of the participation of plant-based chemicals in the green synthesis process. More specifically, these chemicals were associated with the reduction and stability of Ag-NPs.

2.2.3. Morphological and Elemental Composition Investigation

The physicochemical characterization of Ag-NPs is an important tool for understanding and optimizing their biological properties. To reveal the size, shape, and elemental composition of Ag-NPs, transmission electron microscopy (TEM) and energy-dispersive X-ray spectroscopy (EDX) are crucial instruments. In the present investigation, it was found that the water extract of *P. oleracea* leaves possesses the capability to produce spherical Ag-NPs with diameters ranging from 5 to 40 nm, with an average particle size of 13.75 $\pm$ 8.7 nm (as depicted in Figure 2A,B). Furthermore, as shown in Figure 2A, the TEM investigation shows that the green-produced NPs are neatly distributed and free of aggregation. Similarly, using TEM, the shape and size of the Ag-NPs that were produced by aqueous extract of *Eugenia roxburghii* are spherical, with sizes ranging from 19 to 39 nm with an average of 24 nm [7]. Furthermore, the shape of synthesized Ag-NPs using cell-free supernatant of *Aspergillus flavus* was spherical with a size of 12.5 based on the TEM image [42].

The detection of sizes and shapes of Ag-NPs is an important analysis due to the association between these parameters and biological activity. The surface area and reactivity are both affected by size, while the exposed facets are determined by form. Both of these factors have a substantial impact on the interactions that occur with biological organisms [43]. This finding was consistent with the findings that were recorded by Kambale et al. [20]. Those authors were able to fabricate Ag-NPs using the aqueous extract for three plants, *Senna siamea*, *Crossopteryx febrifuga*, and *Brillantaisia patula*, with sizes of 115 nm, 47 nm, and 45 nm, respectively, based on TEM analysis. *Staphylococcus aureus*, *Pseudomonas aeruginosa*, and *Escherichia coli* are the three bacteria that the authors analyze in order to determine the antibacterial activity of three different Ag-NPs that were created. The data showed that the Ag-NPs formed using an aqueous extract of *B. patula* showed promising antibacterial activity, which was greater than those recorded by *C. febrifuga* and *S. siamea*. The authors suggested that this activity could be related to the smaller size of Ag-NPs formed by *B. patula* than others. In addition, this activity could be attributed to the capping agents which varied between plants. On the other hand, Acharya and co-authors successfully formed spherical and rod-shaped Ag-NPs and investigated their antibacterial activity against different Gram-positive (G+ve) strains and Gram-negative (G-ve) strains [44]. Interestingly, the activity of the spherical shape against pathogenic bacterial strains was greater than the activity recorded by the rod shape.

The EDX analysis was utilized to evaluate the composition of the Ag-NPs that were produced through plant-mediated biosynthesis. As shown, identical absorption peaks were observed at bending energies of 2.8, 3.0, and 3.2 KeV [20]. The EDX analysis reveals that the silver peaks were the most dominant in the sample with weight and atomic percentages of 65.86% and 54.95%, respectively (Figure 2C). The absence of an N peak indicates that the activity of plant aqueous extract reduces all metal precursors ($AgNO_3$) and forms metallic

Ag-NPs. One possible explanation for the appearance of other peaks, such as O, C, and Cl, is that they are caused by the scattering of capping agents that coat the produced Ag-NPs [45].

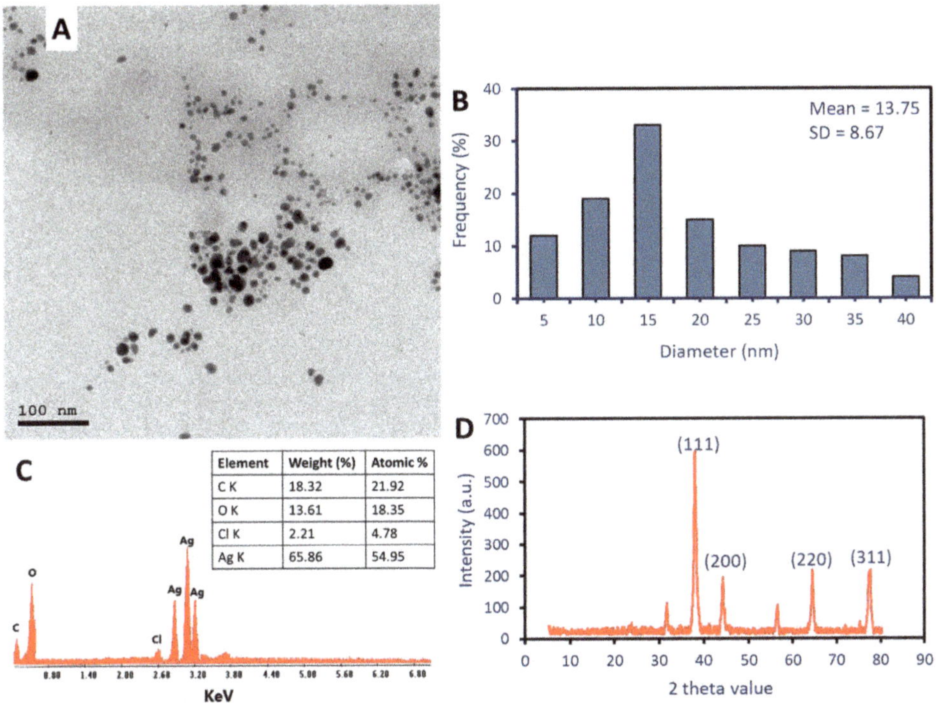

Figure 2. Study of Ag-NPs Profile. The spherical and well-arranged shape of the Ag-NPs is shown in (**A**), the size distribution in (**B**), the composition of the as-formed Ag-NPs is shown in (**C**), and the crystalline nature of the Ag-NPs is validated in (**D**) through XRD.

2.2.4. X-ray Diffraction (XRD)

Analysis using XRD is an essential method for determining the characteristics of Ag-NPs and acquiring an understanding of the structural properties of these particles. At two theta values of 38.14°, 44.19°, 64.45°, and 77.37°, Figure 2D displays four diffraction peaks. These peaks correspond to the Bragg's reflection of (111), (200), (220), and (311), respectively. In accordance with the standard of JCPDS-file No-04-0783, the XRD patterns that were obtained are consistent with the face-centered cubic (FCC) structure of metallic Ag-NPs [20]. These data confirmed the green synthesized Ag-NPs were crystalline in nature [46]. Consistent with the results of the EDX investigation, the presence of extra XRD peaks suggests the presence of impurities originating from the plant extract. The crystallite size of Ag-NPs was determined by employing the Debye–Scherrer equation, which was derived from the XRD examination. The analysis of the data revealed that the typical size of the crystallites was 38 nm. The collected data are consistent with those that determine the average crystallite size of Ag-NPs manufactured by the aqueous extract of *Eugenia roxburghii* to be 35 nm. This calculation is based on the Debye–Scherrer formula [7].

2.2.5. Dynamic Light Scattering (DLS)

DLS analysis indicated that the biosynthesized Ag-NPs in the colloidal fluid had a diameter of 83.5 nm (Figure 3A). As shown, the obtained Ag-NP diameter by DLS was greater than the sizes obtained by TEM and XRD. Similarly, the particle sizes of formed Ag-NPs by the water extract of *Phaseolus vulgaris* were in the ranges of 12–15 nm as detected by TEM, whereas it increased to 188 nm after detection by DLS analysis [18]. These differences could be attributed to a wide range of factors. For instance, the calculation of particle size using DLS is affected by capping agents that originated from plant extract and coated the NPs. Additionally, the DLS measures the hydrodynamic residue of NPs in the hydrated state whereas the TEM measures the particle size as a solid state. Furthermore, the effect of the colloidal fluid's non-uniform distribution of produced nanoparticles on DLS observations is another reason why TEM and DLS computations differ [47].

The mono-dispersity or polydispersity of Ag-NPs in the colloidal fluid was detected using DLS analysis by measuring the polydispersity index (PDI). Honary et al. reported that the particles were described as polydisperse and monodisperse when the PDI value was greater or less than 0.7, respectively [48]. In this investigation, the produced Ag-NPs have a PDI value of 0.37 which indicates the mono-dispersity nature. The obtained results were matched with those reported that the PDI value of Ag-NPs synthesized by *Eucalyptus camaldulensis* was 0.399 which confirmed the mono-dispersity nature [25]. The utilization of monodisperse silver nanoparticles demonstrated superior performance and novel applications in comparison to their polydisperse counterparts.

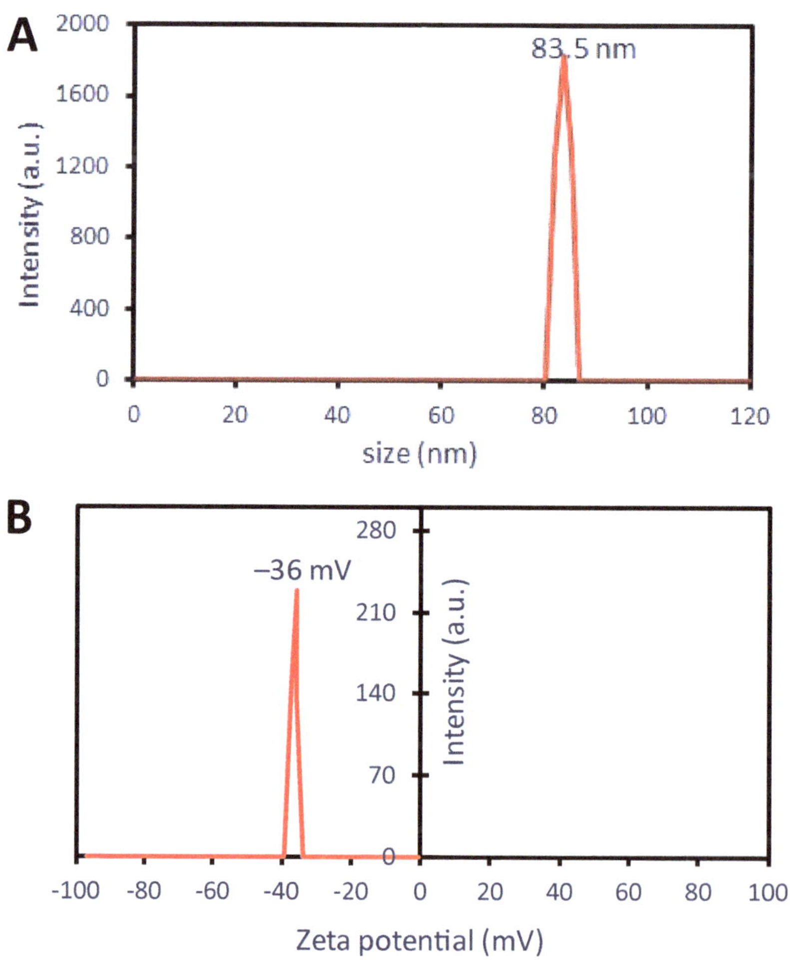

Figure 3. The stability and surface charge of produced Ag-NPs as assessed by dynamic light scattering (**A**), and zeta potential (**B**).

2.2.6. Zeta Potential (ζ)

More investigation about the NPs' stability and surface charge were assessed using ζ-potential analysis. Based on a ζ-potential study, the following information was given as the criteria for classifying the stability of nanoparticles (NPs): ±0–10 mV is a range that correlates to highly unstable particles, whereas ±10–20 mV is considered to be generally stable. On the other hand, ±20–30 mV is considered to be moderate, whereas a value greater than ± 30 mV is considered to be highly stable, respectively [49]. The ζ-value of the Ag-NPs derived from *P. oleracea* plants was −36 mV (Figure 3B), demonstrating that the synthesized NPs are highly stable. In a related work, the ζ-potential of Ag-NPs produced by a water leaves' extract of *Eugenia roxburghii* was found to be −37.8 mV, indicating excellent stability [7]. Capping agents, such as polyphenolic and flavonoid compounds found in water-based extracts, may be responsible for the Ag-NPs surface's negative charge [7]. Curiously, the absence of agglomeration or aggregation over time is prevented by the presence of a single charge, a negative charge, on the surface of the NPs.

2.3. *Antimicrobial Activity*

The agar well diffusion method was used to assess the effectiveness of manufactured Ag-NPs in inhibiting the development of several pathogenic microorganisms, such as *Staphylococcus aureus, Bacillus subtilis, Pseudomonas aeruginosa, Escherichia coli, Candida albicans*, and *Aspergillus brasiliensis.* Results showed that the action of Ag-NPs against several bacteria was concentration-dependent. Consistent with previously published research, Ag-NPs synthesized using aqueous *Psidium guajava* leaf extract had a concentration-dependent antimicrobial effect against a variety of bacteria, including *Bacillus megaterium, B. subtilis, Arthrobacter creatinolyticus, E. coli, Alcaligenes faecalis, Saccharomyces cerevisiae, Aspergillus niger, Acinetobacter baumannii*, and *Rhizopus oryzae* [23]. Additionally, the antimicrobial efficacy of produced Ag-NPs using fruit water extract of *Prosopis farcta* against *Streptococcus pneumonia, Staphylococcus aureus, Salmonella typhi*, and *E. coli* was dose-dependent [11].

In this investigation, the topmost activity was verified for a concentration of 100 μg mL^{-1} with clear zones of 20.7 ± 0.5, 18.7 ± 0.7, 15.3 ± 0.5, 17.4 ± 1.02, 16.3 ± 0.5, and 15.5 ± 0.6 mm for *P. aeruginosa, E. coli, B. subtilis, S. aureus, C. albicans*, and *A. brasiliensis*, respectively ($p \leq 0.001$) (Figure 4). At low concentrations, the diameter of these transparent zones diminished. Clear zones measuring 9.3 ± 0.5, 12.5 ± 0.6, 13.7 ± 0.6, 11.7 ± 0.5, 11.0 ± 0.5, and 10.3 ± 0.6 mm were reduced for the same sequence of microorganisms when the concentration was 12.5 μg mL^{-1}. It is worth noting that for G-ve and *S. aureus* (G+ve), the activity of the produced Ag-NPs remained at a low concentration (6.25 μg mL^{-1}). Likewise, the Ag-NPs produced by the callus aqueous extract of *Solanum incanum* exhibited their maximum antimicrobial activity at a concentration of 200 μg mL^{-1}, inhibiting the growth of *S. aureus, B. subtilis, Klebsiella pneumoniae, E. coli, P. aeruginosa*, and *C. albicans* with zone inhibition values ranging from 19.8 to 24.2 mm. The min imum activity was achieved at a concentration of 12.5 μg mL^{-1} [50].

The min imum inhibitory concentration (MIC) value is a critical point that should be detected before integrating the Ag-NPs into medication. Herein, synthesized Ag-NPs had a MIC value of 12.5 μg mL^{-1} against *B. subtilis* and fungi, with clear zones ranging from 9.3 to 11 mm, and 6.25 μg mL^{-1} against *S. aureus* and G-ve (*P. aeruginosa* and *E. coli*), with clear zones ranging from 9.7 to 11.3 mm (Table 1). The collected data were compared to the MIC of Ag-NPs produced by *Streptomyces antimycoticus*, which was 25 μg mL^{-1} for *B. subtilis* and *E. coli* and 12.5 μg mL^{-1} for *S. aureus* and *Salmonella typhi* [51].

It was found that the produced Ag-NPs had better activity against G-ve bacteria than G+ve. Bacterial cell walls differ in structure, which is associated with this action. G+ve bacteria are unable to absorb Ag-NPs because their cell walls are thick with peptidoglycan. In contrast, G-ve bacteria cell walls contain just thin coatings of peptidoglycan, which allows them to facilitate NP ingress and, ultimately, renders nearly all intracellular macromolecules inoperable [25]. This phenomenon is considered one of the antibacterial mechanisms of NPs. Furthermore, the superior antibacterial activity of Ag-NPs toward G-ve bacteria could be related to the presence of more lipopolysaccharides that increase the negatively charged on the surface of G-ve bacteria and hence enhance the electrostatic attraction with Ag-NPs that are positively charged [52]. Moreover, the efflux pump that is responsible for the removal of harmful compounds from the inside of the cells may differ in G-ve bacteria compared to G+ve. The green formed Ag-NPs can overcome the efflux pump mechanism in G-ve bacteria, leading to accumulation inside the cells and hence enhance their antibacterial activity [53].

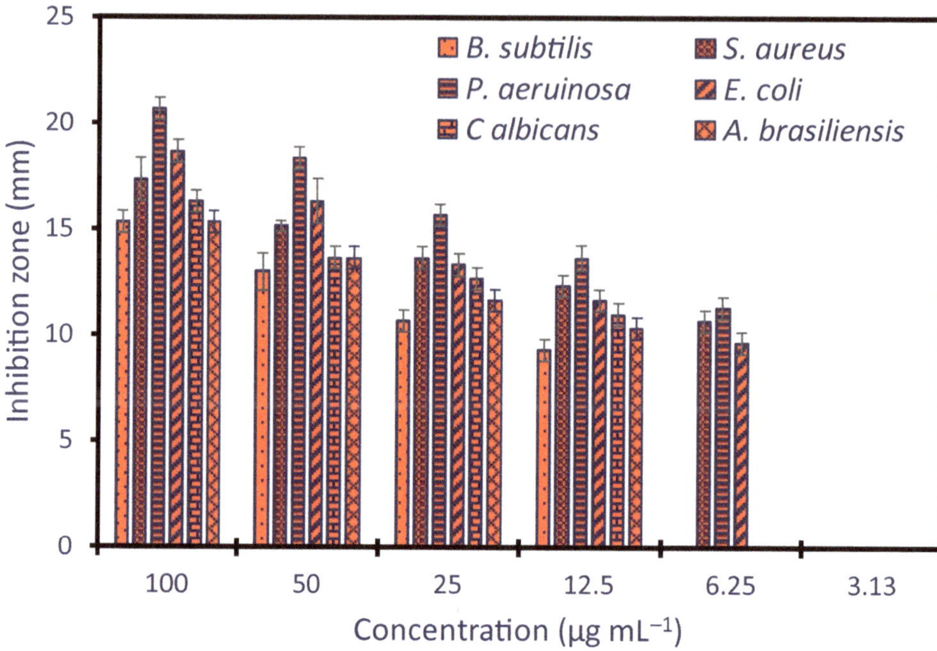

Figure 4. The antimicrobial efficacy of Ag-NPs derived from plants against G+ve bacteria (*B. subtilis* and *S. aureus*), G-ve bacteria (*P. aeruginosa* and *E. coli*), as well as unicellular (*C. albicans*) and multicellular (*A. brasiliensis*) fungi.

Table 1. The MIC values with inhibition clear zones of Ag-NPs against different test organisms.

Test Organism	MIC Value ($\mu g\ mL^{-1}$)	Clear Zone (mm)
B. subtilis	12.5	9.3 ± 0.5
S. aureus	6.25	10.7 ± 0.6
P. aeruginosa	6.25	11.3 ± 0.5
E. coli	6.25	9.7 ± 0.5
C. albicans	12.5	11.0 ± 0.5
A. brasiliensis	12.5	10.3 ± 0.5

Another antimicrobial mechanism is the release of Ag^+ ions inside the cells upon Ag-NP entrance. Reactive oxygen species (ROS) are produced more readily as a result, which can harm the respiratory system of cells and cause cell death [30]. Furthermore, interacting with NPs damages the cytoplasmic membrane's selective permeability function [1]. Ag-NPs can rupture the sterol that is present in the cell wall of *Candida* by blocking the ergosterol pathway synthesis leading death of the cells [54]. The activity of Ag-NPs against multicellular fungi could be attributed to various mechanisms such as the detachment of the toxic ions (Ag^+) and their deleterious impact on macromolecules and cytoplasmic membrane function, inhibition of the germination of conidia due to the reaction of NPs with it, disrupt the chain of electron transport as a result of dysfunction of selective permeability function, and destroy the mitochondria due to high production of ROS (oxidative stress) [1].

2.4. Antioxidant Activity

Discovery novel substances exhibiting antioxidant action is of utmost significance in the health and medicine sectors. Cancer, heart disease, and neurological disorders are just a few of the many diseases that free radicals can cause [55]. Therefore, finding new antioxidant molecules is vital in the development of new treatments and new strategies to prevent these diseases. NPs are candidates as promising antioxidant compounds due to their uncommon physicochemical features, such as small sizes and the ratio between their surface and volume, which improve their activity and enhance their interaction with biological systems to scavenge free radicals [32,56]. In this investigation, two methods, namely DPPH and H_2O_2 assay methods, were used to evaluate the efficacy of green synthesized Ag-NPs in scavenging the free radicals (Figure 5), the antioxidant capacity of Ag-NPs was concentration-dependent, the activity was increased with high NP concentration and vice versa [17].

Using the DPPH assay method, the highest scavenging activity was recorded for 200 $\mu g\ mL^{-1}$ of Ag-NPs with percentages of 88.5 ± 2.3% which is not significant ($p \geq 0.001$) as compared with ascorbic acid (89.3 ± 2.1%) as a positive control (Figure 5A). Additionally, this finding was recorded for a concentration of 100 $\mu g\ mL^{-1}$, the antioxidant activity between Ag-NPs and ascorbic acid was not significant with scavenging percentages of 84.0 ± 1.5% and 85.1 ± 1.1%, respectively. The lowest scavenging activity was recorded for a concentration of 0.78 $\mu g\ mL^{-1}$ with a percentage of 6.2 ± 1.1% followed by a concentration of 1.56 $\mu g\ mL^{-1}$ with a percentage of 33.5 ± 1.5% as compared to ascorbic acid at the same concentrations (10.8 ±2.3% and 40.6 ± 2.7%, respectively) (Figure 5A). The antioxidant activity of Ag-NPs fabricated by *Psidium guajava* water extract was assessed by DPPH and did not show any significant differences at concentrations 100 and 120 $\mu g\ mL^{-1}$ as compared to the control (ascorbic acid) [23]. The authors reported that the scavenging percentages due to 100 and 120 $\mu g\ mL^{-1}$ of Ag-NPs were 83.6% and 89.0%, respectively as compared to ascorbic acid showed scavenging percentages of 89.0% and 90% at the same concentrations. Interestingly, the results of our investigation (83.9%) were higher than those recorded by Ravichandran et al., who found that Ag-NPs manufactured using the leaf extract of *Atrocarpus altilis* had radical scavenging capabilities for DPPH of 79.79% [22].

The H_2O_2 scavenging assay method (Figure 5B) was matched with the DPPH assay method in the concentration-dependent phenomenon, but it differs in that there are significant differences between the scavenging activity of Ag-NPs and ascorbic acid in all treatments. As shown, the highest Ag-NPs scavenging activity was recorded for a concentration of 200 $\mu g\ mL^{-1}$ with percentages of 76.5 ± 1.7%, and the lowest activity was showed at a concentration of 0.78 with percentages of 5.3 ± 1.1% as compared with ascorbic acid (81.6 ± 1.3% and 11.3 ± 2.7% for the same concentrations, respectively). At a concentration of 100 $\mu g\ mL^{-1}$, our findings were in line with those that previously indicated that the H_2O_2 scavenging activity for Ag-NPs produced using the aqueous extract of *Calophyllum tomentosum's* leaves was 83.9% and that of ascorbic acid was 79.7% [17].

The concentration of active compounds to scavenging 50% is defined as effective concentration (EC_{50}). The detection of EC50 is an important factor for investigating and comparing the antioxidant activity of different molecules, optimizing therapeutic concentrations, safety assessment, and cost-effectiveness for the development of a new drug [57]. Herein, the EC50 of green synthesized Ag-NPs and ascorbic acid were (10.4 and 5.7 $\mu g\ mL^{-1}$) and (23.9 and 11.9 $\mu g\ mL^{-1}$) for DPPH and H_2O_2 assay methods, respectively. Recently, the EC50 value of Ag-NPs formed using *Erythrina suberosa* was 30.04 $\mu g\ mL^{-1}$ based on the DPPH method [21].

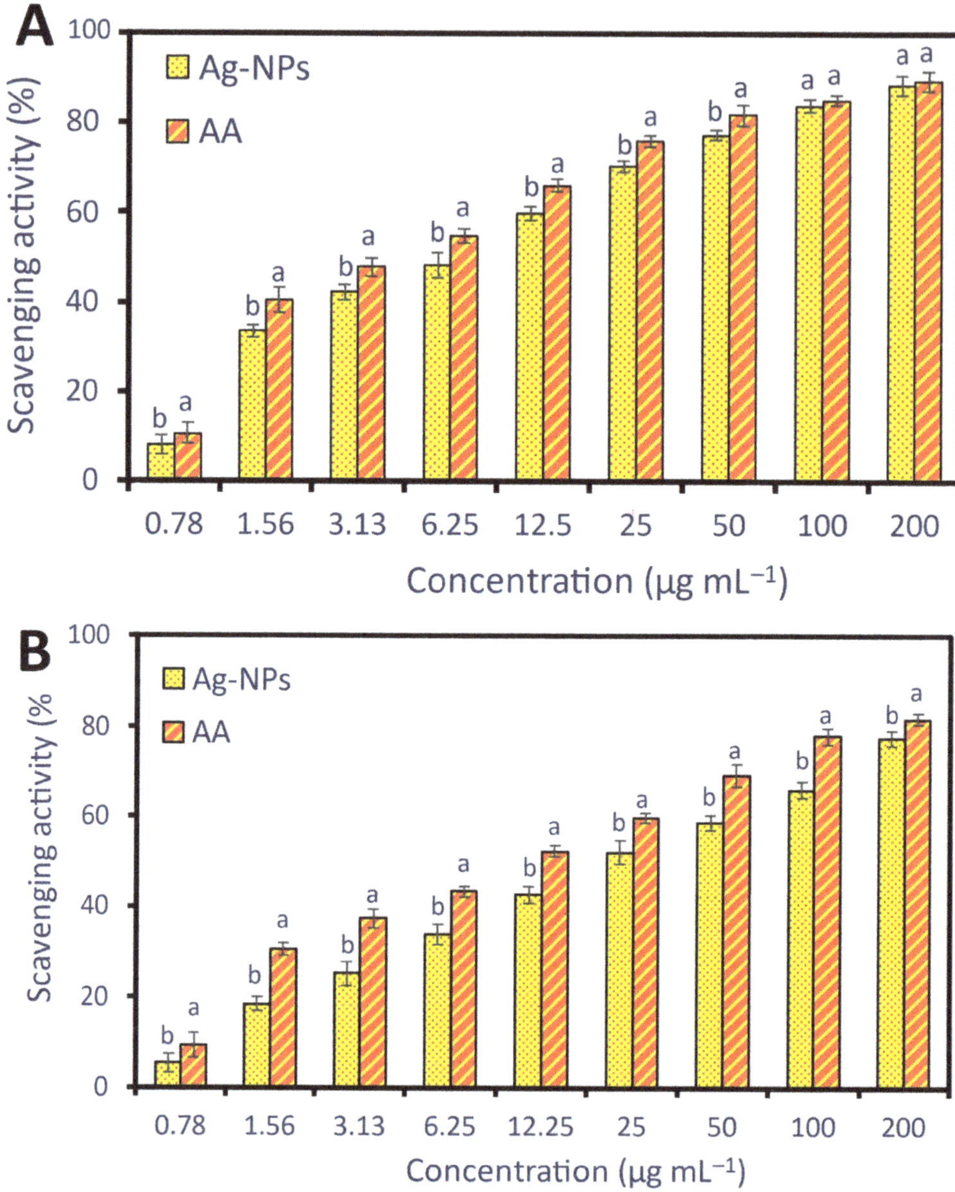

Figure 5. Antioxidant activity of plant-based Ag-NPs assessed using DPPH assay method (**A**) and H_2O_2 assay method (**B**). AA denotes the ascorbic acid (control). Different letters in the same concentration indicate the data are significant ($p \leq 0.05$).

The antioxidant activity of fabricated NPs using biological methods, especially plant extracts, is better than the activity of those synthesized by chemical and physical methods. It is possible that this phenomenon is due to the capping agent that is derived from the plant extract. This capping agent includes phenolic chemicals, flavonoids, alkaloids, and polysaccharides, all of which enhance and multiply the antioxidant capacity of NPs [23,24]. The antioxidant potential of Ag-NPs can be explained by their ability to quench or scavenge free radicals by donating or accepting electrons. The reason behind this is that, depending on the circumstances of the reaction, silver can exist in two oxidation states: Ag^+ and Ag^{2+} [58]. Overall, the green synthesized Ag-NPs can be utilized as an antioxidant agent for safe protecting human health against degenerative disease caused by various oxidative stresses.

2.5. Antiviral Activity

In this investigation, the efficacy of *P. oleracea*-based Ag-NPs to fight the growth of HAV and Coxsackie B virus was evaluated. First, the cytotoxic potential of Ag-NPs against normal Vero cell lines, as host cells, was investigated to detect the MNTC which is 250 μg mL^{-1}. In another investigation, the MNTC value of Ag-NPs formed using an aqueous extract of *Lampranthus coccineus* and *Malephora lutea* was detected by investigating the cytotoxic efficacy against Vero cells [19]. The authors reported that the MNTC was 260.3 and 520.6 and μg mL^{-1} for Ag-NPs produced by *M. lutea* and *L. coccineus*, respectively.

The MTT antiviral assay method showed that the viability of Vero cells inoculated with viruses and treated with Ag-NPs was increased from (34.25 ± 1.4% and 23.85 ± 0.5%) to (86.3 ± 0.8% and 79.89 ± 0.7%) for HAV and Cox-B4, respectively (Figure 6). The obtained results mean the Vero cell viability after being treated with HAV or Cox-B4 viruses in the presence of green synthesized Ag-NPs was increased with the value of 2.52- and 3.35-fold as compared with the viability in the presence of viruses and absence of NPs. On the other hand, data analysis reveals that the as-formed Ag-NPs have antiviral effects with percentages of 79.16% and 73.59% for HAV and Cox-B4, respectively (Figure 6).

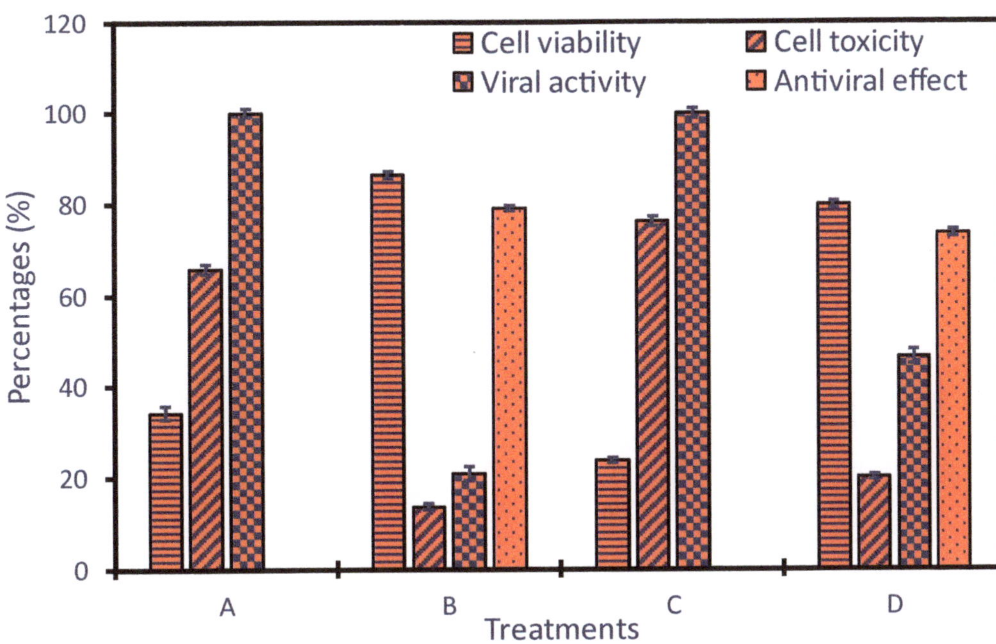

Figure 6. Hepatitis A (HAV) and Cox-B4 virus antiviral activities of Ag-NPs produced using plant extract. (**A**) is the Vero host cells treated with HAV, (**B**) is Vero cells treated with HAV in the presence of Ag-NPs, (**C**) is the Vero cells treated with Cox-B4, and (**D**) is the Vero cells inoculated with Cox-B4 in the presence of Ag-NPs.

The antiviral efficacy of NPs can be attributed to different mechanisms such as the interaction between viruses and cells leading to prohibiting the infection, preventing the entrance of viruses to the host cells through the interact of NPs with cell surfaces or specific receptors, inhibiting the viruses' replications, prevent the spread of viruses, enhance the oxidative stress through production of ROS, cell apoptosis, and enhance the immune response of the host cells [59,60]. The ability of Ag-NPs to block virus attachment to host cells and hence cell damage is achieved by their interaction with the viral envelope, receptors, or surface proteins. NPs have the potential to block virus replications inside the host cells by the function of nucleic acids (DNA or RNA) and blocking the essential enzymes needed for virus replications [61]. In addition, when exposed to NPs, infected cells may release ROS which has damage effects on viral DNA, proteins, and lipid membranes, ultimately hindering the virus's capacity to multiply and infect cells [62]. It is also possible for Ag-NPs to influence the host's immunological response and boost the host's immunity by increasing the synthesis of interferons and proinflammatory cytokines that are used to identify and react to viral infections [63]. With the help of this enhanced immune response, infected cells can be eliminated, and the spread of viruses can be controlled. Ag-NPs can hinder the apoptotic pathways and hence give more time to the immune system to combat the pathogens [63]. Some authors reported that the antiviral activity of green synthesized NPs can be affected by coating agents such as flavonoids, alkaloids, and terpenoids that enhance the antiviral potential [64].

3. Materials and Methods

3.1. Materials

To synthesize Ag-NPs in an eco-friendly manner, analytical grade (99%) silver nitrate ($AgNO_3$) obtained from Sigma Aldrich (Darmstadt, Germany) was used. For the antimicrobial assay, coded test strains were obtained from the ATCC. Cox-B4 and HAV, obtained from the Holding Company for Biological Products and Vaccines (VACSERA) in Doki, Giza, Egypt, were the viruses tested in the anti-viral assay.

3.2. Plant-Synthesized Ag-NPs

The *P. oleracea* plant leaves were collected, washed with tap water, and left to dry and then grinded to form powder. Following this, the formed powder was mixed with distilled H_2O (5 g/100 mL) and subjected to heating for 60 min at 40 °C under agitation conditions (150 rpm). To obtain the supernatant for the production of Ag-NPs, the mixture was centrifuged at 10,000 rpm for 7 min . For biosynthesis, $AgNO_3$ (16.9 mg) was mixed with 80 mL dH_2O followed by adding 20 mL of plant water extract to achieve a final concentration of 1 mM of Ag-NPs. The previous solution underwent stirring conditions for one hour at 150 rpm and the pH of the mixture was 8 by adding NaOH (1 M) drop-by-drop. After that, the solution remained at room temperature overnight to confirm a complete reduction of metal precursor to form a nanostructure which was detected by color change from colorless to yellowish brown.

3.3. Characterization

To detect the surface plasmon resonance (SPR) of the produced Ag-NPs, ultraviolet-visible spectroscopy (JENWAY 6305, Cole-Parmer, Stafford, UK) was used to measure the absorbance of the resultant color from 200 to 600 nm. Furthermore, the plant water extract's functional groups and their contributions to the bio-reduction of $AgNO_3$ to Ag-NPs were determined using Fourier transform infrared (FT-IR, Cary 630, Tokyo, Japan). Here, a disk containing 300 mg of the Ag-NPs was compressed into a mixture of KBr and scanned over a broad spectrum of wavenumbers (400–4000 cm^{-1}) [7]. Transmission electron microscopy (TEM, JEOL 1010, Tokyo, Japan) was used to characterize the size and shape of the NPs. The carbon/copper TEM grid was filled with the NPs solution until full adsorption occurred. Before analysis, gent touched of the loaded grid with blotting paper was performed to remove any surplus solution. Energy-dispersive X-ray (EDX, JEOL, JSM6360LA, Tokyo, Japan) was used to map the elemental composition of the produced Ag-NPs [65].

An X-ray diffraction pattern (XRD, X' Pert Pro, Philips, Eindhoven, The Netherlands) was employed to investigate the crystalline structure of the Ag-NPs that were produced.

Under the settings of 40 kV voltage, 30 mA current, and a Cu-Kα radiation source with a λ value of 1.54 Å, the 2θ values of the XRD pattern were observed within the range of 5–80°. In addition, the average crystallite size of the Ag-NPs was calculated using the Debye–Scherrer equation utilized during the XRD investigation as follows:

$$D = \frac{0.9 \times 1.54}{\beta \cos \theta} \quad (1)$$

where 0.9 is the constant of Scherrer's, 1.54 is the radiation value, β is half of the maximum intensity, and θ is the Bragg's angle.

Zeta potential (ζ) analysis and dynamic light scattering (DLS) were used to determine the surface charge and size distribution of Ag-NPs in the colloidal solution, respectively. To avoid any shadows from appearing during the examination, the produced Ag-NPs were dissolved in high pure water [47]. The surface charge of the Ag-NPs was measured using the Malvern Zetasizer, an instrument manufactured by Nano-ZS and located in Malvern, UK.

3.4. *Pharmacological Activities*

3.4.1. Antimicrobial Activity

Different prokaryotic pathogenic strains designated as G+ve bacteria (*Staphylococcus aureus* ATCC6528 and *Bacillus subtilis* ATCC6533) and G-ve bacteria (*Pseudomonas aeruginosa* ATCC9027 and *Escherichia coli* ATCC8739) as well as eukaryotic strains represented by unicellular fungi (*Candida albicans* ATCC10231), and multicellular fungi (*Aspergillus brasiliensis* ATCC16404), were employed to investigate the antimicrobial potential of plant-based Ag-NPs. The agar well diffusion method was used to investigate this efficacy [66]. At first, nutrient agar, sabouraud dextrose agar, and Capek's Dox agar plates were used to refresh the growth of selected bacterial, yeast, and *Aspergillus* strains, respectively. The inoculated plates were put in an incubator for 24 h at 35 ± 2 °C/or 72 h at 28 °C for bacteria/yeast and *A. brasiliensis*, respectively. After that, the newly cultured bacterial and yeast strains were reinoculated on the surface of plates containing Muller–Hinton agar media for bacteria and yeast, and Capek's Dox agar media for *Aspergillus* strain. Using a sterile cork borer, four wells of 0.6 mm in diameter were made on each agar plate. After that, 100 µL of various Ag-NP concentrations (200, 100, 50, 25, and 12.5 µg mL^{-1}) were added to these wells. The plates were then placed in the refrigerator for an hour before being incubated at a temperature of 35 ± 2 °C for 24 h. A well was then treated with DMSO (a solvent system, $\geq$ 99.7%, Merck, Darmstadt, Germany) to serve as a control. As part of the data collection process, the diameter of the clear zone around each well was measured in millimeters (mm). A distinct zone surrounding the well-formed by the lowest concentration of green-synthesized Ag-NPs was used to determine the min imum inhibitory concentration (MIC) value. The experiment was achieved in triplicate.

3.4.2. Antioxidant Activity

DPPH Assay Method

The DPPH (2,2-diphenyl-1-picrylhydrazyl (2,2-diphenyl-1-picrylhydrazyl) technique was utilized to evaluate the antioxidant potential of produced Ag-NPs. By employing this particular technique, a range of quantities (ranging from 0.78 to 200 µg mL^{-1}) of Ag-NPs were prepared in Milli-Q H_2O. A test tube containing one mL of DPPH (dissolved in methanol), 450 µL of Tris-HCl buffer (pH of 7.4), and one mL of the Ag-NPs solution has been made to achieve the analysis. The mixture was thoroughly mixed and put in an incubator for 30 min ., at 37 °C, and with a shaken condition of 100 rpm in the dark condition. The same conditions and concentrations were used in an additional series of experiments with ascorbic acid serving as the positive control. In the same experimental setup, a test tube containing DPPH and tris-buffer in the absence of any treatment (Ag-NPs or ascorbic acid) was used as a negative control. At the end of the incubation period, the absorbance of the generated color was determined at 517 nm. To determine the free radical scavenging percentages, the following formulae were utilized [57]:

$$\text{DPPH scavenging \%} = \frac{\text{absorbance of control} - \text{absorbance of treatment}}{\text{absorbance of control}} \times 100 \quad (2)$$

H_2O_2 Assay Method

The antioxidant efficacy of formed Ag-NPs was also evaluated using hydrogen peroxide [H_2O_2, 10 mM, dissolved in phosphate buffer (pH = 7.4 and 0.1 M)]. Different Ag-NP concentrations were prepared as follows: 0.78 to 200 μg mL^{-1}. In this method, one mL of Ag-NP solution was mixed well with 2 mL of the prepared H_2O_2 before incubated for 10 min at 37 °C. The JENWAY 6305 spectrophotometer was used to monitor the absorbance of the produced color at 230 nm. The experiment was conducted with the control, which was an Ag-NPs solution devoid of H_2O_2. The following formula was used to compute the H_2O_2 scavenging activity:

$$H_2O_2\text{scavenging \%} = \frac{A - B}{A} \times 100 \quad (3)$$

where A and B were the absorbances of control and treatment, respectively.

3.4.3. Antiviral Activity

Detection of Maximum Non-Toxic Concentration (MNTC) of Biosynthesized Ag-NPs

The biosynthesized Ag-NPs were integrated into a 96-well plate with a normal Vero cell which displayed as host cells to calculate the MNTC using MTT assay. To create a confluent sheet of Vero cells, 10^4 cells/well in 100 μL growth media were cultured in a CO_2 incubator (5%) at 37 °C for 24 h. Post-growth media removal before being treated the Vero cells with Ag-NPs concentrations (1000, 500, 250, 125, 62.5, and 31.25 μg mL^{-1}). DMSO-dissolved generated NPs were tested in triplicate at each concentration. Untreated cells were used as the control. The treated plates were kept in a CO_2 incubator for 48 h at 37 °C in a 5%. Afterward, 20 μL of MTT solution (5 mg mL^{-1}/phosphate buffer) was added to each well, stirred for 5 min at 150 rpm, and then placed in a CO_2 incubator at 37 °C for 5 h. Final step: the well contents were discarded, and 200 μL DMSO were added per well to dissolve formazan crystals (MTT metabolic product). ELIZA microplate readers were used to measure the treated plates' OD at 570 nm.

The viability of the cells was measured using the next equation:

$$\text{Cell viability (\%)} = \frac{A}{B} \times 100 \quad (4)$$

where A and B are the absorbance of treatment and control, respectively.

On the other hand, the toxicity of the cells was measured using the next equation:

$$\text{Cell toxicity (\%)} = \text{cell viability} - 100 \quad (5)$$

Then, the MNTC was calculated by graphing the relationship between the toxicity percentages and various Ag-NP concentrations. Additionally, the CC50, which is defined as the Ag-NP concentration needed for 50% growth inhibition of Vero cells was measured by regression analysis.

Antiviral Activity

Ag-NPs were tested for antiviral activity against the hepatitis A virus (HAV) and Coxsackie B virus. First, host Vero cells were grown into a confluent sheet. In parallel, the viral suspension was incubated with non-toxic NPs (1:1, v/v) at 35 ± 2 °C for one hour. Finally, 100 μL of the virus-Ag-NPs mixture was applied to each Vero cell well. Three independent wells with only Vero cells represented the control (non-infected cells). Shaking for 5 min at 150 rpm was performed to mix the content of the plate, which was then incubated overnight at 37 °C with 5% CO_2. After applying the MTT solution, formazan crystal absorbance was measured to determine Vero cell viability. The antiviral activity was determined by comparing the optical density of infected and uninfected cellular viabilities [67].

3.5. Data Analysis

Statistical analysis was performed on the collected data using SPSS version 18 (SPSS Inc., Chicago, IL, USA). Before using Tukey's multiple comparison test, an analysis of variance (ANOVA) was performed to compare different samples.

4. Conclusions

The "green synthesis" of Ag-NPs from the *P. oleracea* water extract provides an environmentally friendly and efficient process for safe NP production. The morphological study confirms the presence of homogeneous Ag-NPs with 5–40 nm sizes. Silver plays a dominant role, according to EDX. The XRD confirms that they are crystals. The effect of capping agents on dynamic light scattering reveals a bigger hydrodynamic diameter. The results of the zeta potential test show that the material is very stable and has a negative surface charge. The formed Ag-NPs are particularly effective against G-ve bacteria, the antibacterial action of the Ag-NPs is concentration-dependent. Furthermore, they can scavenge free radicals and show antioxidant characteristics. The antiviral effects of Ag-NPs against hepatitis A and Coxsackie B viruses are also encouraging. While these findings are promising, the current study needs more investigation to explore the role of plant active metabolites in the fabrication of Ag-NPs. The antimicrobial activity against wide range of multicellular fungi needs more studies. In addition, other methods to clarify the antioxidant activity and investigate their antiviral against other human viruses need more explanations.

Author Contributions: Conceptualization, A.M.E., S.E.-D.H. and A.F.; methodology, A.M.E., M.F.H. and A.F.; software, K.S.A., A.M.E., S.E.-D.H., M.A.A.-R., M.S. and A.F.; validation, K.S.A., M.A.A.-R., M.S. and A.F.; formal analysis, K.S.A., A.M.E., S.E.-D.H., M.A.A.-R., M.S., M.F.H. and A.F.; investigation, A.M.E., S.E.-D.H., M.A.A.-R. and A.F.; resources, K.S.A., M.S., M.F.H. and A.F.; data curation, K.S.A., A.M.E., S.E.-D.H., M.A.A.-R., M.F.H. and A.F.; writing—original draft preparation, K.S.A., A.M.E., S.E.-D.H., M.A.A.-R., M.S., M.F.H. and A.F.; writing—review and editing, K.S.A., A.M.E., S.E.-D.H., M.A.A.-R., M.F.H. and A.F.; supervision, K.S.A., S.E.-D.H., M.A.A.-R. and A.F.; project administration, K.S.A., A.M.E., S.E.-D.H., M.A.A.-R., M.S., M.F.H. and A.F.; funding acquisition, K.S.A., M.S. and A.F.; All authors have read and agreed to the published version of the manuscript.

Funding: This work was supported and funded by the Deanship of Scientific Research at Imam Mohammad Ibn Saud Islamic University (IMSIU) (grant number IMSIU-RP23027).

Institutional Review Board Statement: Not applicable.

Informed Consent Statement: Not applicable.

Data Availability Statement: The data presented in this study are available on request from the corresponding authors.

Acknowledgments: The authors extend their appreciation to the Botany and Microbiology Department, Faculty of Science, Al-Azhar University, Cairo, Egypt, for the great support in the achievement and publication of this research work. Furthermore, the authors acknowledge the support from Imam Mohammad Ibn Saud Islamic University Riyadh, Saudi Arabia.

Conflicts of Interest: The authors declare no conflicts of interest.

References

1. Cruz-Luna, A.R.; Cruz-Martínez, H.; Vásquez-López, A.; Medina, D.I. Metal nanoparticles as novel antifungal agents for sustainable agriculture: Current advances and future directions. *J. Fungi* **2021**, *7*, 1033. [CrossRef] [PubMed]
2. Malik, S.; Muhammad, K.; Waheed, Y. Nanotechnology: A Revolution in Modern Industry. *Molecules* **2023**, *28*, 661. [CrossRef] [PubMed]
3. Alhalili, Z. Metal Oxides Nanoparticles: General Structural Description, Chemical, Physical, and Biological Synthesis Methods, Role in Pesticides and Heavy Metal Removal through Wastewater Treatment. *Molecules* **2023**, *28*, 3086. [CrossRef]
4. Khan, I.; Saeed, K.; Khan, I. Nanoparticles: Properties, applications and toxicities. *Arab. J. Chem.* **2019**, *12*, 908–931. [CrossRef]

5. Kulkarni, A.G.; De Britto, S.; Jogaiah, S. 18—Economic considerations and limitations of green synthesis vs chemical synthesis of nanomaterials. In *Advances in Nano-Fertilizers and Nano-Pesticides in Agriculture*; Jogaiah, S., Singh, H.B., Fraceto, L.F., Lima, R.D., Eds.; Woodhead Publishing: Sawston, UK, 2021; pp. 459–468.
6. Abdo, A.M.; Fouda, A.; Eid, A.M.; Fahmy, N.M.; Elsayed, A.M.; Khalil, A.M.A.; Alzahrani, O.M.; Ahmed, A.F.; Soliman, A.M. Green synthesis of Zinc Oxide Nanoparticles (ZnO-NPs) by Pseudomonas aeruginosa and their activity against pathogenic microbes and common house mosquito, *Culex pipiens*. *Materials* **2021**, *14*, 6983. [CrossRef] [PubMed]
7. Giri, A.K.; Jena, B.; Biswal, B.; Pradhan, A.K.; Arakha, M.; Acharya, S.; Acharya, L. Green synthesis and characterization of silver nanoparticles using *Eugenia roxburghii* DC. extract and activity against biofilm-producing bacteria. *Sci. Rep.* **2022**, *12*, 8383. [CrossRef]
8. Singh, J.; Dutta, T.; Kim, K.-H.; Rawat, M.; Samddar, P.; Kumar, P. 'Green' synthesis of metals and their oxide nanoparticles: Applications for environmental remediation. *J. Nanobiotechnology* **2018**, *16*, 84. [CrossRef]
9. Amin, M.A.; Abu-Elsaoud, A.M.; Nowwar, A.I.; Abdelwahab, A.T.; Awad, M.A.; Hassan, S.E.-D.; Boufahja, F.; Fouda, A.; Elkelish, A. Green synthesis of magnesium oxide nanoparticles using endophytic fungal strain to improve the growth, metabolic activities, yield traits, and phenolic compounds content of *Nigella sativa* L. *Green Process. Synth.* **2024**, *13*, 20230215. [CrossRef]
10. Radulescu, D.M.; Surdu, V.A.; Ficai, A.; Ficai, D.; Grumezescu, A.M.; Andronescu, E. Green Synthesis of Metal and Metal Oxide Nanoparticles: A Review of the Principles and Biomedical Applications. *Int. J. Mol. Sci.* **2023**, *24*, 15397. [CrossRef]
11. Salari, S.; Esmaeilzadeh Bahabadi, S.; Samzadeh-Kermani, A.; Yosefzaei, F. In-vitro Evaluation of Antioxidant and Antibacterial Potential of GreenSynthesized Silver Nanoparticles Using *Prosopis farcta* Fruit Extract. *Iran. J. Pharm. Res. IJPR* **2019**, *18*, 430–455.
12. Uddin, M.K.; Juraimi, A.S.; Hossain, M.S.; Nahar, M.; Un, A.; Ali, M.E.; Rahman, M. Purslane weed (*Portulaca oleracea*): A prospective plant source of nutrition, omega-3 fatty acid, and antioxidant attributes. *Sci. World J.* **2014**, *2014*, 951019. [CrossRef] [PubMed]
13. Ghorani, V.; Saadat, S.; Khazdair, M.R.; Gholamnezhad, Z.; El-Seedi, H.; Boskabady, M.H. Phytochemical Characteristics and Anti-Inflammatory, Immunoregulatory, and Antioxidant Effects of *Portulaca oleracea* L.: A Comprehensive Review. *Evid.-Based Complement. Altern. Med.* **2023**, *2023*, 2075444. [CrossRef] [PubMed]
14. Eid, A.M.; Fouda, A.; Hassan, S.E.; Hamza, M.F.; Alharbi, N.K.; Elkelish, A.; Alharthi, A.; Salem, W.M. Plant-Based Copper Oxide Nanoparticles; Biosynthesis, Characterization, Antibacterial Activity, Tanning Wastewater Treatment, and Heavy Metals Sorption. *Catalysts* **2023**, *13*, 348. [CrossRef]
15. Aboulthana, W.M.; Omar, N.I.; Hasan, E.A.; Ahmed, K.A.; Youssef, A.M. Assessment of the Biological Activities of Egyptian Purslane (*Portulaca oleracea*) Extract after Incorporating Metal Nanoparticles, in Vitro and in Vivo Study. *Asian Pac. J. Cancer Prev. APJCP* **2022**, *23*, 287–310. [CrossRef] [PubMed]
16. Hussain, I.; Singh, N.; Singh, A.; Singh, H.; Singh, S. Green synthesis of nanoparticles and its potential application. *Biotechnol. Lett.* **2016**, *38*, 545–560. [CrossRef] [PubMed]
17. Govindappa, M.; Hemashekhar, B.; Arthikala, M.-K.; Rai, V.R.; Ramachandra, Y. Characterization, antibacterial, antioxidant, antidiabetic, anti-inflammatory and antityrosinase activity of green synthesized silver nanoparticles using *Calophyllum tomentosum* leaves extract. *Results Phys.* **2018**, *9*, 400–408. [CrossRef]
18. Ege, E.; Kurtay, G.; Karaca, B.; Büyük, İ.; Gökdemir, F.Ş.; Sumer, A. Green synthesis of silver nanoparticles from *Phaseolus vulgaris* L. extracts and investigation of their antifungal activities. *Hacet. J. Biol. Chem.* **2020**, *49*, 11–23.
19. Haggag, E.G.; Elshamy, A.M.; Rabeh, M.A.; Gabr, N.M.; Salem, M.; Youssif, K.A.; Samir, A.; Bin Muhsinah, A.; Alsayari, A.; Abdelmohsen, U.R. Antiviral potential of green synthesized silver nanoparticles of *Lampranthus coccineus* and *Malephora lutea*. *Int. J. Nanomed.* **2019**, *14*, 6217–6229. [CrossRef]
20. Kambale, E.K.; Nkanga, C.I.; Mutonkole, B.-P.I.; Bapolisi, A.M.; Tassa, D.O.; Liesse, J.-M.I.; Krause, R.W.M.; Memvanga, P.B. Green synthesis of antimicrobial silver nanoparticles using aqueous leaf extracts from three Congolese plant species (Brillantaisia patula, *Crossopteryx febrifuga* and *Senna siamea*). *Heliyon* **2020**, *6*, e04493. [CrossRef]
21. Mohanta, Y.K.; Panda, S.K.; Jayabalan, R.; Sharma, N.; Bastia, A.K.; Mohanta, T.K. Antimicrobial, Antioxidant and Cytotoxic Activity of Silver Nanoparticles Synthesized by Leaf Extract of *Erythrina suberosa* (Roxb.). *Front. Mol. Biosci.* **2017**, *4*, 14. [CrossRef]
22. Ravichandran, V.; Vasanthi, S.; Shalini, S.; Shah, S.A.A.; Harish, R. Green synthesis of silver nanoparticles using *Atrocarpus altilis* leaf extract and the study of their antimicrobial and antioxidant activity. *Mater. Lett.* **2016**, *180*, 264–267. [CrossRef]
23. Wang, L.; Wu, Y.; Xie, J.; Wu, S.; Wu, Z. Characterization, antioxidant and antimicrobial activities of green synthesized silver nanoparticles from *Psidium guajava* L. leaf aqueous extracts. *Mater. Sci. Eng. C* **2018**, *86*, 1–8. [CrossRef] [PubMed]
24. Keshari, A.K.; Srivastava, R.; Singh, P.; Yadav, V.B.; Nath, G. Antioxidant and antibacterial activity of silver nanoparticles synthesized by Cestrum nocturnum. *J. Ayurveda Integr. Med.* **2020**, *11*, 37–44. [CrossRef] [PubMed]
25. Liaqat, N.; Jahan, N.; Khalil Ur, R.; Anwar, T.; Qureshi, H. Green synthesized silver nanoparticles: Optimization, characterization, antimicrobial activity, and cytotoxicity study by hemolysis assay. *Front. Chem.* **2022**, *10*, 952006. [CrossRef]
26. Fernández-Poyatos, M.D.P.; Llorent-Martínez, E.J.; Ruiz-Medina, A. Phytochemical Composition and Antioxidant Activity of *Portulaca oleracea*: Influence of the Steaming Cooking Process. *Foods* **2021**, *10*, 94. [CrossRef]
27. Kate, S.; Sahasrabudhe, M.; Pethe, A. Biogenic Silver Nanoparticle Synthesis, Characterization and its Antibacterial activity against Leather Deteriorates. *Jordan J. Biol. Sci.* **2020**, *13*, 493–498.
28. Lee, Y.J.; Park, Y. Graphene oxide grafted gold nanoparticles and silver/silver chloride nanoparticles green-synthesized by a *Portulaca oleracea* extract: Assessment of catalytic activity. *Colloids Surf. A Physicochem. Eng. Asp.* **2020**, *607*, 125527. [CrossRef]

29. Li, Y.; Liao, Q.; Hou, W.; Qin, L. Silver-Based Surface Plasmon Sensors: Fabrication and Applications. *Int. J. Mol. Sci.* **2023**, *24*, 4142. [CrossRef]
30. Dong, Z.-Y.; Narsing Rao, M.P.; Xiao, M.; Wang, H.-F.; Hozzein, W.N.; Chen, W.; Li, W.-J. Antibacterial activity of silver nanoparticles against Staphylococcus warneri synthesized using endophytic bacteria by photo-irradiation. *Front. Microbiol.* **2017**, *8*, 1090. [CrossRef]
31. Lee, K.-C.; Lin, S.-J.; Lin, C.-H.; Tsai, C.-S.; Lu, Y.-J. Size effect of Ag nanoparticles on surface plasmon resonance. *Surf. Coat. Technol.* **2008**, *202*, 5339–5342. [CrossRef]
32. Taha, Z.K.; Hawar, S.N.; Sulaiman, G.M. Extracellular biosynthesis of silver nanoparticles from Penicillium italicum and its antioxidant, antimicrobial and cytotoxicity activities. *Biotechnol. Lett.* **2019**, *41*, 899–914. [CrossRef] [PubMed]
33. Hamza, M.F.; Mira, H.; Wei, Y.; Ning, S.; Guibal, E.; El-Etrawy, A.-A.S.; El Dakkony, S.R. Chitosan functionalized with pyrazolinone derivative for water treatment: Application to Hg (II) removal. *J. Water Process Eng.* **2023**, *56*, 104258. [CrossRef]
34. Khademi-Azandehi, P.; Moghaddam, J. Green synthesis, characterization and physiological stability of gold nanoparticles from Stachys lavandulifolia Vahl extract. *Particuology* **2015**, *19*, 22–26. [CrossRef]
35. Hamza, M.F.; Guibal, E.; Wei, Y.; Fouda, A.; Althumayri, K.; Khoziem, H.A.A.; Mashaal, N.M. Functionalization of thiosemicarbazide/gellan gum for the enhancement of cadmium removal from aqueous solutions–Grafting of tributyl phosphate derivative. *J. Water Process Eng.* **2023**, *54*, 103928. [CrossRef]
36. Coury, C.; Dillner, A.M. A method to quantify organic functional groups and inorganic compounds in ambient aerosols using attenuated total reflectance FTIR spectroscopy and multivariate chemometric techniques. *Atmos. Environ.* **2008**, *42*, 5923–5932. [CrossRef]
37. Ghoshal, G.; Kaur, M. Optimization of extraction of starch from sweet potato and its application in making edible film. *Food Chem. Adv.* **2023**, *3*, 100356. [CrossRef]
38. Coates, J. Interpretation of infrared spectra, a practical approach. In *Encyclopedia of Analytical Chemistry: Applications, Theory, and Instrumentation*; Wiley: Hoboken, NJ, USA, 2000; pp. 10881–10882.
39. Awwad, M.A.; Salem, M.N.; Abdeen, O.A. Biosynthesis of silver nanoparticles using Loquat leaf extract and its antibacterial activity. *Adv. Mater. Lett.* **2013**, *4*, 338–342. [CrossRef]
40. Zhao, M.; Salih, K.A.; Wei, Y.; Guibal, E.; Ning, S.; Goda, A.E.-S.; Hamza, M.F. Novel method for synthesizing high S-bearing hybrid sorbent for efficient silver binding–Characterization, testing, and application to metal recovery from X-ray films. *Chem. Eng. J.* **2023**, *477*, 147010. [CrossRef]
41. Murillo-Rábago, E.I.; Vilchis-Nestor, A.R.; Juarez-Moreno, K.; Garcia-Marin, L.E.; Quester, K.; Castro-Longoria, E. Optimized Synthesis of Small and Stable Silver Nanoparticles Using Intracellular and Extracellular Components of Fungi: An Alternative for Bacterial Inhibition. *Antibiotics* **2022**, *11*, 800. [CrossRef]
42. Fouda, A.; Awad, M.A.; Al-Faifi, Z.E.; Gad, M.E.; Al-Khalaf, A.A.; Yahya, R.; Hamza, M.F. Aspergillus flavus-mediated green synthesis of silver nanoparticles and evaluation of their antibacterial, anti-candida, acaricides, and photocatalytic activities. *Catalysts* **2022**, *12*, 462. [CrossRef]
43. Moreno-Martin, G.; León-González, M.E.; Madrid, Y. Simultaneous determination of the size and concentration of AgNPs in water samples by UV–vis spectrophotometry and chemometrics tools. *Talanta* **2018**, *188*, 393–403. [CrossRef] [PubMed]
44. Acharya, D.; Singha, K.M.; Pandey, P.; Mohanta, B.; Rajkumari, J.; Singha, L.P. Shape dependent physical mutilation and lethal effects of silver nanoparticles on bacteria. *Sci. Rep.* **2018**, *8*, 201. [CrossRef] [PubMed]
45. Bagur, H.; Poojari, C.C.; Melappa, G.; Rangappa, R.; Chandrasekhar, N.; Somu, P. Biogenically synthesized silver nanoparticles using endophyte fungal extract of Ocimum tenuiflorum and evaluation of biomedical properties. *J. Clust. Sci.* **2020**, *31*, 1241–1255. [CrossRef]
46. Rónavári, A.; Kovács, D.; Igaz, N.; Vágvölgyi, C.; Boros, I.M.; Kónya, Z.; Pfeiffer, I.; Kiricsi, M. Biological activity of green-synthesized silver nanoparticles depends on the applied natural extracts: A comprehensive study. *Int. J. Nanomed.* **2017**, *12*, 871–883. [CrossRef] [PubMed]
47. Tomaszewska, E.; Soliwoda, K.; Kadziola, K.; Tkacz-Szczesna, B.; Celichowski, G.; Cichomski, M.; Szmaja, W.; Grobelny, J. Detection Limits of DLS and UV-Vis Spectroscopy in Characterization of Polydisperse Nanoparticles Colloids. *J. Nanomater.* **2013**, *2013*, 313081. [CrossRef]
48. Honary, S.; Barabadi, H.; Gharaei-Fathabad, E.; Naghibi, F. Green synthesis of silver nanoparticles induced by the fungus Penicillium citrinum. *Trop. J. Pharm. Res.* **2013**, *12*, 7–11. [CrossRef]
49. Bhattacharjee, S. DLS and zeta potential–what they are and what they are not? *J. Control. Release* **2016**, *235*, 337–351. [CrossRef] [PubMed]
50. Lashin, I.; Fouda, A.; Gobouri, A.A.; Azab, E.; Mohammedsaleh, Z.M.; Makharita, R.R. Antimicrobial and in vitro cytotoxic efficacy of biogenic silver nanoparticles (Ag-NPs) fabricated by callus extract of *Solanum incanum* L. *Biomolecules* **2021**, *11*, 341. [CrossRef]
51. Salem, S.S.; El-Belely, E.F.; Niedbała, G.; Alnoman, M.M.; Hassan, S.E.-D.; Eid, A.M.; Shaheen, T.I.; Elkelish, A.; Fouda, A. Bactericidal and in-vitro cytotoxic efficacy of silver nanoparticles (Ag-NPs) fabricated by endophytic actinomycetes and their use as coating for the textile fabrics. *Nanomaterials* **2020**, *10*, 2082. [CrossRef]
52. More, P.R.; Pandit, S.; Filippis, A.; Franci, G.; Mijakovic, I.; Galdiero, M. Silver Nanoparticles: Bactericidal and Mechanistic Approach against Drug Resistant Pathogens. *Microorganisms* **2023**, *11*, 369. [CrossRef]

53. Gaurav, A.; Bakht, P.; Saini, M.; Pandey, S.; Pathania, R. Role of bacterial efflux pumps in antibiotic resistance, virulence, and strategies to discover novel efflux pump inhibitors. *Microbiology* **2023**, *169*, 001333. [CrossRef] [PubMed]
54. Yadav, T.C.; Gupta, P.; Saini, S.; Mohiyuddin, S.; Pruthi, V.; Prasad, R. Plausible mechanistic insights in biofilm eradication potential against Candida spp. using in situ-synthesized tyrosol-functionalized chitosan gold nanoparticles as a versatile antifouling coating on implant surfaces. *ACS Omega* **2022**, *7*, 8350–8363. [CrossRef] [PubMed]
55. Flieger, J.; Flieger, W.; Baj, J.; Maciejewski, R. Antioxidants: Classification, Natural Sources, Activity/Capacity Measurements, and Usefulness for the Synthesis of Nanoparticles. *Materials* **2021**, *14*, 4135. [CrossRef] [PubMed]
56. Nassar, A.-R.A.; Atta, H.M.; Abdel-Rahman, M.A.; El Naghy, W.S.; Fouda, A. Myco-synthesized copper oxide nanoparticles using harnessing metabolites of endophytic fungal strain Aspergillus terreus: An insight into antibacterial, anti-Candida, biocompatibility, anticancer, and antioxidant activities. *BMC Complement. Med. Ther.* **2023**, *23*, 261. [CrossRef] [PubMed]
57. Munteanu, I.G.; Apetrei, C. Analytical Methods Used in Determining Antioxidant Activity: A Review. *Int. J. Mol. Sci.* **2021**, *22*, 3380. [CrossRef]
58. Bedlovičová, Z.; Strapáč, I.; Baláž, M.; Salayová, A. A brief overview on antioxidant activity determination of silver nanoparticles. *Molecules* **2020**, *25*, 3191. [CrossRef] [PubMed]
59. Bhatti, A.; DeLong, R.K. Nanoscale Interaction Mechanisms of Antiviral Activity. *ACS Pharmacol. Transl. Sci.* **2023**, *6*, 220–228. [CrossRef] [PubMed]
60. Fouda, A.; Hassan, S.E.-D.; Eid, A.M.; Abdel-Rahman, M.A.; Hamza, M.F. Light enhanced the antimicrobial, anticancer, and catalytic activities of selenium nanoparticles fabricated by endophytic fungal strain, Penicillium crustosum EP-1. *Sci. Rep.* **2022**, *12*, 11834. [CrossRef]
61. Louten, J. Virus Replication. In *Essential Human Virology*; Academic Press: Cambridge, MA, USA, 2016; pp. 49–70. [CrossRef]
62. Luceri, A.; Francese, R.; Lembo, D.; Ferraris, M.; Balagna, C. Silver Nanoparticles: Review of Antiviral Properties, Mechanism of Action and Applications. *Microorganisms* **2023**, *11*, 629. [CrossRef]
63. Khatun, S.; Putta, C.L.; Hak, A.; Rengan, A.K. Immunomodulatory nanosystems: An emerging strategy to combat viral infections. *Biomater. Biosyst.* **2023**, *9*, 100073. [CrossRef]
64. Kamli, M.R.; Srivastava, V.; Hajrah, N.H.; Sabir, J.S.; Ali, A.; Malik, M.A.; Ahmad, A. Phytogenic fabrication of Ag–Fe Bimetallic nanoparticles for cell cycle arrest and apoptosis signaling pathways in Candida auris by generating oxidative stress. *Antioxidants* **2021**, *10*, 182. [CrossRef]
65. Hamza, M.F.; Mira, H.; Khalafalla, M.S.; Wang, J.; Wei, Y.; Yin, X.; Ning, S.; Althumayri, K.; Fouda, A. Photocatalytic Performance of Functionalized Biopolymer for Neodymium (III) Sorption and the Recovery from Leachate Solution. *Catalysts* **2023**, *13*, 672. [CrossRef]
66. Humphries, R.M.; Ambler, J.; Mitchell, S.L.; Castanheira, M.; Dingle, T.; Hindler, J.A.; Koeth, L.; Sei, K. CLSI Methods Development and Standardization Working Group Best Practices for Evaluation of Antimicrobial Susceptibility Tests. *J. Clin. Microbiol.* **2018**, *56*, e01934-17. [CrossRef]
67. Ratan, Z.A.; Mashrur, F.R.; Chhoan, A.P.; Shahriar, S.M.; Haidere, M.F.; Runa, N.J.; Kim, S.; Kweon, D.H.; Hosseinzadeh, H.; Cho, J.Y. Silver Nanoparticles as Potential Antiviral Agents. *Pharmaceutics* **2021**, *13*, 2034. [CrossRef]

pharmaceuticals

MDPI

Article

Synthesis and Characterization of Chemically and Green-Synthesized Silver Oxide Particles for Evaluation of Antiviral and Anticancer Activity

Muhammad Asif [1], Wajeeha Iqbal [1], Muhammad Fakhar-e-Alam [1,*], Zahid Hussain [1], Malik Saadullah [2], Mudassir Hassan [3], Javed Rehman [4,5], Kholood A. Dahlous [6,*] and Noora H. Al-Qahtani [7]

1 Department of Physics, Government College University Faisalabad, Faisalabad 38000, Pakistan
2 Department of Pharmaceutical Chemistry, Government College University Faisalabad, Faisalabad 38000, Pakistan
3 Department of Zoology, Government College University Faisalabad, Faisalabad 38000, Pakistan
4 State Key Laboratory of Metastable Materials Science and Technology, School of Materials Science and Engineering, Yanshan University, Qinhuangdao 066004, China
5 MEU Research Unit, Middle East University, Amman 11831, Jordan
6 Department of Chemistry, College of Science, King Saud University, Riyadh 11451, Saudi Arabia
7 Center for Advanced Materials, Qatar University, Doha P.O. Box 2713, Qatar
* Correspondence: fakharphy@gmail.com (M.F.-e.-A.); kdahloos@ksu.edu.sa (K.A.D.)

Abstract: Silver oxide (Ag_2O) particles are wonderful candidates due to their unique properties, and their use in a wide range of research, industrial and biomedical applications is rapidly increasing. This makes it fundamental to develop simple, environmentally friendly methods with possible scaling. Herein, sodium borohydride and *Datura innoxia* leaf extract were applied as chemical and biological stabilizing and reducing agents to develop Ag_2O particles. The primary aim was to evaluate the anticancer and antiviral activity of Ag_2O particles prepared via two methods. XRD, UV-visible and SEM analyses were used to examine the crystallite structure, optical properties and morphology, respectively. The resulting green-synthesized Ag_2O particles exhibited small size, spherically agglomerated shape, and high anticancer and antiviral activities compared to chemically synthesized Ag_2O particles. The MTT (3-(4,5-dimethylthiazol-2-yl)-2,5 diphenyltetrazolium-bromide) assay of green-synthesized Ag_2O particles showed high anticancer activity against MCF-7 cells with IC_{50} = 17.908 μg/mL compared to chemically synthesized Ag_2O particles with IC_{50} = 23.856 μg/mL. The antiviral activity of green-synthesized Ag_2O particles and chemically synthesized Ag_2O particles was also evaluated by a plaque-forming assay, and green-synthesized Ag_2O particles showed higher antiviral ability with IC_{50} = 0.618 μg/mL as compared to chemically synthesized Ag_2O particles with IC_{50} = 6.129 μg/mL. We propose the use of green-synthesized Ag_2O particles in cancer treatment and drug delivery.

Keywords: silver oxide particles; *Datura innoxia*; anticancer activity; antiviral activity

1. Introduction

The global cancer problem is progressively increasing every year [1]. According to the World Health Organization (WHO) 2020 reports, there were 9.9 million deaths globally, with breast cancer mortality (2.26 million) being particularly high in developing countries, especially in Pakistan [2–4].

Metal oxide particles have been leading the way in materials research for industrial, energy, and biomedical applications over the last few decades.

A number of benefits, including ease of use, environmental friendliness, and ease of scaling, have generated considerable interest in green nanotechnology. Herbals are ingredients (extracts) that are derived from plants, either in combination or alone, and are used to treat and prevent many diseases. Many plant extracts have shown anticancer activity against several cancer cells without harming the growth of healthy cells. Plants are widely considered the optimal choice of material due to their stabilizing capabilities and bio-reducing properties [5,6].

Silver oxide particles have attracted significant interest among metal oxide particles, including gold, silver, manganese, zinc, and copper particles, because of their diverse range of uses in sectors such as textiles, cancer treatment, antiviral medications, electronics, food production, optical instruments, and rechargeable batteries and especially in biomedical applications [7–10]. Ag_2O particles have antifungal [10], anticancer [11], antiviral [12], anticancer [13], anti-inflammatory [5], and antioxidant properties [14]. Ag_2O particles can be prepared using a variety of techniques, including chemical, physical, and green-synthesis techniques [15–17]. Ag_2O particles have high efficiency due to their outstanding antimicrobial activity towards viruses, bacteria, and other eukaryotic microorganisms [18,19]. Some important viruses are *influenza virus* [20], human *immunodeficiency virus (HIV)*, *human parainfluenza virus* [21], *dengue virus* [22], and *herpes simplex virus 1 (HSV1)* [23]. These viral infections are causing current epidemics and threaten the lives of humans on this planet [24,25].

In the current study, Ag_2O particles were prepared via a green synthesis process by using *Datura innoxia* leaf extract. The extract effectively decreased and stabilized the ions present in the silver nitrate solution, resulting in Ag_2O particle synthesis without requiring any chemical reducing or stabilizing agent. However, in the chemical synthesis process, sodium borohydride was used to prepare the Ag_2O particles, which is a very strong stabilizing/reducing agent. The green and chemically prepared Ag_2O particles were characterized. Finally, the anticancer and antiviral efficacy of green and chemically prepared Ag_2O particles were explored. We suggest that further in vivo anticancer and antiviral studies of *Datura innoxia* Ag_2O particles should be performed.

2. Results and Discussions

2.1. X-ray Diffraction Analysis

An X-ray diffraction (XRD) study was used to determine the crystal structure and calculate the crystallite size of Ag_2O particles prepared using chemical and green synthesis processes. Figure 1a,b present the crystal structure patterns of the chemical and green synthesis of Ag_2O particles prepared by coprecipitation processes and annealed at 400 °C for 12 h for refinement. The crystal structure of chemically and green-prepared Ag_2O particles was investigated and calculated as cubic crystal structure and justified while comparing JCPDS No. 01-087-0719.The miller indices of maximum intensity peak are labeled with the (111) reflection/lattice plane at a diffraction angle of 38.4°, while the remaining lattice planes appeared in the following order: peaks at two thetas (2θ) = 44.5°, 64.6°, 77.6° and 82.3° labeled, and with respective indices of (200), (220), (311) and (222) in both chemical and green processes, respectively. The XRD pattern was similar in both conditions. In addition, it was observed that the maximum intensity peak had a broad size, which confirmed the growth of the particles. The average crystallite sizes of chemically and green-synthesized Ag_2O particles were ~63 and ~54 nm, respectively, as shown in Table 1. Moreover, the crystallite size was calculated from X-ray diffraction (XRD) data using the given formulas [26–29].

$$C.S = \frac{k\lambda}{\beta cos\theta} \tag{1}$$

Here, the crystallite size is ($C.S$), Scherrer constant (k), wavelength (λ), full width half maximum (β), and angle (θ).

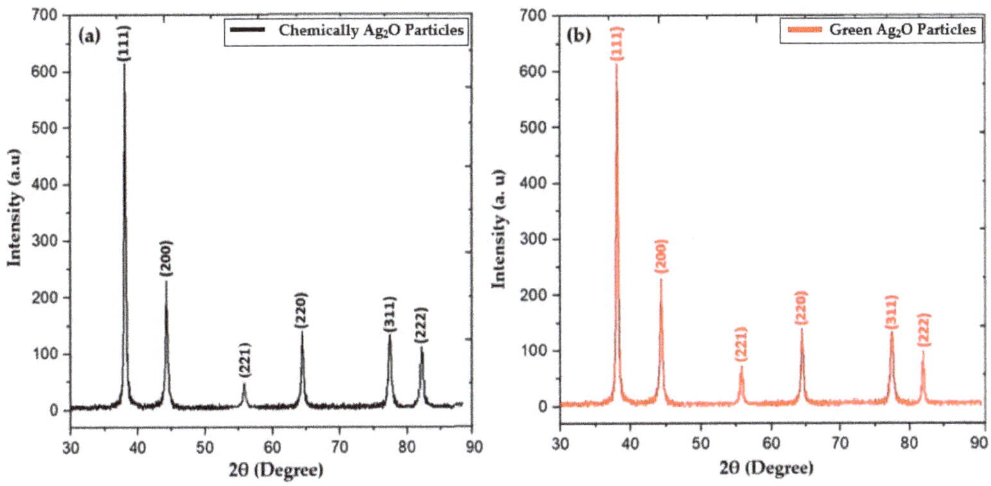

Figure 1. XRD graph of (**a**) chemically synthesized Ag_2O particles and (**b**) green-synthesized Ag_2O particles.

Table 1. (**a**) shows the parameters, miller indices, diffraction angle, and crystallite size of chemically synthesized Ag_2O particles. (**b**) shows the parameters, miller indices, diffraction angle, and crystallite size of the green-synthesized Ag_2O particles.

Miller Indices (h,k,l)	Diffraction Angle 2θ (Theta)	Crystallite Size "*C.S*" (nm)
	(a)	
(111)	38.1	41.3
(200)	44.3	55.7
(220)	64.5	75.6
(311)	77.4	81.2
	(b)	
(111)	38.1	32.2
(200)	44.3	46.6
(220)	64.8	66.6
(311)	77.7	69.9

2.2. FTIR Analysis

The chemical bond and functional groups of both chemically and green-synthesized Ag_2O particles were investigated using Fourier transform infrared spectroscopy (FTIR) in the wavelength range of 500–4000 cm^{-1}. In Figure 2a,b, it can be observed that the FTIR spectra of chemically synthesized Ag_2O particles exhibited a shift in the bands compared to those synthesized using *Datura innoxia* plant extract. The addition of *Datura innoxia* plant extract to silver nitrate resulted in a change in the functional groups of Ag_2O particles. The green-synthesized Ag_2O particles showed several peaks corresponding to major functional groups at 3357, 2347, and 1631 cm^{-1}, while the chemically synthesized Ag_2O particles showed a shift in the bands at 3390, 2364, and 1620 cm^{-1}. These peaks are associated with the stretching vibration of the hydroxyl group (H-bonded O-H stretch) [30–32]. Additionally, the O-H bending vibration of water molecules absorbed on the surface of Ag_2O particles, which may be crucial for biomedical assays such as anticancer and antimicrobial activities [30,31], and a weak stretching vibration of C=C [17], were observed. The weak peaks at 1395 and 1387 cm^{-1}

of Ag_2O correspond to NO^{3-} ions (nitrates). Furthermore, the presence of an O-Ag-O bending mode of vibration at 611 cm^{-1} confirmed the formation of metal–oxygen bonding [9,30,31]. Moreover, the FTIR spectra of *Datura innoxia* leaf extract are shown in Figure 2c, which are quite similar to those in the previously published article [17].

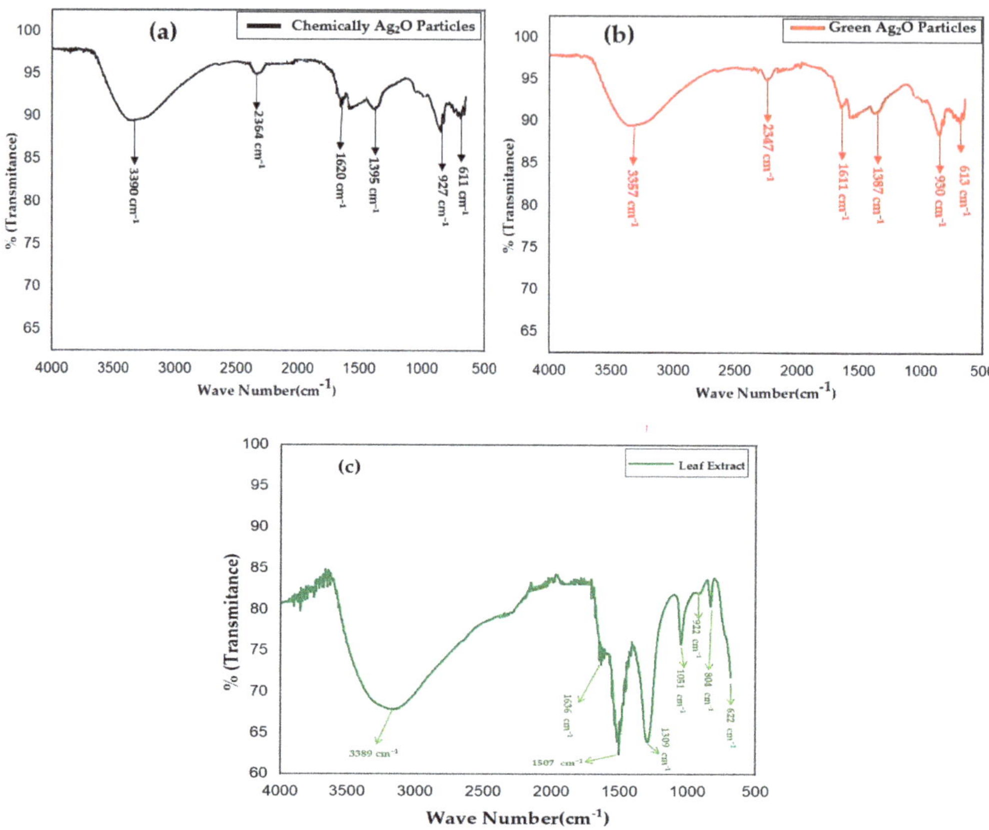

Figure 2. FTIR graph of (**a**) chemically synthesized Ag_2O particles, (**b**) green-synthesized Ag_2O particles, and (**c**) *Datura innoxia* leaf extract.

2.3. UV–Visible Analysis

UV–visible spectroscopy was employed to analyze the optical density or absorption spectra of both chemically and green-synthesized particles. In the current experimental strategy, chemically and green-synthesized Ag_2O particles were carefully examined. When chemically and green-synthesized Ag_2O particle samples were dispersed in deionized water to find the absorption spectra in the range of 350 nm to 850 nm, we revealed a sharp absorption band at 410 nm in the absorption spectra of chemically synthesized Ag_2O particles, as depicted in Figure 3a. This might indicate the presence of chemically synthesized Ag_2O particles such as in [17]. The absorption spectra of green-synthesized Ag_2O particles are depicted in Figure 3b, where the presence of Ag_2O particles is confirmed from the green-synthesized Ag_2O sample using these spectra. Generally, green-synthesized Ag_2O particles in deionized water absorbed radiation near the wavelength of 414.7 nm. It was observed from the UV–visible graph that the confirmation of the surface plasmon resonance peak near 425 nm indicates the presence of green-synthesized Ag_2O particles, as shown in Figure 3b. On the metallic surface of green-synthesized Ag_2O particles, there are resonant oscillations of free electrons through interbond transitions and surface plasmon resonance (SPR) bands [33]. In the graph, the surface plasmon peak indicates the presence of Ag_2O particles with different sizes, and the spherical shape is confirmed in SEM. The absorption spectra of *Datura innoxia* leaf extract is depicted in Figure 3c, which shows a peak at ~220 nm. For more details about the absorbance of the *Datura innoxia* leaf extract, see the previously published paper [34].

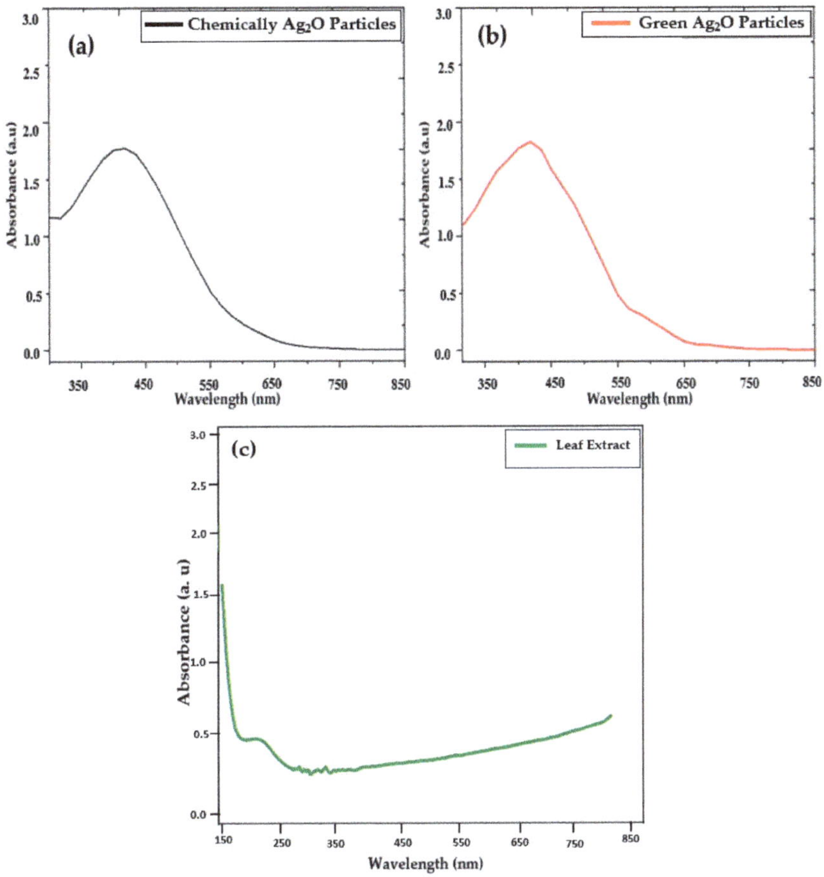

Figure 3. UV–visible graph of (**a**) chemically synthesized Ag_2O particles, (**b**) green-synthesized Ag_2O particles, and (**c**) *Datura innoxia* leaf extract.

2.4. SEM and EDX Analysis

The surface morphology of both chemically and green-synthesized Ag_2O particles was analyzed using scanning electron microscopy (SEM). The SEM images of chemically and green-synthesized Ag_2O particles are shown in Figure 4a,b at a scale of 3 μm scale, respectively. Spherical grains of the chemically and green-synthesized Ag_2O particles can be seen in Figure 4, with some non-uniformly distributed aggregates present. The SEM micrographs confirmed that the chemically and green-synthesized Ag_2O particles mostly have spherical shapes of various sizes. In Figure 4b, the bioagents of *Datura innoxia* leaf extract strongly interact with Ag ions to produce uniform spherical shapes with small sizes. The green-synthesized Ag_2O particles had spherical shapes of dissimilar sizes but were smaller than the chemically synthesized Ag_2O particles. The spherical grains were circulated with red circles. Hence, the SEM results of green-synthesized Ag_2O particles were much better than those of the chemical Ag_2O particles. The energy-dispersive X-ray spectroscopy (EDX) technique was employed to conduct an elemental compositional analysis of both chemically and green-synthesized Ag_2O particles. The results from the EDX analysis verified the existence of Ag as a main element and O and C as the primary elements in the samples, as depicted in Figure 4c,d. The negligible percentage of carbon is due to lab environment or lab equipment. Kasthuri et al. [17] and Gajendaran et al. [35] also reported similar results, where elemental silver was detected in the graph obtained by EDX analysis, confirming the reduction of silver ions to elemental silver.

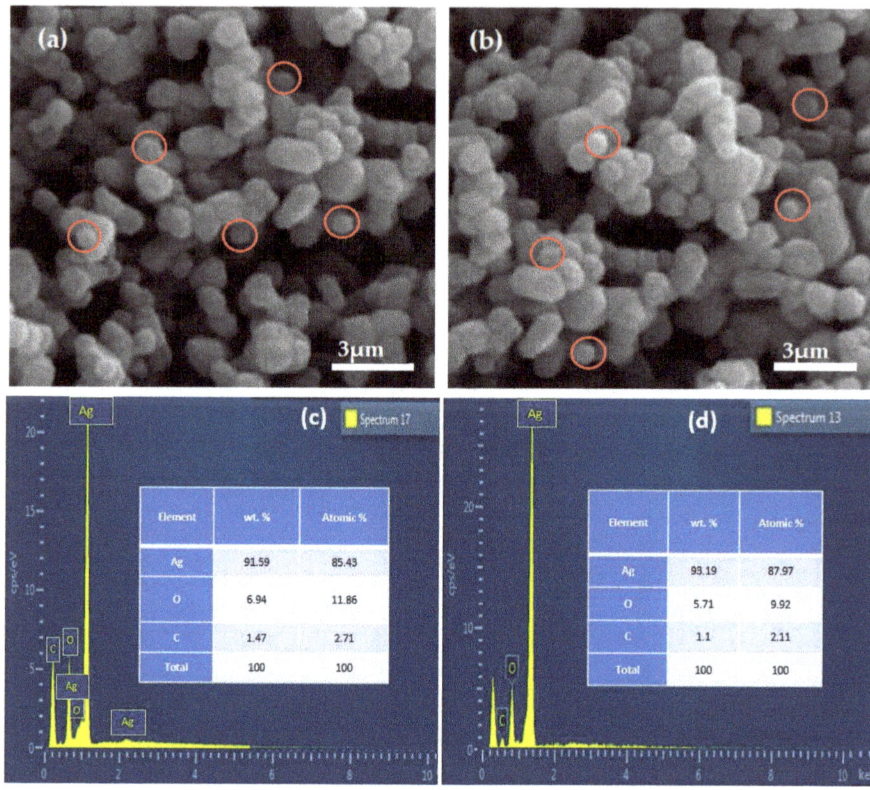

Figure 4. SEM images and EDX spectrum of (**a**) chemically synthesized Ag_2O particles, (**b**) green-synthesized Ag_2O particles at 3 μm, (**c**) chemically synthesized Ag_2O particles, and (**d**) green-synthesized Ag_2O particles.

2.5. Anticancer Activity against MCF-7 Cells

The results of the cytotoxicity investigation of both types of Ag_2O particles on the breast cancer (MCF-7) cell line revealed that both particles were cytotoxic against the cancer cell line and were less toxic towards the Vero cell line. Maximum cell death was detected for the green-synthesized Ag_2O particles with an IC_{50} of 17.908 μg/mL, compared to chemically synthesized Ag_2O particles with an IC_{50} of 23.856 μg/mL against MCF-7 cells after 48 h of exposure. As can be seen in Figure 5, the cytotoxicity of both Ag_2O particles is concentration-dependent [36].

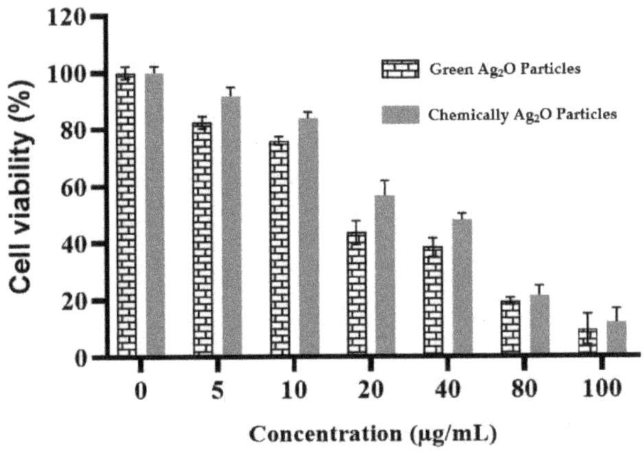

Figure 5. Cytotoxicity evaluation of both green- and chemically synthesized Ag_2O particles against MCF-7 cell lines.

2.6. Cytotoxicity Activity against Vero Cells

To rule out the possibility that cellular toxicity may be the cause of the decline in infectivity, a range of concentrations (1, 5, 10, 50, and 100 μg/mL) were incubated with Vero cell monolayers, as shown in Figure 6. Each concentration of Ag_2O particles was incubated for various time periods (48 h), and cell viability was measured using the 3-(4,5-dimethyllthiazol-2-yl)-2,5 diphenyl-tetrazolium-bromide (MTT) assay. Chemically prepared Ag_2O particles had toxic effects in the concentration range of 10–50 μg/mL. However, green-synthesized Ag_2O particles within the range were shown/found to have low cytotoxicity in Vero cells. These statistics were valuable for determining concentrations for testing in antiviral assays. We used concentrations that were significantly below the cytotoxic threshold, ranging from 0.5 to 10 μg/mL.

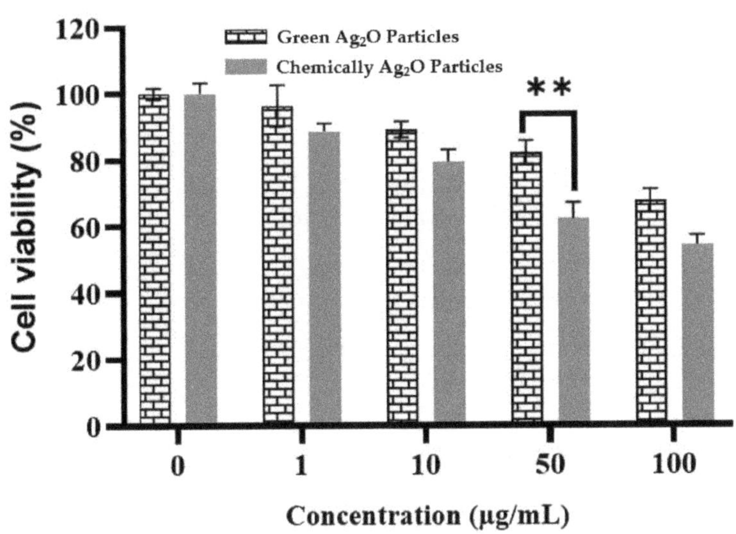

Figure 6. Cytotoxicity evaluation of both green and chemical Ag_2O particles against normal (Vero) cell. ** $p \leq 0.01$.

2.7. Antiviral Activity

A stock solution of silver oxide particles was prepared via a chemical-synthesis process as well as a green-synthesis process with a concentration solution of 10 mg/L by dispersing the working solution of silver oxide particles (0.1, 0.5, 1, 2, 4, 8 and 10 μg/mL) into Newcastle disease virus (NDV)-incorporated Vero cells. The solution was then removed, washed and inoculated with 0.5% methyl cellulose for 72 h. The medium was aspirated, and the cells were fixed with 10% formaldehyde and stained with 1% crystal violet; then, the plaques were counted. The plaque analysis formation was calculated. Green-synthesized Ag_2O particles showed significant toxicity against NDV virus compared to chemically synthesized Ag_2O particles (Figure 7).

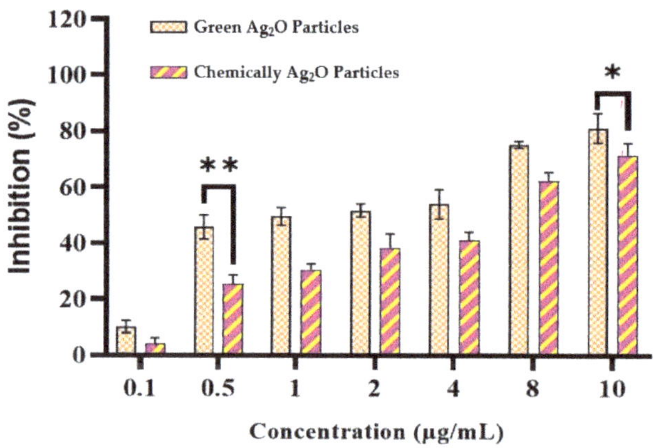

Figure 7. Green-synthesized Ag_2O particles showed higher antiviral activity as compared to chemical-based Ag_2O particles in a dose-dependent manner, where * is $p \leq 0.05$, ** $p \leq 0.01$.

2.8. Properties of Green-Synthesized Ag_2O Particles

The Ag_2O particles prepared using the green-synthesis process, which utilizes plant extracts, showed distinct properties compared to those prepared through traditional chemical methods. Some of the new properties of green-synthesized Ag_2O particles are mentioned, such as smaller crystallite size, higher surface area, improved stability, increased antimicrobial and antioxidant potential, anticancer and antiviral properties, reduced toxicity and environmental impact, unique crystal structures and morphologies, potential for large-scale production, and cost-effectiveness. The green-synthesis method offers a sustainable and eco-friendly approach to producing Ag_2O particles with advanced properties for various applications [6,12,13,16,17]. For more information on the properties of green-synthesized particles, see Table 2.

Table 2. Previous reported study of different plant extracts, nanoparticles, and their applications.

Sr#	Materials and Plants Name	Applications	IC_{50} (μg/mL)	References
1	Green-synthesized AgNPs (*Datura innoxia* leaf extract)	anticancer	15.2 and 8.5	[37]
2	Biosynthesis of AgNPs with *Datura innoxia*	anticancer	20	[28]
3	Green-synthesized AgNPs (*Baccaurea ramiflora*)	anticancer	110 and 140	[38]
4	AgNPs with *Syzygium aromaicum*	anticancer	60 and 50	[39]
5	Green-synthesized AgNPs (*Ctenolepis garcini*)	anticancer	33.78	[40]
6	Green-synthesized gold nanoparticles (AuNPs) with (leaf extracts of *Ocimum gratissimum Linn*)	anticancer	10 and 25	[41]
7	Green copper nanoparticles (CuNPs) with *Eclipta prostrata*	anticancer	1.71 and 1.81	[42]

Table 2. *Cont.*

Sr#	Materials and Plants Name	Applications	IC_{50} (μg/mL)	References
8	PVP-coated AgNPs	antiviral	0.44	[43]
9	*Datura innoxia* leaf extract	anticancer	0.6	[44]
10	Green (*Datura innoxia* extract) and chemically synthesized Ag NPs	Anticancer, antibacterial and antioxidant	--	[17]

3. Materials and Methods

3.1. Materials

Silver nitrate ($AgNO_3$), sodium borohydride ($NaBH_4$), ethanol, polyvinylpyrrolidone, deionized water, dimethyl sulfoxide (DMSO), fetal bovine serum (FBS), Dulbecco's modified eagle medium (DMEM), phosphate-buffered saline (PBS), and antibiotics (penicillin + streptomycin) were purchased from Sigma-Aldrich (St. Louis, MO, USA). In addition, the *Datura innoxia* plant was collected from the garden of the Department of Botany, Government College University, Faisalabad).

3.2. Preparation of Extract

Fresh leaves of *Datura innoxia* were cut into small pieces, washed twice with distilled water and dried [17]. In the next step, 200 g of powdered *Datura innoxia* was mixed with 750 mL of distilled water and heated at 80 °C for 3 h. Then, the obtained solution was filtered and scraped to obtain a dark yellow colored extract. Next, 0.407 g of extract was dissolved in 50 mL of deionized water and stirred continuously for 10 min for homogeneity.

3.3. Green Synthesis Method

An amount of 3.5 g of $AgNO_3$ was dissolved in 200 mL of distilled water. The prepared extract was added dropwise into the $AgNO_3$ solution until the color of the solution turned dark brown and maintained its pH (9–11), and finally, we obtained the precipitates. The solution was centrifuged at 7000 rpm for 10 min and dried. Then, it was annealed at 400 °C for 12 h. Finally, the prepared precipitate was ground to obtain a fine powder [17,18,45]. A schematic flow chart is depicted in Figure 8.

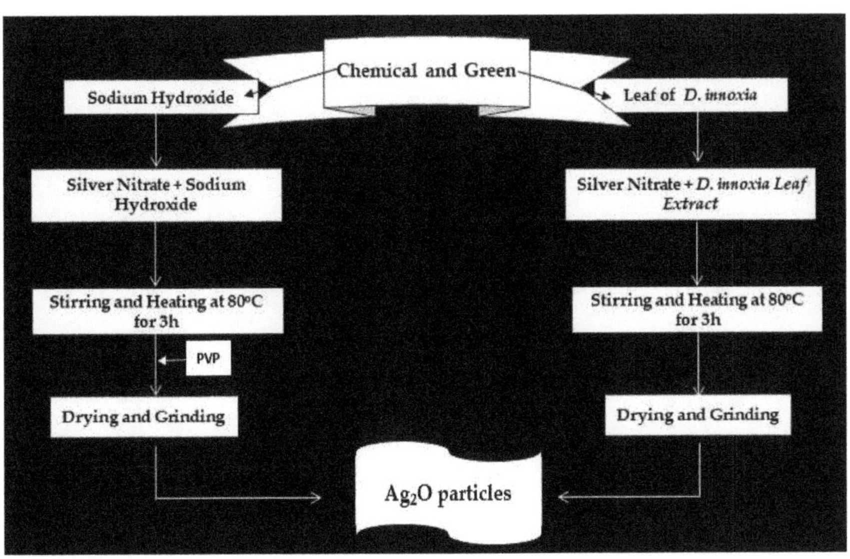

Figure 8. Schematic flow chart of chemically and green-synthesized Ag_2O particles.

3.4. Chemical Synthesis Method

An amount of 0.407 g of $NaBH_4$ was dissolved in 50 mL of deionized water and kept in an ice bath for 3 h. In the next step, 3.5 g of $AgNO_3$ was taken and dissolved in 200 mL of distilled water and kept under continuous stirring on a magnetic stirrer for 40 min to obtain a homogeneous solution [46]. Next, the $NaBH_4$ solution was removed from the ice bath and placed in a magnetic stirrer, and then the $AgNO_3$ solution was added dropwise. The solution was constantly stirred for 3 h to obtain dark-colored precipitates; then, 0.3 g Polyvinylpyrrolidone was mixed in 10 mL of water, and precipitates were prepared. The solution was centrifuged at 7000 rpm for 10 min and dried. Then, it was annealed at 400 °C for 12 h, and finally, the dark precipitate was ground to obtain a fine powder [27,47]. A schematic flow chart is depicted in Figure 8.

3.5. Characterization of the Synthesized Nanomaterial

X-ray diffraction (D8 advance Bruker, Karlsruhe, Germany) was used to confirm the crystal structure of the prepared particles. UV–visible spectroscopy (BK-UV1800PC DB, Bio-base, Jinan, China) was employed to compute the optical density, and FTIR (Spectrum 2, Perkin Elmer, Waltham, MA, USA) was used to study the functional groups (stretching and vibrational). The surface morphology of both chemically and green-synthesized Ag_2O particles was analyzed using scanning electron microscopy (Cube 10 Emcraft, Hanam, Republic of Korea) analysis. An energy-dispersive X-ray (EDX) spectrometer was used to confirm the elemental composition of the synthesized materials.

3.6. Bioassay

3.6.1. Cell Lines and Viruses

MCF-7 and green African monkey kidney (Vero) cell lines were gifted from the National Institute of Biotechnology and Genetic Engineering (NIBGE) in Faisalabad, Pakistan. MCF-7 and Vero cells were cultivated in DMEM/F-12 medium containing 1% (*v*/*v*) antibiotics and 10% (*v*/*v*) FBS. The flasks were kept at 37 °C in a humidified atmosphere with 5% CO_2. NDV was grown in 9-day-old chicken embryo eggs. Before use, stock viruses were collected, titrated, and stored [46].

3.6.2. Cytotoxicity Assay

MTT assays were used to measure the cytotoxicity of the chemically and green-synthesized Ag_2O particles. MCF-7 cells were seeded in 96-well plates. Cells were incubated with increasing concentrations of particles at 37 °C and 5% CO_2 for 48 h. The cells were treated with a 5 mg/mL MTT solution and then incubated for 4 h. After removing the MTT, 150 μL of DMSO was added and left for 5 min. The optical density was calculated using a microplate reader. Each experiment was performed in triplicate. The cytotoxicity level was quantified by determining the IC_{50} value, representing the concentration of particles that suppressed the growth of MCF-7 cells by half (50%) in comparison to untreated cells. Due to chemically synthesized Ag_2O particles, the basicity of the solution may increase and hence become toxic towards the cell line. On the other hand, green-synthesized Ag_2O particles were synthesized in a water-based extract, so they exhibited low toxicity. The percentage viability of Ag_2O particles was calculated using the following formula [48,49].

$$\%age\ Cell\ Viability = \frac{Abs\ of\ control - Abs\ of\ treated\ cells}{Abs\ of\ control} \times 100\% \quad (2)$$

3.6.3. Antiviral Activity

Chemically and green-synthesized Ag_2O particles were dissolved in DMEM without serum and used at concentrations of 0.5, 1, 2, 4, 8 and 10 μg/mL. The percentage (%) inhibition was calculated by dividing the number of plaques acquired in the positive control, which had 0% inhibition (no antiviral compounds added to the cell monolayers). A plaque-forming assay was performed to check the antiviral activity of both chemically and green-synthesized Ag_2O particles. For this, confluent Vero cell monolayers (12-well plates) were cleaned with phosphate-buffered saline and infected with NDV for 1 h at 37 °C, with an infection diversity of 0.02 plaque-forming units per cell. The virus inoculum was mixed with Ag_2O particles to perform the test. Unencapsulated virus was inactivated using citrate buffer at pH 3. After being washed in PBS, the samples were incubated for 48 h in fresh growing medium with carboxymethylcellulose. Monolayers infected with NDV were fixed and stained with 10% formaldehyde. The plates were then stained with crystal violet after fixation. Microscopically, the plaques were counted. The mean plaque count for each drug concentration was expressed as a percentage of the mean plaque count of the control virus, using the formula shown below. The plaques were quantified under a microscope. The mean plaque count for every drug concentration was calculated as a ratio to the mean plaque count of the control virus, using the formula below. A graph was plotted to show the relationship between the number of plaques and the drug concentration [29,49].

$$Inhibition\ (\%) = \frac{(Mean\ no.\ of\ Plaques\ in\ control - Mean\ no.\ of\ Plaques\ in\ samples)}{(Mean\ no.\ of\ Plaques\ in\ control)} \times 100\% \quad (3)$$

3.7. Statistical Analysis (S.A)

Statistical analysis (S.A) was performed using Student's *t*-test. All cytotoxic results on MCF-7 and Vero cell line experiments were reported as mean ± SD (standard deviation). A value of $p \leq 0.05$ was statistically significant (indicated by *), and a value of $p \leq 0.01$ was considered highly significant (indicated by **).

4. Conclusions

Silver oxide (Ag_2O) particles were synthesized via a chemical- and green-synthesis approach. The XRD results revealed a cubic crystal structure. UV–visible spectroscopy results gave maximum absorption spectra at 410 nm and 414.7 nm, respectively, confirming the growth of chemically and green-synthesized Ag_2O particles. An in vitro MTT assay of the green and chemically Ag_2O particles revealed that both possess significant anticancer activity against MCF-7 cells with IC_{50} 17.908 µg/mL and IC_{50} 23.856 µg/mL, respectively. The antiviral activity of both particles was also evaluated by plaque-forming assay, and the green-synthesized Ag_2O particles exhibited a higher antiviral ability with IC_{50} 0.618 µg/mL compared to chemically synthesized Ag_2O particles with IC_{50} 6.129 µg/mL. These results revealed that green-synthesized Ag_2O particles proved to be better than chemically synthesized Ag_2O particles against cancer and viral infections. In the case of chemically synthesized Ag_2O particles, toxicity (toxic behavior) was observed against normal (Vero) cells, unlike green-synthesized Ag_2O particles. This observation further supports the idea that green-synthesized Ag_2O particles are safer than chemically synthesized Ag_2O particles. This research could potentially play a role in biomedical applications, particularly in the field of nanomedicine in the near future. We also suggest that in vivo anticancer and antiviral studies of green-synthesized Ag_2O particles should be performed.

Author Contributions: Conceptualization, M.F.-e.-A., M.A. and W.I.; methodology, M.A. and W.I.; software, M.A.; validation, M.F.-e.-A., M.H. and J.R.; formal analysis, Z.H.; investigation, M.A. and M.S.; resources, M.S.; data curation, M.A. and M.H.; writing—original draft preparation, M.A. and W.I.; writing—review and editing, M.F.-e.-A., J.R. and K.A.D.; visualization, M.F.-e.-A., M.S. and N.H.A.-Q.; supervision, M.F.-e.-A.; project administration, M.F.-e.-A. and K.A.D.; funding acquisition, K.A.D. All authors have read and agreed to the published version of the manuscript.

Funding: This work was funded by researchers Supporting Project Number (RSP2024R388) King Saud University, Riyadh, Saudi Arabia.

Institutional Review Board Statement: Not applicable.

Informed Consent Statement: Not applicable.

Data Availability Statement: Data is contained within the article.

Acknowledgments: This work was funded by researchers Supporting Project Number (RSP2024R388) King Saud University, Riyadh, Saudi Arabia.

Conflicts of Interest: The authors declare no conflict of interest.

References

1. Bray, F.; Parkin, D.M. Cancer in sub-Saharan Africa in 2020: A review of current estimates of the national burden, data gaps, and future needs. *Lancet Oncol.* **2022**, *23*, 719–728. [CrossRef] [PubMed]
2. Sung, H.; Ferlay, J.; Siegel, R.L.; Laversanne, M.; Soerjomataram, I.; Jemal, A.; Bray, F. Global Cancer Statistics 2020: GLOBOCAN Estimates of Incidence and Mortality Worldwide for 36 Cancers in 185 Countries. *CA Cancer J. Clin.* **2021**, *71*, 209–249. [CrossRef]
3. Mettlin, C. Global breast cancer mortality statistics. *CA Cancer J. Clin.* **1999**, *49*, 138–144. [CrossRef] [PubMed]
4. Khan, N.H.; Duan, S.F.; Wu, D.D.; Ji, X.Y. Better reporting and awareness campaigns needed for breast cancer in Pakistani women. *Cancer Manag. Res.* **2021**, *13*, 2125–2129. [CrossRef] [PubMed]
5. Iqbal, S.; Fakhar-e-Alam, M.; Akbar, F.; Shafiq, M.; Atif, M.; Amin, N.; Ismail, M.; Hanif, A.; Farooq, W.A. Application of silver oxide nanoparticles for the treatment of cancer. *J. Mol. Struct.* **2019**, *1189*, 203–209. [CrossRef]
6. Bonam, S.R.; Wu, Y.S.; Tunki, L.; Chellian, R.; Halmuthur, M.S.K.; Muller, S.; Pandy, V. What has come out from phytomedicines and herbal edibles for the treatment of cancer? *ChemMedChem* **2018**, *13*, 1854–1872. [CrossRef]
7. Zargar, M.; Shameli, K.; Najafi, G.R.; Farahani, F. Plant mediated green biosynthesis of silver nanoparticles using *Vitex negundo* L. extract. *J. Ind. Eng. Chem.* **2014**, *20*, 4169–4175. [CrossRef]
8. Wiley, B.J.; Im, S.H.; McLellan, J.; Siekkinen, A.; Xia, Y. Maneuvering the surface plasmon resonance of silver nanostructures through shape-controlled synthesis. *J. Phys. Chem. B* **2006**, *110*, 15666–15675. [CrossRef]
9. Sondi, I.; Salopek-Sondi, B. Silver nanoparticles as antimicrobial agent: A case study on *E. coli* as a model for Gram-negative bacteria. *J. Colloid Interface Sci.* **2004**, *275*, 177–182. [CrossRef]
10. Yao, J.; Yang, M.; Duan, Y. Chemistry, biology, and medicine of fluorescent nanomaterials and related systems: New insights into biosensing, bioimaging, genomics, diagnostics, and therapy. *Chem. Rev.* **2014**, *114*, 6130–6178. [CrossRef]
11. Pryshchepa, O.; Pomastowski, P.; Buszewski, B. Silver nanoparticles: Synthesis, investigation techniques, and properties. *Adv. Colloid Interface Sci.* **2020**, *284*, 102246. [CrossRef]
12. Danish, M.S.S.; Estrella-Pajulas, L.L.; Alemaida, I.M.; Grilli, M.L.; Mikhaylov, A.; Senjyu, T. Green synthesis of silver oxide nanoparticles for photocatalytic environmental remediation and biomedical applications. *Metals* **2022**, *12*, 769. [CrossRef]
13. Ismail, G.A.; El-Sheekh, M.M.; Samy, R.M.; Gheda, S.F. Antimicrobial, antioxidant, and antiviral activities of biosynthesized silver nanoparticles by phycobiliprotein crude extract of the cyanobacteria *Spirulina platensis* and *Nostoc linckia*. *Bionanoscience* **2021**, *11*, 355–370. [CrossRef]
14. Islam, T.; Ara, I.; Islam, T.; Sah, P.K.; de Almeida, R.S.; Matias, E.F.F.; Ramalho, C.L.G.; Coutinho, H.D.M.; Islam, M.T. Ethnobotanical uses and phytochemical, biological, and toxicological profiles of *Datura metel* L.: A review. *Curr. Res. Toxicol.* **2023**, *4*, 100106. [CrossRef] [PubMed]
15. Khan, Z.; Al-Thabaiti, S.A.; Obaid, A.Y.; Al-Youbi, A. Preparation and characterization of silver nanoparticles by chemical reduction method. *Colloids Surf. B Biointerfaces* **2011**, *82*, 513–517. [CrossRef]
16. Moond, M.; Singh, S.; Sangwan, S.; Devi, R.; Beniwal, R. Green synthesis and applications of silver nanoparticles: A systematic review. *AATCC J. Res.* **2022**, *9*, 272–285. [CrossRef]
17. Mousavi-Khattat, M.; Keyhanfar, M.; Razmjou, A. A comparative study of stability, antioxidant, DNA cleavage and antibacterial activities of green and chemically synthesized silver nanoparticles. *Artif. Cells Nanomed. Biotechnol.* **2018**, *46* (Suppl. 3), 1022–1031. [CrossRef]
18. Flieger, J.; Franus, W.; Panek, R.; Szymańska-Chargot, M.; Flieger, W.; Flieger, M.; Kołodziej, P. Green synthesis of silver nanoparticles using natural extracts with proven antioxidant activity. *Molecules* **2021**, *26*, 4986. [CrossRef] [PubMed]
19. Martina, B.E.E.; Koraka, P.; Osterhaus, A.D.M.E. Dengue virus pathogenesis: An integrated view. *Clin. Microbiol. Rev.* **2009**, *22*, 564–581. [CrossRef]
20. Gaikwad, S.; Ingle, A.; Gade, A.; Rai, M.; Falanga, A.; Incoronato, N.; Russo, L.; Galdiero, S.; Galdiero, M. Antiviral activity of mycosynthesized silver nanoparticles against herpes simplex virus and human parainfluenza virus type 3. *Int. J. Nanomed.* **2013**, *8*, 4303–4314.
21. Scaturro, P.; Cortese, M.; Chatel-Chaix, L.; Fischl, W.; Bartenschlager, R. Dengue virus non-structural protein 1 modulates infectious particle production via interaction with the structural proteins. *PLoS Pathog.* **2015**, *11*, e1005277. [CrossRef] [PubMed]
22. Shen, Y.; Nemunaitis, J. Herpes simplex virus 1 (HSV-1) for cancer treatment. *Cancer Gene Ther.* **2006**, *13*, 975–992. [CrossRef] [PubMed]
23. Pierson, T.C.; Diamond, M.S. The continued threat of emerging flaviviruses. *Nat. Microbiol.* **2020**, *5*, 796–812. [CrossRef] [PubMed]
24. Wasik, B.R.; de Wit, E.; Munster, V.; Lloyd-Smith, J.O.; Martinez-Sobrido, L.; Parrish, C.R. Onward transmission of viruses: How do viruses emerge to cause epidemics after spillover? *Philos. Trans. R. Soc. B* **2019**, *374*, 20190017. [CrossRef] [PubMed]
25. Panáček, A.; Kolář, M.; Večeřová, R.; Prucek, R.; Soukupová, J.; Kryštof, V.; Hamal, P.; Zbořil, R.; Kvítek, L. Antifungal activity of silver nanoparticles against *Candida* spp. *Biomaterials* **2009**, *30*, 6333–6340. [CrossRef] [PubMed]
26. Shankar, S.; Rhim, J.W. Amino acid mediated synthesis of silver nanoparticles and preparation of antimicrobial agar/silver nanoparticles composite films. *Carbohydr. Polym.* **2015**, *130*, 353–363. [CrossRef] [PubMed]

27. Mani, M.; Harikrishnan, R.; Purushothaman, P.; Pavithra, S.; Rajkumar, P.; Kumaresan, S.; Al Farraj, D.A.; Elshikh, M.S.; Balasubramanian, B.; Kaviyarasu, K. Systematic green synthesis of silver oxide nanoparticles for antimicrobial activity. *Environ. Res.* **2021**, *202*, 111627. [CrossRef] [PubMed]
28. Gajendran, B.; Chinnasamy, A.; Durai, P.; Raman, J.; Ramar, M. Biosynthesis and characterization of silver nanoparticles from Datura inoxia and its apoptotic effect on human breast cancer cell line MCF7. *Mater. Lett.* **2014**, *122*, 98–102. [CrossRef]
29. Al-Khedhairy, A.A.; Wahab, R. Silver nanoparticles: An instantaneous solution for anticancer activity against human liver (HepG2) and breast (MCF-7) cancer cells. *Metals* **2022**, *12*, 148. [CrossRef]
30. Allahverdiyev, A.M.; Abamor, E.S.; Bagirova, M.; Rafailovich, M. Antimicrobial effects of TiO_2 and Ag_2O nanoparticles against drug-resistant bacteria and leishmania parasites. *Future Microbiol.* **2011**, *6*, 933–940. [CrossRef]
31. Fayyadh, A.A.; Jaduaa Alzubaidy, M.H. Green-synthesis of Ag_2O nanoparticles for antimicrobial assays. *J. Mech. Behav. Mater.* **2021**, *30*, 228–236. [CrossRef]
32. Stoimenov, P.K.; Klinger, R.L.; Marchin, G.L.; Klabunde, K.J. Metal oxide nanoparticles as bactericidal agents. *Langmuir* **2002**, *18*, 6679–6686. [CrossRef]
33. Chandirika, J.U.; Annadurai, G. Biosynthesis and characterization of silver nanoparticles using leaf extract Abutilon indicum. *Glob. J. Biotechnol. Biochem* **2018**, *13*, 7–11.
34. Mardare, G.; Lazar, L.; Malutan, T. Potential Application of Invasive Plant Species Datura innoxia for the Scopolamine Extracts of the Plant Organs and Analysis Using UV–VIS Spectrophotometry. *Forests* **2022**, *13*, 1555. [CrossRef]
35. Kasthuri, J.; Veerapandian, S.; Rajendiran, N. Biological synthesis of silver and gold nanoparticles using apiin as reducing agent. *Colloids Surf. B Biointerfaces* **2009**, *68*, 55–60. [CrossRef]
36. Rogers, J.V.; Parkinson, C.V.; Choi, Y.W.; Speshock, J.L.; Hussain, S.M. A preliminary assessment of silver nanoparticle inhibition of monkeypox virus plaque formation. *Nanoscale Res. Lett.* **2008**, *3*, 129–133. [CrossRef]
37. Patil, S.; Chandrasekaran, R. Biogenic nanoparticles: A comprehensive perspective in synthesis, characterization, application and its challenges. *J. Genet. Eng. Biotechnol.* **2020**, *18*, 67. [CrossRef]
38. Banerjee, S.; Islam, S.; Chattopadhyay, A.; Sen, A.; Kar, P. Synthesis of silver nanoparticles using underutilized fruit *Baccaurea ramiflora* (Latka) juice and its biological and cytotoxic efficacy against MCF-7 and MDA-MB 231 cancer cell lines. *S. Afr. J. Bot.* **2022**, *145*, 228–235. [CrossRef]
39. Venugopal, K.; Rather, H.A.; Rajagopal, K.; Shanthi, M.P.; Sheriff, K.; Illiyas, M.; Rather, R.A.; Manikandan, E.; Uvarajan, S.; Bhaskar, M.; et al. Synthesis of silver nanoparticles (Ag NPs) for anticancer activities (MCF 7 breast and A549 lung cell lines) of the crude extract of *Syzygium aromaticum*. *J. Photochem. Photobiol. B Biol.* **2017**, *167*, 282–289. [CrossRef]
40. Narayanan, M.; Divya, S.; Natarajan, D.; Senthil-Nathan, S.; Kandasamy, S.; Chinnathambi, A.; Alahmadi, T.A.; Pugazhendhi, A. Green synthesis of silver nanoparticles from aqueous extract of *Ctenolepis garcini* L. and assess their possible biological applications. *Process Biochem.* **2021**, *107*, 91–99. [CrossRef]
41. Gupta, A.; Pandey, S.; Variya, B.; Shah, S.; Yadav, J.S. Green synthesis of gold nanoparticles using different leaf extracts of *Ocimum gratissimum* Linn for anti-tubercular activity. *Curr. Nanomed.* **2019**, *9*, 146–157. [CrossRef]
42. Akintelu, S.A.; Oyebamiji, A.K.; Olugbeko, S.C.; Latona, D.F. Green chemistry approach towards the synthesis of copper nanoparticles and its potential applications as therapeutic agents and environmental control. *Curr. Res. Green Sustain. Chem.* **2021**, *4*, 100176. [CrossRef]
43. Lara, H.H.; Ayala-Nuñez, N.V.; Ixtepan-Turrent, L.; Rodriguez-Padilla, C. Mode of antiviral action of silver nanoparticles against HIV-1. *J. Nanobiotechnology* **2010**, *8*, 1. [CrossRef]
44. Chamani, E.; Ebrahimi, R.; Khorsandi, K.; Meshkini, A.; Zarban, A.; Sharifzadeh, G. In vitro cytotoxicity of polyphenols from *Datura innoxia* aqueous leaf-extract on human leukemia K562 cells: DNA and nuclear proteins as targets. *Drug Chem. Toxicol.* **2020**, *43*, 138–148. [CrossRef]
45. Tahir, M.; Fakhar-e-Alam, M.; Asif, M.; Iqbal, M.J.; Abbas, A.; Hassan, M.; Rehman, J.; Bhatti, Q.A.; Mustafa, G.; Alothman, A.A.; et al. Investigation of gadolinium doped manganese nano spinel ferrites via magnetic hypothermia therapy effect towards MCF-7 breast cancer. *Heliyon* **2024**, *10*, E24792. [CrossRef]
46. Rhim, J.W.; Wang, L.F.; Hong, S.I. Preparation and characterization of agar/silver nanoparticles composite films with antimicrobial activity. *Food Hydrocoll.* **2013**, *33*, 327–335. [CrossRef]
47. Sadiqa, A.; Rasul, A.; Hassan, M.; Sultana, S.; Jabeen, F. Identification of Novel Natural Inhibitors to Human 3-Phosphoglycerate Dehydrogenase (PHGDH) for Cancer Treatment. *Molecules* **2022**, *27*, 6108. [CrossRef]
48. Fakhar-e-Alam, M.; Amjad, I.; Saadullah, M.; Tahir, M.; Jawad, M.; Asif, M.; Atif, M.; Zara, S.; Rashad, M. Antitumor activity of Zinc oxide nanoparticles fused with Green Extract of *Nigella Sativa*. *J. Saudi Chem. Soc.* **2024**, *28*, 101814. [CrossRef]
49. Shetti, N.P.; Mishra, A.; Bukkitgar, S.D.; Basu, S.; Narang, J.; Raghava Reddy, K.; Aminabhavi, T.M. Conventional and nanotechnology-based sensing methods for SARS coronavirus (2019-nCoV). *ACS Appl. Bio Mater.* **2021**, *4*, 1178–1190. [CrossRef] [PubMed]

pharmaceuticals

MDPI

Article

Exploring the Potential of Halotolerant Actinomycetes from Rann of Kutch, India: A Study on the Synthesis, Characterization, and Biomedical Applications of Silver Nanoparticles

Paras Dayma [1,†], Nisha Choudhary [2,†], Daoud Ali [3], Saud Alarifi [3], Pravin Dudhagara [1], Kuldeep Luhana [4], Virendra Kumar Yadav [3,*], Ashish Patel [3,*] and Rajesh Patel [1,*]

1 Department of Biosciences, Veer Narmad South Gujarat University, Surat 395007, Gujarat, India; paras_dayma@yahoo.com (P.D.); dudhagarapr@gmail.com (P.D.)

2 Department of Life Sciences, Hemchandracharya North Gujarat University, Patan 384265, Gujarat, India; nishanaseer03@gmail.com

3 Department of Zoology, College of Science, King Saud University, P.O. Box 2455, Riyadh 11451, Saudi Arabia

4 Department of Biotechnology, Hemchandracharya North Gujarat University, Patan 384265, Gujarat, India; kuldeep.dnatech@gmail.com

* Correspondence: yadava94@gmail.com (V.K.Y.); uni.ashish@gmail.com (A.P.); rkpatel@vnsgu.ac.in (R.P.)

† These authors contributed equally to this work.

Abstract: A tremendous increase in the green synthesis of metallic nanoparticles has been noticed in the last decades, which is due to their unique properties at the nano dimension. The present research work deals with synthesis mediated by the actinomycete *Streptomyces tendae* of silver nanoparticles (AgNPs), isolated from Little and Greater Rann of Kutch, India. The confirmation of the formation of AgNPs by the actinomycetes was carried out by using a UV-Vis spectrophotometer where an absorbance peak was obtained at 420 nm. The X-ray diffraction pattern demonstrated five characteristic diffraction peaks indexed at the lattice plane (111), (200), (231), (222), and (220). Fourier transform infrared showed typical bands at 531 to 1635, 2111, and 3328 cm^{-1}. Scanning electron microscopy shows that the spherical-shaped AgNPs particles have diameters in the range of 40 to 90 nm. The particle size analysis displayed the mean particle size of AgNPs in aqueous medium, which was about 55 nm (±27 nm), bearing a negative charge on their surfaces. The potential of the *S. tendae*-mediated synthesized AgNPs was evaluated for their antimicrobial, anti-methicillin-resistant *Staphylococcus aureus* (MRSA), anti-biofilm, and anti-oxidant activity. The maximum inhibitory effect was observed against *Pseudomonas aeruginosa* at (8 μg/mL), followed by *Escherichia coli* and *Aspergillus niger* at (32 μg/mL), and against *Candida albicans* (64 μg/mL), whereas *Bacillus subtilis* (128 μg/mL) and *Staphylococcus aureus* (256 μg/mL) were much less sensitive to AgNPs. The biosynthesized AgNPs displayed activity against MRSA, and the free radical scavenging activity was observed with an increase in the dosage of AgNPs from 25 to 200 μg/mL. AgNPs in combination with ampicillin displayed inhibition of the development of biofilm in *Pseudomonas aeruginosa* and *Streptococcus pneumoniae* at 98% and 83%, respectively. AgNPs were also successfully coated on the surface of cotton to prepare antimicrobial surgical cotton, which demonstrated inhibitory action against *Bacillus subtilis* (15 mm) and *Escherichia coli* (12 mm). The present research integrates microbiology, nanotechnology, and biomedical science to formulate environmentally friendly antimicrobial materials using halotolerant actinomycetes, evolving green nanotechnology in the biomedical field. Moreover, this study broadens the understanding of halotolerant actinomycetes and their potential and opens possibilities for formulating new antimicrobial products and therapies.

Keywords: actinomycete; halotolerant; silver nanoparticles; multidrug resistance; Rann of Kutch

1. Introduction

Actinomycetes are a diverse category of Gram-positive, filamentous bacteria that have higher guanine + cytosine content [1]. It is widely distributed in terrestrial and aquatic ecosystems and plays a significant biological and ecological role in the environment, including the degradation and recycling of substances, and the generation of bioactive molecules [2,3]. Prokaryotes and eukaryotes both can produce antimicrobial compounds whereas the prokaryotic group of organisms, actinomycetes are the prolific producers of bioactive substances [4]. Approximately 70% of the total antibiotics that are used today for the treatment of various diseases are alone obtained from actinomycetes, especially *Streptomyces* [5] in addition to taromycin A [6], retimycin A [7,8], and tetrocarcins [9,10]. *Streptomyces*, a well-known genus, which produces diverse bioactive secondary metabolites like antibiotics, anticancer [11], antiviral, anti-malarial agents [12,13], etc. contributing significantly to medically important antibiotics [14,15], while other unexplored actinomycetes genera hold potential for bioactive metabolites [16,17]. In the last decade, microbial infections have increased tremendously [18–20], leading to antibiotic resistance due to misuse [21–23]; resistance mechanisms include genetic changes and metabolic pathways [24], demanding the formulation of new compounds to combat multidrug resistance [25–27].

The high salinity and alkalinity are the uniqueness of the desert, which leads to distinct microbial compositions and structures [28]. The defense potential of these microorganisms is exhibited by producing bioactive molecules against drug-resistant bacteria [29,30]. These microorganisms have the potential for antibiotic production and nanoparticle synthesis, increasing stability and biocidal action through surface modification by biological macromolecules [31,32].

Noble metallic nanoparticles (NPs) like silver, gold, and platinum, synthesized biologically, are biocompatible [33,34]. These NPs are effective against drug-resistant bacteria, which offers safer solutions for biomedical applications [35]. Biocompatibility remains a major issue among the NPs synthesized by chemical and physical routes. Recently silver nanoparticles (AgNPs) have been widely used in biomedicine, textiles, etc. due to their effectiveness and antimicrobial activity [36]. To date, several types of microorganisms have been used for the synthesis of AgNPs like bacteria [37], fungi [38], algae [39], and actinomycetes. However halotolerant actinomycetes along with antimicrobial activity have been rarely used for the synthesis of AgNPs, Nevertheless, actinomycetes have received relatively a little attention regarding their potential for synthesizing nanoparticles [40]. Synthesis and characterization of AgNPs [41] have been documented from *Streptomyces* sp., *Nocardia sp.* [42–44], *Thermomonospora sp.* [45], and *Rhodococcus sp.* Among *Streptomyces, Streptomyces sp.* VITBT7, *Streptomyces. sp.* MBRC-91, *Streptomyces parvulus* SSNP11, *Streptomyces rochei, Streptomyces aureofaciens* MTCC356, *Streptomyces spp.* I, II; *Streptomyces albidoflavus* CNP10, *Streptomyces parvulus* DPUA1549, *Streptomyces seoulensis* DPUA 1747, *Streptomyces owasiensis* DPUA 1748, *Streptomyces spp.* 09 PBT 005, *Streptomyces narbonensis* SSHH-1E and *Streptomyces xinghaiensis* OF1 [46] have been explored to date for the formation of AgNPs.

Wypij et al. synthesized AgNPs by using an acidophilic actinobacterial SH11 strain isolated from pine forest soil which was polydisperse and spherical in shape whose mean size was 13.2 nm. The AgNPs exhibited antibacterial activity in *Staphylococcus aureus, Bacillus subtilis,* and *Escherichia coli* by using the disc diffusion minimum inhibitory concentration (MIC) method [47]. Otari et al. also synthesized 5–50 nm AgNPs by using *Rhodococcus* spp. and assessed their antimicrobial activity against pathogenic microorganisms [48]. Recently, Enain synthesized AgNPs from *Streptomyces avermitilis* Azhar A.4 E and assessed their larvicidal effect on the black cutworm, *Agrotis ipsilon* [49].

Out of all these investigations, hardly any attempts were made at the synthesis of AgNPs from the halotolerant actinomycetes isolated from the desert area. So, the current investigation reports the synthesis of AgNPs from desert-isolated halotolerant actinomycetes which also have activity against methicillin-resistant *Staphylococcus aureus* (MRSA) pathogens.

The major aim of this current study was to synthesize AgNPs using actinomycetes isolated from the salty desert of Kutch, i.e., Rann of Kutch. One of the objectives was to isolate and characterize the halotolerant actinomycetes from the saline desert area. The second objective was to observe the antibiotic production and antimicrobial activity profile of the isolated strain. Thirdly, we aimed to screen, identify, and design applications for the development of AgNPs from the potential strain of actinomycetes. Another objective was to characterize the developed AgNPs by using analytical instruments. Lastly, our goal was to evaluate the biomedical applications, including the antimicrobial activity of the AgNPs. Such a greener approach will play a crucial role in material science and it will also prove valuable in combating drug-resistant bacteria.

2. Results

2.1. Extracellular Biosynthesis of AgNPs from Saline Desert Actinomycetes

For the reduction of Ag^+ to Ag^0, different ratios of cell-free supernatant to $AgNO_3$ were examined. The reaction mixture, having an equal amount of $AgNO_3$ and culture supernatant, showed a rapid color change compared to other reactions. The synthesis of AgNPs using actinomycete was examined mainly through the observation of the color change in the reaction mixture in the presence of 1 mM $AgNO_3$. The difference in color change indicates the difference in the size of the AgNPs. Control experiments without actinomycete showed no color change. The transformation of color from pale yellow to dark brown occurred after 4 to 24 h of incubation.

2.2. UV-Vis Spectroscopic Analysis of AgNPs Synthesized by S. tendae (GR-CHA-4)

UV-Vis spectra of AgNPs synthesized by actinobacteria and control are shown in Figure 1; these were recorded immediately after the color change (within 1 h) from pale yellow to brown. An uninoculated MGYP medium was used as a control. Homogenous AgNPs have been known to produce a Surface Plasmon Resonance (SPR) band in the range of 420–450 nm [50]. The absorbance peak reflects the size and shape of silver NPs and a shift in the SPR peak to longer wavelengths with an increase in particle size could suggest that AgNPs produced by actinomycete isolate are smaller in size with a spherical shape [51]. The AgNPs synthesized within 4 h represented rapid synthesis [52]. The AgNPs synthesized by *S. tendae* showed an absorption peak at 405 nm, confirming the formation of AgNPs.

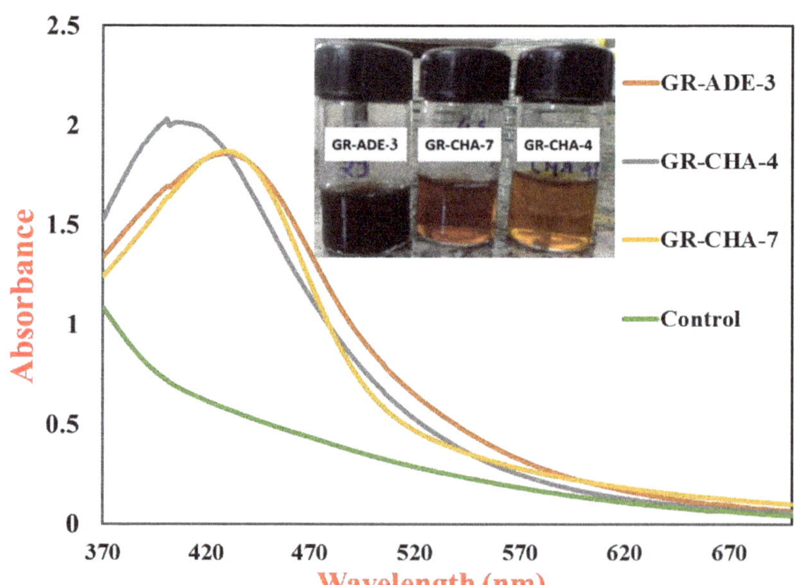

Figure 1. UV-Vis spectra of the AgNPs synthesized by three isolates along with the control reaction.

2.3. Effect of Reaction Parameters on AgNP Synthesis Using Isolate S. tendae (GR-CHA-4)

2.3.1. Medium Optimization for Nanoparticle Synthesis

Based on the literature survey, the nanoparticle-producing ability of the isolate *S. tendae*-GR-CHA-4 was further optimized by using different growth media such as MGYP, ISP Medium No 1, starch casein broth, casein glycerol broth, and M9 minimal medium (sodium acetate as carbon source). The rapid AgNP synthesis was observed after 4 **h** using MGYP. Furthermore, AgNPs did not show clumping out of five media. MGYP was best for AgNP synthesis using isolate GR-CHA-4. The other four media were not suitable for AgNP formation using GR-CHA-4 isolate due to slow synthesis (after 24 h) and the presence of aggregation.

2.3.2. Synthesis of AgNPs under Normal, Alkaline, Saline, and Saline + Alkaline Conditions

To optimize the effect of pH and NaCl concentration together with the nanoparticle production ability of the selected isolate, the isolate was grown on an MGYP medium in the presence of four different conditions, i.e., normal (0.0% *w/v* salt, 7.0 pH), alkaline (0.0% *w/v* salt, 9.0 pH), saline (5.0% *w/v* salt, 7.0 pH), and saline + alkaline (5% *w/v* salt, 9.0 pH) condition. Among all the four conditions used, the combination of 0% *w/v* salt and pH 7 supported the nanoparticle synthesis, while no synthesis occurred in other conditions.

2.3.3. Effect of $AgNO_3$ Concentration on Nanoparticle Synthesis

AgNP formation is highly influenced by the concentration of the parental compound. Low concentration will not produce applicable AgNPs, while high concentration will cause clumping and aggregation. Therefore, optimization is required for the formation of stable AgNPs. The formation of AgNPs took place in the presence of all the $AgNO_3$ concentrations starting from 1 mM to 5 mM. From the tested concentrations, 2 mM was found to be the optimum one, as it showed the absorption peak with the highest intensity (Figure 2a).

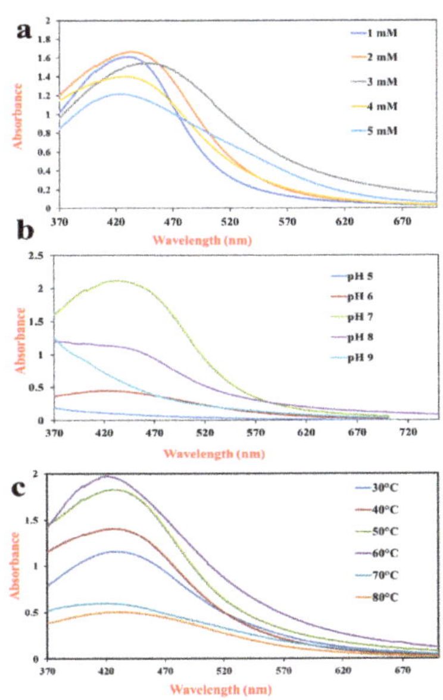

Figure 2. Effect of (**a**) $AgNO_3$ concentration, (**b**) pH, and (**c**) temperature on AgNPs synthesis by *S. tendae* GR-CHA-4.

2.3.4. Effect of pH on AgNP Synthesis

Variations in the pH of the reaction mixture influence the functionality of the enzymes and metabolites, thereby affecting the synthesis of NPs. This can lead to changes in the morphology and distribution of NPs. To check the relationship between pH and AgNP synthesis, the reaction mixture was allowed to react at pH 5.0, 6.0, 7.0, 8.0, and 9.0. The maximum synthesis of NPs occurred at pH 7.0, followed by pH 8.0 and pH 6.0, which showed much less bioreduction of $AgNO_3$ (Figure 2b), while pH 5.0 and pH 9.0 did not support the reduction of $AgNO_3$ to AgNPs.

2.3.5. Effect of Temperature on AgNP Synthesis

Biosynthesis of AgNPs was observed at 30 °C, 40 °C, 50 °C, 60 °C, 70 °C, and 80 °C. AgNPs were formulated at all six temperatures, but the rate of synthesis and the yield obtained were different. There was a gradual increase in the velocity of the reaction as well as the concentration of AgNPs from 30 °C to 60 °C, which can be observed from UV-Vis spectra. Above 60 °C, there was a sharp decrease in the synthesis of AgNPs (Figure 2c).

2.3.6. AgNP Synthesis under Optimized Conditions Using *S. tendae* (GR-CHA-4)

All the optimized factors were put together in the experiment to study the nanoparticle synthesis under optimized conditions. The MGYP was used as a growth medium for the growth of the selected strain (GR-CHA-4). The parameters applied during nanoparticle synthesis were pH 7.0, temperature 60 °C, and 2 mM $AgNO_3$. After incubation, color change from pale yellow to brown was observed within 1 h. So, based on various factors, the optimized medium is favorable for synthesizing AgNPs on a large scale.

2.3.7. Particle Size Analysis (PSA) and Zeta Potential of Synthesized AgNPs

The size distribution, average particle size, and concentration of synthesized AgNPs were measured by Nanoparticle Tracking Analysis (Figure 3a). The NTA is based on two properties of particles, light scattering and Brownian motion, and in comparison, to the Dynamic Light Scattering (DLS) method, NTA is more accurate. The results of PSA displayed the mean particle size of about 55 nm (±27 nm). The concentration of AgNPs was 2.70 × 10^8 particles/mL. The zeta potential (ZP) of the AgNPs was −20.4 mV, while conductivity was 0.0443 mS/cm (Figure 3b).

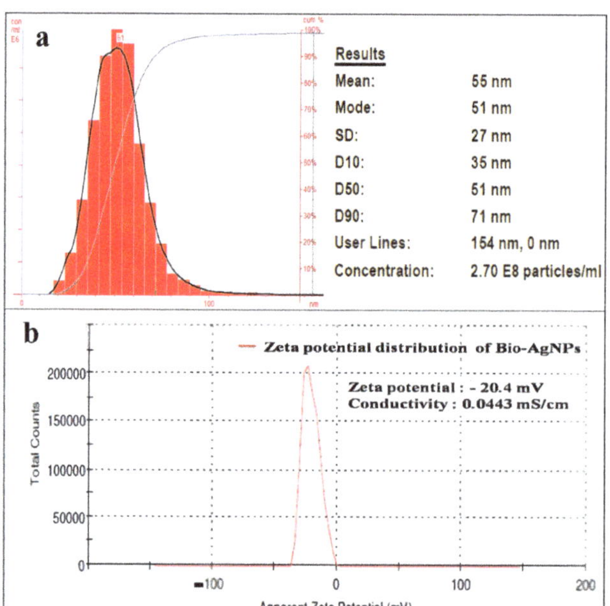

Figure 3. Particle size distribution analysis of AgNPs synthesized by *S. tendae* GR-CHA-4, and (**a**) zeta potential (**b**).

2.3.8. Fourier Transform Infrared (FT-IR) Spectroscopy of AgNPs for the Identification of Functional Groups

FTIR spectroscopy was used to identify the surface chemistry of biosynthesized AgNPs. FTIR measurements are also used to study the possible interaction between AgNPs and protein molecules, which is responsible for the synthesis and stabilization of well-dispersed AgNPs in the reaction mixture [53]. Figure 4 shows the presence of four major functional groups recorded between wave numbers 531 and 3328 cm^{-1}.

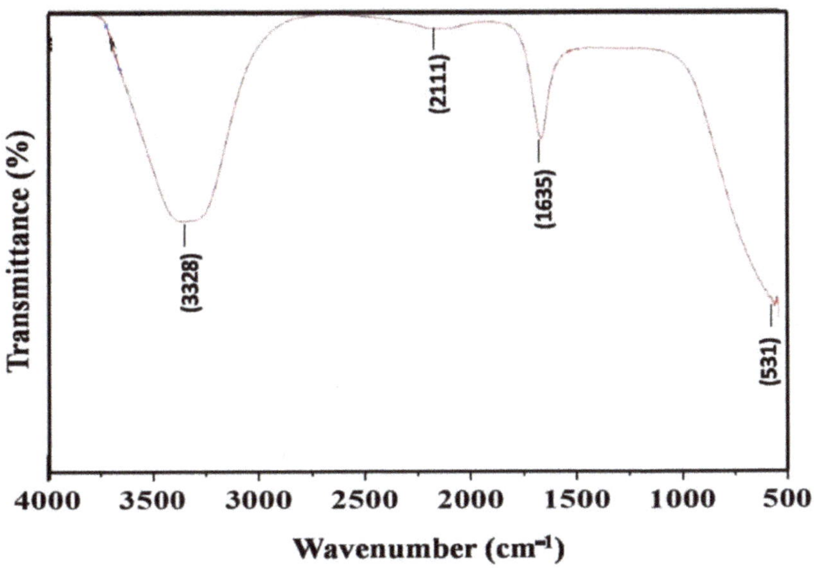

Figure 4. FTIR spectroscopy of AgNPs synthesized by *S. tendae* GR-CHA-4.

2.3.9. X-ray Diffraction (XRD) Analysis for Phase Identification

The exact nature of the AgNPs can be deduced from the XRD analysis. The XRD pattern (Figure 5) revealed the crystalline nature of synthesized AgNPs. The XRD pattern for AgNPs showed diffraction peaks at 27.06, 35.7, 37.8, 40.9, 43.8, 54.1, 56.5, and 68.8°. Out of all these peaks, the highest and sharpest peaks were at 27.06 and 54.1°.

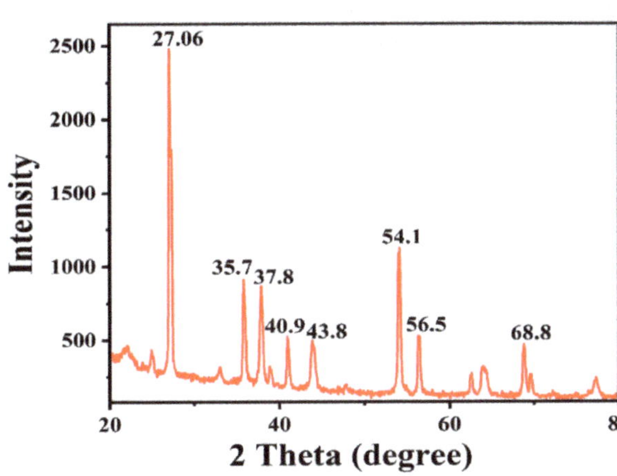

Figure 5. XRD pattern of AgNPs synthesized by *S. tendae* GR-CHA-4.

2.3.10. Morphological Analysis of AgNPs Synthesized by *S. tendae* by Using Scanning Electron Microscope (SEM)

The SEM image of the dried AgNPs shows the spherical-shaped NPs in scattered form (Figure 6a). The SEM micrograph clearly showed the presence of spherical-shaped particles having diameters in the range of 40 to 90 nm.

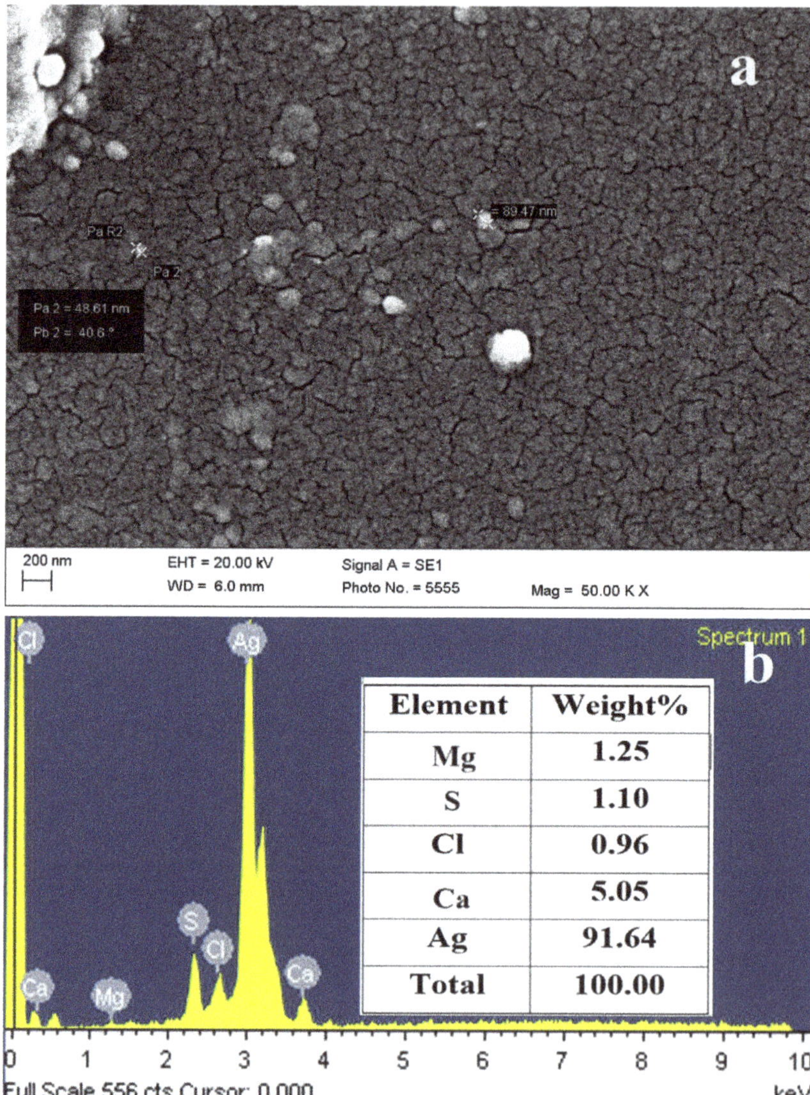

Figure 6. SEM micrograph (**a**) and EDS spectra (**b**) of AgNPs synthesized by *S. tendae* GR-CHA-4.

The energy dispersive X-ray spectroscopy (EDS) spectra of AgNPs shown in Figure 6b reveal peaks for Ag, Cl, S, Mg, and Ca. Out of all these elements, Ag was 91.64 (wt.%), Ca was (5.05%), Mg (1.25%), Cl (0.96%), and S (1.1%).

2.3.11. Three-Dimensional Analysis of AgNPs Using an Atomic Force Microscope (AFM)

AFM allows 2D and 3D characterization of nanomaterials, and the topographical features were analyzed using the AFM microscope for better visualization of surface morphology. AFM analysis provides information about the morphology and surface roughness of the materials. The AFM characterization shows two- and three-dimensional AFM images of AgNPs (Figure 7a). The 2D surface topographical images (Figure 7b) reveal the spherical nature of particles, whereas the 3D AFM micrograph shows the height and surface roughness of the AgNPs.

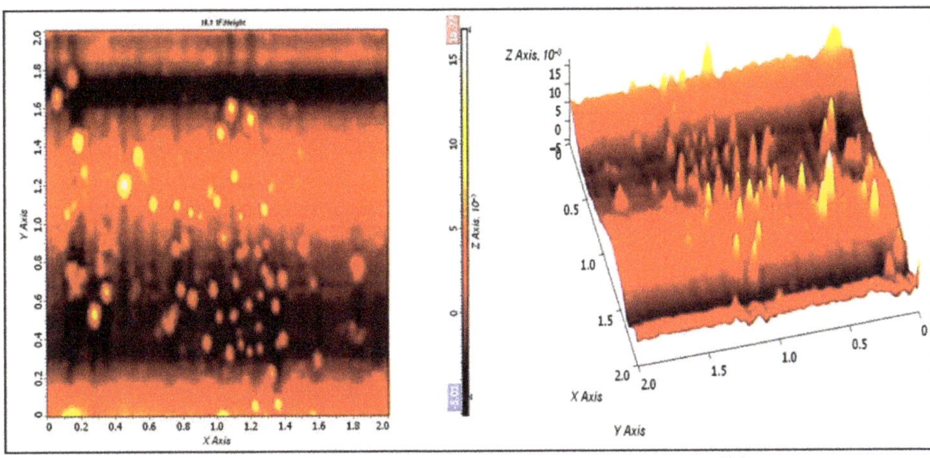

(a) (b)

Figure 7. Two-dimensional (**a**) and three-dimensional (**b**) AFM images of AgNPs synthesized by *S. tendae* GR-CHA-4.

2.3.12. Antimicrobial Activity of AgNPs (MIC)

Table 1 shows the MIC and MBC values of AgNPs and standard antibiotics against bacterial and fungal test cultures. Due to the smaller size and high concentration of AgNPs, it is worth using formulated AgNPs to control and kill pathogenic bacteria and fungi. The developed AgNPs from the GR-CHA-4 strain exhibited the highest inhibitory activity against *P. aeruginosa* (8 µg/mL), followed by *E. coli* and *A. niger* (32 µg/mL), then against *C. albicans* (64 µg/mL). *B. subtilis* (128 µg/mL) and *S. aureus* (256 µg/mL) were much less sensitive to AgNPs.

Table 1. Antimicrobial activity of AgNPs (MIC and MBC).

S. No.	Tested Microorganism	MIC of AgNPs (µg/mL)	MBC of AgNP (µg/mL)	MIC of Antibiotic (µg/mL)		
				AMP	K	TE
1	*B. subtilis* MTCC 441	128	128	128	8	4
2	*P. aeruginosa* MTCC 1688	8	16	512	12	64
3	*S. aureus* MTCC 737	256	256	128	3	64
4	*E. coli* MTCC 1687	32	64	512	128	64
				AMB	FLU	
5	*C. albicans* MTCC 183	32	64	8	256	
6	*A. niger* MTCC 1344	64	64	4	512	

AMP—ampicillin, K—kanamycin, TE—tetracycline, AMB—amphotericin B, FLU—fluconazole.

2.3.13. Synergistic Effect of AgNPs

The strategy of combining metal NPs with conventional antibiotics is a good alternative to combat growing bacterial resistance. The synergistic effect of NPs was studied against bacterial and fungal test cultures, and the FIC index and their interpretation values are shown in Table 2.

Table 2. Synergistic effect of AgNPs with conventional antibiotics.

S. No.	Tested Microorganism	AgNPs + Ampicillin (μg/mL)	FIC	AgNPs +Tetracycline (μg/mL)	FIC	AgNPs+ Amphotericin B (μg/mL)	FIC
1	*Bacillus subtilis* (MTCC 441)	64 + 64	1	16 + 0.5	0.25		
2	*P. aeruginosa* (MTCC 1688)	2 + 128	0.5	1 + 8	0.25		
3	*S. aureus* (MTCC 737)	128 + 64	1	64 + 16	0.5		
4	*E. coli* (MTCC 1687)	8 + 128	0.5	4 + 8	0.375		
5	*C. albicans* (MTCC 183)					16 + 4	1
6	*A. niger* (MTCC 1344)					32 + 2	1

FIC index	Interpretation
≤0.5	Synergistic
>0.5–1.0	Additive or non-synergistic
1.0–4.0	In different
>4	Antagonistic

2.3.14. AgNP Activity against MRSA

The rise of multi-drug resistance has necessitated the creation of a novel category of antimicrobial drugs. The biosynthesized AgNPs showed a good amount of activity against MRSA, with zone inhibition of 16 mm and 12 mm against MRSA 2 and MRSA 7, respectively.

2.3.15. Anti-Biofilm Activity of AgNPs Synthesized with *S. tendae*

Generation of the sessile communities and their inborn multi-drug resistance is the basis of several chronic and relentless bacterial infections [54]. The anti-biofilm efficacy of AgNPs was evaluated against *P. aeruginosa* and *S. pneumoniae* by applying a crystal violet assay (Table 3).

Table 3. Anti-biofilm activity of AgNPs.

Tested Microbes	Percentage Inhibition						
	AgNPs Dose (μg/mL)					AMP	AgNPs + AMP
	10	20	30	40	50	50	30 μg/mL+ 30 μg/mL
P. aeruginosa	15	22	30	46	60	35	98
S. pneumoniae	12	20	25	32	44	28	83

2.3.16. Anti-Oxidant Activity of AgNPs

An incremental rise in the percentage of free radical scavenging activity was noted (40.14, 52.12, 64.23, and 80.44%) as the quantity of AgNPs increased from 25 μg/mL to 200 μg/mL (Figure 8).

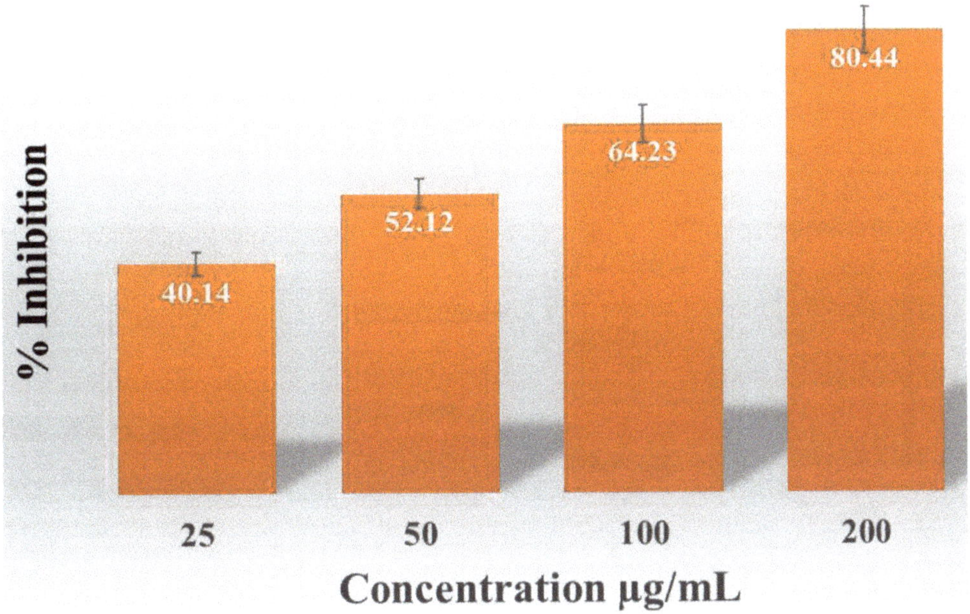

Figure 8. Anti-oxidant activity of AgNPs produced from *S. tendae*.

2.3.17. Preparation of Anti-Microbial Cotton

The AgNP-treated cotton effectively suppressed the growth of *Bacillus subtilis* and *E. coli*, resulting in the formation of ZOI of 15 mm and 12 mm, respectively.

3. Discussion

The change in color from pale yellow to dark brown was noticed after 4 to 24 h of incubation, as shown in Figure 9a,b. The color change suggested that actinomycete played a significant role in the development of AgNPs. Similar observations have been reported for *Bacillus licheniformis* [55], *P. aeruginosa* [56], *E. coli* [57], and *Bacillus megaterium* [58]. The mechanism of formation of AgNPs by the actinomycetes is well described in the literature. The actinomycetes, being metal-tolerant, take the Ag^+ ions from the aqueous medium into the cell and cytoplasm (Figure 9b). The Ag^+ ions are further reduced by the various biological molecules present inside the actinomycetes. Further, these reduced AgNPs are capped by biological molecules and released into the medium if the nature of the actinomycetes is extracellular, and the AgNPs have to be extracted by applying sonication and another approach to extract the AgNPs inside actinomycetes. Alkaliphilic actinomycetes *Nocardiopsis valliformis* from an alkaline Lonar crater were reported for the extracellular synthesis of AgNPs by Rathod and their group [59]. Extracellular biogenic synthesis of AgNPs was also found in the actinomycete isolated from marine sediment [60]. From the two sites of ROK, three potential actinomycetes were screened out for the synthesis of AgNPs. The three strains were coded as GR-CHA-4, GR-ADE-3, and GR-CHA-7, where the GR stands for Greater Rann of Kutch, CHA stands for Charanka Solar Park, and ADE stands for Adesar region. GR-CHA-4 and GR-CHA-7 were isolated from the Charanka solar park region, while GR-ADE-3 was isolated from the Adesar region of ROK. Out of all the three potential organisms, the AgNPs synthesized by GR-CHA-4 were of the desired shape and property.

So, the synthesis of AgNPs from GR-CHA-4 was selected for further optimization based on spectral analysis (UV-Vis) of AgNPs, reaction time, and color change. Physico-chemical parameters such as growth medium, pH, temperature, and precursor ($AgNO_3$)

concentration were optimized for AgNP synthesis. The narrow surface plasmon peak obtained at 428 nm indicated the lower aggregation of particles. The SPR of NPs is affected by the morphology, concentration, and interparticle distance, which indicates its efficiency in monitoring the aggregation of NPs [61].

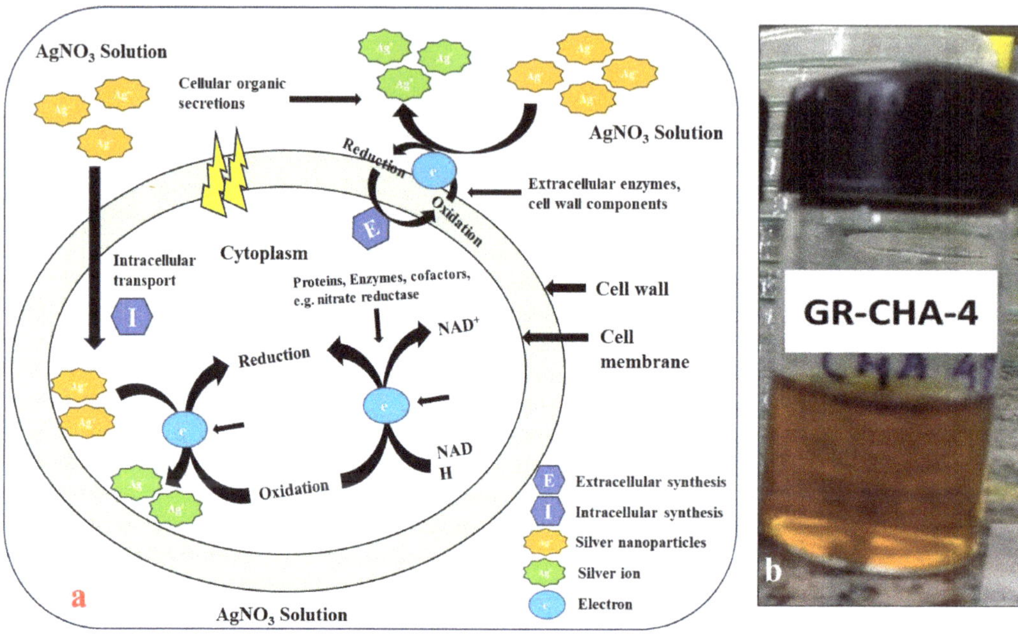

Figure 9. Mechanism of formation of AgNPs by actinomycetes (**a**) and color change for AgNP synthesis using actinomycete isolates (**b**).

The results obtained for the optimization of the media for AgNPs proved that differences in the medium components affect the production of secondary metabolites and ultimately influence nanoparticle production using the isolates. Similar reports on MGYP for the biosynthesis of various NPs have been found [62]. So, there is a need to optimize the medium components using statistical design [63].

The results obtained for the synthesis of AgNPs under normal, alkaline, saline, and saline + alkaline conditions are discussed here. The results showed that the NaCl concentration interferes with the formation of NPs. The growth of NPs due to nucleation is not possible in the presence of salt, so 5% NaCl interferes with the AgNP formation. Our results are in agreement with the earlier report which showed silver nanoparticle synthesis in MGYP at pH 7 [52]. Waghmare et al. (2014) also showed that neutral pH is optimum for AuNP biosynthesis using *Streptomyces hygroscopicus* [64]. In contrast, Skladanowski et al. (2017) synthesized gold and AgNPs from *Streptomyces* sp. strain NH21 by growing in a medium having pH 5.5 [65].

A vast literature exists favoring the influence of a range of substrate concentrations on nanoparticle synthesis. Most of the investigations reported the use of 1 mM $AgNO_3$ for AgNP synthesis from actinomycetes [66,67].

Thirumurugan et al. (2020) documented the synthesis of AgNPs from actinobacteria at a very low concentration [68]. Giri et al. found a very high concentration of $AgNO_3$ as the optimum concentration to support nanoparticle synthesis [69]. AgNP synthesis using a high concentration of parental compounds (i.e., $AgNO_3$) is beneficial in biomedical sector applications. The concentrated AgNPs can be diluted for the applicable formulation, so it is desirable to formulate AgNPs using a high concentration of $AgNO_3$. The important parameter that influences the size and shape of NPs is the pH of the reaction mixture. This factor can alter the charge of secondary metabolites and bio-molecules involved in the formation of NPs, which may affect their stability and capping properties [70,71].

The above-mentioned results are from the recent study conducted on the synthesis of AgNPs from actinobacteria. Their findings showed the synthesis of comparatively smaller NPs with highly negative ZP (−26.2) values at pH 7. Contrary to these reports, acidic and alkaline pH also proved to support the biosynthesis of NPs [72]. The pH from acidic (pH 4.0) to neutral (pH 7.0) led to the formation of smaller and spherical NPs. Acidic or alkaline pH favors the formation of irregularly shaped NPs with agglomeration [73]. The shape of AgNPs at pH 7.0 is usually spherical, but acidic pH causes the formation of hexagonal or irregularly shaped NPs [74]. So, neutral pH is the best for the synthesis of stable and spherical NPs.

From the results obtained for the effect of temperature on AgNP synthesis, it was found that 60 °C was considered as an optimum temperature for AgNP synthesis. Beyond 60 °C, synthesis occurred, but at a slower rate with a lesser yield. Similar observations are reported on the synthesis of NPs in the presence of high temperatures. In one such investigation, investigators biosynthesized AgNPs in a boiling water bath at a much higher rate, where the investigators hypothesized the role of thermo-stable compounds in nanoparticle formation [72]. Similarly, an increase in yield concerning an increase in temperature was observed by Kiran et al., where the investigators found the synthesis of AgNPs at a temperature range of 40–100 °C, with maximum absorbance at 100 °C. The rate of reaction and kinetic energy in the reaction at high temperatures are increased, so rapid formation is found [75].

The Particle Size Analysis (PSA) and zeta potential (ZP) of the *S. tendae*-mediated synthesized AgNPs showed a resemblance to the results reported by Skladanowski et al. [65]. The small-sized spherical-shaped AgNPs (45 nm) from *Streptomyces* sp. have been reported. Furthermore, the biological synthesis of NPs with different shapes and sizes depends on the biological entity involved, reaction time, and metal ion concentration. For instance, *Streptomyces griseorubens* synthesized spherical-shaped AgNPs with 5–20 nm size [76]. Smaller particles show a larger surface area to volume ratio; hence, the size of NPs affects the bactericidal action of NPs.

The ZP value of the AgNPs was −20.4 mV (Figure 3b) and the present results were similar to the recent findings of Vijayabharathi et al. [77]. The author reported a negatively charged surface of AgNPs synthesized by *Streptomyces griseoplanus* with a ZP value of −20.4 mV. The negative ZP value could be assigned to the negatively charged functional groups present on the surface of NPs acquired from cellular metabolites [78]. Further, the narrow and centered ZP shows the stability of NPs in a colloidal suspension [79]. Furthermore, such negatively charged NPs are more suitable to use for drug antibiotic complex formation, which is valuable for biomedical applications.

FT-IR spectra of AgNPs exhibited bands in the region of 531 to 3328 cm^{-1}. The vibration located at 3328 and 2111 cm^{-1} corresponds to the stretching vibration of the alcohol (ROH) group and C-O stretching mode [80,81], respectively. Furthermore, the FTIR spectrum also revealed a peak at 1635 cm^{-1}, attributed to the C=O stretching vibrations in amide linkages (amide II) of protein present in cell-free supernatant [82,83]. Proteins contain several functional groups, like OH from amino acid side chains, like serine, threonine, and tyrosine, amide groups (from the peptide backbone), and C=O groups (from acidic side chains such as aspartic and glutamic acid) [84]. The microbially synthesized (*Streptomyces*) AgNPs cap and stabilize the developed NPs, preventing their aggregation. The capped protein molecules could involve amino acid residues with OH groups, along with H_2O molecules associated with the protein structure. Previous FTIR analysis of AgNPs showed that proteins such as amide I (around 1650 cm^{-1}) and amide II (around 1550 cm^{-1}) are likely involved in the synthesis and stabilization of AgNPs [85].

Similarly, Muthusamy et al. reported AgNPs of *Streptomyces olivaceus* having six functional groups, C=C-H, ROH, C=N-OH, C-C, R-NH_2, and RCOOH, in the range of

455.20 to 3294.42 cm^{-1} [86]. The characteristic spectrum obtained indicates the presence of protein-like compounds attached to the synthesized NPs, confirming the role of metabolically produced proteins as capping agents during production and also interrupting the particle aggregation. Furthermore, the carbonyl groups are known for their silver-binding properties [87].

The sharp intensity peak in the XRD pattern indicates the crystalline nature and small crystallite size of the developed AgNPs. The typical five characteristic diffraction peaks indexed at the lattice plane were (111), (200), (231), (222), and (220). Apart from these, the recorded XRD pattern shows additional unassigned intense peaks that may be due to the formation of the crystalline bio-organic compounds/metalloproteins that are present in the culture broth. All the peaks were analyzed through the Joint Committee on Powder Diffraction Standards (JCPDS) and the pattern was in agreement with the standard values file number 89-3722. These data are in agreement with the previously conducted analysis by Składanowski et al., which documented the peaks at 2θ values (38.1°, 44.6°, 64.6°, 77.5°, 81.5°, and 115.0°) of crystalline AgNPs [65]. Likewise, Muthusamy et al. (2018) obtained the XRD pattern of synthesized AgNPs from *Streptomyces olivaceus* (MSU3), showing four intense peaks with 2θ values around 38.12°, 44.30°, 64.45°, and 77.41, with the lattice plane (111), (200), (220), and (311), respectively [86].

A team led by Manikprabhu and Lingappa (2013) performed the XRD characterization of AgNPs produced from *Streptomyces coelicolour* with the spectrum peak values of 75.41° and 40.21° [88]. Recently, Pallavi et al. documented the crystalline nature of AgNPs along with strong peaks in the range of 30 to 80° 2θ values from the *Streptomyces hirsutuS* strain SNPGA-8 [89].

The SEM images suggested the monodispersed nature of the AgNPs in the solution. Much literature is available on the use of SEM imaging in knowing the size and shape of bio-synthesized AgNPs. Spherical-shaped AgNPs with a diameter of 19.5–20.9 nm have been synthesized by Vijayabharathi et al. by using *Streptomyces griseoplanus* SAI-25 [77].

Recently, Ghany et al. synthesized monodispersed spherical AgNPs having an average size of 8.48 ± 1.72 nm and 9.67 ± 2.64 nm from actinomycetes *Glutamicibacter nicotianae* SNPRA1 and *Leucobacter aridicollis* SNPRA2, respectively [90]. Further, Nayka and their team also reported the formation of spherical and polydisperse AgNPs of size 32.40 nm from *Streptomyces* sp. NS-33 [91]. The majority of the studies show the formation of spherical-shaped AgNPs from actinomycetes isolates. However, several studies also reported the formation of rod-shaped AgNPs from *Nocardia mediterranei* [46,92].

The EDS clearly shows a high amount of Ag, which indicates the purity of the sample, while S and Cl are due to the media used for the halotolerant actinomycetes. Ca and Mg are present as an impurity, which is again from the media used for the actinomycetes.

The AFM images were in close agreement with Zarina et al., who synthesized spherical and polydisperse AgNPs from 50 to 76 nm in size, and also observed the height and surface roughness properties of NPs using a 3D AFM micrograph. Likewise, the average size of AgNPs (68.13 nm) synthesized from actinomycetes was reported by Chauhan et al. [93]. Further, Sadhasivam et al. studied the spherical shape and homogenous nature of AgNPs [94]. Recently, AFM technique-based histogram analysis and surface roughness of the AgNPs were observed by Iniyan et al., who showed the presence of very small-sized NPs in the range of 6 to 7 nm [95].

From the antimicrobial activity of AgNPs, the MIC values showed that GNB was more sensitive to AgNPs than GPB. This might be due to the thinner cell wall of GNB than that of Gram-positive bacteria [96]. Similarly, Wypij et al. (2018) also reported the highest inhibitory action of AgNPs against *P. aeruginosa* (16 µg/mL), and *S. aureus* was the least sensitive among all the tested organisms (256 µg/mL) [73]. In contrast, Sivasankar et al. reported the MIC values of AgNPs synthesized from *Streptomyces violaceus* against Gram-positive bacteria (*S. aureus* and *B. subtilis*) and GNB (*E. coli* and *P. aeruginosa*) and found that *P. aeruginosa* (MIC 111.6 µg/mL) was the least sensitive of the tested bacteria [96].

Immanuel et al. (2018) demonstrated much lower MIC values in the range of 0.5 to 3.0 μg/mL against clinical pathogens. When tested against clinical pathogens, namely *E. coli*, *Enterococcus faecalis*, *Klebsiella pneumoniae*, *Streptococcus mutant*, and *S. pneumoniae*, the AgNPs fabricated by *Streptomyces olivaceus* exhibited MIC values of 1.25, 1.25, 2.5, 0.625, and 0.625 μg/mL, respectively [96].

The MIC value of anti-fungal activity reported by Manivasagan et al. against *A. niger* (16 μg/mL) and *C. albicans* (10 μg/mL) was lower than the MIC value [44] reported in our study, whereas our results are better than the latest study on the antifungal activity of actinomycetes conducted by Wypij et al. (2018), which showed MIC values of 64 μg/mL and 96 μg/mL against *C. albicans* [73]. Further, the anti-fungal potential of AgNPs synthesized from acidophilic actinomycetes was evaluated against a panel of fungal pathogens causing superficial mycoses, such as *C. albicans*, *C. tropicalis*, *Malassezia furfur*, and *Trichophyton rubrum*, with MIC values of 15, 16, 16, and 26 μg/mL, respectively.

Among the commercial antibiotics, tetracycline demonstrated the highest inhibitory activity against bacteria, followed by kanamycin and ampicillin. AgNPs exhibited higher inhibitory action against bacterial growth than ampicillin. In the case of kanamycin, the growth of GPB was inhibited at a much lower concentration than in the presence of AgNPs, while the GNB was found to be more sensitive to AgNPs than kanamycin. Similarly, a study reported higher bactericidal activity of the synthesized AgNPs in comparison to ampicillin, tetracycline, and kanamycin when tested against *Bacillus subtilis*, *E. coli*, *K. pneumoniae*, *P. aeruginosa*, *Proteus mirabilis*, *S. aureus*, and *Salmonella infantis* [97]. So, the synthesized AgNPs revealed more potentiality against GNB as compared to commercial antibiotics. The anti-fungal affectivity of AgNPs was also higher than fluconazole, except for amphotericin-B.

As mentioned in earlier reports, the biocidal activity of AgNPs depends on the size and stability of particles. The findings are supported by various investigations that studied the size-dependent antimicrobial activity of AgNPs [73] and also demonstrated the microbicidal activity of AgNPs formulated by two different haloalkaliphilic actinobacteria and found that smaller-sized particles exhibited better antimicrobial activity [98].

Several mechanisms have been proposed for the biocidal activity of AgNPs. Several targets of AgNPs in the bacterial cell have been identified. (i) Disruption of the cell wall and cell membrane affects the regulation of the transport mechanism [99], (ii) increased permeability of the cell membrane leads to leakage of vital cell constituents and nutrients [100], and (iii) penetration of AgNPs inside the microorganisms is followed by interaction with biomolecules (lipids, proteins, and nucleic acid) [101].

The synergistic action of tetracycline and AgNPs was significant against both Gram-positive and Gram-negative test cultures. A combination of ampicillin and AgNPs demonstrated synergistic efficacy against GPB, and in Gram-negative bacteria, an indifferent effect was observed. Anti-fungal antibiotic fluconazole in combination with AgNPs also exhibited an indifferent effect against *C. albicans* and *A. niger*. The findings obtained in this study are consistent with the research conducted by Wypij et al. (2018) [73]. Anasane et al. conducted a study on the combined effectiveness of AgNPs, ketoconazole, and fluconazole against fungal infections [78]. Enhancement in the antibacterial activity of penicillin, streptomycin, ampicillin, and cephalexin against bacterial pathogens has been shown by various investigators [102,103]. The coadministration of AgNPs with antibiotics showed significantly increased antibacterial efficacy, while also resulting in reduced dosage requirements for both substances. Utilizing smaller concentrations of compounds can mitigate their toxicity while still achieving the desired outcome [104]. Additionally, investigators asserted that this combination effectively restores the ability of the medicine to kill microorganisms that have become resistant to it. For instance, *S. mutans* was found to be sensitive towards vancomycin treatment in the presence of AgNPs [105]. Likewise, the resistant strain of *P. mirabilis* showed sensitivity toward the same antibiotics in the presence of biologically synthesized AgNPs [106].

The results obtained for the MRSA activity of AgNPs were in close agreement with the previous results. In one of the investigations, the activity against MRSA by AgNPs synthesized by actinobacterium *Sinomonas mesophila* was reported. AgNPs synthesized by marine *Micromonospora* exhibited excellent bactericidal activity against a range of pathogens [88]. The efficacy reported was much higher than the standard antibiotic cefotaxime. Apart from silver, other NPs such as MgO and CuNPs from actinomycetes also exhibited their bactericidal action against MDR and MRSA strain [107,108].

The biofilm formation by *P. aeruginosa* showed more sensitivity towards AgNPs and standard antibiotic ampicillin compared to *S. pneumoniae*. In addition, the combinational approach showed remarkable inhibition of biofilm formation in both the tested cultures. About 98% inhibition was observed in the case of *P. aeruginosa*, whereas biofilm formation by *S. pneumoniae* decreased up to 83% in the presence of AgNPs and ampicillin. The results obtained by the biogenic AgNPs were shown to disrupt the biofilm growth mode of bacteria and fungi. Potential anti-biofilm activity (95% inhibition) of AgNPs synthesized by *B. licheniformis* was noticed in contradiction to *P. aeruginosa* and *S. epidermidis* [109].

The scavenging effect of vitamin C was 45.6% at 100 μg/mL concentration. Antioxidant activity of AgNPs is well-studied and well-known [110]. Due to good anti-oxidant activity, AgNPs are now commercially used in skin lotion and anti-aging creams.

The application of AgNPs onto cotton fabric is attributed to the presence of a negative charge on the surface of the AgNPs. The positive functional group on the cotton fiber ties up with negatively charged AgNPs. The data obtained are very close to the work reported by Yan et al., [111]. Likewise, textile fabric loaded with copper NPs was also evaluated for antimicrobial efficiency against *S. aureus* and *E. coli* [112]. The utilization of ZnNPs has also been suggested in the production of antimicrobial packaging to enhance the durability of packaged materials [113,114].

4. Materials and Methods

4.1. Materials

The collection of the soil samples was carried out from Greater Rann of Kutch, i.e., Charanka Solar Park and Adesar (Kutch, India), Starch Casein Agar (SCA) (HI-media Mumbai, India, Analytical grade), NaCl, and $AgNO_3$ (98%, AR grade, Rankem, Mumbai, India), and double distilled water (ddw). Microbial strains *Bacillus subtilis* MTCC 441, *Staphylococcus aureus* MTCC 737, *Escherichia coli* MTCC 1687, *Pseudomonas aeruginosa* MTCC 1688, *Candida albicans* MTCC 183, and *Aspergillus niger* MTCC 1344 were procured from Microbial Type Culture Collection Center (MTCC), Chandigarh, India. MRSA 2 and MRSA 7 were isolated from the laboratory with Whatman filter paper No 1 (Merck, Mumbai, India).

4.2. Methods

4.2.1. Sample Collection Site

The soil sample was collected from the greater Rann of Kutch from Kutch district of Gujarat, India, which is shown below in Figure 10. Samples were collected from two sites, one from Charanka Solar Park (latitude: 23.8952° N and longitude: 71.2261° E, Code: GR-CHA), and another from Adesar region (latitude: 23.5581° N and 70.9814° E), and code GR-ADE.

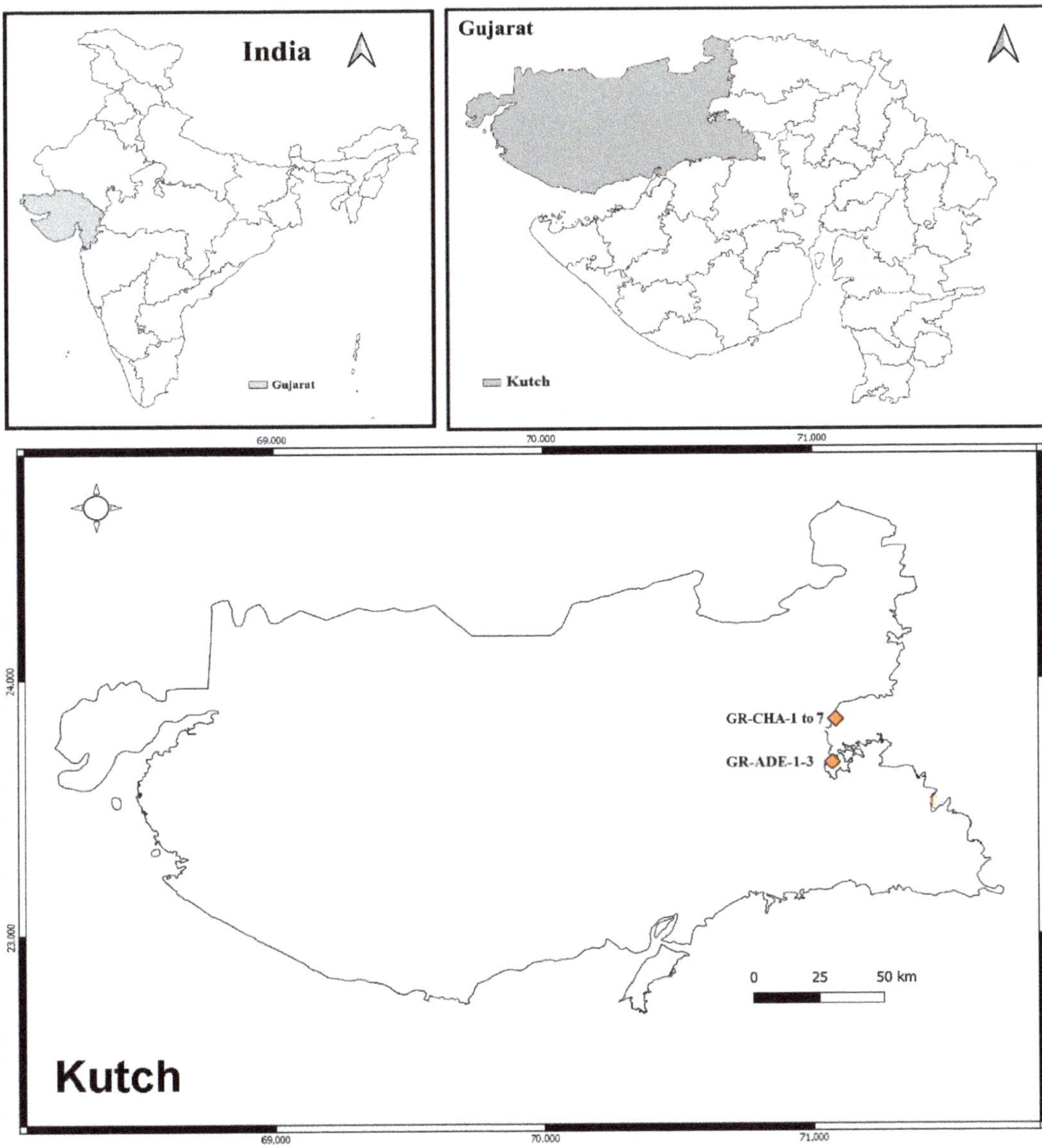

Figure 10. Soil sample collection site from Kutch: Greater Rann of Kutch.

4.2.2. Enrichment and Isolation of Actinomycetes

The enrichment and isolation of actinomycetes were carried out in the following sequence order, as shown in Figure 11 [115].

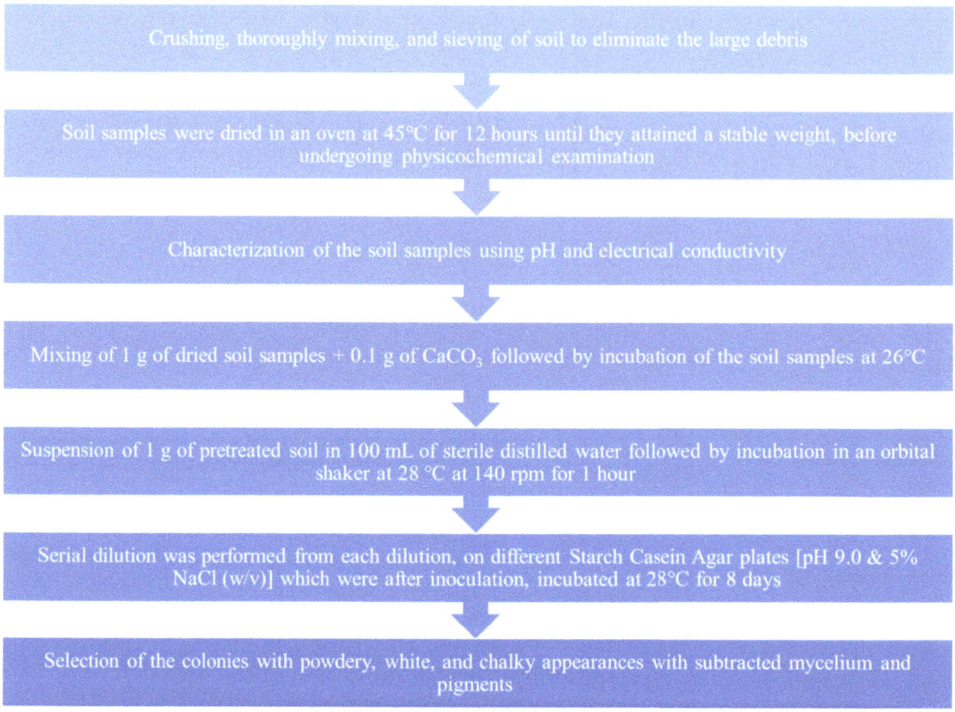

Figure 11. Steps involved in the enrichment and isolation of actinomycetes from desert soil.

4.2.3. Effect of Salt Concentration on the Growth of Isolate

The effect of salt concentration on growth was studied by supplying the isolates with a range of NaCl concentrations of 0.0, 2.5, 5.0, and 10.0 (% *w*/*v*) on SCA plates. After 7 days of incubation, the tolerance limits of actinomycetes to NaCl were determined and analyzed comparatively. Incubation was carried out as per the optimum temperature observed in the earlier study [116].

4.2.4. Effect of pH on the Growth of Isolates

The influence of pH on growth was demonstrated by using SCA plates having different pHs, from 5.0 to 9.0. The acidic pH was adjusted with 5% sterile CH_3COOH solution, and the alkaline pH was adjusted with 20% sterile Na_2CO_3 solution after separate autoclaving. After 7 days of incubation, the tolerance limits of the isolate to pH were determined and analyzed comparatively. Salt and temperature were used for each isolate as per the results of the growth of isolates under normal, alkaline, saline, and saline + alkaline conditions. Growth response was also investigated with the stress-supplemented condition, i.e., alkaline, saline, and saline + alkaline. Four different combinations (Table 4) of pH and salt were used to study the haloalkaliphilic nature of the isolates. Control was kept without any stress [117].

Table 4. Combination of stress conditions.

Condition	pH	NaCl (%, *w*/*v*)
Normal	7.0	0.0
Alkaline	9.0	0.0
Saline	7.0	5.0
Saline + alkaline	9.0	5.0

4.2.5. Screening for the Presence of Antagonistic Substances

Actinomycetes are excellent elaborators of pharmaceutical products and are well known for finding novel biologically active secondary metabolite [118,119]. The primary screening of antibiotics was conducted using the top agar method. Isolates were grown on SCA (5.0%, *w*/*v*, NaCl, pH 9.0) for one week. After incubation, the top agar was mixed with the test culture overlaid on the base agar and incubated for one day. The zone of inhibition (ZOI) surrounding the actinobacterial colony was observed, and results were recorded in mm. The screening of all the isolated strains for their antimicrobial activity against MTCC strains was performed.

4.2.6. Molecular Identification of the Actinomycete Isolates

The identification of the isolated actinomycete was carried out by using 16S rRNA gene sequencing where pure culture strain on SCA slants was outsourced (Chromous Biotech Pvt. Ltd., Bangalore, India). The 16s rRNA sequence alignment was carried out manually with the available nucleotide sequence retrieved from EzTaxon [120,121]. The isolate was identified using the EzTaxon database (Table 5). Tylosin and nikkomycin-like compounds have been reported from *Streptomyces tendae* [122].

Table 5. Identification of isolates using the EzTaxon database.

S. No.	EzTaxon Database Suggested Species	Selected Species	Hit Strain Name	Similarity (%)
1	*S. tendae*	*S. tendae*	ATCC 19812(T)	98.46
2	*Streptomyces violaceorubidus*		LMG 20319(T)	98.46
3	*Streptomyces gougerotii*		NBRC 3198(T)	98.46

4.2.7. Biosynthesis of AgNPs

About 30 mL of malt, glucose, yeast peptone (MGYP) medium made up of malt and yeast extract each (0.3%), glucose (1.0%), and peptone (0.5%) (pH-7.0, NaCl 0.0% *w*/*v*) was inoculated from a 1-week-old culture grown on an SCA plate (pH-9.0; NaCl 5.0% *w*/*v*). The incubation of all the flasks was carried out along with shaking at 120 rpm at 30 °C for 72 h. About 10 mL of inoculum was inoculated into 50 mL MGYP (pH 7) after that incubation of the flasks was carried out at 30 °C along with shaking at 100 rpm and for 96 h. After incubation, the filtration of the biomass was carried out using Whatman filter paper No. 1, where the filtrate containing crude nitrate reductase (NR) was subsequently used for biosynthesis. The supernatant was exposed to 1 mM of $AgNO_3$ aqueous solution in equal amounts and the mixture was left undisturbed under static conditions in the dark at 30 °C, while the control had only $AgNO_3$ aqueous solution and no actinomycete supernatant culture [123,124].

4.2.8. Optimization of Physicochemical Parameters

The isolated actinomycete was further optimized for extracellular nanoparticle synthesis using pH, temperature, $AgNO_3$ concentration, medium composition, and under-stress conditions.

Medium Optimization for AgNP Synthesis

To reveal the effect of components of the media on the production of secondary metabolites involved in the formation of NPs, the isolate was grown in starch casein broth, ISP medium No 1, M9 (sodium acetate as a carbon source), casein glycerol broth, and MGYP medium. NaCl was not added in any medium and pH was set to 7.0. The biosynthesis of AgNPs was carried out according to the protocol described in 3.19.

Nanoparticle Synthesis under Normal, Alkaline, Saline, and Saline + Alkaline Conditions

To optimize the pH effect and concentration of NaCl on the ability of AgNP production of the selected isolate, all the isolated strains were grown in the presence of 4 different conditions, i.e., normal (0.0% *w/v* salt, 7.0 pH), alkaline (0.0% *w/v* salt, 9.0 pH), saline (5.0% *w/v* salt, 7.0 pH), and saline + alkaline (5.0% *w/v* salt, 9.0 pH).

Effect of $AgNO_3$ Concentration on AgNP Synthesis

The effect of $AgNO_3$ on the formation of AgNPs was observed using 1 mM to 5 mM $AgNO_3$ concentration at pH 7.0 and 30 °C. During incubation, the color change of the reaction solution was observed at different time intervals. Further confirmation was carried out based on UV–visible spectra.

Effect of pH on AgNP Synthesis

The influence of pH on the biosynthesis of NPs was studied in the presence of pH 5.0, 6.0, 7.0, 8.0, and 9.0. The reaction mixture was set to different pHs followed by incubation at 30 °C in the dark. During incubation, the color change of the reaction mixture was observed at different time intervals. Further confirmation was carried out based on UV–visible spectra.

Effect of Temperature on AgNP Synthesis

The relationship between temperature and nanoparticle formation was evaluated at different temperatures from 30 to 80 °C. The confirmation of the synthesis of AgNPs was revealed by the color change of the mixture (pale yellow to brown). Further confirmation was carried out by performing UV–visible spectroscopy.

4.2.9. In Vitro Antimicrobial Activity of AgNPs

The antimicrobial activity of the synthesized AgNPs was assessed against *S. aureus* MTCC 737, *B. subtilis* MTCC 441, *E. coli* MTCC 1687, *P. aeruginosa* MTCC 1688, *C. albicans* MTCC 183, and *A. niger* MTCC 1344. To determine the MIC of AgNPs, the microtiter broth dilution technique was used as per the guidelines given by the Clinical Laboratory Standards Institute (CLSI) using 96-well ELISA microtiter plates. Muller–Hinton (MH) broth and Sabouraud dextrose (SD) broth were utilized for growing bacteria and fungi, respectively. Test cultures were grown in respective mediums and diluted to 0.4 McFarland standards for MIC testing. To each well (capacity 300 µL), 185 µL medium and 10 µL of AgNPs suspended in distilled water were added. Contents in the well were mixed properly and the following concentrations of AgNPs were prepared (1024, 512, 256, 128, 64, 32, 16, 8, 4, and 2 µg/mL) using a two-fold dilution method, which was followed by the addition of 5 µL of test culture to each well. The positive control (broth + microbial inoculums without AgNPs) and negative control (sterile un-inoculated broth) were also kept along with the experimental sets. Tetracycline, kanamycin, and ampicillin were used as standard anti-bacterial antibiotics, while amphotericin-B and fluconazole were used as anti-fungal antibiotics. The plates were incubated at 37 °C for bacteria and 28 °C for fungi for 2–3 days. After incubation, plates were read for absorbance at 600 nm using a spectrophotometer. MIC was estimated from the lowest concentration that inhibited the 100% growth of the test culture by comparing it with the negative control. The 5 µL aliquot of the sample showing complete inhibition of microbial growth was spotted on the respective medium for the estimation of the Minimum Bactericidal Concentration (MBC) of AgNPs against bacterial and fungal test cultures. The lowest concentration without bacterial colony on the agar plate was considered as MBC of AgNPs.

4.2.10. Synergistic Activity of AgNPs with Commercial Antibiotics

To evaluate the synergistic role of AgNPs with commercial antibiotics, the MIC value of individual agents (AgNPs and antibiotics) was combined in a single well and serially diluted to achieve the 1/2 MIC, 1/4, 1/8, and 1/16 MIC concentrations in the subsequent wells. Tetracycline and ampicillin were taken as anti-bacterial antibiotics and amphotericin B was used as an anti-fungal agent. The microtiter plate well with no turbidity was used to calculate the fractional inhibitory concentration (FIC) index. To calculate the FIC index, Equation (1) was used:

$$\text{FIC} = \frac{\text{MIC of AgNPs in combination with antibiotic}}{\text{MIC of AgNPs alone}} + \frac{\text{MIC of antibiotic in combination with AgNPs}}{\text{MIC of antibiotic alone}} \quad (1)$$

4.2.11. Activity against MRSA

MRSA strains isolated from the clinical samples were used in the study. The activity of the synthesized AgNPs against MRSA was evaluated by utilizing the agar well diffusion method with some modifications [125]. Briefly, MRSA strain grown in Mueller–Hinton broth having turbidity equal to 0.4 McFarland was spread heavily onto Mueller–Hinton plates. With the help of the sterile borer, wells were formed on the plate. Then, 50 µL of AgNPs sample was added into their respective cups. Plates were incubated at 20 °C for 30 min to facilitate the diffusion followed by incubation at 37 °C overnight. The next day, the ZOI was measured in mm and results were recorded. The isolate inhibited the growth of the MRSA strain with a ZOI of 12 mm against MRSA-7.

Metabolites against MRSA have been reported from saline desert isolates by Damavandi et al. [126]. Recently, inhibition of the staphyloxanthin-based activity against MRSA has been demonstrated from Streptomyces by a team led by Charousova [127].

4.2.12. Anti-Biofilm Activity

Inhibition of biofilm formation by *P. aeruginosa* and *S. pneumoniae* was investigated in the presence of AgNPs alone and in combination with the standard antibiotic ampicillin using the tissue culture plate method [128,129]. Individual wells of the plates were poured, with the 190 µL of testing culture having 1×10^6/mL concentration, and the incubation of the plates was carried out at 37 °C for 6 h, which was followed by washing with Phosphate Buffer Saline (PBS) to eliminate planktonic forms of bacteria. The biofilm developed on the surface of the well was fixed using sodium acetate (2%) followed by staining with crystal violet (0.1% *w*/*v*) and rinsing off the excess strain, followed by washing with Milli-Q water and air drying. After drying, wells were filled with 95% ethanol to make a suspension of adherent bacteria of the biofilm. The measurement of optical density (O.D) was carried out by an ELISA plate reader at 595 nm. The inhibition percentage of biofilm development was estimated by using Equation (2) [130].

$$1 = \frac{OD_{595} \text{ of cells treated with AgNPs}}{OD_{595} \text{ of non-treated control}} \times 100 \quad (2)$$

4.2.13. Antioxidant Activity of Synthesized AgNPs

Antioxidants protect the cell by neutralizing the free radicals and thereby play a significant role in biomedical applications [131]. About 1 mL of different concentrations of AgNPs (25, 50, 100, and 200 µg/mL) was added to 0.5 mL 1, 1-diphenyl-2-picrylhydrazyl (DPPH) (1 mM). The mixture was placed under dark conditions for half an hour followed by UV-Vis measurement at 517 nm. A control containing DPPH without AgNPs was used, and vitamin C (ascorbic acid) was considered as standard. Lower absorbance of the reaction mixture suggests a higher DPPH radical scavenging activity. The percentage of scavenging activity was estimated by applying Equation (3).

$$\% \text{ of RSA} = \frac{\text{Abs control} - \text{Abs sample}}{\text{Abs control}} \times 100 \quad (3)$$

where:

RSA = Radical scavenging activity;
Abs control = absorbance of DPPH radical + ethanol;
Abs sample = absorbance of DPPH radical + AgNPs.

4.2.14. Biosynthesis of AgNPs on Cotton Fabrics

The antimicrobial activity of AgNP-coated cotton fabrics was evaluated by utilizing the disc diffusion process. Before being used, cotton textiles were cleaned, sterilized, and dried, according to Shilpa et al. (2023) [132]. AgNPs were applied onto the surface of cotton cloths measuring 1 cm × 1 cm and then left to dry in the air. The effectiveness of silver nanoparticle (AgNP)-treated cotton fabrics in killing bacteria was assessed by examining their antibacterial potential against both the Gram-positive bacteria (GPB) and the Gram-negative bacteria (GNB) on Mueller–Hinton Agar (MHA) plates at various time intervals. A control was established using a cell-free supernatant that did not contain AgNPs. ZOI was detected on the plates after they had been incubated for one day at 37 °C [133].

4.3. Characterization of the Synthesized AgNPs

All the optimized conditions were put together in one experiment, and the AgNPs developed were analyzed using the following instruments.

4.3.1. UV-Vis Spectral Analysis

The synthesis of the AgNPs in the supernatant was confirmed by withdrawing 3 mL of the colloidal sample at regular time intervals. Surface Plasmon Resonance (SPR) spectra were measured in the range of 250 nm to 750 nm with a 10 mm path length quartz cuvette using a UV-Vis spectrophotometer (Shimadzu, Tokyo, Japan, UV-1800).

4.3.2. Nanoparticle Tracking Analysis (NTA) and Zeta Potential of AgNPs

The particle size distribution of the synthesized AgNPs was measured using NTA, Version 2.3 Build 0034. The sample was prepared by adding 1–2 mg powder sample in a 10 mL Milli-Q water in a tube followed by sonication for 10 min to obtain finely dispersed particles. The confirmation of the stability of AgNPs was carried out using zeta potential (ZP) analysis (ZS 90; Malvern Instruments Ltd., Malvern, UK).

4.3.3. Fourier Transform Infra-Red (FT-IR) Analysis

The analysis of functional groups on the surface of AgNPs was conducted using FT-IR. The FT-IR spectroscopic investigation was conducted using a Tensor-27 instrument (Bruker, Ettlingen, Germany) with a scan range of 400–4000 cm^{-1} at a scanning speed of 2 mm/S. The thoroughly desiccated AgNPs powders were processed with high-quality KBr for consolidation in a ratio of 1:50 for the analysis.

4.3.4. SEM

The surface features of the synthesized AgNPs were analyzed using a SEM-Zeiss Evo MA 15, (Cambridge, UK), instrument, operating at an accelerating voltage of 20 kV. The AgNP sample was placed on the carbon tape, which in turn was fixed on an aluminum stub, and micrographs were taken. The elemental analysis of the sample was carried out using EDS attached along with the SEM. The elemental analysis was carried out with the help of an Oxford Instruments (Abingdon, Oxfordshire, UK) EDS analyzer.

4.3.5. X-ray Diffraction (XRD) Analysis

The fingerprint characterization of crystalline metallic silver and its structure determination was performed by XRD by using a Rigaku D/max 2550 X-ray diffractometer (Tokyo, Japan). The measurement of the powder sample was carried out in the range of 2θ, ranging from 20° to 70°, with a 0.05°/S scan rate.

4.3.6. AFM

The 3D and 2D images were taken by AFM, by using Multiview 1000 Nanonics, (Malcha Jerusalem, Israel), instrument. The dispersed mixture of AgNPs prepared above during UV was spread on a fresh mica sheet with the help of a micropipette. Further, the slide was allowed to dry, followed by washing with Milli-Q water to remove unattached particles.

5. Conclusions

The present study successfully explored the potential of the halotolerant actinomycetes, *Streptomyces tendae*, isolated from the Rann of Kutch, India, for the green synthesis of AgNPs in a single step. The supernatant of *S. tendae* possesses several secondary metabolites and extracellular enzymes that are responsible for the reduction of silver salt into NPs. The confirmation of the synthesized AgNPs by analytical instruments showed the formation of 20–90 nm by SEM and an average particle size of 50 nm by PSA. The size, shape, and yield of AgNPs by the *Streptomyces* spp. are influenced by various parameters like types of microorganisms used, pH, temperature, nutrient medium, etc. The highest antimicrobial activity of the AgNPs was observed against *Pseudomonas aeruginosa*, and they also showed anti-MRSA activity. The capability of the AgNPs in inhibiting biofilm development and antioxidant activity suggests the synthesized AgNPs as having a potential therapeutic role. The synergistic effect of AgNPs with antibiotics like penicillin demonstrated a significant reduction in the formation of biofilm, suggesting their potential application in increasing antibiotic efficacy. The application of AgNPs in the preparation of antimicrobial surgical cotton showcases their practical application in the biomedical field. In brief, the investigation combines microbiology, nanotechnology, and biomedical sciences to construct eco-friendly antimicrobial compounds from halotolerant actinomycetes to address multidrug-resistant pathogens. Finally, this investigation showcases the various applications of AgNPs and lays the groundwork for in-depth investigations into the biomedical potential of halotolerant actinomycetes from desert environments.

6. Future Prospects and Limitations

The present study could be further used to enhance antimicrobial therapies, by using novel antibiotic combinations (synergism) and targeted drug delivery. Moreover, the applications of the developed AgNPs will be analyzed for the in vivo studies. In addition to this, the developed AgNPs could be applied for wound healing, cancer therapy, and other biomedical applications. By addressing all these limitations and expanding the scope of the applications, the present investigation and the developed AgNPs has the potential to contribute significantly to the field of biomedicine and the environment.

Author Contributions: Conceptualization, P.D. (Paras Dayma), P.D. (Pravin Dudhagara), and R.P.; methodology, R.P.; software, D.A. and S.A.; validation, N.C. and K.L., formal analysis, K.L, P.D. (Paras Dayma), D.A. and N.C.; investigation, P.D. (Paras Dayma), R.P., A.P., P.D. (Pravin Dudhagara) and V.K.Y.; resources, D.A. and S.A.; data curation, K.L., P.D. (Pravin Dudhagara), S.A. and A.P., writing—original draft preparation, P.D. (Paras Dayma), N.C., V.K.Y., A.P. and R.P.; writing—review and editing, N.C., V.K.Y., P.D. (Pravin Dudhagara), K.L., D.A. and S.A; visualization, R.P., N.C., K.L. and S.A.; supervision, R.P., A.P. and V.K.Y.; project administration, R.P., A.P. and V.K.Y., funding acquisition, D.A. and S.A. All authors have read and agreed to the published version of the manuscript.

Funding: This research received no external funding.

Institutional Review Board Statement: Not applicable.

Informed Consent Statement: Not applicable.

Data Availability Statement: Data is contained within the article.

Acknowledgments: This research was supported by Researchers Supporting Project number (RSP2024R27), King Saud University, Riyadh, Saudi Arabia.

Conflicts of Interest: The authors declare no conflict of interest associated with the publication of this article.

References

1. De Simeis, D.; Serra, S. Actinomycetes: A Never-Ending Source of Bioactive Compounds—An Overview on Antibiotics Production. *Antibiotics* **2021**, *10*, 483. [CrossRef] [PubMed]
2. Sarkar, G.; Suthindhiran, K. Diversity and Biotechnological Potential of Marine Actinomycetes from India. *Indian J. Microbiol.* **2022**, *62*, 475–493. [CrossRef]
3. Selim, M.S.M.; Abdelhamid, S.A.; Mohamed, S.S. Secondary Metabolites and Biodiversity of Actinomycetes. *J. Genet. Eng. Biotechnol.* **2021**, *19*, 72. [CrossRef] [PubMed]
4. Subathra Devi, C.; Merlyn Keziah, S.; Jemimah Naine, S.; Mohanasrinivasan, V. Actinomycetes: Microbiology to Systems Biology. In *Actinobacteria*; Springer: Singapore, 2022; pp. 1–35.
5. Atanasov, A.G.; Zotchev, S.B.; Dirsch, V.M.; Supuran, C.T. Natural Products in Drug Discovery: Advances and Opportunities. *Nat. Rev. Drug Discov.* **2021**, *20*, 200–216. [CrossRef]
6. Duan, C.; Yu, M.; Xu, J.; Li, B.-Y.; Zhao, Y.; Kankala, R.K. Overcoming Cancer Multi-Drug Resistance (MDR): Reasons, Mechanisms, Nanotherapeutic Solutions, and Challenges. *Biomed. Pharmacother.* **2023**, *162*, 114643. [CrossRef] [PubMed]
7. Duncan, K.R.; Crüsemann, M.; Lechner, A.; Sarkar, A.; Li, J.; Ziemert, N.; Wang, M.; Bandeira, N.; Moore, B.S.; Dorrestein, P.C.; et al. Molecular Networking and Pattern-Based Genome Mining Improves Discovery of Biosynthetic Gene Clusters and Their Products from *Salinispora* Species. *Chem. Biol.* **2015**, *22*, 460–471. [CrossRef]
8. Kim, H.; Kim, S.; Kim, M.; Lee, C.; Yang, I.; Nam, S.-J. Bioactive Natural Products from the Genus *Salinospora*: A Review. *Arch. Pharm. Res.* **2020**, *43*, 1230–1258. [CrossRef] [PubMed]
9. Tan, Y.; Hu, Y.; Wang, Q.; Zhou, H.; Wang, Y.; Gan, M. Tetrocarcins N and O, Glycosidic Spirotetronates from a Marine-Derived Micromonospora Sp. Identified by PCR-Based Screening. *RSC Adv.* **2016**, *6*, 91773–91778. [CrossRef]
10. Motallebirad, T.; Mardanshah, O.; Safarabadi, M.; Ghaffari, K.; Orouji, M.A.; Abedi, B.; Azadi, D. Screening, Molecular Identification, Population Diversity, and Antibiotic Susceptibility Pattern of Actinomycetes Species Isolated from Meat and Meat Products of Slaughterhouses, Restaurants, and Meat Stores of a Developing Country, Iran. *Front. Microbiol.* **2023**, *14*, 1134368. [CrossRef]
11. Liu, K.; Jiang, Z.; Lalancette, R.A.; Tang, X.; Jäkle, F. Near-Infrared-Absorbing B–N Lewis Pair-Functionalized Anthracenes: Electronic Structure Tuning, Conformational Isomerism, and Applications in Photothermal Cancer Therapy. *J. Am. Chem. Soc.* **2022**, *144*, 18908–18917. [CrossRef]
12. Kronheim, S.; Solomon, E.; Ho, L.; Glossop, M.; Davidson, A.R.; Maxwell, K.L. Complete Genomes and Comparative Analyses of Streptomyces Phages That Influence Secondary Metabolism and Sporulation. *Sci. Rep.* **2023**, *13*, 9820. [CrossRef] [PubMed]
13. Liu, F.; Liu, X.; Huang, Q.; Arai, T. Recent Progress of Magnetically Actuated DNA Micro/Nanorobots. *Cyborg Bionic Syst.* **2022**, *2022*, 9758460. [CrossRef] [PubMed]
14. Alam, K.; Mazumder, A.; Sikdar, S.; Zhao, Y.-M.; Hao, J.; Song, C.; Wang, Y.; Sarkar, R.; Islam, S.; Zhang, Y.; et al. Streptomyces: The Biofactory of Secondary Metabolites. *Front. Microbiol.* **2022**, *13*, 968053. [CrossRef] [PubMed]
15. Caicedo-Montoya, C.; Manzo-Ruiz, M.; Ríos-Estepa, R. Pan-Genome of the Genus Streptomyces and Prioritization of Biosynthetic Gene Clusters With Potential to Produce Antibiotic Compounds. *Front. Microbiol.* **2021**, *12*, 677558. [CrossRef] [PubMed]
16. Parra, J.; Beaton, A.; Seipke, R.F.; Wilkinson, B.; Hutchings, M.I.; Duncan, K.R. Antibiotics from Rare Actinomycetes, beyond the Genus Streptomyces. *Curr. Opin. Microbiol.* **2023**, *76*, 102385. [CrossRef] [PubMed]
17. Barbuto Ferraiuolo, S.; Cammarota, M.; Schiraldi, C.; Restaino, O.F. Streptomycetes as Platform for Biotechnological Production Processes of Drugs. *Appl. Microbiol. Biotechnol.* **2021**, *105*, 551–568. [CrossRef] [PubMed]
18. Darby, E.M.; Trampari, E.; Siasat, P.; Gaya, M.S.; Alav, I.; Webber, M.A.; Blair, J.M.A. Molecular Mechanisms of Antibiotic Resistance Revisited. *Nat. Rev. Microbiol.* **2023**, *21*, 280–295. [CrossRef] [PubMed]
19. Hu, B.; Das, P.; Lv, X.; Shi, M.; Aa, J.; Wang, K.; Duan, L.; Gilbert, J.A.; Nie, Y.; Wu, X.-L. Effects of 'Healthy' Fecal Microbiota Transplantation against the Deterioration of Depression in Fawn-Hooded Rats. *mSystems* **2022**, *7*, e0021822. [CrossRef] [PubMed]
20. He, X.; Jiang, Z.; Akakuru, O.U.; Li, J.; Wu, A. Nanoscale Covalent Organic Frameworks: From Controlled Synthesis to Cancer Therapy. *Chem. Commun.* **2021**, *57*, 12417–12435. [CrossRef]
21. Mancuso, G.; Midiri, A.; Gerace, E.; Biondo, C. Bacterial Antibiotic Resistance: The Most Critical Pathogens. *Pathogens* **2021**, *10*, 1310. [CrossRef]
22. Liu, K.; Jiang, Z.; Zhao, F.; Wang, W.; Jäkle, F.; Wang, N.; Tang, X.; Yin, X.; Chen, P. Triarylboron-Doped Acenethiophenes as Organic Sonosensitizers for Highly Efficient Sonodynamic Therapy with Low Phototoxicity. *Adv. Mater.* **2022**, *34*, 202206594. [CrossRef] [PubMed]
23. Zhang, L.; Shi, H.; Tan, X.; Jiang, Z.; Wang, P.; Qin, J. Ten-Gram-Scale Mechanochemical Synthesis of Ternary Lanthanum Coordination Polymers for Antibacterial and Antitumor Activities. *Front. Chem.* **2022**, *1*, 898324. [CrossRef] [PubMed]
24. Pulingam, T.; Parumasivam, T.; Gazzali, A.M.; Sulaiman, A.M.; Chee, J.Y.; Lakshmanan, M.; Chin, C.F.; Sudesh, K. Antimicrobial Resistance: Prevalence, Economic Burden, Mechanisms of Resistance and Strategies to Overcome. *Eur. J. Pharm. Sci.* **2022**, *170*, 106103. [CrossRef]
25. Salam, M.A.; Al-Amin, M.Y.; Salam, M.T.; Pawar, J.S.; Akhter, N.; Rabaan, A.A.; Alqumber, M.A.A. Antimicrobial Resistance: A Growing Serious Threat for Global Public Health. *Healthcare* **2023**, *11*, 1946. [CrossRef] [PubMed]
26. Zhang, H.; Fu, R.; Zheng, Q.; Song, X.; Wu, J.; Ren, Y. Continuous Mode of Color and Functionality Construction for Cotton by Bacterial Pigment Based on Nano-Suspension System. *Ind. Crops Prod.* **2024**, *214*, 118510. [CrossRef]

27. Wang, Y.; Zhai, W.; Cheng, S.; Li, J.; Zhang, H. Surface-Functionalized Design of Blood-Contacting Biomaterials for Preventing Coagulation and Promoting Hemostasis. *Friction* **2023**, *11*, 1371–1394. [CrossRef]
28. Zhang, G.; Bai, J.; Zhai, Y.; Jia, J.; Zhao, Q.; Wang, W.; Hu, X. Microbial Diversity and Functions in Saline Soils: A Review from a Biogeochemical Perspective. *J. Adv. Res.* **2023**, *59*, 129–140. [CrossRef] [PubMed]
29. Han, X.; Zhao, C.; Wang, S.; Pan, Z.; Jiang, Z.; Tang, X. Multifunctional TiO_2/C Nanosheets Derived from 3D Metal–Organic Frameworks for Mild-Temperature-Photothermal-Sonodynamic-Chemodynamic Therapy under Photoacoustic Image Guidance. *J. Colloid. Interface Sci.* **2022**, *621*, 360–373. [CrossRef]
30. Jiang, Z.; Han, X.; Zhao, C.; Wang, S.; Tang, X. Recent Advance in Biological Responsive Nanomaterials for Biosensing and Molecular Imaging Application. *Int. J. Mol. Sci.* **2022**, *23*, 1923. [CrossRef]
31. Salem, S.S.; Mekky, A.E. Biogenic Nanomaterials: Synthesis, Characterization, and Applications. In *Biogenic Nanomaterials for Environmental Sustainability: Principles, Practices, and Opportunities. Environmental Science and Engineering*; Springer: Cham, Switzerland, 2024; pp. 13–43.
32. Yadav, V.K.; Choudhary, N.; Ali, D.; Alarifi, S.; Dwivedi, V.; Patel, A.; Fulekar, M.H. A Novel and Economical Approach for the *Fusarium Oxysporum* Mediated Myco-Synthesis of Mesoporous Floral-Shaped Silica Nanoparticles from Coal Fly Ash Waste. *Part. Part. Syst. Charact.* **2024**, 2400007. [CrossRef]
33. Habibullah, G.; Viktorova, J.; Ruml, T. Current Strategies for Noble Metal Nanoparticle Synthesis. *Nanoscale Res. Lett.* **2021**, *16*, 47. [CrossRef] [PubMed]
34. Choudhary, N.; Chaudhari, J.; Mochi, V.; Patel, P.; Ali, D.; Alarifi, S.; Sahoo, D.K.; Patel, A.; Kumar Yadav, V. Phytonanofabrication of Copper Oxide by Albizia Saman and Their Potential as an Antimicrobial Agent and Remediation of Congo Red Dye from Wastewater. *Water* **2023**, *15*, 3787. [CrossRef]
35. Rabiee, N.; Ahmadi, S.; Akhavan, O.; Luque, R. Silver and Gold Nanoparticles for Antimicrobial Purposes against Multi-Drug Resistance Bacteria. *Materials* **2022**, *15*, 1799. [CrossRef]
36. Kaushal, A.; Khurana, I.; Yadav, P.; Allawadhi, P.; Banothu, A.K.; Neeradi, D.; Thalugula, S.; Barani, P.J.; Naik, R.R.; Navik, U.; et al. Advances in Therapeutic Applications of Silver Nanoparticles. *Chem. Biol. Interact.* **2023**, *382*, 110590. [CrossRef]
37. Ibrahim, E.; Fouad, H.; Zhang, M.; Zhang, Y.; Qiu, W.; Yan, C.; Li, B.; Mo, J.; Chen, J. Biosynthesis of Silver Nanoparticles Using Endophytic Bacteria and Their Role in Inhibition of Rice Pathogenic Bacteria and Plant Growth Promotion. *RSC Adv.* **2019**, *9*, 29293–29299. [CrossRef]
38. Nasr Azadani, F.; Madani, M.; Karimi, J.; Sepahvand, S. Green Synthesis of Silver Nanoparticles by Fusarium Oxysporum and Its Function Against Aspergillus and Fusarium Fungi. *Indian J. Microbiol.* **2024**, *64*, 213–224. [CrossRef] [PubMed]
39. El Ouardy, K.; Lbouhmadi, R.; Attaoui, H.; Mouzaki, M.; Mouine, H.; Lemkhente, Z.; Mir, Y. Biosynthesis and Characterization of Silver Nanoparticles Produced by Parachlorella Kessleri and Cyclotella Spp., and the Evaluation of Their Antibacterial Activity. *Int. J. Mol. Sci.* **2023**, *24*, 10599. [CrossRef]
40. Golinska, P.; Wypij, M.; Ingle, A.P.A.; Gupta, I.; Dahm, H.; Rai, M. Biogenic Synthesis of Metal Nanoparticles from Actinomycetes: Biomedical Applications and Cytotoxicity. *Appl. Microbiol. Biotechnol.* **2014**, *98*, 8083–8097. [CrossRef] [PubMed]
41. Paterlini, P.; Rodríguez, C.; Ledesma, A.; Pereyra, J.; Dávila Costa, J.S.; Álvarez, A.; Romero, C.M. Characterization of Biosynthesized Silver Nanoparticles from Streptomyces Aqueous Extract and Evaluation of Surface-Capping Proteins Involved in the Process. *Nano-Struct. Nano-Objects* **2021**, *26*, 100755. [CrossRef]
42. Subbaiya, R.; Selvam, M.M.; Sundar, K. Biological Synthesis of Silver Nanorods from Nocardia Mediterranei -5016 and Its Antitumor Activity against Non-Small Cell Lung Carcinoma Cell Line. *Int. J. Pharmtech Res.* **2015**, *8*, 298–307.
43. Oza, G.; Pandey, S.; Gupta, A.; Kesarkar, R.; Sharon, M.; Ambernath, W. Biosynthetic Reduction of Gold Ions to Gold Nanoparticles by Nocardia Farcinica. *J. Microbiol. Biotech.* **2012**, *2*, 511–515.
44. Manivasagan, P.; Alam, M.S.; Kang, K.-H.; Kwak, M.; Kim, S.-K. Extracellular Synthesis of Gold Bionanoparticles by Nocardiopsis Sp. and Evaluation of Its Antimicrobial, Antioxidant and Cytotoxic Activities. *Bioprocess Biosyst. Eng.* **2015**, *38*, 1167–1177. [CrossRef] [PubMed]
45. Roy, A.; Pandit, C.; Gacem, A.; Alqahtani, M.S.; Bilal, M.; Islam, S.; Hossain, M.d.J.; Jameel, M. Biologically Derived Gold Nanoparticles and Their Applications. *Bioinorg. Chem. Appl.* **2022**, *2022*, 1–13. [CrossRef] [PubMed]
46. Kumari, S.; Tehri, N.; Gahlaut, A.; Hooda, V. Actinomycetes Mediated Synthesis, Characterization, and Applications of Metallic Nanoparticles. *Inorg. Nano-Met. Chem.* **2021**, *51*, 1386–1395. [CrossRef]
47. Wypij, M.; Golinska, P.; Dahm, H.; Rai, M. Actinobacterial-mediated Synthesis of Silver Nanoparticles and Their Activity against Pathogenic Bacteria. *IET Nanobiotechnol.* **2017**, *11*, 336–342. [CrossRef] [PubMed]
48. Otari, S.V.; Patil, R.M.; Ghosh, S.J.; Thorat, N.D.; Pawar, S.H. Intracellular Synthesis of Silver Nanoparticle by Actinobacteria and Its Antimicrobial Activity. *Spectrochim. Acta A Mol. Biomol. Spectrosc.* **2015**, *136*, 1175–1180. [CrossRef] [PubMed]
49. Abou El-Enain, I.M.; Elqady, E.M.; El-said, E.; Salem, H.H.A.; Badr, N.F.; Abd-Allah, G.E.; Rezk, M.M. Biosynthesized Silver Nanoparticles (Ag NPs) from Isolated Actinomycetes Strains and Their Impact on the Black Cutworm, Agrotis Ipsilon. *Pestic. Biochem. Physiol.* **2023**, *194*, 105492. [CrossRef]
50. Asif, M.; Yasmin, R.; Asif, R.; Ambreen, A.; Mustafa, M.; Umbreen, S. Green Synthesis of Silver Nanoparticles (AgNPs), Structural Characterization, and Their Antibacterial Potential. *Dose-Response* **2022**, *20*, 155932582210887. [CrossRef]
51. Kaur, H.; Kaur, H.; Sharma, A. Study of SPR Peak Shifting of Silver Nanoparticles with Change in Surrounding Medium. *Mater. Today Proc.* **2021**, *37*, 3574–3576. [CrossRef]

52. Ejaz, U.; Afzal, M.; Mazhar, M.; Riaz, M.; Ahmed, N.; Rizg, W.Y.; Alahmadi, A.A.; Badr, M.Y.; Mushtaq, R.Y.; Yean, C.Y. Characterization, Synthesis, and Biological Activities of Silver Nanoparticles Produced via Green Synthesis Method Using Thymus Vulgaris Aqueous Extract. *Int. J. Nanomed.* **2024**, *19*, 453–469. [CrossRef]
53. Jini, D.; Sharmila, S.; Anitha, A.; Pandian, M.; Rajapaksha, R.M.H. In Vitro and in Silico Studies of Silver Nanoparticles (AgNPs) from Allium Sativum against Diabetes. *Sci. Rep.* **2022**, *12*, 22109. [CrossRef] [PubMed]
54. Fang, P.; Gao, K.; Yang, J.; Li, T.; Gong, W.; Sun, Q.; Wang, Y. Prevalence of Multidrug-Resistant Pathogens Causing Neonatal Early and Late Onset Sepsis, a Retrospective Study from the Tertiary Referral Children's Hospital. *Infect. Drug Resist.* **2023**, *16*, 4213–4225. [CrossRef] [PubMed]
55. Kalimuthu, K.; Suresh Babu, R.; Venkataraman, D.; Bilal, M.; Gurunathan, S. Biosynthesis of Silver Nanocrystals by Bacillus Licheniformis. *Colloids Surf. B Biointerfaces* **2008**, *65*, 150–153. [CrossRef] [PubMed]
56. Paul, D.; Sinha, S.N. Isolation and Characterization of Phosphate Solubilizing Bacterium Pseudomonas Aeruginosa KUPSB12 with Antibacterial Potential from River Ganga, India. *Ann. Agrar. Sci.* **2017**, *15*, 130–136. [CrossRef]
57. Koilparambil, D.; Liya, C.; Smitha, V.; Shaikmoideen, M. Green Synthesis of Silver Nanoparticles by Escherichia Coli: Analysis of Antibacterial Activity. *J. Water Environ. Nanotechnol.* **2016**, *1*, 63–74. [CrossRef]
58. Saravanan, M.; Vemu, A.K.; Barik, S.K. Rapid Biosynthesis of Silver Nanoparticles from Bacillus Megaterium (NCIM 2326) and Their Antibacterial Activity on Multi Drug Resistant Clinical Pathogens. *Colloids Surf. B Biointerfaces* **2011**, *88*, 325–331. [CrossRef] [PubMed]
59. Rathod, D.; Golinska, P.; Wypij, M.; Dahm, H.; Rai, M. A New Report of Nocardiopsis Valliformis Strain OT1 from Alkaline Lonar Crater of India and Its Use in Synthesis of Silver Nanoparticles with Special Reference to Evaluation of Antibacterial Activity and Cytotoxicity. *Med. Microbiol. Immunol.* **2016**, *205*, 435–447. [CrossRef] [PubMed]
60. Abd-Elnaby, H.M.; Abo-Elala, G.M.; Abdel-Raouf, U.M.; Hamed, M.M. Antibacterial and Anticancer Activity of Extracellular Synthesized Silver Nanoparticles from Marine Streptomyces Rochei MHM13. *Egypt. J. Aquat. Res.* **2016**, *42*, 301–312. [CrossRef]
61. Chandran, N.; Bayal, M.; Pilankatta, R.; Nair, S.S. Tuning of Surface Plasmon Resonance (SPR) in Metallic Nanoparticles for Their Applications in SERS. In *Nanomaterials for Luminescent Devices, Sensors, and Bio-imaging Applications. Progress in Optical Science and Photonics*; Springer: Singapore, 2021; pp. 39–66.
62. Selwal, N.; Rahayu, F.; Herwati, A.; Latifah, E.; Supriyono; Suhara, C.; Kade Suastika, I.B.; Mahayu, W.M.; Wani, A.K. Enhancing Secondary Metabolite Production in Plants: Exploring Traditional and Modern Strategies. *J. Agric. Food Res.* **2023**, *14*, 100702. [CrossRef]
63. Singh, V.; Haque, S.; Niwas, R.; Srivastava, A.; Pasupuleti, M.; Tripathi, C.K.M. Strategies for Fermentation Medium Optimization: An In-Depth Review. *Front. Microbiol.* **2017**, *7*, 02087. [CrossRef]
64. Waghmare, S.S.; Deshmukh, M.A.; Sadowski, Z. Biosynthesis, Optimization, Purification and Characterization of Gold Nanoparticles. *Afr. J. Microbiol. Res.* **2014**, *8*, 138–146. [CrossRef]
65. Składanowski, M.; Wypij, M.; Laskowski, D.; Golińska, P.; Dahm, H.; Rai, M. Silver and Gold Nanoparticles Synthesized from *Streptomyces* Sp. Isolated from Acid Forest Soil with Special Reference to Its Antibacterial Activity against Pathogens. *J. Clust. Sci.* **2017**, *28*, 59–79. [CrossRef]
66. Khodashenas, B.; Ghorbani, H.R. Synthesis of Silver Nanoparticles with Different Shapes. *Arab. J. Chem.* **2019**, *12*, 1823–1838. [CrossRef]
67. Shaikh, W.A.; Chakraborty, S.; Owens, G.; Islam, R.U. A Review of the Phytochemical Mediated Synthesis of AgNP (Silver Nanoparticle): The Wonder Particle of the Past Decade. *Appl. Nanosci.* **2021**, *11*, 2625–2660. [CrossRef]
68. Alqahtani, M.A.; Al Othman, M.R.; Mohammed, A.E. Bio Fabrication of Silver Nanoparticles with Antibacterial and Cytotoxic Abilities Using Lichens. *Sci. Rep.* **2020**, *10*, 16781. [CrossRef]
69. Giri, A.K.; Jena, B.; Biswal, B.; Pradhan, A.K.; Arakha, M.; Acharya, S.; Acharya, L. Green Synthesis and Characterization of Silver Nanoparticles Using Eugenia Roxburghii DC. Extract and Activity against Biofilm-Producing Bacteria. *Sci. Rep.* **2022**, *12*, 8383. [CrossRef]
70. Shiraz, M.; Imtiaz, H.; Azam, A.; Hayat, S. Phytogenic Nanoparticles: Synthesis, Characterization, and Their Roles in Physiology and Biochemistry of Plants. *BioMetals* **2023**, *37*, 23–70. [CrossRef]
71. Zhang, X.; Ma, G.; Wei, W. Simulation of Nanoparticles Interacting with a Cell Membrane: Probing the Structural Basis and Potential Biomedical Application. *NPG Asia Mater.* **2021**, *13*, 52. [CrossRef]
72. Sowani, H.; Mohite, P.; Damale, S.; Kulkarni, M.; Zinjarde, S. Carotenoid Stabilized Gold and Silver Nanoparticles Derived from the Actinomycete Gordonia Amicalis HS-11 as Effective Free Radical Scavengers. *Enzym. Microb. Technol.* **2016**, *95*, 164–173. [CrossRef]
73. Wypij, M.; Czarnecka, J.; Świecimska, M.; Dahm, H.; Rai, M.; Golinska, P. Synthesis, Characterization and Evaluation of Antimicrobial and Cytotoxic Activities of Biogenic Silver Nanoparticles Synthesized from Streptomyces Xinghaiensis OF1 Strain. *World J. Microbiol. Biotechnol.* **2018**, *34*, 23. [CrossRef]
74. Shalaby, E.A. Algae-Mediated Silver Nanoparticles: Synthesis, Properties, and Biological Activities. In *Green Synthesis of Silver Nanomaterials*; Elsevier: Amsterdam, The Netherlands, 2022; pp. 525–545.
75. Kiran Manam, V.; Murugesan, S. Biological Synthesis of Silver Nanoparticles from Marine Alga Copomenia Sinuosa and Its Invitro Ant-Diabetic Efficacy Biological Synthesis of Silver Nanoparticles from Marine Alga Colpomenia Sinuosa and Its in Vitro Anti-Diabetic Activity. *Am. J. Bio-Pharmacol. Biochem. Life Sci.* **2014**, *3*, 01–07.

76. Baygar, T.; Ugur, A. Biosynthesis of Silver Nanoparticles by Streptomyces Griseorubens Isolated from Soil and Their Antioxidant Activity. *IET Nanobiotechnol.* **2017**, *11*, 286–291. [CrossRef] [PubMed]
77. Vijayabharathi, R.; Sathya, A.; Gopalakrishnan, S. Extracellular Biosynthesis of Silver Nanoparticles Using Streptomyces Griseoplanus SAI-25 and Its Antifungal Activity against Macrophomina Phaseolina, the Charcoal Rot Pathogen of Sorghum. *Biocatal. Agric. Biotechnol.* **2018**, *14*, 166–171. [CrossRef]
78. Anasane, N.; Golińska, P.; Wypij, M.; Rathod, D.; Dahm, H.; Rai, M. Acidophilic Actinobacteria Synthesised Silver Nanoparticles Showed Remarkable Activity against Fungi-causing Superficial Mycoses in Humans. *Mycoses* **2016**, *59*, 157–166. [CrossRef]
79. Potara, M.; Bawaskar, M.; Simon, T.; Gaikwad, S.; Licarete, E.; Ingle, A.; Banciu, M.; Vulpoi, A.; Astilean, S.; Rai, M. Biosynthesized Silver Nanoparticles Performing as Biogenic SERS-Nanotags for Investigation of C26 Colon Carcinoma Cells. *Colloids Surf. B Biointerfaces* **2015**, *133*, 296–303. [CrossRef] [PubMed]
80. Abd-Elhady, H.M.; Ashor, M.A.; Hazem, A.; Saleh, F.M.; Selim, S.; El Nahhas, N.; Abdel-Hafez, S.H.; Sayed, S.; Hassan, E.A. Biosynthesis and Characterization of Extracellular Silver Nanoparticles from Streptomyces Aizuneusis: Antimicrobial, Anti Larval, and Anticancer Activities. *Molecules* **2021**, *27*, 212. [CrossRef] [PubMed]
81. Marathe, K.; Naik, J.; Maheshwari, V. Biogenic Synthesis of Silver Nanoparticles Using Streptomyces Spp. and Their Antifungal Activity Against Fusarium Verticillioides. *J. Clust. Sci.* **2021**, *32*, 1299–1309. [CrossRef]
82. Devaraj, P.; Kumari, P.; Aarti, C.; Renganathan, A. Synthesis and Characterization of Silver Nanoparticles Using Cannonball Leaves and Their Cytotoxic Activity against MCF-7 Cell Line. *J. Nanotechnol.* **2013**, *2013*, 1–5. [CrossRef]
83. Urnukhsaikhan, E.; Bold, B.-E.; Gunbileg, A.; Sukhbaatar, N.; Mishig-Ochir, T. Antibacterial Activity and Characteristics of Silver Nanoparticles Biosynthesized from Carduus Crispus. *Sci. Rep.* **2021**, *11*, 21047. [CrossRef] [PubMed]
84. Hayes, H.C.; Luk, L.Y.P.; Tsai, Y.-H. Approaches for Peptide and Protein Cyclisation. *Org. Biomol. Chem.* **2021**, *19*, 3983–4001. [CrossRef]
85. Sahoo, S.; Shivani, K.; Padhy, A.A.; Kumari, V.; Mishra, P. Principles, Methods, and Applications of Protein Folding Inside Cells. In *Protein Folding Dynamics and Stability*; Springer: Singapore, 2023; pp. 251–284.
86. Muthusamy, S.; Vaishnavi, R.; Neelakannan, M.; Kannan, D.; Silambarasan, T.; Immanuel, G. Investigation on Characterization and Biomedical Properties of Silver Nanoparticles Synthesized by an Actinobacterium Streptomyces Olivaceus (MSU3). *Biocatal. Agric. Biotechnol.* **2019**, *17*, 151–159. [CrossRef]
87. Jain, A.S.; Pawar, P.S.; Sarkar, A.; Junnuthula, V.; Dyawanapelly, S. Bionanofactories for Green Synthesis of Silver Nanoparticles: Toward Antimicrobial Applications. *Int. J. Mol. Sci.* **2021**, *22*, 11993. [CrossRef] [PubMed]
88. Manikprabhu, D.; Lingappa, K. Microwave Assisted Rapid and Green Synthesis of Silver Nanoparticles Using a Pigment Produced by Streptomyces Coelicolor Klmp33. *Bioinorg. Chem. Appl.* **2013**, *2013*, 1–5. [CrossRef] [PubMed]
89. Pallavi, S.S.; Rudayni, H.A.; Bepari, A.; Niazi, S.K.; Nayaka, S. Green Synthesis of Silver Nanoparticles Using Streptomyces Hirsutus Strain SNPGA-8 and Their Characterization, Antimicrobial Activity, and Anticancer Activity against Human Lung Carcinoma Cell Line A549. *Saudi J. Biol. Sci.* **2022**, *29*, 228–238. [CrossRef] [PubMed]
90. Abd El-Ghany, M.N.; Hamdi, S.A.; Korany, S.M.; Elbaz, R.M.; Emam, A.N.; Farahat, M.G. Biogenic Silver Nanoparticles Produced by Soil Rare Actinomycetes and Their Significant Effect on Aspergillus-Derived Mycotoxins. *Microorganisms* **2023**, *11*, 1006. [CrossRef]
91. Nayaka, S.; Chakraborty, B.; Bhat, M.P.; Nagaraja, S.K.; Airodagi, D.; Swamy, P.S.; Rudrappa, M.; Hiremath, H.; Basavarajappa, D.S.; Kanakannanavar, B. Biosynthesis, Characterization, and in Vitro Assessment on Cytotoxicity of Actinomycete-Synthesized Silver Nanoparticles on Allium Cepa Root Tip Cells. *Beni Suef Univ. J. Basic. Appl. Sci.* **2020**, *9*, 51. [CrossRef]
92. Subbaiya, R.; Saravanan, M.; Priya, A.R.; Shankar, K.R.; Selvam, M.; Ovais, M.; Balajee, R.; Barabadi, H. Biomimetic Synthesis of Silver Nanoparticles from *Streptomyces Atrovirens* and Their Potential Anticancer Activity against Human Breast Cancer Cells. *IET Nanobiotechnol.* **2017**, *11*, 965–972. [CrossRef] [PubMed]
93. Chauhan, S.; Arora, M.; Sati, P.C.; Chhoker, S.; Katyal, S.C.; Kumar, M. Structural, Vibrational, Optical, Magnetic and Dielectric Properties of $Bi_{1-x}Ba_xFeO_3$ Nanoparticles. *Ceram. Int.* **2013**, *39*, 6399–6405. [CrossRef]
94. Sadhasivam, S.; Shanmugam, P.; Yun, K. Biosynthesis of Silver Nanoparticles by Streptomyces Hygroscopicus and Antimicrobial Activity against Medically Important Pathogenic Microorganisms. *Colloids Surf. B Biointerfaces* **2010**, *81*, 358–362. [CrossRef]
95. Iniyan, A.M.; Kannan, R.R.; Joseph, F.-J.R.S.; Mary, T.R.J.; Rajasekar, M.; Sumy, P.C.; Rabel, A.M.; Ramachandran, D.; Vincent, S.G.P. In Vivo Safety Evaluation of Antibacterial Silver Chloride Nanoparticles from Streptomyces Exfoliatus ICN25 in Zebrafish Embryos. *Microb. Pathog.* **2017**, *112*, 76–82. [CrossRef]
96. Sivasankar, P.; Seedevi, P.; Poongodi, S.; Sivakumar, M.; Murugan, T.; Sivakumar, L.; Sivakumar, K.; Balasubramanian, T. Characterization, Antimicrobial and Antioxidant Property of Exopolysaccharide Mediated Silver Nanoparticles Synthesized by Streptomyces Violaceus MM72. *Carbohydr. Polym.* **2018**, *181*, 752–759. [CrossRef] [PubMed]
97. Railean-Plugaru, V.; Pomastowski, P.; Wypij, M.; Szultka-Mlynska, M.; Rafinska, K.; Golinska, P.; Dahm, H.; Buszewski, B. Study of Silver Nanoparticles Synthesized by Acidophilic Strain of Actinobacteria Isolated from the of Picea Sitchensis Forest Soil. *J. Appl. Microbiol.* **2016**, *120*, 1250–1263. [CrossRef]
98. Shahid, M.; Naeem-Ullah, U.; Khan, W.S.; Saeed, S.; Razzaq, K. Biocidal Activity of Green Synthesized Silver Nanoformulation by Azadirachta Indica Extract a Biorational Approach against Notorious Cotton Pest Whitefly, Bemisia Tabaci (Homoptera; Aleyrodidae). *Int. J. Trop. Insect Sci.* **2022**, *42*, 2443–2454. [CrossRef]

99. Matras, E.; Gorczyca, A.; Przemieniecki, S.W.; Oćwieja, M. Surface Properties-Dependent Antifungal Activity of Silver Nanoparticles. *Sci. Rep.* **2022**, *12*, 18046. [CrossRef]
100. Mikhailova, E.O. Silver Nanoparticles: Mechanism of Action and Probable Bio-Application. *J. Funct. Biomater.* **2020**, *11*, 84. [CrossRef] [PubMed]
101. Liao, C.; Li, Y.; Tjong, S. Bactericidal and Cytotoxic Properties of Silver Nanoparticles. *Int. J. Mol. Sci.* **2019**, *20*, 449. [CrossRef]
102. Aremu, O.S.; Qwebani-Ogunleye, T.; Katata-Seru, L.; Mkhize, Z.; Trant, J.F. Synergistic Broad-Spectrum Antibacterial Activity of Hypoxis Hemerocallidea-Derived Silver Nanoparticles and Streptomycin against Respiratory Pathobionts. *Sci. Rep.* **2021**, *11*, 15222. [CrossRef] [PubMed]
103. Al-Ansari, M.; Alkubaisi, N.; Vijayaragavan, P.; Murugan, K. Antimicrobial Potential of Streptomyces Sp. to the Gram Positive and Gram Negative Pathogens. *J. Infect. Public Health* **2019**, *12*, 861–866. [CrossRef] [PubMed]
104. Bruna, T.; Maldonado-Bravo, F.; Jara, P.; Caro, N. Silver Nanoparticles and Their Antibacterial Applications. *Int. J. Mol. Sci.* **2021**, *22*, 7202. [CrossRef]
105. Gao, Z.; Chen, X.; Wang, C.; Song, J.; Xu, J.; Liu, X.; Qian, Y.; Suo, H. New Strategies and Mechanisms for Targeting Streptococcus Mutans Biofilm Formation to Prevent Dental Caries: A Review. *Microbiol. Res.* **2024**, *278*, 127526. [CrossRef]
106. Buszewski, B.; Railean-Plugaru, V.; Pomastowski, P.; Rafińska, K.; Szultka-Mlynska, M.; Golinska, P.; Wypij, M.; Laskowski, D.; Dahm, H. Antimicrobial Activity of Biosilver Nanoparticles Produced by a Novel Streptacidiphilus Durhamensis Strain. *J. Microbiol. Immunol. Infect.* **2018**, *51*, 45–54. [CrossRef] [PubMed]
107. El-Sayyad, G.S.; Mosallam, F.M.; El-Batal, A.I. One-Pot Green Synthesis of Magnesium Oxide Nanoparticles Using Penicillium Chrysogenum Melanin Pigment and Gamma Rays with Antimicrobial Activity against Multidrug-Resistant Microbes. *Adv. Powder Technol.* **2018**, *29*, 2616–2625. [CrossRef]
108. Rasool, U.; Hemalatha, S. Marine Endophytic Actinomycetes Assisted Synthesis of Copper Nanoparticles (CuNPs): Characterization and Antibacterial Efficacy against Human Pathogens. *Mater. Lett.* **2017**, *194*, 176–180. [CrossRef]
109. Kalishwaralal, K.; BarathManiKanth, S.; Pandian, S.R.K.; Deepak, V.; Gurunathan, S. Silver Nanoparticles Impede the Biofilm Formation by Pseudomonas Aeruginosa and Staphylococcus Epidermidis. *Colloids Surf. B Biointerfaces* **2010**, *79*, 340–344. [CrossRef] [PubMed]
110. AboElmaaty, S.A.; Shati, A.A.; Alfaifi, M.Y.; Elbehairi, S.E.I.; Sheraba, N.S.; Hassan, M.G.; Badawy, M.S.E.M.; Ghareeb, A.; Hamed, A.A.; Gabr, E.Z. Biofilm Inhibitory Activity of Actinomycete-Synthesized AgNPs with Low Cytotoxic Effect: Experimental and In Silico Study. *Microorganisms* **2022**, *11*, 102. [CrossRef] [PubMed]
111. Yan, J.; Abdelgawad, A.M.; El-Naggar, M.E.; Rojas, O.J. Antibacterial Activity of Silver Nanoparticles Synthesized In-Situ by Solution Spraying onto Cellulose. *Carbohydr. Polym.* **2016**, *147*, 500–508. [CrossRef] [PubMed]
112. Sharma, V.; Basak, S.; Ali, S.W. Synthesis of Copper Nanoparticles on Cellulosic Fabrics and Evaluation of Their Multifunctional Performances. *Cellulose* **2022**, *29*, 7973–7988. [CrossRef]
113. Kim, I.; Viswanathan, K.; Kasi, G.; Thanakkasaranee, S.; Sadeghi, K.; Seo, J. ZnO Nanostructures in Active Antibacterial Food Packaging: Preparation Methods, Antimicrobial Mechanisms, Safety Issues, Future Prospects, and Challenges. *Food Rev. Int.* **2022**, *38*, 537–565. [CrossRef]
114. Kalia, A.; Kaur, M.; Shami, A.; Jawandha, S.K.; Alghuthaymi, M.A.; Thakur, A.; Abd-Elsalam, K.A. Nettle-Leaf Extract Derived ZnO/CuO Nanoparticle-Biopolymer-Based Antioxidant and Antimicrobial Nanocomposite Packaging Films and Their Impact on Extending the Post-Harvest Shelf Life of Guava Fruit. *Biomolecules* **2021**, *11*, 224. [CrossRef]
115. Huynh, N.T.N.; Pham, N.T.; Van Tran, C.; Nguyen, D.T.; Dinh, M.T.N.; Nguyen, V.T.; Nguyen, M.H.; Van Ngo, H.; Ho, A.N.; Cheng, J.; et al. Screening for Antimycobacterial Activity of Actinomycetes Collected in Vietnam—Isolation and Activity of Metabolites from Streptomyces Alboniger (A121). *Nat. Prod. Commun.* **2024**, *19*, 1934578X231224994. [CrossRef]
116. Sharma, A.; Dev, K.; Sourirajan, A.; Choudhary, M. Isolation and Characterization of Salt-Tolerant Bacteria with Plant Growth-Promoting Activities from Saline Agricultural Fields of Haryana, India. *J. Genet. Eng. Biotechnol.* **2021**, *19*, 99. [CrossRef] [PubMed]
117. Racchi, I.; Scaramuzza, N.; Hidalgo, A.; Berni, E. Combined Effect of Water Activity and PH on the Growth of Food-Related Ascospore-Forming Molds. *Ann. Microbiol.* **2020**, *70*, 69. [CrossRef]
118. El Karkouri, A.; Assou, S.A.; El Hassouni, M. Isolation and Screening of Actinomycetes Producing Antimicrobial Substances from an Extreme Moroccan Biotope. *Pan Afr. Med. J.* **2019**, *33*, 329. [CrossRef] [PubMed]
119. Goodfellow, M.; Fiedler, H.-P. A Guide to Successful Bioprospecting: Informed by Actinobacterial Systematics. *Antonie Van. Leeuwenhoek* **2010**, *98*, 119–142. [CrossRef] [PubMed]
120. Bizuye, A.; Gedamu, L.; Bii, C.; Gatebe, E.; Maina, N. Molecular-Based Identification of Actinomycetes Species That Synthesize Antibacterial Silver Nanoparticles. *Int. J. Microbiol.* **2020**, *2020*, 1–17. [CrossRef]
121. Pathalam, G.; Rajendran, H.A.D.; Appadurai, D.R.; Gandhi, M.R.; Michael, G.P.; Savarimuthu, I.; Naif, A.A.-D. Isolation and Molecular Characterization of Actinomycetes with Antimicrobial and Mosquito Larvicidal Properties. *Beni Suef Univ. J. Basic. Appl. Sci.* **2017**, *6*, 209–217. [CrossRef]
122. Veelken, M.; Pape, H. Production of Tylosin and Nikkomycin by Immobilized Streptomyces Cells. *Eur. J. Appl. Microbiol. Biotechnol.* **1982**, *15*, 206–210. [CrossRef]
123. Zhang, Y.; Douglas, G.B.; Kaksonen, A.H.; Cui, L.; Ye, Z. Microbial Reduction of Nitrate in the Presence of Zero-Valent Iron. *Sci. Total Environ.* **2019**, *646*, 1195–1203. [CrossRef] [PubMed]

124. Hamedi, S.; Ghaseminezhad, M.; Shokrollahzadeh, S.; Shojaosadati, S.A. Controlled Biosynthesis of Silver Nanoparticles Using Nitrate Reductase Enzyme Induction of Filamentous Fungus and Their Antibacterial Evaluation. *Artif. Cells Nanomed. Biotechnol.* **2017**, *45*, 1588–1596. [CrossRef]
125. Mechouche, M.S.; Merouane, F.; Messaad, C.E.H.; Golzadeh, N.; Vasseghian, Y.; Berkani, M. Biosynthesis, Characterization, and Evaluation of Antibacterial and Photocatalytic Methylene Blue Dye Degradation Activities of Silver Nanoparticles from Streptomyces Tuirus Strain. *Envron. Res.* **2022**, *204*, 112360. [CrossRef]
126. Damavandi, M.S.; Shojaei, H.; Esfahani, B.N. The Anticancer and Antibacterial Potential of Bioactive Secondary Metabolites Derived From Bacterial Endophytes in Association with Artemisia Absinthium. *Sci. Rep.* **2023**, *13*, 18473. [CrossRef]
127. Charousová, I.; Medo, J.; Hleba, L.; Javoreková, S. Streptomyces Globosus DK15 and Streptomyces Ederensis ST13 as New Producers of Factumycin and Tetrangomycin Antibiotics. *Braz. J. Microbiol.* **2018**, *49*, 816–822. [CrossRef]
128. Oliveira, A.; Cunha, M. de L.R. Comparison of Methods for the Detection of Biofilm Production in Coagulase-Negative Staphylococci. *BMC Res. Notes* **2010**, *3*, 260. [CrossRef]
129. Chen, H.; Wubbolts, R.W.; Haagsman, H.P.; Veldhuizen, E.J.A. Inhibition and Eradication of Pseudomonas Aeruginosa Biofilms by Host Defence Peptides. *Sci. Rep.* **2018**, *8*, 10446. [CrossRef]
130. Wei, G.-X.; Campagna, A.N.; Bobek, L.A. Effect of MUC7 Peptides on the Growth of Bacteria and on Streptococcus Mutans Biofilm. *J. Antimicrob. Chemother.* **2006**, *57*, 1100–1109. [CrossRef]
131. Losada-Barreiro, S.; Sezgin-Bayindir, Z.; Paiva-Martins, F.; Bravo-Díaz, C. Biochemistry of Antioxidants: Mechanisms and Pharmaceutical Applications. *Biomedicines* **2022**, *10*, 3051. [CrossRef]
132. Shilpa, S.A.; Pavithra, A.J.; Hikku, G.S.; Jeyasubramanian, K.; Veluswamy, P.; Ikeda, H. Imparting Efficient Antibacterial Activity to Cotton Fabrics by Coating with Green Synthesized Nano-Ag/PMMA Composite. *Bionanoscience* **2023**, *13*, 2180–2194. [CrossRef]
133. Ibrahim, H.M.M.; Hassan, M.S. Characterization and Antimicrobial Properties of Cotton Fabric Loaded with Green Synthesized Silver Nanoparticles. *Carbohydr. Polym.* **2016**, *151*, 841–850. [CrossRef]

pharmaceuticals

MDPI

Article

Synthesis and Characterization of Multifunctional Chitosan–Silver Nanoparticles: An In-Vitro Approach for Biomedical Applications

Gulamnabi Vanti [1], Naresh Poondla [2,3,4], Prasath Manogaran [5], Nagappa Teradal [6], Veeresh S [1], Ram Kaulgud [1] and Mahantesh Kurjogi [1,*]

1 Multidisciplinary Research Unit, Karnataka Medical College and Research Institute, Hubli 580021, India; nabisam1@gmail.com (G.V.); vshugar@gmail.com (V.S.); mrukimshubli@gmail.com (R.K.)
2 Department of Neurology, Icahn School of Medicine at Mount Sinai, New York, NY 10029, USA; naresh.poondla@mssm.edu
3 Center for Global Health Research, Saveetha Medical College& Hospital, Chennai 602105, India
4 Department of Applied Chemistry, Saveetha School of Engineering, Saveetha Institute of Medical and Technical Science (SIMATS), Chennai 602105, India
5 Department of Clinical and Translational Sciences, Marshall University, Huntington, WV 25755, USA; prasathbiomed@gmail.com
6 Department of Chemistry, J. S. S. Arts, Science and Commerce College, Gokak 591307, India; nlteradal@gmail.com
* Correspondence: mahantesh.kurjogi@gmail.com

Abstract: Antibiotics are successful in promoting health quality by preventing various infectious diseases and minimizing mortality and morbidity all over the world. However, the indiscriminate use of antibiotics has led to the emergence of multi-drug-resistant bacteria, which pose a serious threat to health care sector. Therefore, it is necessary to develop novel antimicrobial agents with versatile characteristics, such as antibacterial activity, low toxicity, wound healing potency, and antioxidant property. In this context, silver chitosan nanoparticles were synthesized in the present study, and their physical characterization revealed that the size of synthesized chitosan–silver nanoparticles was 14–25 nm, with positive surface charge. The functional groups and crystalline nature of the nanoparticles were confirmed by FT-IR and XRD analysis. Further, the silver chitosan nanoparticles showed antibacterial activity against two important clinical pathogens, *S. aureus* and *E. coli*. The MTT assay carried out in the present study showed that the synthesized nanoparticles are non-toxic to host cells. A scratch assay on fibroblast cells (L292) demonstrated that the silver chitosan nanoparticles showed promising wound healing activity. A fluorescent DCFH-DA staining assay revealed anantioxidant property of the synthesized nanoparticles. Overall, the study emphasizes the versatile nature of synthesized chitosan–silver nanoparticles, suggesting their great compatibility for biomedical applications.

Keywords: silver nanoparticles; chitosan; antibacterial activity; antioxidant activity; wound healing activity

1. Introduction

Antibiotics play a crucial role in enhancing health by preventing numerous infectious diseases and reducing mortality and morbidity worldwide. However, their overuse has led to the rise of multi-drug-resistant bacteria, presenting a significant challenge to the health care sector [1,2]. The continued rise in antibiotic-resistant bacteria may be driven by the high frequency of spontaneous mutations and the exchange of genetic material between microbial strains [3]. On the other hand, an inadequate blood circulation and increased inflammation in the wound area complicate the treatment process, especially in surface wound infections. In addition, wound recovery and the wound–healing process may also lead to increased health care expenses. *Staphylococcus aureus* is one of the most common ESKAPE pathogens (*Enterococcus faecium, S. aureus, Klebsiella pneumoniae, Acinetobacter baumannii, Pseudomonas aeruginosa,* and *Enterobacter* spp.) that interrupt the wound healing process by biofilm formation [4]. Wound healing is a complex process involving the interaction between immune cells and the extracellular matrix to halt bleeding and prevent infection. Additionally, wounds increase the levels of reactive oxygen species, which further activate transcriptional signals and trigger caspase-3-dependent apoptosis, leading to cell death [5]. However, systemic antibiotics can barely penetrate into wound biofilms and topically applied antibiotics can easily lead to sensitization. Therefore, it is essential to explore novel antimicrobial agents with multifunctional properties, including antimicrobial activity, wound healing capabilities, low toxicity, and excellent compatibility. In this regard, nanotechnology has gathered worldwide interest due to the versatile characteristics of nanoparticles. Additionally, chitosan, a natural biopolymer, has demonstrated significant potential in controlled drug delivery and wound healing. Its biocompatibility and non-toxic nature further enhance its appeal for biomedical applications. In recent years, chitosan-based nanomaterials have been extensively studied for wound healing applications due to their antibacterial properties and biocompatibility. Additionally, chitosan is recognized for its ability to enhance the proliferative phase of wound healing and reduce inflammation by stimulating inflammatory cells, macrophages, and fibroblasts in the wound area [6]. Several researchers have adopted a combination of chitosan and metal nanoparticles in the synthesis of chitosan-based nanoparticles in order to enhance antimicrobial activity and biological safety for clinical application. Numerous studies have explored various strategies for preparing these chitosan-based metal nanoparticles, including hydrogels, fibers, sponges, films, membranes, and scaffolds, all of which are utilized in wound healing assays [7–13]. Despite numerous reports on various chitosan-based formulations for wound healing assays, several major challenges persist. These include issues with controlled drug delivery, the sterilization of chitosan-based formulations, and the scalability of manufacturing processes for commercial production [14]. Moreover, there is a lack of information regarding the powdered form of chitosan-based silver nanoparticles and their application in wound treatment [15]. Silver, on the other hand, is one of the most extensively studied metals, historically known for its broad-spectrum antimicrobial activity. Silver nanoparticles are able to penetrate bacterial cell walls, disrupt cell membrane structure, and overall improve the healing process, particularly in topical wound infections.

Chitosan and silver each address infection and wound healing through distinct mechanisms. Therefore, it is crucial to develop an effective, biocompatible therapeutic that combines these two agents to leverage their synergistic effects on microbes and the wound healing process. In this study, a novel, cost-effective, and sustainable method was utilized to fabricate silver on chitosan, aiming to exhibit antibacterial properties, enhance wound healing, and scavenge reactive oxygen species.

2. Results

2.1. Nanoparticles Characterization

The reaction conditions and reducing agents used in the preparation of nanoparticles play a crucial role in the synthesis of nanoparticles. In the current study, chitosan and silver nitrate were efficiently reduced to nano size using hydrazine as a reducing agent. A change in color was observed visually and confirmed by an absorption peak at ~455 nm (Figure 1a), suggesting the transition of Ag^0 from $AgNO_3$ substrate. Dynamic Light Scattering (DLS) results revealed that the synthesized NPs were in the range of 16–190 nm, with an average diameter of 55 $\pm$ 19.5 nm, by Gaussian distribution (Figure 1b).

Particle size distribution analysis in aqueous solution showed a 0.64 reading, suggesting that the nanoparticles were highly dispersive inaqueous medium. The surface charge of the NPs was confirmed by the zeta potential, which showed a positive (+19.2 mV) surface charge (Figure 2a). Further, the crystal structure was observed by diffraction peaks in XRD at 38.008°, 44.211°, 64.012°, and 78.54°, which correspond to the planes of 111, 200, 220, and

320, respectively, suggesting the simple cubic phase of silver nanoparticles with crystalline nature (JCPDS file no. 89-3722). The broadening of Bragg's peaks presents the successful formation of Ch-AgNPs. The average crystalline size of silver was calculated using the Scherrer formula, as below:

$$D = 0.94\,\lambda/\beta\mathrm{Cos}\theta$$

Whereby D is the average crystallite domain size perpendicular to the reflecting planes, λ is the X-ray wavelength, β is the full width at half maximum (FWHM), and θ is the diffraction angle.

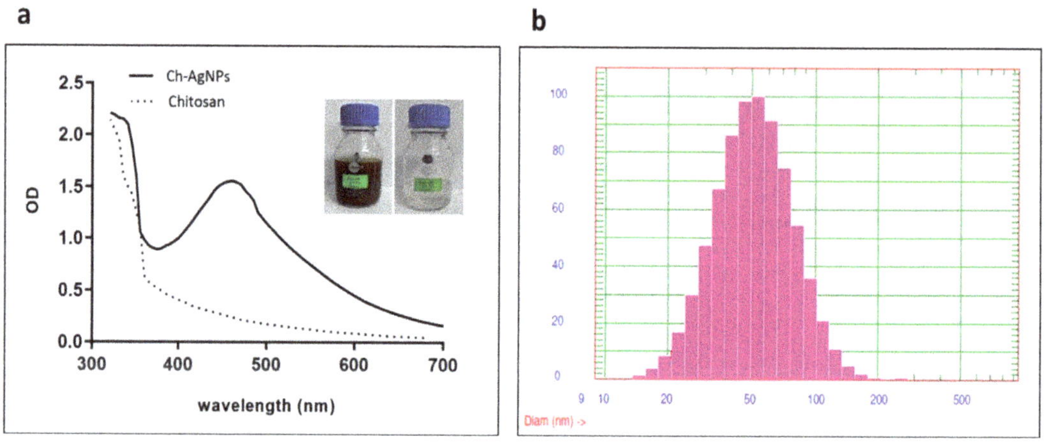

Figure 1. (**a**) The color change and the UV-Vis spectra of synthesized Ch-AgNPs. (**b**) Gaussian distribution analysis of the synthesized Ch-AgNPs.

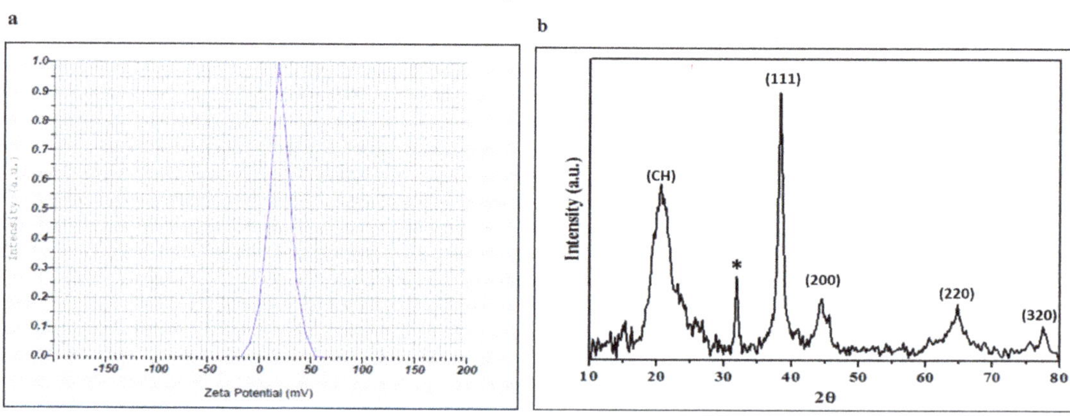

Figure 2. (**a**) The zeta potential of the synthesized nanoparticles (**b**) XRD characterization of synthesized nanoparticles, * Unassigned peak.

The average crystalline size was calculated to be 23.82 nm, and unassigned peaks (32.004°) were also observed (marked with asterisks), suggesting that the crystallization of the bio-organic phase occurs on the Ag nanoparticles (Figure 2b).

The FT-IR spectra of bulk chitosan alone indicated a band at 3451.33 cm^{-1}, which was basically due to the stretching of hydroxyl and amino groups. However, in the same position, more stretching was observed in the NPs with a band length of 3456.24 cm^{-1}, which was slightly higher compared to bulk chitosan. Further, NPs witnessed a sharp peak at 1384.26 cm^{-1} and 1640.93 cm^{-1}, whereas these peaks were found at 1384.11 cm^{-1} and

1647.83 cm^{-1} in bulk chitosan, suggesting a stretching of the functional groups -$CONH_2$ (Figure 3). Other peak variations such as 1500–1000 cm^{-1} in the NPs observed in the present study might be due to –OH, C-O, and C-H bending, which help to stabilize and redistribute the vibrational frequencies in NPs.

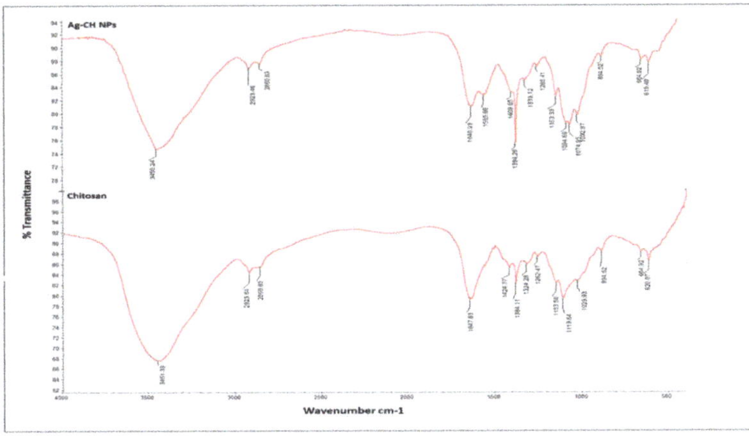

Figure 3. FT-IR spectra of synthesized Ch-AgNPs.

2.2. Electron Microscopy and EDS Analysis of NPs

Observation under SEM revealed the morphology of the NPs, which were spherical in shape and ranged from 20 to 50 nm in size (Figure 4a). Additionally, X-ray studies showed the presence of the silver element at its 2.98 KeV (Lα) energy level by EDS analysis (Figure 4b). Other observed peaks in the spectra might have been due to deposition during sample preparation. In support of SEM, the morphology of NPs was further validated with TEM, and the analysis confirmed the spherical shape of the NPs; the observed NPs were in the range of 14 to 25 nm in diameter (Figure 4c).

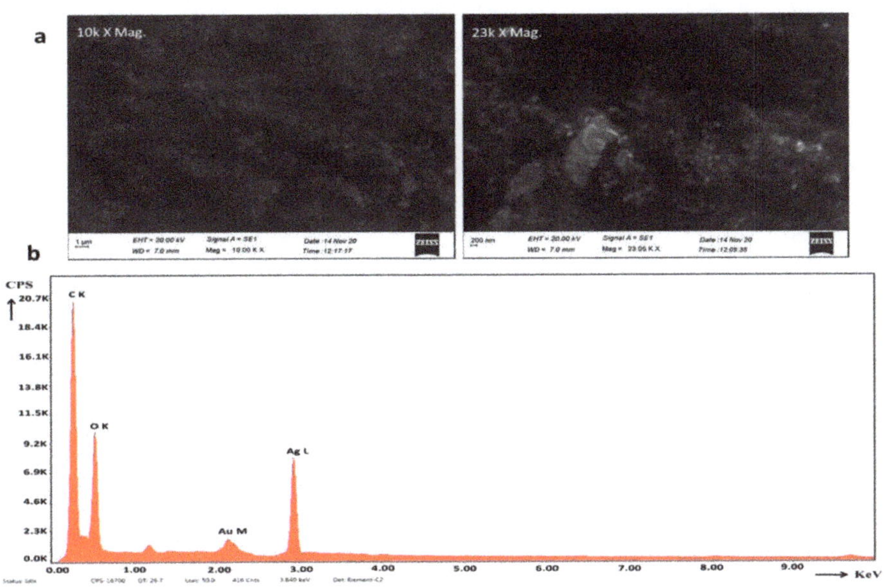

Figure 4. *Cont.*

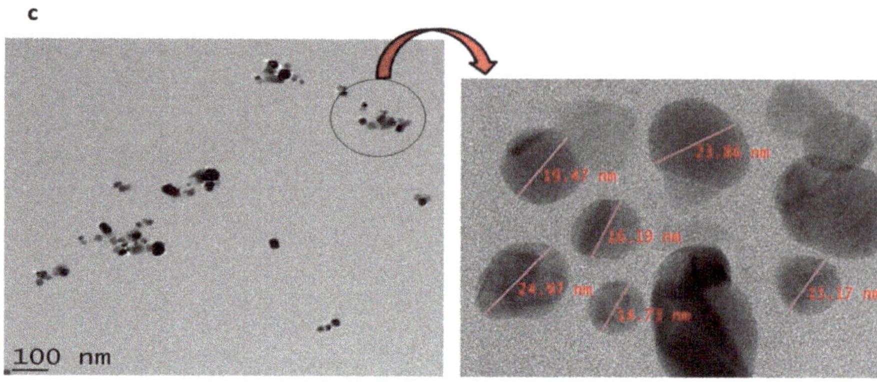

Figure 4. (**a**) Shape and size of synthesized NPs as depicted by SEM. (**b**) Elemental analysis of nano Ag by EDS. (**c**) Morphology confirmation of synthesized nanoparticles by TEM.

2.3. Efficacy of NPs on Clinical Pathogens

In the present study, the synthesized Ch-AgNPs showed antibacterial activity, with MIC values of 0.8 μg/mL and 1.6 μg/mL against Gram-positive *S. aureus* and Gram-negative *E. coli*, respectively, when compared with that of standard Streptomycin and Ampicillin antibiotics, respectively, with MIC 0.8 μg/mL (Figure 5).

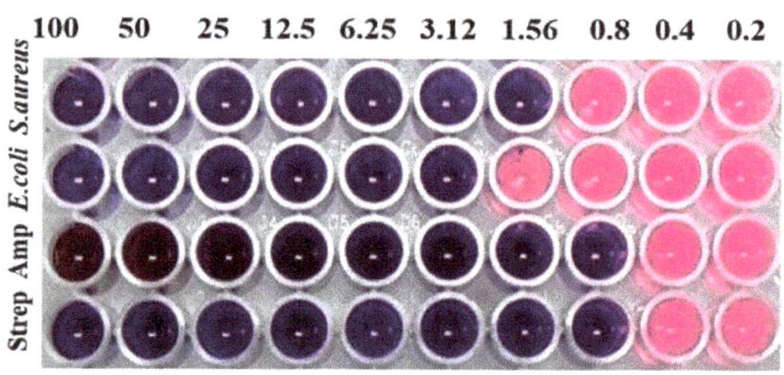

Figure 5. MIC of Ch-AgNPs against *S. aureus* and *E. coli*.

2.4. Toxicity and WoundHealing Assay

The MTT assay showed that HEK-293 cells (NCL Pune, India) were viable up to 82% at 1.5 μg/mL NP concentrations; however, as the concentration of the NPs increased, the HEK-293 cells viability decreased, and at 6 μg/mL of NPs concentration, the HEK-293 cell viability was 51.2 ± 0.9%. On the other hand, the standard drug cisplatin at 6 μg/mL showed 38.1 ± 0.5% HEK-293 cell viability (Figure 6a,b). Furthermore, the 50% inhibitory concentration (IC_{50}) of synthesized NP was calculated and estimated to be 5.53 μg/mL.

Further, the wound healing activity of NPs assayed by the artificial scratch assay method on normal fibroblast cells (L292 cells) showed 97% wound closure with 18.9 μM cell migrations at 0.55 μg/mL of NPs. Meanwhile, buffer-incubated cells showed 14% wound closure at 24 h of incubation. However, standard ascorbic acid used in this study showed 98.8% wound healing activity when tested on fibroblast cells (Figure 7a,b).

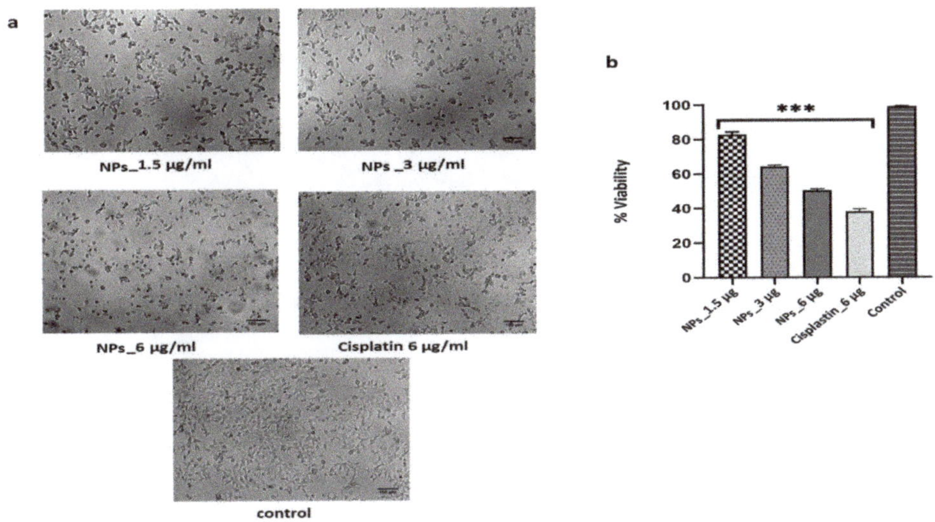

Figure 6. (**a**) Toxicity assay of Ch-AgNPs. (**b**) IC_{50} value of Ch-AgNPs, as determined by the MTT assay *** $p < 0.01$.

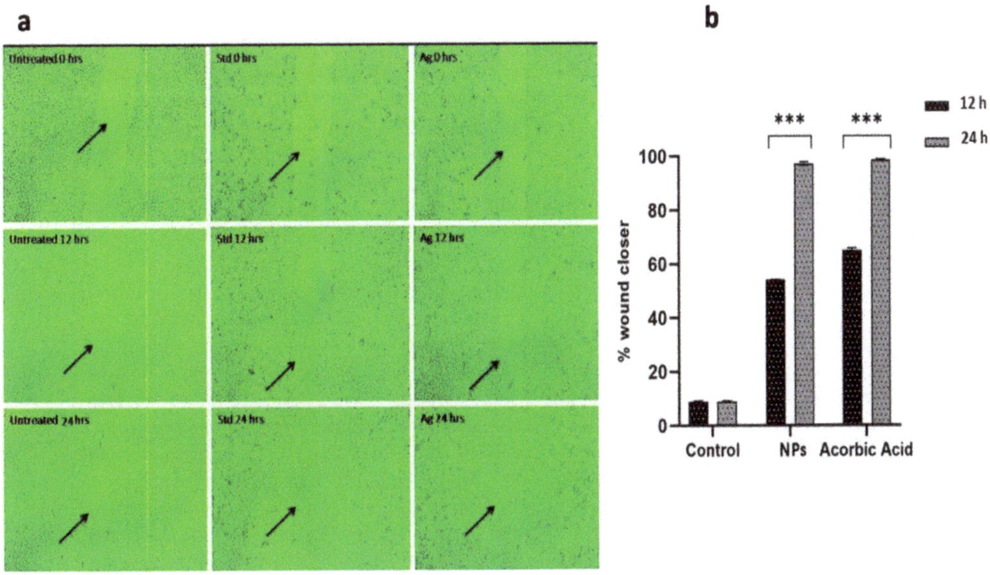

Figure 7. (**a**) Scratch assay depicting wound healing activity of synthesized nanoparticles. (**b**) Graph illustrating 97% wound closure when treated with Ch-AgNPs at 24 h, *** $p < 0.001$.

2.5. Antioxidant Activity of NPs

T-47D breast cells were induced with exogenous ROS generator DOX and treated with nanoparticles to assess their antioxidant property. Oxidative stress was assessed using dichloro-dihydro-fluorescein diacetate (DCFH-DA). The fluorescence emission in DOX-treated samples was significantly high when compared with that of the control and treated samples (DOX + NPs). The decreased fluorescence emission in the treated sample indicates the quenching effect of the synthesized nanoparticles in the DCFH-DA assay (Figure 8a,b).

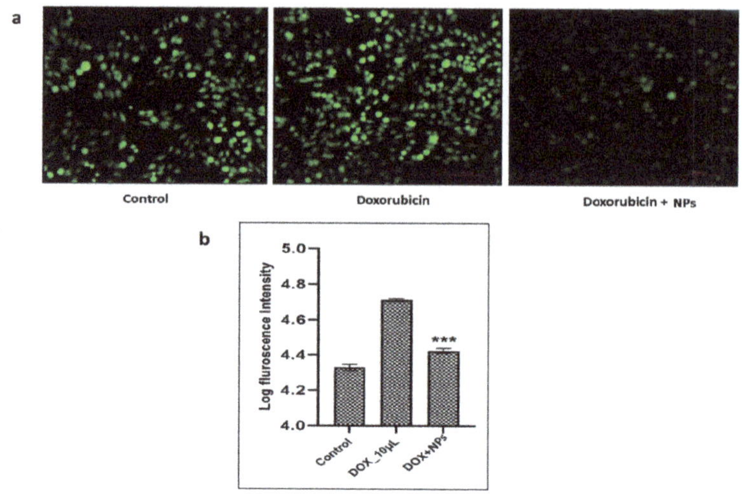

Figure 8. (**a**) Quenching effect in cells treated with nanoparticles compared to the control and DOX alone. (**b**) Graph showing the logarithmic fluorescence intensity of cells treated with DCFH-DA, *** $p < 0.001$.

3. Discussion

In the last few years, chitosan application in medical research have significantly increased due to its high specificity, sensitivity, and reduced toxicity to mammalian cells [16,17]. Recently, chitosan application in the biomedical field for tissue engineering and drug delivery was also approved by the US FDA [18]. The interactive amino and hydroxyl groups of chitosan play a vital role in enhancing cell-to-cell adhesion, promoting low immunogenicity, and enacting bio-tolerability properties, which make chitosan an ideal candidate for biomedical applications [19,20]. However, studies indicate an enhanced synergistic effect of chitosan in biomedical usage when combined with metal nanoparticles [17].

In the present study, we synthesized silver nanoparticles using chitosan as a stabilizing and capping molecule and hydrazine as a reducing agent. During the synthesis process, silver added to the chitosan solution led to the formation of a silver core shell surrounded by the hydroxyl and amine groups of the chitosan, which was responsible for the capping and stability of the NPs [16]. The reducing agent hydrazine hydrate ($N_2H_4{\cdot}H_2O$) at lower concentrations (0.1–0.4%) aids in Ch-AgNPs formation by reducing silver nitrate to silver ions and eliminating nitrogen gas [21]. In the present study, a chitosan–acetic acid suspension was prepared prior to the initiation of the AgNPs synthesis process using hydrazine hydrate as a reducing agent; similarly, 0.2 g of chitosan was dissolved into 10 mL of 1% (v/v) acetic acid and used as a substrate for the preparation of silver nanoparticle–chitosan composite spheres [22]. Whilst in other studies chitosan pellets have been produced with optimal AgNPs using chitosan suspension in 0.2 M acetic acid [23], a similar methodology was also followed in our previous study, where hydrazine hydrate was used as a reducing agent for the preparation of chitosan copper nanoparticles [24]. In the present study, the zeta potential of synthesized nanoparticles was+19.2 mV, which is in corroboration with the available literature, in which the zeta potential value of silver nanoparticles was +36.0 mV, suggesting that the zeta potential value is highly dependent on the concentration of reducing or capping agent [22]. On the contrary, it has been stated that the zeta potential values of Ch-AgNPs range between − 0.0695 and − 0.225 mV, indicating the negative charge of zeta potential values [25]. The spectrophotometer peak recorded at 455 nm was known to be due to the surface plasmon resonance (SPR) of the NPs and its precursors in the dielectric environment of the solution [26]. Previous findings also support that the interaction of the amino and hydroxyl groups of chitosan polymer with silver ions occurs due to peak observed at this particular range [27]. Furthermore, the NPs synthesized in the current study had a positive surface charge which was directly related to the higher electrostatic repulsion between the NPs. The functional group of chitosan involved in the formation of Ag NPs was confirmed by FT-IR analysis, and the changes in the corresponding vibration band were related to the interaction between the Ag NPs and the chitosan amino and hydroxyl groups [28–32]. The stretching peak of an aliphatic primary amine (3344.41 cm^{-1}) and a normal hydroxyl (−OH) group (3400−3200 cm^{-1}) of chitosan coexisted due to their overlapping stretching frequencies, and this is well documented in the literature [33]. Further, bulk chitosan exhibited stretching peaks at 1384.11 cm^{-1} and 1647.83 cm^{-1} due to the presence of the -$CONH_2$ group. The prepared Ch-AgNPs also showed peaks at 1384.26 cm^{-1} and 1640.93 cm^{-1}, corresponding to the stretching of the functional group -$CONH_2$ [28], suggesting the successful surface passivation of chitosan.

In addition, the XRD diffraction peak at 20.519° corresponds to chitosan, which confirms the successful passivation of Ag NPs with chitosan molecules; moreover, the observed 2θ values are in good agreement with reported values [25]. Further, FT-IR analysis showed a peak at 1565.66 cm^{-1} in the NPs compared to bulk chitosan, which may be due to amide functional involvement in the NP formation [34,35]. Thus, in our study, the sustainable fabrication of hybrid chitosan–silver nanoparticles was accomplished by using a simple and cost-effective reducing agent.

The application of antibiotics for the management of bacterial infections has been practiced for many years. However, in the present era, the use of conventional antibiotics has led to mediocre results due to the rapid development of resistant bacteria among nosocomial infections. In recent years, nanoparticles were found to be effective against several plant pathogens and are now garnering considerable attention for their use against clinical pathogens. In the present study, the synthesized Ch-AgNPs were screened for their antibacterial activity against two economically important clinical pathogens, namely *S. aureus* and *E. coli*, showing successful inhibition of both the pathogens. Similarly, our previous reports also support the antibacterial activity of silver nanoparticles against *S. aureus* and *E. coli* using the agar disk diffusion method [36]. Further, the role of chitosan in the release of metal nanoparticles at the infection site was highlighted in our previous study [24]. Likewise, another study also demonstrated that the silver nanoparticle-loaded collagen–chitosan dressing material could show 100% antibacterial activity at 3000 $\mu g/cm^2$ [37].

Furthermore, synthesized Ch-AgNPs were used for an invitro cytotoxicity study, which are often used to characterize the biological response to nanoparticles. The results of such studies are helpful in identifying the toxic nature associated with nanoparticle exposure at higher concentration. HEK-293 is a robust and fast-growing cell linethat is highly reproducible and consistent. Moreover, HEK cells provide relevant information on human-specific responses to toxic substances, making them more suitable for assessing potential human health risks. Therefore, in the present study, cytotoxicity was carried out against normal HEK-293 cells at three different concentrations (1.5–6 $\mu g\ mL^{-1}$) with appropriate controls. The toxicity study revealed that the IC_{50} value of the synthesized nanoparticles was 5.53 μg/mL, suggesting the biocompatible nature of the Ch-AgNPs when used at lower concentrations (<5.53 μg/mL). A study by Xue et al. also demonstrated that AgNPs are able to decrease the viability of HepG2 cells when exposed for 24 and 48 h at higher concentrations [38]. On the contrary, another study reported the variable toxicity of chitosan–silver nanocomposite particles, indicating that the toxicity of the nanoparticles is not only concentration-dependent but also highly dependent on the morphology of the nanoparticles [39]. Similarly, another comprehensive study on toxicity with various substrates using zebrafish embryos showed low-to-moderate toxicity, demonstrating that toxicity of is also dependent on the substrate composition used in the synthesized nanoparticles [40].

Several articles have reported the usage of chitosan-based nanoparticles in different forms, such as hydrogels, fibers, sponges, films, membranes and scaffolds, for wound healing assays [7–13]. However, information on chitosan-based silver nanoparticles in powdered form, which are quite effective in wound treatment, is very limited 15]. Therefore, the present study endeavored to evaluate the wound healing property of synthesized NPs on fibroblast cells (L292). The outcome of wound healing activity was promising, and we found a 97% recovery of wound with 0.55 μg/mL of NPs. The concentration used for wound healing activity was 10-times less than that of the IC_{50} value, which suggests the potential role of Ch-AgNPs in the management of wound infections. This enhanced activity might be due to the synergistic effect of chitosan and AgNPs, which accelerates the wound healing process by triggering inflammatory cells, macrophages, and fibroblast cells that help proliferate cells during the wound healing process [6,35,41]. Similarly, the available literature suggests that chitosan is one of the important biopolymers not only used in wound dressings for to enhance the wound healing process but also to inhibit bacterial infection in the wound area [42]. An adequate number of clinical trials (ongoing and completed) evaluating the safety and efficacy of chitosan for wound healing activity was also reported in another study [43]. Further, the wound healing activity of chitosan was found to be evident in both medical and veterinary domains [44].

In eukaryotic cells, ROS-induced apoptosis is generally escorted by the loss of mitochondrial membrane potential [45]. Oxidative stress can occur when ROS overcome the detoxifying ability of individual cells, which further leads to comorbidities such as-inflammation, cancer, and neurodegenerative disease [45,46]. In our study, T-47D breast cells induced with exogenous ROS generator DOX increased florescence intensity 2.4-fold higher compared to a control. Meanwhile, T-47D breast cells treated with synthesized nanoparticles showed a reduced florescence intensity by 1.2-fold. The observed ROS scavenging property of synthesized Ch-AgNPs could be due to the hydroxyl (-OH) and amino (-NH_2) groups in the biopolymer [47]. In addition, free amino groups present in the biopolymer (NH_2) chitosan can react with OH to form stable macromolecule radicals, which are further degraded [48]. It was proven that the degraded products of biopolymer chitosan are non-toxic and cause no immunogenic reaction in the cells [49,50].

4. Conclusions

In the present investigations, chitosan solution was used as a stabilizing agent for the synthesis of silver nanoparticles, while hydrazine hydrate was used as reducing agent. Further characterization of the synthesized nanoparticles presented an absorption peak at ~455 nm with UV–Vis spectroscopy, and the morphology of the synthesized nanoparticles was found to be spherical, with a size of 15–30 nm, as confirmed by SEM and TEM analysis. The functional groups and crystalline nature of the synthesized nanoparticles were revealed by FTIR and XRD analysis. Furthermore, the chitosan–silver nanoparticles synthesized in the present study showed various biological activities, such as antibacterial activity against *S. aureus* and *E. coli*, wound healing activity, and antioxidant activity. Moreover, the MTT assay carried out in the present study also showed that the synthesized nanoparticles were non-toxic to host cells. Despite the usage of advanced antiseptics, wound infections remain a major concern in the health care sector due to the emergence of antibiotic-resistant microorganisms. Therefore, our study suggests that biocompatible polymer-based multifunctional silver nanoparticles could be more reliable for biomedical applications.

5. Materials and Methods

Silver nitrate ($AgNO_3$, 99.98%), low-molecular-weight (LMW) chitosan, acetic acid (glacial, 99–100%), and hydrazine hydrate were procured from Sigma-Aldrich, St. Louis, MO, USA. Milli Q water was used throughout the experiment. Nutrient broth was purchased from Himedia Chemicals (Mumbai, India). *S. aureus* and *E. coli* cultures were grown and maintained at the Multi-Disciplinary Research Unit, Karnataka Medical College and Research Institute (KMCRI), Hubli, Karnataka, India.

5.1. Synthesis of Chitosan–Silver Nanoparticles (Ch-AgNPs)

The chitosan–silver nanoparticles were synthesized, with little modification of the previously reported procedures [22,24].

A chitosan suspension was prepared by dissolving 0.1 g of low-molecular-weight chitosan (75% deacetylated) into 10 mL of 1% (*v*/*v*) acetic acid with constant stirring for 18 h at room temperature. Further, chitosan–silver nanoparticles were synthesized using0.2% chitosan suspension and $AgNO_3$ (1 mM) with constant stirring on a hot plate at 80 °C for 2 h; the reducing agent hydrazine hydrate (0.2%) was gradually added to this solution until the color changed to brown, indicating the conversion of $AgNO_3$ to AgNps. The reduced nanoparticles (NPs) were centrifuged (8000× *g* for 10 min) with three washes. Further, they were dried in a hot air oven at 50 °C before they were subjected to physical and chemical characterization.

5.2. Characterization of the Nanoparticles

5.2.1. Spectroscopic Studies

The synthesized NPs were initially observed using a UV-visible spectrophotometer (SP-UV 500DB; Uberlingen, Germany), with a 200–700 nm wavelength scan. Further, the NPs were subjected to Dynamic Light Scattering (DLS) to obtain the average particle size and polydispersity index using a high-performance particle size analyzer Z3000 (Nicomp, San Francisco, CA, USA). The surface charge was obtained by using zeta potential readings with a 7.4 pH graphite electrode at room temperature (SZ-100 particle size analyzer; Horiba; Koyoto, Japan). In addition, the bond vibrations of the functional groups involved in the NPs' formation was recorded by Fourier transform infrared spectroscopy (FTIR; Nicolet 6700 Thermo Scientific, Waltham MA, USA) at 400–4000 cm^{-1}. The cubic nature of the metal and chitosan, and silver passivation were recorded by X-ray diffraction studies using an AXS D8 X-ray diffraction system (Bruker; Billerica, MA, USA), with the Cu Kα line (1.5406 Å) employed to generate X-rays (40 kV/35 mA).

5.2.2. Electron Microscopy Studies

The surface morphology of the NPs was studied by scanning electron microscopy(SEM) (Carl Zeiss EV018; Oberkohen, Germany). A thin smear of 10 µL (1:5; *v*/*v*) NCs suspension was placed on a microscopy stub to obtain a fine film, dried, and sputter-coated with a gold layer under high vacuum. Images were captured at a 7 mm working distance at different magnifications (10 K and 23 K). X-rays from the sample were captured by employing EDS with 5 kV energy. To obtain an accurate particle size, the NCs were subjected to transmission electron microscopy (TEM; Jeol Model JM 2100, Tokyo, Japan) and the images were recorded at different magnifications.

5.3. Antibacterial Activity of Ch-AgNPs

The antibacterial activity of the synthesized Ch-AgNPs was studied against Gram-positive *S. aureus* and Gram-negative *E. coli* by the broth dilution method [51]. *S. aureus* and *E. coli* were inoculated in 10 mL of nutrient broth (Hi-Media, Mumbai, India) and incubated at 37 °C for 16 h, and then they were sub-cultured in 10 mL of the same medium under the same conditions for 3 h to obtain the active growth phase. Different concentrations of NPs were serially diluted (100–0.2 µg mL^{-1}) into each well; further, microbial inoculum (1:1000) was added and the final volume was made to 200 µL. Similarly, control antibiotics streptomycin and ampicillin were pipetted (100–0.2 µg mL^{-1}) into the next two rows and serially diluted, and microbial inoculum was added to this. After 24 h of incubation at 37 °C, aqueous resazurin (30 µL) solution was added to each well and any change in color was recorded.

5.4. Cytotoxicity Assay of Ch-AgNPs by MTT

In the present study, normal HEK 293 (Human Embryonic Kidney) cells were used for the cyotoxicity assay, and they were procured from the National Chemical Laboratory (NCL), Pune. The cells were maintained in optimum condition at the Multi-Disciplinary Research Unit, KMCRI Hubli (minimum essential medium (MEM) supplemented with 10% fetal bovine serum at 37 °C, 5% CO_2 with 100% relative humidity). The cells were centrifuged in a 15 mL tube at 1500 rpm for 5 min after trypsinization. The cell count of approximately 10,000 cells was adjusted using MEM, and 200 µL of the cell suspension was added into each 96-well plate, which was further incubated under the same conditions for 24 h. The media seeded with HEK-293 cells were treated with different concentrations (1.5, 3, and 6 µg/mL) of NPs and incubated under the same conditions for 24 h. Media without NPs and media with 6 µg/mL cisplatin were used as negative and positive controls, and the experiment was carried out three times. The averagesof the viable cells were plotted on agraph. After the incubation period, the rates of cell growth and inhibition was determined by 3-(4,5-dimethylthiazol-2-yl)-2,5-diphenyltetrazolium bromide (MTT). MTT reagent (0.5 mg/mL) was added to each well and incubated under the same conditions for 4 h. Inside the metabolically active cells, MTT was reduced to an insoluble, dark purple formazan. The medium was removed completely without disturbing the crystals formed, the formazan crystals were dissolved in 100 µL DMSO (dimethyl sulfoxide), and the plate was gently shaken to solubilize the formed formazan. The absorbance was measured using a microplate reader (Thermo Scientific, Multiskan Sky High Microplate Spectrophotometer, Waltham MA, USA) at 570 nm and 630 nm, and the percentage of cell inhibition was calculated using the following formula:

$$\%\text{ cell inhibition} = 100 - \text{Absorbance (treatment)}/\text{Absorbance (Control)} \times 100$$

The concentration of NPs needed to inhibit cell growth by 50% (IC_{50}) was then generated from the dose–response curve of the cell lines.

5.5. Wound Healing Property of Ch-AgNPs

A wound healing assay was carried out as per the protocol by [52], with minor changes. Normal fibroblast cells (L292 cells) were grown in DMEM with 10% FBS, and after confluence the cells were detached from the flask by trypsin, aspirated into a 15 mL falcon tube, and centrifuged at 1500 rpm for 5 min at RT. The known number of cells were suspended in 100 µL DMEM with supplement in a sterile 12-well plate and incubated for 24 h to reach ~100% confluence as a monolayer at 37 °C with 5% CO_2. A scratch was made to the monolayer, and the wells were gently washed with DMEM to remove the detached cells; then, they were further washed with 1× phosphate-buffer saline (PBS). Media containing NPs were added (0.5 µg/mL) to each well and further incubated for 24 h. Ascorbic acid was used as a positive control. The wound gap distance was quantitatively evaluated using MagVision measurement tool at 4 × resolution. The cell migration rate was calculated using the following formula:

$$M_R = (W_i - W_t)/T$$

Whereby M_R is the cell migration rate in micrometer scale (µM/h), W_i is the initial wound width (µM), W_t is the final wound width (µM), and T is the duration of migration (in hours).

5.6. Antioxidant Property of Ch-AgNPs

The antioxidantproperty of the Ch-AgNPs was evaluated by measuring the total reactive oxygen species (ROS) using a fluorescent dye 2′,7′-dichlorodihydrofluorescein diacetate (DCFH-DA) in adherent breast cancer cells by employing the Vanti et al. method, with somemodification [53].

This assay was carried out in 24-well sterile plates by using T-47D breast cells procured from the National Chemical Laboratory (NCL), Pune, India. In each well, cells were seeded (2×10^5 cells) in Roswell Park Memorial Institute (RPMI) 1640 medium with supplements and incubated 48 h instandard conditions. Further, 48 h grown culture media were replaced with exogenous ROS generator doxorubicin (DOX) (10 μM) in RPMI medium and incubated for 4 h with the same conditions. Subsequent to the incubation period, media were replaced by 3 μg/mL NPs in 1×phosphate-buffer saline (PBS), control wells were incubated without NPs, and the experiment plate was incubated for 1h at standard conditions. After incubation, the medium from the each well was removed and the plate was washed twice with cold PBS (pH 7.4). To this, 500 μL of DCFH-DA working solution (10 μM) was added and the plate was incubated at 37 °C for 30 min in dark conditions. PBS from each well was removed, and RIPA lysis and extraction buffer (Thermo scientific) were added (300 μL) to each well; the plate was then incubated on ice for 5 min. Cell lysate was collected in tubes and cold centrifuged was conducted at 12,000 rpm for 10 min. The supernatant was carefully transferred (100 μL) to a black 96-well plate and the fluorescence was measured with 485 nm excitation and 530 nm emission wavelengths in a fluorometer (plate reader) (Tecan Infinite 200 PRO, Crailsheim, Germany). Fluorescence images were captured at 40× magnification using EVOS™ M7000 Thermo Fisher.

5.7. Statistical Analysis

All the experiments in the present study were carried out in triplicate, and the obtained results are presented as mean ± standard deviation. The analysis of data was carried out statistically using analysis of variance (ANOVA) with Prism version 8 software. Differences were deemed significant at the 0.001% level.

Author Contributions: Conception of the study was conducted by G.V. and M.K. designed and conducted the experiments. G.V. and M.K. wrote the manuscript, V.S., P.M. and N.T. helped to analyze the XRD and FT-IR data. M.K., R.K. and N.P. guided and reviewed the manuscript. All authors have read and agreed to the published version of the manuscript.

Funding: This research received no external funding.

Institutional Review Board Statement: Not applicable.

Informed Consent Statement: Not Applicable.

Data Availability Statement: Data are contained within the article.

Acknowledgments: The authors would like to thank the Department of Health Research, Government of India New Delhi, and Multi-Disciplinary Research Unit, Karnataka Medical College and Research Institute, Hubli, Karnataka, India.

Conflicts of Interest: All contributing authors declare no conflicts of interest.

References

1. Browne, A.J.; Chipeta, M.G.; Haines-Woodhouse, G.; Kumaran, E.P.; Hamadani, B.H.; Zaraa, S.; Henry, N.J.; Deshpande, A.; Reiner, R.C.; Day, N.P.; et al. Global antibiotic consumption and usage in humans, 2000–2018: A spatial modelling study. *Lancet Planet. Health* **2021**, *5*, e893–e904. [CrossRef] [PubMed]
2. Ayukekbong, J.A.; Ntemgwa, M.; Atabe, A.N. The threat of antimicrobial resistance in developing countries: Causes and control strategies. *Antimicrob. Resist. Infect. Control* **2017**, *6*, 47. [CrossRef]
3. Terreni, M.; Taccani, M.; Pregnolato, M. New Antibiotics for Multidrug-Resistant Bacterial Strains: Latest Research Developments and Future Perspectives. *Molecules* **2021**, *26*, 2671. [CrossRef] [PubMed]
4. Goswami, A.G.; Basu, S.; Banerjee, T.; Shukla, V.K. Biofilm and wound healing: From bench to bedside. *Eur. J. Med. Res.* **2023**, *28*, 157. [CrossRef] [PubMed]
5. Villalpando-Rodriguez, G.E.; Gibson, S.B. Reactive Oxygen Species (ROS) Regulates Different Types of Cell Death by Acting as a Rheostat. *Oxid. Med. Cell. Longev.* **2021**, *2021*, 9912436. [CrossRef]
6. Liu, H.; Wang, C.; Li, C.; Qin, Y.; Wang, Z.; Yang, F.; Li, Z.; Wang, J. A functional chitosan-based hydrogel as a wound dressing and drug delivery system in the treatment of wound healing. *RSC Adv.* **2018**, *8*, 7533–7549. [CrossRef]

7. Hajji, S.; Khedir, S.B.; Hamza-Mnif, I.; Hamdi, M.; Jedidi, I.; Kallel, R.; Nasri, M. Biomedical potential of chitosan-silver nanoparticles with special reference to antioxidant, antibacterial, hemolytic and in vivo cutaneous wound healing effects. *Biochim. Biophys. Acta Gen. Subj.* **2019**, *1863*, 241–254. [CrossRef]
8. Kharaghani, D.; Khan, M.Q.; Tamada, Y.; Ogasawara, H.; Inoue, Y.; Saito, Y.; Kim, I.S. Fabrication of electrospun antibacterial PVA/Cs nanofibers loaded with CuNPs and AgNPs by an *in-situ* method. *Polym. Test.* **2018**, *72*, 315–321. [CrossRef]
9. Ahmed, R.; Tariq, M.; Ali, I.; Asghar, R.; Khanam, P.N.; Augustine, R.; Hasan, A. Novel electrospun chitosan/polyvinyl alcohol/zinc oxide nanofibrous mats with antibacterial and antioxidant properties for diabetic wound healing. *Int. J. Biol. Macromol.* **2018**, *20*, 385–393. [CrossRef]
10. Ran, L.; Zou, Y.; Cheng, J.; Lu, F. Silver nanoparticles in situ synthesized by polysaccharides from *Sanghuangporussanghuang* and composites with chitosan to prepare scaffolds for the regeneration of infected full-thickness skin defects. *Int. J. Biol. Macromol.* **2019**, *125*, 392–403. [CrossRef]
11. Wichai, S.; Chuysinuan, P.; Chaiarwut, S.; Ekabutr, P.; Supaphol, P. Development of bacterial cellulose/alginate/chitosan composites incorporating copper (II) sulfate as an antibacterial wound dressing. *Int. J. Drug Deliv. Technol.* **2019**, *51*, 662–671. [CrossRef]
12. Shah, A.; Yameen, M.A.; Fatima, N.; Murtaza, G. Chemical synthesis of chitosan/silver nanocomposites films loaded with moxifloxacin: Their characterization and potential antibacterial activity. *Int. J. Pharm.* **2019**, *561*, 19–34. [CrossRef] [PubMed]
13. Ye, H.; Cheng, J.; Yu, K. In situ reduction of silver nanoparticles by gelatin to obtain porous silver nanoparticle/chitosan composites with enhanced antimicrobial and wound-healing activity. *Int. J. Biol. Macromol.* **2019**, *121*, 633–642. [CrossRef] [PubMed]
14. Patrulea, V.; Ostafe, V.; Borchard, G.; Jordan, O. Chitosan as a starting material for wound healing applications. *Eur. J. Pharm. Biopharm.* **2015**, *97*, 417–426. [CrossRef]
15. Shehabeldine, A.M.; Salem, S.S.; Ali, O.M.; Abd-Elsalam, K.A.; Elkady, F.M.; Hashem, A.H. Multifunctional silver nanoparticles based on chitosan: Antibacterial, antibiofilm, antifungal, antioxidant, and wound-healing activities. *J. Fungi.* **2022**, *8*, 612. [CrossRef]
16. Sharifi-Rad, J.; Quispe, C.; Butnariu, M.; Rotariu, L.S.; Sytar, O.; Sestito, S.; Rapposelli, S.; Akram, M.; Iqbal, M.; Krishna, A.; et al. Chitosan nanoparticles as a promising tool in nanomedicine with particular emphasis on oncological treatment. *Cancer Cell Int.* **2021**, *21*, 1–21. [CrossRef]
17. Yadav, M.; Kaushik, B.; Rao, G.K.; Srivastava, C.M.; Vaya, D. Advances and challenges in the use of chitosan and its derivatives in biomedical fields: A Review. *Carbohydr. Polym.* **2023**, *26*, 100323. [CrossRef]
18. Gagliardi, A.; Giuliano, E.; Venkateswararao, E.; Fresta, M.; Bulotta, S.; Awasthi, V.; Cosco, D. Biodegradable polymeric nanoparticles for drug delivery to solid tumors. *Front. Pharmacol.* **2021**, *12*, 601–626. [CrossRef]
19. Bravo-Osuna, I.; Vauthier, C.; Farabollini, A.; Palmieri, G.; Ponchel, G. Mucoadhesion mechanism of chitosan and thiolated chitosan-poly (isobutyl cyanoacrylate) core-shell nanoparticles. *Biomater. Res.* **2007**, *28*, 2233–2243. [CrossRef]
20. Ali, A.; Ahmed, S.A. Review on chitosan and its nanocomposites in drug delivery. *Int. J. Biol. Macromol.* **2018**, *109*, 273–286. [CrossRef]
21. Shah, M.; Fawcett, D.; Sharma, S.; Tripathy, S.K.; Poinern, G.E.J. Green synthesis of metallic nanoparticles via biological entities. *J. Mater.* **2015**, *8*, 7278–7308. [CrossRef]
22. Mirda, E.; Idroes, R.; Khairan, K.; Tallei, T.E.; Ramli, M.; Earlia, N.; Maulana, A.; Idroes, G.M.; Muslem, M.; Jalil, Z. Synthesis of chitosan-silver nanoparticle composite spheres and their antimicrobial activities. *Polymers* **2021**, *13*, 3990. [CrossRef] [PubMed]
23. Sartori, P.; Delamare, A.P.; Machado, G.; Devine, D.M.; Crespo, J.S.; Giovanela, M. Synthesis and characterization of silver nanoparticles for the preparation of chitosan pellets and their application in industrial wastewater disinfection. *Water* **2023**, *15*, 190. [CrossRef]
24. Vanti, G.L.; Masaphy, S.; Kurjogi, M.; Chakrasali, S.; Nargunda, V.B. Synthesis and application of chitosan-copper nanoparticle on dampping off causing plant pathogenic Fungi. *Int. J. Biol. Macromol.* **2020**, *156*, 1387–1395. [CrossRef]
25. Badawy, M.E.I.; Lotfy, T.M.R.; Shawir, S.M.S. Preparation and antibacterial activity of chitosan-silver nanoparticles for application in preservation of minced meat. *Bull Natl. Res. Cent.* **2019**, *43*, 83. [CrossRef]
26. Singha, D.; Sahu, D.; Sahu, K. Coupling of molecular transition with the surface plasmon resonance of silver nanoparticles inside the restricted environment of reverse micelles. *ACS Omega.* **2017**, *2*, 5494–5503. [CrossRef] [PubMed]
27. Sanpui, P.; Murugadoss, A.; Prasad, P.D.; Ghosh, S.S.; Chattopadhyay, A. The antibacterial properties of a novel chitosan-ag nanoparticle composite. *Int. J. Food. Microbiol.* **2008**, *124*, 142–146. [CrossRef]
28. Govindan, S.; Nivethaa, E.A.; Saravanan, R.; Narayanan, V.; Stephen, A. Synthesis and of chitosan-silver nanocomposite. *Appl. Nanosci.* **2012**, *2*, 299–303. [CrossRef]
29. Vanlalveni, C.; Lallianrawna, S.; Biswas, A.; Selvaraj, M.; Changmai, B.; Rokhum, S.L. Green synthesis of silver nanoparticles using plant extracts and their antimicrobial activities: A review of recent literature. *RSC Adv.* **2021**, *11*, 2804–2837. [CrossRef]
30. Giri, A.K.; Jena, B.; Biswal, B.; Pradhan, A.K.; Arakha, M.; Acharya, S.; Acharya, L. Green synthesis and characterization of silver nanoparticles using Eugenia roxburghii DC. extract and activity against biofilm-producing bacteria. *Sci. Rep.* **2022**, *12*, 8383. [CrossRef]

31. Shah, M.Z.; Guan, Z.H.; Din, A.U.; Ali, A.; Rehman, A.U.; Jan, K.; Faisal, S.; Saud, S.; Adnan, M.; Wahid, F.; et al. Synthesis of silver nanoparticles using Plantago lanceolata extract and assessing their antibacterial and antioxidant activities. *Sci. Rep.* **2021**, *11*, 20754. [CrossRef] [PubMed]
32. Meena, P.R.; Singh, A.P.; Tejavath, K.K. Biosynthesis of silver nanoparticles using Cucumis prophetarum aqueous leaf extract and their antibacterial and antiproliferative activity against cancer cell lines. *ACS Omega.* **2020**, *5*, 5520.
33. Nandiyanto, A.B.D.; Oktiani, R.; Ragadhita, R. How to Read and Interpret FTIR Spectroscope of Organic Material. *Indones. J. Sci. Technol.* **2019**, *4*, 97–118. [CrossRef]
34. Ji, Y.; Yang, X.; Ji, Z.; Zhu, L.; Ma, N.; Chen, D.; Jia, X.; Tang, J.; Cao, Y. DFT-calculated IR spectrum amide I, II, and III band contributions of N-methylacetamide fine components. *ACS Omega.* **2020**, *5*, 8572–8578. [CrossRef] [PubMed]
35. Shinde, S.; Folliero, V.; Chianese, A.; Zannella, C.; De Filippis, A.; Rosati, L.; Prisco, M.; Falanga, A.; Mali, A.; Galdiero, M.; et al. Synthesis of chitosan-coated silver nanoparticle bioconjugates and their antimicrobial activity against multidrug-resistant bacteria. *Appl. Sci.* **2021**, *11*, 9340. [CrossRef]
36. Jogaiah, S.; Kurjogi, M.; Abdelrahman, M.; Hanumanthappa, N.; Tran, L.S. *Ganoderma applanatum*- mediated green synthesis of silver nanoparticles: Structural characterisation, and in vitro and in vivo biomedical and agrochemical properties. *Arab. J. Chem.* **2019**, *12*, 1108–1120. [CrossRef]
37. Li, R.; Xu, Z.; Jiang, Q.; Heng, Y.; Chen, Z.; Chen, X. Characterization and biological evaluation of a novel silver nanoparticle-loaded collagen-chitosan dressing. *Regen. Biomat.* **2020**, *7*, 371–380. [CrossRef]
38. Xue, Y.; Zhang, T.; Zhang, B.; Gong, F.; Huang, Y.; Tang, M. Cytotoxicity and apoptosis induced by silver nanoparticles in human liver HepG2 cells in different dispersion media. *J. Appl. Toxicol.* **2016**, *36*, 352–360. [CrossRef]
39. Freire, P.L.; Albuquerque, A.J.; Farias, I.A.; da Silva, T.G.; Aguiar, J.S.; Galembeck, A.; Flores, M.A.; Sampaio, F.C.; Stamford, T.C.M.; Rosenblatt, A. Antimicrobial and cytotoxicity evaluation of colloidal chitosan–silver nanoparticles–fluoride nanocomposites. *Int. J. Biol. Macromol.* **2016**, *93*, 896–903. [CrossRef]
40. Wahab, S.; Ali, H.M.; Khan, M.; Khan, T.; Krishnaraj, C.; Yun, S.I. Green synthesis and antibacterial assessment of chitosan/silver nanocomposite conjugated with tobramycin against antibiotic resistant Pseudomonas aeruginosa. *Arab. J. Ch.* **2024**, *17*, 105458. [CrossRef]
41. Potara, M.; Jakab, E.; Damert, A.; Popescu, O.; Canpean, V.; Astilean, S. Synergistic antibacterial activity of chitosan–silver nanocomposites on *Staphylococcus aureus*. *Nanotechnology* **2011**, *22*, 135101. [CrossRef] [PubMed]
42. Matica, M.A.; Aachmann, F.L.; Tondervik, A.; Sletta, H.; Ostafe, V. Chitosan as a wound dressing starting material: Antimicrobial properties and mode of action. *Inter. J. Mol. Sci.* **2019**, *20*, 5889. [CrossRef] [PubMed]
43. Shivakumar, P.; Gupta, M.S.; Jayakumar, R.; Gowda, D.V. Prospection of chitosan and its derivatives in wound healing: Proof of patent analysis (2010–2020). *Int. J. Biol. Macromol.* **2021**, *184*, 701–712. [CrossRef] [PubMed]
44. Ueno, H.; Mori, T.; Fujinaga, T. Topical formulations and wound healing applications of chitosan. *Adv. Drug Deliv. Rev.* **2001**, *52*, 105–115. [CrossRef]
45. Liu, Y.; Liu, H.; Wang, L.; Wang, Y.; Zhang, C.; Wang, C.; Yan, Y.; Fan, J.; Xu, G.; Zhang, Q. Amplification of oxidative stress via intracellular ROS production and antioxidant consumption by two natural drug-encapsulated nanoagents for efficient anticancer therapy. *Nanoscale Adv.* **2020**, *2*, 3872–3881. [CrossRef]
46. Formentini, L.; Santacatterina, F.; de Arenas, C.N.; Stamatakis, K.; López-Martínez, D.; Logan, A.; Fresno, M.; Smits, R.; Murphy, M.P.; Cuezva, J.M. Mitochondrial ROS production protects the intestine from inflammation through functional M2 macrophage polarization. *Cell Rep.* **2017**, *19*, 1202–1213. [CrossRef]
47. Lin, W.; Qi, X.; Guo, W. A barrier against reactive oxygen species: Chitosan/acellular dermal matrix scaffold enhances stem cell retention and improves cutaneous wound healing. *Stem Cell Res. Ther.* **2020**, *11*, 383. [CrossRef]
48. Tamer, T.; Aacute, K.; Mohyeldin, M.; Soltes, L. Free radical scavenger activity of chitosan and its aminated derivative. *J. Appl. Pharm. Sci.* **2016**, *6*, 195–201. [CrossRef]
49. Muzzarelli, R.A. Biochemical significance of exogenous chitins, chitosan in animals, patients. *Carbohydr. Polym.* **2019**, *93*, 7–16. [CrossRef]
50. Hattori, H.; Ishihara, M. Changes in blood aggregation with differences in molecular weight and degree of deacetylation of chitosan. *Biomed. Mater.* **2015**, *10*, 015014. [CrossRef]
51. Palomino, J.C.; Martin, A.; Camacho, M.; Guerra, H.; Swings, J.; Portaels, F. Resazurin microtiter assay plate: Simple and inexpensive method for detection of drug resistance in Mycobacterium tuberculosis. *Antimicrob. Agents Chemother.* **2002**, *46*, 2720–2722. [CrossRef] [PubMed]
52. Liang, C.C.; Park, A.Y.; Guan, J.L. In vitro scratch assay: A convenient and inexpensive method for analysis of cell migration in vitro. *Nat. Protoc.* **2007**, *2*, 329–333. [CrossRef] [PubMed]
53. Vanti, G.L.; Kurjogi, M.; Basavesha, K.; Teradal, N.L.; Masaphy, S.; Nargund, V.B. Synthesis and antibacterial activity of solanum torvum mediated silver nanoparticle against Xxanthomonasaxonopodis *pv. Punicae* and *Ralstonia solanacearum*. *J. Biotech.* **2020**, *309*, 20–28. [CrossRef] [PubMed]

pharmaceuticals

MDPI

Article

Therapeutic Efficacy of *Helianthemum lippii* Extract and Silver Nanoparticles Synthesized from the Extract against Cadmium-Induced Renal Nephrotoxicity in Wistar Rats

Ibtissam Laib [1,2,3], Boutlilis Djahra Ali [1,2], Ali Alsalme [4], David Cornu [5], Mikhael Bechelany [5,6] and Ahmed Barhoum [7,*]

1 Department of Cellular and Molecular Biology, Faculty of Natural and Life Sciences, El Oued University, El Oued 39000, Algeria; laib-ibtissam@univ-eloued.dz (I.L.); djahra@yahoo.fr (B.D.A.)

2 Laboratory of Biology, Environment and Health, Faculty of Natural and Life Sciences, El Oued University, El-Oued 39000, Algeria

3 Higher School of Saharan Agriculture, El Oued 39000, Algeria

4 Department of Chemistry, College of Science, King Saud University, Riyadh 11451, Saudi Arabia; aalsalme@ksu.edu.sa

5 Institut Européen des Membranes (IEM), UMR 5635, University of Montpellier, ENSCM, CNRS, 34095 Montpellier, France; david.cornu@umontpellier.fr (D.C.); mikhael.bechelany@umontpellier.fr (M.B.)

6 Functional Materials Group, Gulf University for Science and Technology (GUST), Mubarak Al-Abdullah 32093, Kuwait

7 NanoStruc Research Group, Chemistry Department, Faculty of Science, Helwan University, Cairo 11795, Egypt

* Correspondence: ahmed.barhoum@science.helwan.edu.eg

Abstract: This study explored the therapeutic efficacy of *Helianthemum lippii* and silver nanoparticles (Ag NPs) synthesized using a *H. lippii* extract to alleviate cadmium-induced nephrotoxicity in Wistar rats. Sub-acute toxicity assessments of *H. lippii* (100 mg/kg, 1000 mg/kg, and 4000 mg/kg) and Ag NPs (2 mg/kg and 10 mg/kg) did not find any significant difference, compared with untreated control rats (n = 3 animals/group). Then, the adult Wistar rats were divided into one control (untreated/unexposed) and six experimental groups (n = 5/group): Ag NPs alone, *H. lippii* alone, exposure to 50 mg/kg $CdCl_2$ in drinking water for 35 days, exposure to $CdCl_2$ for 35 days followed by treatment with 0.1 mg/kg/day Ag NPs (intraperitoneal injection) and/or 100 mg/kg/day *H. lippii* by gavage for 15 days. In the $CdCl_2$-exposed group, body weight decreased; urea, creatinine, and uric acid concentrations increased ($p < 0.05$ vs. control), indicative of nephrotoxicity, antioxidant defenses (SOD, GSH, and CAT) were reduced, and malondialdehyde concentration increased. Moreover, the kidney's architecture in $CdCl_2$-exposed rats was altered: fibrosis, inflammatory cell infiltration, glomerular destruction, and tubular dilatation. Treatment with *H. lippii* and/or Ag NPs after $CdCl_2$ exposure improved some of the renal function and architecture alterations induced by $CdCl_2$, and also increased body weight. This study underscores the potential therapeutic applications of *H. lippii* and Ag NPs to decrease oxidative stress and promote xenobiotic detoxification, in line with the growing emphasis on environmentally conscious practices in scientific research and healthcare.

Keywords: *Helianthemum lippii*; silver nanoparticles; cadmium toxicity; nephrotoxicity; biochemical parameters; oxidative stress; histopathology; Wistar rats; intraperitoneal injection; gavage

1. Introduction

Heavy metal contamination in food and feedstuffs poses significant risks to human and animal health, making it a global issue [1]. Cadmium (Cd), a naturally occurring heavy metal with high bioaccumulation potential, is released into the environment, particularly in industrialized areas. Cd is lethal even at extremely low doses. Chronic exposure to low Cd concentrations causes adverse health effects in pediatric and adult populations, including reduced glomerular filtration rate and fecundity [2,3]. The tolerable Cd intake is 0.83 μg/kg body weight/day, and a urinary Cd excretion rate of 5.24 μg/g creatinine is considered the threshold level for toxicity [2]. However, recent studies suggest that these levels may not provide sufficient health protection because adverse health effects are observed at lower Cd accumulation levels. Cadmium chloride ($CdCl_2$) targets various organs, including the bones, lungs, skeletal muscles, heart, and kidneys [4]. Cd toxicity is due to its promotion of reactive oxygen species (ROS) production by reducing the levels of antioxidant enzymes, such as catalase, superoxide dismutase (SOD), and glutathione (GSH) [5]. Chronic Cd exposure often leads to renal damage, resulting in kidney disease. Various pathways contribute to organ damage induced by cadmium exposure, including cell apoptosis, autophagy [6], necrosis, cell–cell junction disruption [7], and cell-signaling pathway disorganization. Cd impact on membrane-dependent functions is often attributed to the induction of lipid peroxidation, which affects many enzymatic activities, possibly through the displacement of beneficial metals from active sites or direct binding to the enzyme-active sites [8]. In kidney tissue, Cd accumulates prominently in the proximal convoluted tubules, leading to glycosuria, proteinuria, and aminoaciduria [9,10].

In recent years, interest has been increasing in alternative and safer therapeutic methods to address Cd-induced renal damage due to the considerable health risks associated with heavy metal toxicity [11]. Previous studies highlighted the susceptibility of vital organs, such as the liver and kidneys, to Cd toxicity [12]. Conventional strategies have explored the use of metals (e.g., zinc, copper, and selenium) as antagonists or antioxidants to mitigate Cd toxicity; however, they must be administered at high doses, and this can pose serious risks [13], such as gastrointestinal disturbances, neurotoxicity, and imbalances in essential minerals within the body. Moreover, the efficacy of these treatments can be inconsistent, sometimes offering only partial protection against Cd-induced damage, which leaves patients at ongoing risk of health complications. Consequently, attention has shifted to plant-based remedies, and many studies have investigated the potential of plant extracts to provide safe and effective protection against Cd-induced nephrotoxicity [14]. The strong antioxidant and protective activities of plant extracts in tissues and membrane lipids are mediated through free radical scavenging in a dose-dependent manner. Therefore, plant extracts have been tested in various experimental models as protective agents against various toxicants [15]. Due to their antioxidant properties and minimal side effects, plant (e.g., green tea, curcumin, and black cumin) extracts have emerged as promising alternatives for managing Cd-induced kidney damage [16–18]. This shift towards plant-based compounds underscores the importance of exploring nature-derived solutions to mitigate the adverse effects of heavy metal exposure on human health.

Simultaneously, nanoparticle-based therapies present innovative solutions for the targeted and effective treatment of heavy-metal-induced nephrotoxicity. Nanoparticles (NPs) can be engineered to deliver therapeutic agents directly to the kidneys, thereby enhancing treatment efficacy while minimizing systemic side effects [19]. Among NPs, silver nanoparticles (Ag NPs) have gained prominence due to their unique physicochemical properties, including a high surface area-to-volume ratio, excellent conductivity, and anti-inflammatory activity, making them versatile for various applications, including heavy metal detoxification [20,21]. Ag NPs synthesized using plant extracts exhibit promising capabilities for targeted antioxidant and anti-inflammatory effects. They also demonstrate a strong affinity for heavy metals like cadmium, effectively binding and sequestering cadmium ions [22]. This dual action of sequestration and antioxidant activity helps mitigate oxidative stress and inflammation in the affected tissues. Furthermore, NPs can enhance the bioavailability of phytochemicals, ensuring higher concentrations reach the affected tissues to exert protective effects, underscoring their potential as therapeutic agents in heavy metal detoxification efforts.

Helianthemum lippii is recognized for its abundance of phytochemicals [23,24]. It presents numerous therapeutic advantages and serves as a promising candidate for nanoparticle (NP) synthesis [21]. Its phytochemical constituents, such as flavonoids, phenolic acids, tannins, and alkaloids [25], are renowned for their robust antioxidant, anti-inflammatory, anti-ulcer, analgesic, anticancer, anti-biofilm, and antimicrobial properties [26]. These compounds are crucial in mitigating oxidative stress, scavenging free radicals, and modulating signaling pathways implicated in various diseases, particularly in heavy-metal-induced nephrotoxicity. Moreover, *H. lippii* phytochemicals are adept in the synthesis of zinc NPs [27] and silver (Ag) NPs [21], where they serve as effective reducing and stabilizing agents in green synthesis processes, ensuring biocompatibility and therapeutic efficacy. Leveraging *H. lippii* phytochemicals for NP synthesis holds immense promise for therapeutic applications, such as targeted delivery, enhanced bioavailability, and reduced cytotoxicity. The synergistic interactions among these phytochemicals further amplify their therapeutic effects, establishing *H. lippii*-based NPs as a compelling option for addressing a range of ailments, including heavy-metal-induced nephrotoxicity.

Several notable studies have demonstrated the efficacy of phytochemicals and NPs for therapeutic applications, affirming the viability of this approach. Recent research on green-synthesized Ag NPs using plant extracts from *Azadirachta indica* and *Moringa oleifera* has shown significant antioxidant and antimicrobial activities, showcasing the potential of phytochemical-mediated NP synthesis [28]. Moreover, investigations into plant-based NPs derived from *Camellia sinensis* (green tea) and aloe vera have revealed promising results in managing oxidative stress and inflammation across various disease models [29,30]. These findings, coupled with the current study, underscore the potential of H. lipid-based NPs in providing effective and environmentally conscious solutions for managing heavy-metal-induced nephrotoxicity. This study explored the therapeutic potential of *H. lippii* and Ag NPs, synthesized using a *H. lippii* extract, for alleviating Cd-induced nephrotoxicity in Wistar rats. Initial sub-acute toxicity assessments of various doses of *H. lippii* and Ag NPs indicated their safety, compared to untreated controls. The adult Wistar rats were then divided into seven groups, including untreated control and experimental groups treated with *H. lippii* or Ag NPs alone, exposed to $CdCl_2$, or exposed to $CdCl_2$ followed by treatment with *H. lippii* and/or Ag NPs. Monitoring of body weight, renal function markers, and oxidative stress indicators provided insights into the nephrotoxic effects of $CdCl_2$ exposure and the potential protective effects of *H. lippii* and Ag NPs. A histological examination revealed $CdCl_2$-induced alterations in the kidney architecture, which were mitigated by treatment with *H. lippii* and Ag NPs, highlighting their promising therapeutic applications in managing oxidative stress and xenobiotic detoxification, and emphasizing environmentally conscious practices in scientific research and healthcare.

2. Results and Discussion

2.1. Phytochemical Screening

Table 1 summarizes the results of the phytochemical analysis of the *H. lippii* aqueous extract. The extract contained polyphenols, catechin and gallic tannins, flavonoids, saponins, anthocyanins, leucoanthocyanins, cardiac glycosides, steroids, terpenoids, and mucilages. Alkaloids were absent when tested with a Mayer reagent, but present according to a Wagner test. These findings highlight the rich diversity of phytochemicals present in the *H. lippii* aqueous extract, suggesting its potential therapeutic value. They also underscore the plant's importance in traditional medicine and its potential applications in pharmaceutical and nutraceutical industries. More studies are needed to explore the specific health benefits and pharmacological activities associated with these different phytochemicals.

2.2. HPLC-Based Quantitative Analysis

An HPLC analysis of the *H. lippii* aqueous extract (Figure 1 and Table 2) allowed for the identification of only six phenolic compounds, despite the presence of many peaks. Gallic acid was the most abundant, followed by chlorogenic acid, quercetin, naringin, p-coumaric acid, and caffeic acid. These findings provide valuable insights into the chemical composition of the *H. lippii* extract and its potential therapeutic applications. The significant presence of gallic acid, chlorogenic acid, and quercetin suggests their potential contribution to the medicinal properties attributed to *H. lippii*. Previous studies highlighted the antioxidant and anticancer properties of gallic acid and catechin [30]. Caffeic acid exhibits antioxidant and iron-chelating activities and reduces acute immune and inflammatory responses [31]. Naringin and quercetin, present at moderate levels in the extract, are potent antioxidants with promising activity against oxidative damage [32]. The existence of these secondary metabolites in the *H. lippii* extract aligns with its traditional use as a remedy for various diseases, providing scientific evidence to support its pharmacological potential. The identification and quantification of these phenolic compounds enrich our understanding of *H. lippii* therapeutic properties and pave the way for future research for medicinal applications. Future studies may elucidate the specific mechanisms of action and the therapeutic efficacy of the *H. lippii* extract's components. However, in the HPLC chromatogram (Figure 1), notable peaks were observed at 10–12 min. These peaks were not identified in the present study but suggest the presence of other significant phytochemicals in the *H. lippii* extract. Future research will identify these compounds using more advanced analytical techniques and additional standards.

Table 1. Results of the phytochemical screening of the *H. lippii* aqueous extract.

Phytochemical Compounds		*H. lippii* (Aqueous Extract)
Polyphenols		(+)
Alkaloids	Mayer	(−)
	Wagner	(+)
Tannins	Catechin	(+)
	Gallic	(+)
Flavonoids		(+)
Saponins		(+)
Anthocyanins		(+)
Leucoanthocyanins		(+)
Cardiac glycosides		(+)
Steroids and terpenoids		(+)
Mucilages		(+)

(−) Absence. (+) Presence.

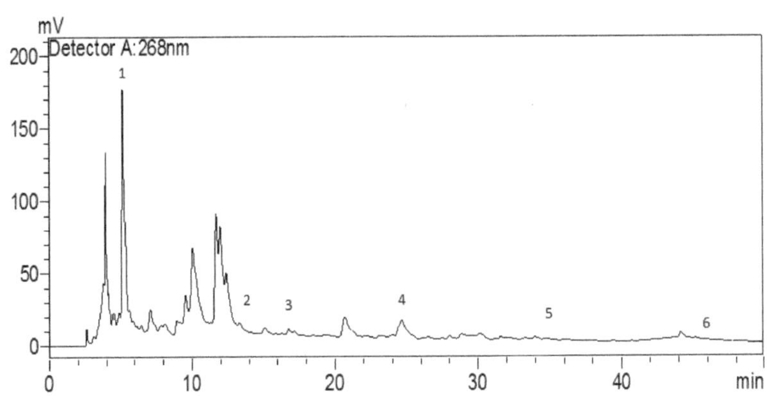

Figure 1. HPLC chromatogram of the *H. lippii* aqueous extract: 1: gallic acid; 2 chlorogenic acid; 3: caffeic acid; 4: p-Coumaric acid; 5: naringin; 6: quercetin.

Table 2. Retention time and concentration of phenolic compounds identified in *H. lippii* aqueous extract.

Phenolic Compound	Retention Time (Min)	Equation	Concentration (μg/g Extract)
Caffeic acid	16.27	y = 42,239x	444.81
p-Coumaric acid	23.81	y = 27,977	663.77
Gallic acid	5.29	y = 54,681x	9495.11
Vanillic acid	15.53	y = 20,674	ND
Chlorogenic acid	13.39	y = 21,665x	7107.24
Naringin	34.78	y = 19,379x	738.19
Rutin	28.37	y = 1649x	ND
Quercetin	45.04	y = 2,142,281x	1118.64
Vanillin	21.46	y = 9286x	ND

y: HPLC peak area. x: concentration (μg/mL), ND: not detected.

2.3. Characteristics of the Ag NPs Fabricated Using the H. lippii Extract

The XRD pattern of the synthesized Ag NPs included distinct diffraction peaks at 38.2°, 44.4°, 64.7°, and 77.5°, corresponding to the (111), (200), (220), and (311) crystallographic planes of the face-centered cubic unit cell, respectively. These peaks were in excellent agreement with the characteristic peaks of metallic silver (JCPDS Card No. 04-0783) [33]. The well-defined features of these peaks indicated the remarkable crystallinity of the Ag NPs. The Scherrer equation and the peak full width at half maximum yielded a crystallite size of 12.84 nm, confirming the nano-scale dimensions and effectiveness of the green synthesis process (Figure 2a). Similar observations were previously reported by other researchers who studied various plant-based synthesis methods. Figure 2c displays particle size ranges from 10 to 90 nm, with an average particle size distribution of 35 nm, highlighting their uniformity and stability (Figure 2b,c). Meanwhile, an SEM analysis revealed the Ag NPs spherical morphology. The Ag NPs elemental composition was confirmed by the SEM-energy-dispersive X-ray spectroscopy analysis that displayed a prominent signal in the silver region and additional peaks corresponding to carbon and oxygen. These additional peaks suggest the presence of residual components from the synthesis process or potential stabilizing agents. These findings are in agreement with the results reported by (Barhoum et al., 2015 [33]; Ghasemi et al., 2024 [34]; Khanal et al., 2022 [35]; Asefian et al., 2024 [36]).

2.4. Sub-Acute Toxicity Study

The sub-acute toxicity test data of the *H. lippii* aqueous extract and Ag NPs in Wistar albino rats indicate no significant adverse effects across all parameters and doses tested. The rats, observed at various intervals (3 h, 24 h, 7 days, and 14 days) after administration, showed no abnormalities in body weight changes, movement, or eye condition and none experienced diarrhea or death (Table 3). Both the control groups and the low-, medium-, and high-dose groups of the *H. lippii* extract (100 mg/kg, 1000 mg/kg, and 4000 mg/kg) and Ag NPs (2 mg/kg and 10 mg/kg) maintained normal conditions throughout the study, suggesting that neither *H. lippii* extract nor Ag NPs exhibit sub-acute toxicity at these doses. This lack of toxicity, even at relatively high doses, is a promising indicator for their potential use as therapeutic agents. Given the observed safety profile, *H. lippii* aqueous extract and Ag NPs have the potential to be developed as therapeutic drugs, specifically for combating Cd-induced renal nephrotoxicity. Cd-induced nephrotoxicity is a serious health concern, and the development of effective treatments with minimal side effects is crucial. The normal health parameters observed in the rats suggest that these compounds could be administered safely without causing harm, a critical consideration in drug development. Further studies, including comprehensive analyses of kidney function parameters, oxidative stress markers, histopathological features, body weight changes, and renal weight changes after exposure to $CdCl_2$ and treatment with *H. lippii* extract and Ag NPs, were conducted and are discussed in the next sections to evaluate the therapeutic efficacy of *H. lippii* extract and Ag NPs in mitigating renal damage caused by cadmium.

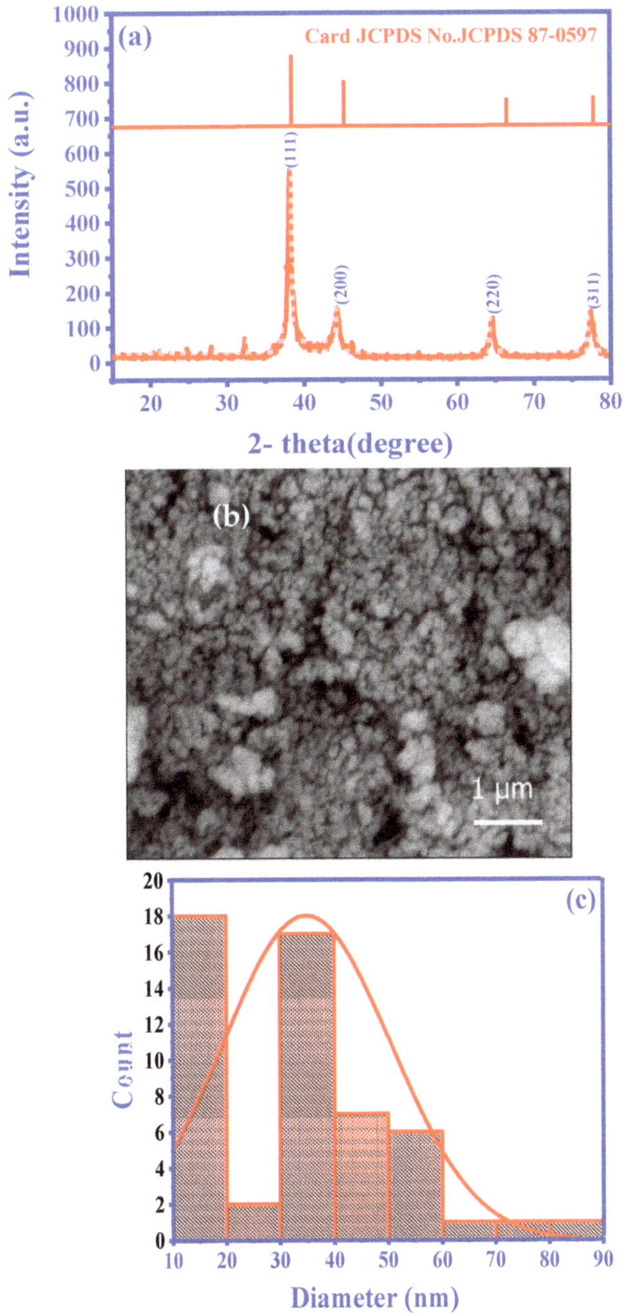

Figure 2. Characteristics of synthesized Ag NPs: (**a**) crystalline structure (XRD data), (**b**) morphology (SEM image), and (**c**) size distribution analysis.

Table 3. The sub-acute toxicity test of the dose of *H. lippii* aqueous extract and of the Ag NPs in Wistar albino rats. The dose was given in the time zero without exposing the Wistar rats to $CdCl_2$, and the observation was made at different time intervales at 3 h, 24 h, 7 days, and 14 days.

Parameters	Dose of *H.lippii*				Dose of Ag NPs		
	Control Group (0 mg/kg)	Low Dose Group (100 mg/kg)	Medium Dose Group (1000 mg/kg)	High Dose Group (4000 mg/kg)	Control Group (0 mg/kg	Low Dose Group (2 mg/kg)	Medium Dose Group (10 mg/kg)
Body weight changes	N	N	N	N	N	N	N
Death	0	0	0	0	0	0	0
Movement	N	N	N	N	N	N	N
Diarrhea	N	N	N	N	N	N	N
Eyes	N	N	N	N	N	N	N

N: Normal.

2.5. *H. lippii and Ag NP Effect on Cadmium-Induced Nephrotoxicity*

Then, the effects of the *H. lippii* extract and Ag NPs on Cd-induced kidney toxicity were investigated in the adult Wistar albino rats (n = 5 animals/group) exposed or not to $CdCl_2$ (50 mg/kg body weight/day) in drinking water for 35 days. Then, the rats that were treated or not treated with the Ag NPs (0.1 mg/kg, body weight/day by intraperitoneal injection) and/or *H. lippii* extract (100 mg/kg, body weight/day by gavage) were investigated for 15 days. Some mice received only the Ag NPs (0.1 mg/kg, body weight/day by intraperitoneal injection) or the *H. lippii* extract (100 mg/kg, body weight/day by gavage) for 35 days.

Body Weight and Relative Kidney Weight

An analysis of the body weight changes and relative kidney weight at the end of the study revealed important insights into the impact of $CdCl_2$ exposure and the potential protective effects of *H. lippii* and Ag NPs. In the control group (Group 1; baseline body weight = 282 $\pm$ 14.7 g), body weight increased by 0.072 $\pm$ 0.02 g/day (Figure 3a,b). Conversely, upon exposure to $CdCl_2$ (Group 2; (baseline body weight = 244.8 $\pm$ 2.69 g), body weight decreased by $-$0.181 $\pm$ 0.06 g/day. According to (Poli et al., 2022) [37], this may be explained by increased lipid degeneration caused by Cd toxicity [38], resulting in a significant decrease in food uptake, food avoidance, or post-food palatability due to Cd toxicity. Moreover, the activation of oxidative stress results in changes in antioxidant status and leads to severe metabolic abnormalities and weight loss [39]. Conversely, exposure to *H. lippii* alone (Group 3; baseline body weight = 244.8 $\pm$ 2.69 g) or Ag NPs alone (Group 5; baseline body weight = 231.8 $\pm$ 15.7 g) did not affect the normal pattern of body weight gain, as indicated by their weight increase by 0.119 $\pm$ 0.09 g/day and 0.042 $\pm$ 0.01 g/day, respectively, further confirming their relative safety. The administration of *H. lippii* or Ag NPs after $CdCl_2$ exposure (Group 4 and Group 6 with baseline body weight = 247.2 $\pm$ 1.1 g and 247.2 $\pm$ 1.1 g, respectively) limited body weight loss ($-$0.05 $\pm$ 0.2 g/day and 0.07 $\pm$ 0.009 g/day, respectively). Moreover, in Group 7 (exposure to $CdCl_2$ followed by administration of both *H. lippii* and Ag NPs; baseline body weight = 234.0 $\pm$ 13.0 g), the body weight increase was comparable to that in the control group (0.072 $\pm$ 0.02 g/day). This suggests a potential protective role of the *H. lippii* extract and Ag NPs against Cd-induced metabolic abnormalities and oxidative stress. These findings underscore the therapeutic potential of *H. lippii* and Ag NPs in mitigating Cd-induced toxicity.

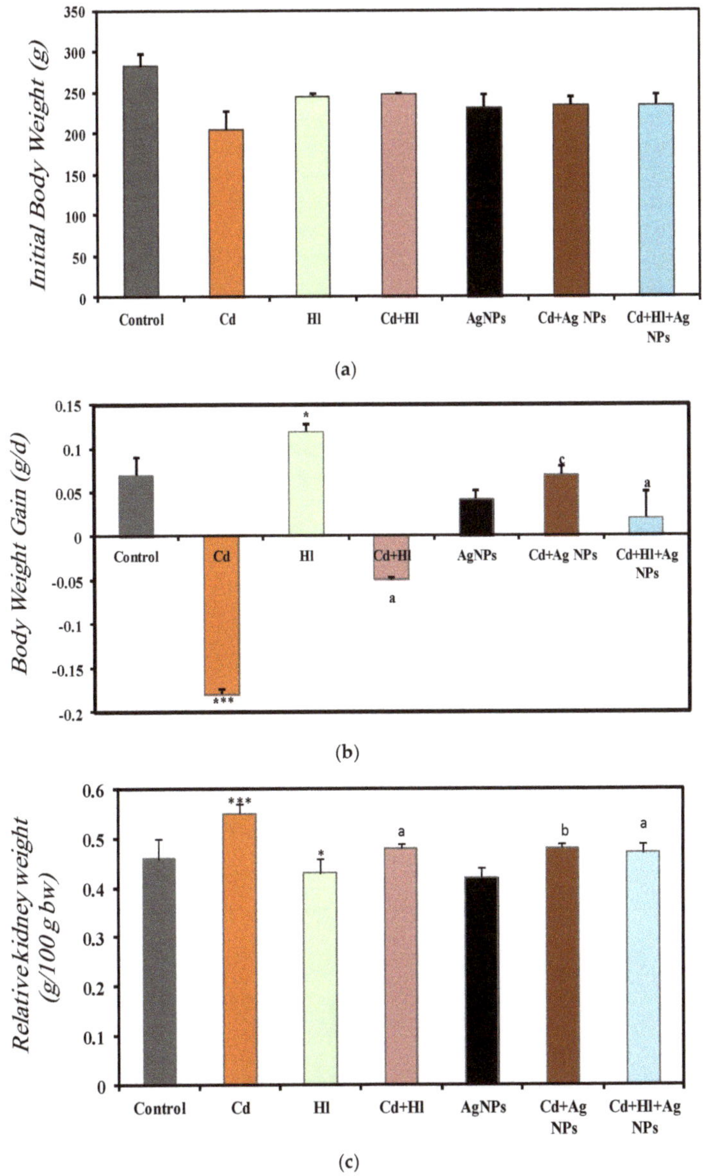

Figure 3. Comparison of baseline body weight (**a**), body weight gain (**b**), and relative kidney weight (**c**) in the seven rat groups. Group 1 (Control): no exposure/treatment. Group 2 (Cd): addition of $CdCl_2$ (50 mg/kg body weight/day) in drinking water for 35 days. Group 3 (*Hl*): *H. lippii* extract (100 mg/kg body weight/day, by gavage, for 35 days). Group 4 (Cd + *Hl*): $CdCl_2$ exposure (like in Group 2) followed by *H. lippii* extract (100 mg/kg body weight/day by gavage) for 15 days. Group 5 (Ag): Ag NPs (100 µg/kg body weight/day, intraperitoneal injection) for 35 days. Group 6 (Cd + Ag): $CdCl_2$ exposure (like in Group 2) followed by Ag NPs (0.1 mg/kg body weight/day by intraperitoneal injection) for 15 days. Group 7 (Cd+ *Hl* +Ag): $CdCl_2$ exposure (like in Group 2) followed by *H. lippii* extract (100 mg/kg body weight/day by gavage) and Ag NPs (0.1 mg/kg body weight/day by intraperitoneal injection) for 15 days. * $p < 0.05$, *** $p < 0.001$ vs. Group 1; a $p < 0.05$, b $p < 0.01$, c $p < 0.001$: vs. Group 2.

The comparison of the relative kidney weight in the different groups at the end of the study (Figure 3c) showed that, compared to Group 1 (control), it was significantly increased in Group 2 (exposure to $CdCl_2$) (0.46 ± 0.04 vs. 0.55 ± 0.02), suggesting a hypertrophic response induced by Cd exposure. Conversely, in Group 3 (*H. lippii* alone) and Group 5 (Ag NPs alone), the relative kidney weights were 0.43 ± 0.03 and 0.42 ± 0.02, respectively, reaffirming their safety profiles (Figure 3c). In Group 4 ($CdCl_2$ + *H. lippii* extract), Group 6 ($CdCl_2$ + Ag NPs), and Group 7 ($CdCl_2$+ *H. lippii* +Ag), the relative kidney weights were significantly decreased, compared with Group 2: 0.48 ± 0.01, 0.48 ± 0.02, and 0.47 ± 0.01, respectively. This suggests a potential reversal of Cd-induced hypertrophy, underscoring the protective effects of the *H. lippii* extract and Ag NPs against Cd toxicity. These results are in agreement with the findings by (Liu et al. 2022) [40], who tested Ag NPs as nanostructures for novel and improved biological uses.

2.6. Biochemical Parameters

Figure 4 summarizes the data on the effect of $CdCl_2$ exposure and treatment with the *H. lippii* extract and/or Ag NPs on different serum markers (Table S2, Supplementary Materials file). In Group 2 ($CdCl_2$ exposure), serum triglycerides (0.79 ± 0.01 g/L) (Figure 4a), cholesterol (0.78 ± 0.02 mg/L) (Figure 4b), and glucose (1.13 ± 0.09 g/L) (Figure 4c) were significantly increased, compared with Group 1 (control). These findings indicate disrupted lipid metabolism and suggest potential liver damage affecting protein synthesis, as evidenced by the reduction in the serum albumin concentration (29.5 ± 0.0131 g/L) (Figure 4d). Conversely, these markers were not significantly different in Group 3 (*H. lippii* extract alone) and Group 5 (Ag NPs alone), compared with the control group, indicating that the *H. lippii* extract and Ag NPs alone do not alter the lipid profiles, glucose metabolism, or albumin levels. In Group 4 (*H. lippii* extract after $CdCl_2$ exposure), Group 6 ($CdCl_2$ exposure + Ag NPs), and Group 7 ($CdCl_2$ exposure + *H. lippii* extract + Ag NPs), these parameters tended to be normalized, suggesting a mitigating effect on $CdCl_2$-induced alterations. Specifically, serum triglycerides, cholesterol, glucose, and albumin levels were within normal ranges, according to controls (triglycerides: 0.63 ± 0.01 g/L, 0.59 ± 0.05 g/L, 0.40 ± 0.01 g/L; cholesterol: 0.75 ± 0.01 mg/L, 0.63 ± 0.03 mg/L, 0.75 ± 0.01 mg/L; glucose: 0.82 ± 0.10 g/L, 1.08 ± 0.009 g/L, 0.88 ± 0.06 g/L; albumin: 31.33 ± 0.44 g/L, 29.66 ± 0.4 g/L, 30.75 ± 0.3 g/L, respectively).

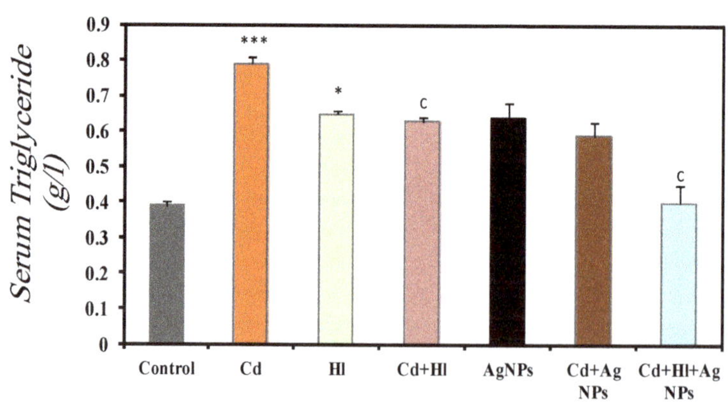

(a)

Figure 4. *Cont.*

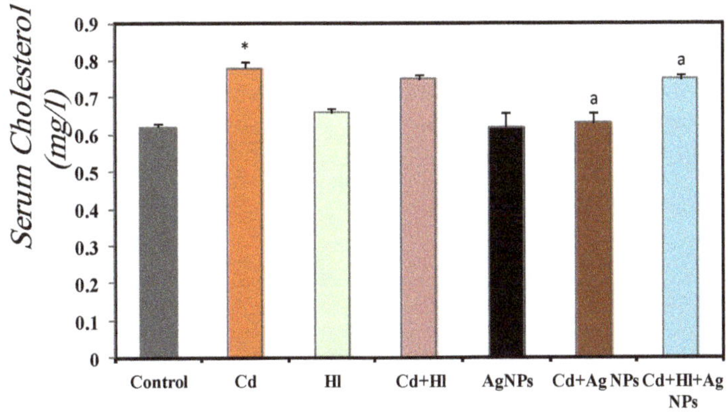

(b)

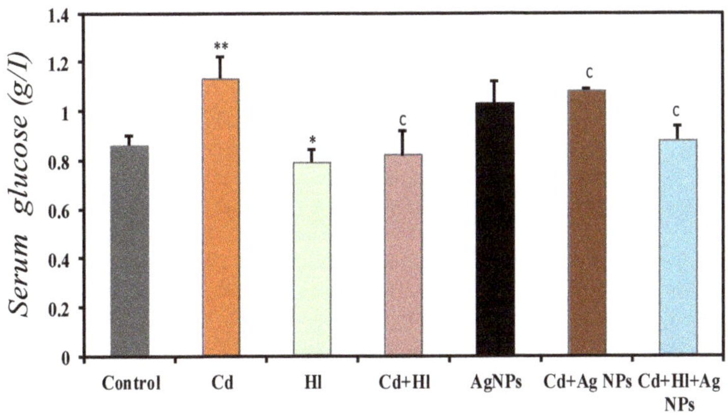

(c)

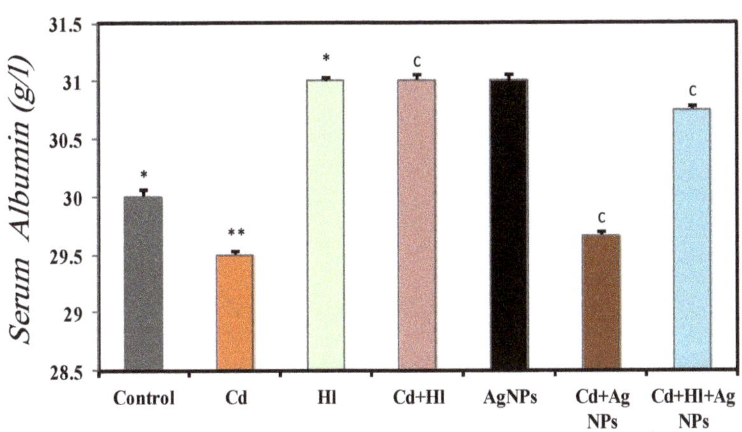

(d)

Figure 4. Comparison of different serum markers in the seven rat groups. Group 1 (Control): no treatment/exposure. Group 2 (Cd): exposure to $CdCl_2$ (50 mg/kg body weight/day) in drinking water for 35 days. Group 3 (*Hl*): *H. lippii* extract (100 mg/kg body weight/day) by gavage for 35 days. Group 4 (Cd + *Hl*): $CdCl_2$ exposure (like in Group 2) followed by *H. lippii* extract (100 mg/kg body weight/day by gavage) for 15 days. Group 5 (Ag): Ag NPs (100 μg/kg body weight/day, intraperitoneal injection) for 35 days. Group 6 (Cd + Ag): $CdCl_2$ exposure (like in Group 2) followed by Ag NPs (0.1 mg/kg body weight/day by intraperitoneal injection) for 15 days. Group 7 (Cd + *Hl* + Ag): $CdCl_2$ exposure (like in Group 2) followed by *H. lippii* extract (100 mg/kg body weight/day by gavage) and Ag NPs (0.1 mg/kg body weight/day by intraperitoneal injection) for 15 days. (**a**) serum triglycerides, (**b**) serum cholesterol, (**c**) serum glucose, (**d**) serum albumin. * $p < 0{,}05$, ** $p < 0.01$, *** $p < 0.001$ vs. Group 1; a $p < 0.05$, c $p < 0.001$: vs. Group 2.

Most biochemical markers in the groups treated with the *H. lippii* extract and/or Ag NPs were restored to levels near those of the control group, likely due to the anti-inflammatory and antioxidant properties of *H. lippii*. The tannic acid in *H. lippii* enhances glucose uptake by tissues, suppresses gluconeogenesis, and activates insulin secretion from β-cells [41], while naringenin protects the islets of Langerhans from degenerative changes. In rats exposed to cadmium and treated with *H. lippii* and/or Ag NPs, lipid parameters, serum albumin levels, protein levels, and calcium concentrations were regulated, attributed to the presence of flavonoids and phenolic compounds in the extract that scavenge superoxide, hydroxyl ions, and peroxyl radicals, preventing lipid peroxidation, lowering lipogenic enzyme activity, and enhancing lipoprotein lipase function [42]. These flavonoids' antioxidant capacities also positively affect protein levels and calcium. Additionally, silver nanoparticles improve lipid profiles, protein levels, and blood glucose levels, consistent with their anti-hyperglycemic, antioxidant, and anti-inflammatory responses [43,44]. The combined treatment of *H. lippii* and Ag NPs significantly restored most biochemical parameters, suggesting that the antioxidants in both treatments synergistically improved these levels against $CdCl_2$ exposure. Ag-based nanomaterials are less toxic to biological systems and have greater therapeutic efficacy when bio-conjugated with plant extracts due to the variety of phytochemicals or capping agents provided by the plant extracts, combined with the small size and large surface area of Ag NPs, which allows for maximum adsorption of these capping agents onto their surfaces. This combined treatment offers a promising strategy for addressing renal abnormalities caused by heavy-metal toxicity [45,46].

These findings underscore the potential therapeutic role of the *H. lippii* extract and Ag NPs in ameliorating $CdCl_2$-induced effects on lipid profiles, glucose metabolism, and protein synthesis, warranting further investigations into their clinical applications in the context of Cd toxicity. Similarly, (Rehman et al., 2023) and El-Baz et al., (2023) [47,48] previously showed Ag NP's restorative activity and ability to improve lipid profiles, protein levels, and blood glucose levels, in line with their anti-hyperglycemic, antioxidant, and inflammatory responses.

2.7. Biochemical Biomarkers of Renal Function

Figure 5 summarizes renal function biomarkers across the seven experimental groups (Table S3, Supplementary Materials File). In Group 2 ($CdCl_2$-treated), the serum urea (0.58 ± 0.02 g/L), creatinine (5.36 ± 0.001 mg/L), uric acid (20.00 ± 0.001 mg/L), and urea-to-creatinine ratio (108.0 ± 11.2) were significantly elevated, compared to Group 1 (control), indicating $CdCl_2$-induced nephrotoxicity, consistent with the findings of (Liu et al., 1998) [49]. Conversely, Group 3 (*H. lippii* extract) and Group 5 (Ag NPs) showed values similar to controls: urea (0.45 ± 0.022 g/L, 0.46 ± 0.025 g/L), creatinine (4.81 ± 0.05 mg/L, 4.010 ± 0.0001 mg/L), uric acid (11.33 ± 1.45 mg/L, 11.67 ± 1.28 mg/L), and urea-to-creatinine ratio (94.87 ± 6.7, 104.74 ± 8.60), indicating biocompatibility under normal conditions. Group 4 ($CdCl_2$ + *H. lippii* extract) showed decreased levels, compared to Group 2: urea (0.47 ± 0.028 g/L), creatinine (4.25 ± 0.001 mg/L), uric acid (16.25 ± 1.50 mg/L), and urea-to-creatinine ratio (110.9 ± 10.0), suggesting that the *H. lippii* extract mitigates $CdCl_2$-induced renal damage via antioxidant compounds. Similarly, Group 6 ($CdCl_2$ + Ag NPs) displayed reduced biomarker levels: urea (0.47 ± 0.01 g/L), creatinine (5.11 ± 0.08 mg/L), uric acid (12.5 ± 0.77 mg/L), and urea-to-creatinine ratio (95.25 ± 6.46), indicating Ag

NPs alleviate $CdCl_2$-induced renal damage. Group 7 ($CdCl_2$ + *H. lippii* extract + Ag NPs) exhibited comparable trends: urea (0.48 ± 0.02 g/L), creatinine (4.81 ± 0.08 mg/L), uric acid (11.75 ± 0.55 mg/L), and urea to creatinine ratio (95.1 ± 11.4), highlighting combined effects in restoring renal function post $CdCl_2$-induced nephrotoxicity.

The protective effect of Ag NPs was evident in the significant reduction in kidney function biomarkers, compared to the Cd-exposed group, consistent with findings by (Rehman et al., 2023) [47]. Ag NPs stabilize membranes, combat oxidative stress, and mitigate inflammatory responses, thereby limiting intracellular enzyme leakage. Studies underscore their cytoprotective activities both in vitro and in vivo [48]. The antioxidant- and free-radical-scavenging properties of Ag NPs likely contribute to restoring biochemical and histological parameters close to normal levels, highlighting their potential therapeutic value for kidney function protection. Group 4 (Cd exposure followed by *H. lippii*) exhibited improved kidney biomarkers due to the extract's high concentration of bioactive compounds (gallic acid, chlorogenic acid, caffeic acid, p-coumaric acid), which protect against cellular injury. Furthermore, *H. lippii*'s bioactive compounds possess potent anti-inflammatory properties by inhibiting cytokine production (TNF-α, IL-1β, IL-6) [48–52], thereby reducing inflammation and supporting renal tissue repair. These findings align with the previous research demonstrating their antioxidant efficacy against Cd-induced cell damage [48–52]. Combining *H. lippii* extract with silver nanoparticles enhanced kidney function, compared to $CdCl_2$ alone, illustrating the synergistic renal protective effects of silver compounds and the antioxidant properties of the plant extract.

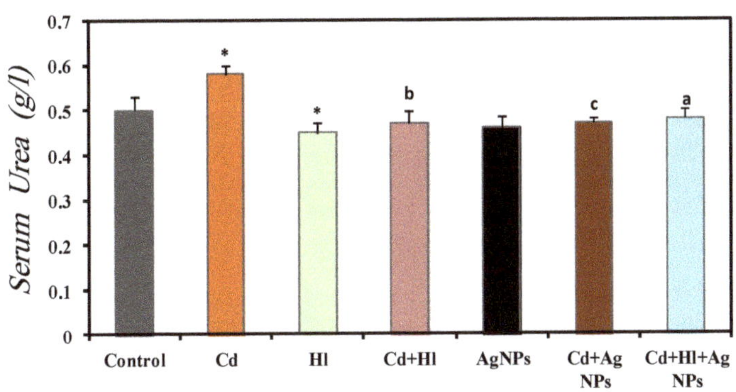

(a)

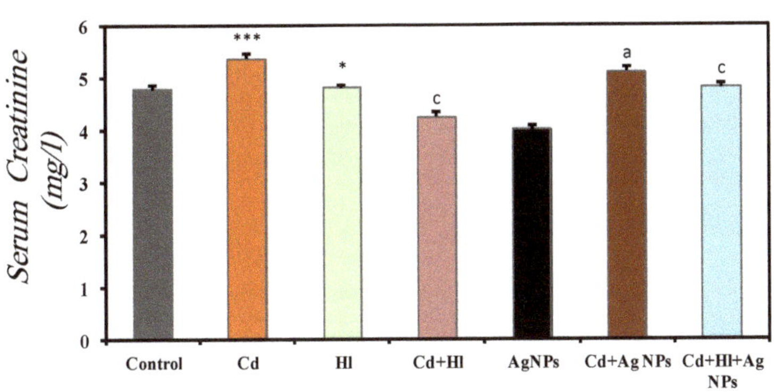

(b)

Figure 5. *Cont.*

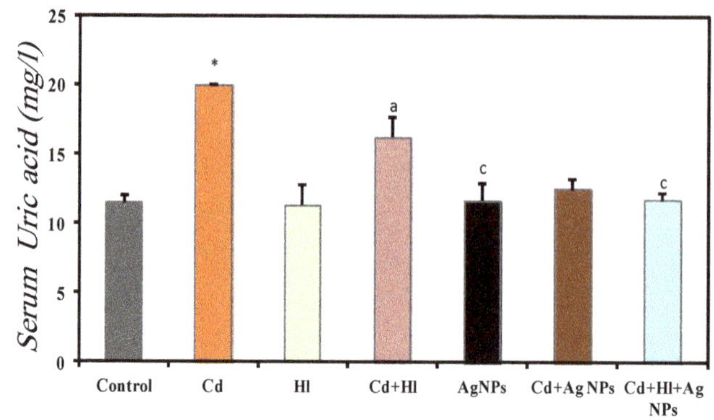

(**c**)

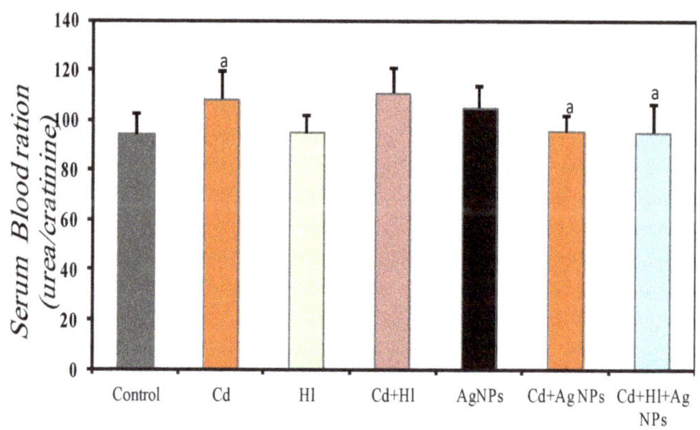

(**d**)

Figure 5. Renal function marker levels in the seven rat groups. Group 1 (Control): no treatment/exposure. Group 2 (Cd): addition of $CdCl_2$ (50 mg/kg body weight/day) in drinking water for 35 days. Group 3 (Hl): *H. lippii* extract (100 mg/kg body weight/day), by gavage for 35 days. Group 4 (Cd + *Hl*): $CdCl_2$ exposure (like in Group 2) followed by *H. lippii* extract (100 mg/kg body weight/day by gavage) for 15 days. Group 5 (Ag): Ag NPs (100 µg/kg body weight/day, intraperitoneal injection) for 35 days. Group 6 (Cd + Ag)/: $CdCl_2$ exposure (like in Group 2) followed by Ag NPs (0.1 mg/kg, body weight/day by intraperitoneal injection) for 15 days. Group 7 (Cd + Hl + Ag): $CdCl_2$ exposure (like in Group 2) followed by *H. lippii* extract (100 mg/kg, body weight/day by gavage) and Ag NPs (0.1 mg/kg, body weight/day by intraperitoneal injection) for 15 days. (**a**) serum urea, (**b**) serum creatinine, (**c**) serum uric acid, (**d**) serum blood ration urea/creatinine. * $p < 0.05$, *** $p < 0.001$ vs. Group 1; a $p < 0.05$, b $p < 0.01$, c $p < 0.001$: vs. Group 2.

2.8. Oxidative Stress Markers

The analysis of the kidney oxidative stress markers in the seven experimental groups (Figure 6) revealed a significant increase in the MDA concentration in $CdCl_2$-exposed rats (Group 2), compared with controls (Group 1) (0.9061 ± 0.0592 vs. 0.403 ± 0.021 nmol/mg protein) (Figure 6a), which is indicative of higher oxidative stress and potential kidney damage (Table S4, Supplementary Materials File). Conversely, antioxidant defense markers were decreased in Group 2, compared with Group 1: SOD activity (0.239 ± 0.00001 vs. 0.26 ± 0.009 U/mg protein) (Figure 6b), GSH levels (0.00022 ± 0.000001 vs. 0.00023 ± 0.001 nmol/g tissue) (Figure 6c), and catalase activity (0.01931 ± 0.0072 vs. 0.04373 ± 0.008 U/g tissue) (Figure 6d). The GSH and catalase are important indicators of oxidative damage to macromolecules, and our findings are compatible with previous findings [53]. (Ijaz et al., 2023) [11] and Albasher et al., (2020) [54] showed that in rats, exposure to Cd in drinking water for 30 days significantly increases the kidney's MDA concentration and significantly decreases catalase and SOD activities, compared with the control group.

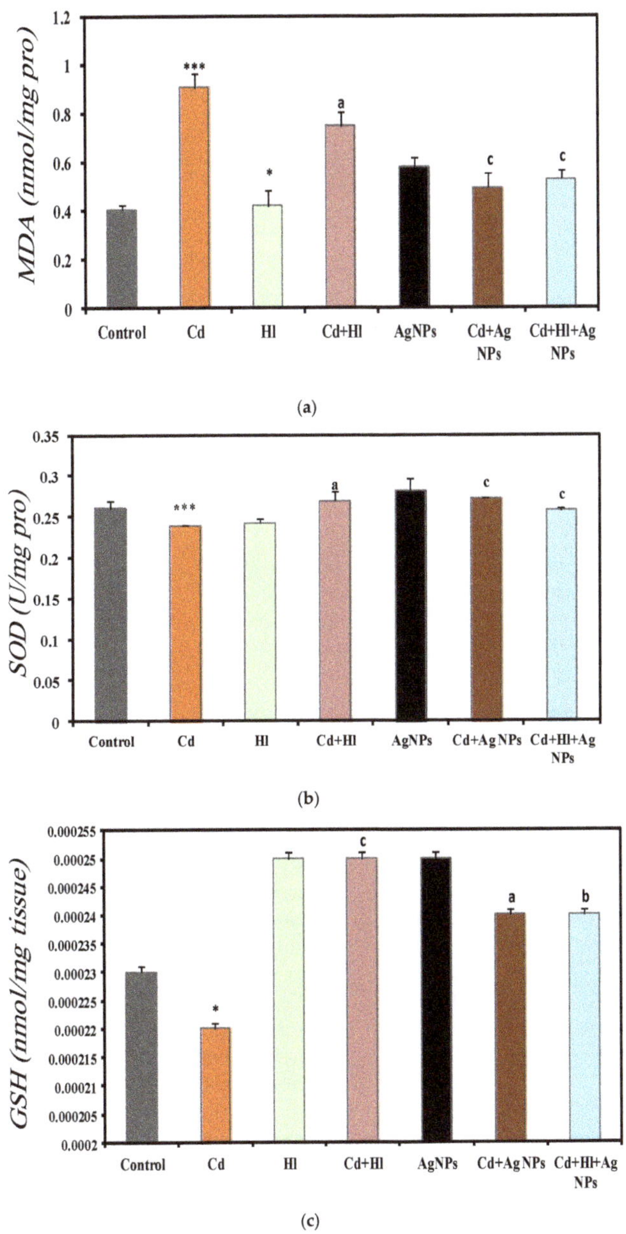

Figure 6. *Cont.*

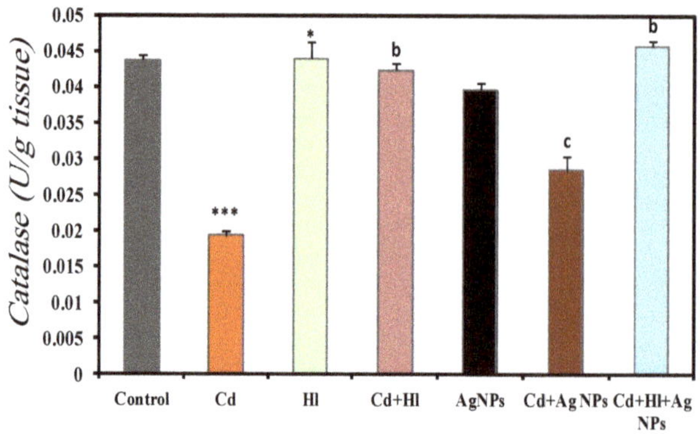

(**d**)

Figure 6. Oxidative stress markers in the seven rat groups. Group 1 (Control): no treatment/exposure. Group 2 (Cd): addition of $CdCl_2$ (50 mg/kg body weight/day) in drinking water for 35 days. Group 3 (*Hl*): *H. lippii* extract (100 mg/kg body weight/day, by gavage for 35 days). Group 4 (Cd + *Hl*): $CdCl_2$ exposure (like in Group II) followed by *H. lippii* extract (100 mg/kg body weight/day by gavage) for 15 days. Group 5 (Ag): Ag NPs (100 µg/kg body weight/day, by intraperitoneal injection) for 35 days. Group 6 (Cd + Ag): $CdCl_2$ exposure (like in Group II) followed by Ag NPs (0.1 mg/kg body weight/day by intraperitoneal injection) for 15 days. Group 7 (Cd + Hl + Ag): $CdCl_2$ exposure (like in Group II) followed by *H. lippii* extract (100 mg/kg body weight/day by gavage) and Ag NPs (0.1 mg/kg body weight/day by intraperitoneal injection) for 15 days. (**a**) MDA, (**b**) SOD, (**c**) GSH, (**d**) Catalase. * $p < 0.05$, *** $p < 0.001$ vs. Group 1; a $p < 0.05$, b $p < 0.01$, c $p < 0.001$: vs. Group 2.

Conversely, these oxidative stress markers did not significantly differ in rats treated only with *H. lippii* extract (Group 3) or Ag NPs (Group 5) compared with controls (Group 1), suggesting no adverse effects on kidney oxidative stress from these treatments alone. Treatment with *H. lippii* following $CdCl_2$ exposure (Group 4) resulted in a reduction in the oxidative stress markers and an increase in antioxidant defenses, compared with Group 2. Specifically, the MDA concentration decreased (0.7469 ± 0.0545 nmol/mg protein), while SOD, GSH, and catalase levels increased, indicating an amelioration of kidney oxidative damage. This beneficial effect can be attributed to the high concentration of bioactive compounds in *H. lippii*, such as gallic acid, chlorogenic acid, caffeic acid, and p-coumaric acid, which are known for their potent antioxidant properties [24,55]. *H. lippii* enhances the kidney's antioxidant defense system by scavenging ROS directly and enhancing the activity of endogenous antioxidant enzymes. These mechanisms play crucial roles in neutralizing oxidative stress and protecting renal cells from damage induced by Cd exposure. Moreover, *H. lippii* facilitates the synthesis of metallothionein, a metal-binding protein that aids in cadmium detoxification and reduces its accumulation in renal tissues, thereby mitigating oxidative-stress-related cellular damage associated with heavy metal toxicity [54–57].

The rats treated with Ag NPs after $CdCl_2$ exposure (Group 6) showed notable reductions in oxidative stress markers and enhanced antioxidant defenses compared to Group 2. Specifically, the MDA concentration decreased (0.4919 ± 0.0594 nmol/mg protein), while the SOD, GSH, and catalase levels increased, indicating that Ag NPs may alleviate kidney oxidative damage through their robust antioxidant and anti-inflammatory properties. Ag NPs exert their protective effects against cadmium toxicity primarily through their potent antioxidant activity [58]. Cadmium exposure triggers the generation of reactive oxygen species (ROS), leading to oxidative stress and renal cell damage [22]. Ag NPs directly scavenge these ROS, thereby mitigating oxidative damage to cellular components such as lipids, proteins, and DNA. Moreover, Ag NPs enhance the activity of endogenous antioxidant enzymes, including SOD, catalase, and GPx [58], and they have been shown to upregulate the expression of Nrf2, a key regulator of cellular defense against oxidative stress, which aids in preventing cadmium-induced cellular damage.

Furthermore, the combined treatment with the *H. lippii* extract and Ag NPs after $CdCl_2$ exposure (Group 7) further enhanced protection against oxidative stress. The MDA concentration was reduced (0.5274 ± 0.0382 nmol/mg protein), while SOD, GSH, and catalase levels were elevated compared to Group 2, underscoring the distinct antioxidant efficacy of each component. These results highlight the synergistic benefits of combining plant extracts and Ag NPs in safeguarding kidney structure and function from $CdCl_2$-induced toxicity. This combined approach capitalizes on the strengths of natural and nanotechnology-derived therapeutic strategies, enhancing bioavailability, improving drug delivery, boosting therapeutic efficacy, minimizing side effects, offering multifaceted therapy, and potentially overcoming drug resistance. The synergistic therapeutic effects observed underscore the promise of this approach for effectively and safely managing a broad spectrum of diseases.

2.9. Histological Alterations in Kidney

The semi-quantitative analysis of kidney tissue samples revealed distinct architectural damage among the experimental groups (Figure 7 and Table S5). In Group 2 ($CdCl_2$ exposure), there were severe histopathological changes, including prominent inflammatory cell infiltration (+++), destroyed glomeruli (+++), and tubular dilation (+++), indicating extensive tissue damage induced by cadmium exposure. These findings align with previous studies reporting Cd-induced structural alterations, such as increased mesangial matrix and glomerular swelling [59]. Cadmium toxicity targets the proximal tubular epithelium, sensitizing it to oxidative stress and leading to kidney cell injury [11]. Elevated nitric oxide and ROS production further exacerbate tissue damage and contribute to kidney dysfunction [60].

Groups 3 and 5, treated with *H. lippii* extract or Ag NPs alone, respectively, exhibited no significant histopathological alterations compared to controls (Group 1), indicating the biocompatibility of these treatments under normal conditions. In Group 4 (*H. lippii* extract after $CdCl_2$ exposure), although tubular dilation persisted, inflammatory infiltration and glomerular destruction were notably absent compared to Group 2. This suggests that *H. lippii* extract mitigates $CdCl_2$-induced histopathological changes by enhancing antioxidant defenses, reducing tissue inflammation, and modulating the NRF_2 transcription factor, crucial for antioxidant protein induction [61]. The extract's flavonoids and phenolic acids scavenge ROS, minimizing lipid peroxidation and preserving renal architecture by attenuating tubular degeneration and interstitial fibrosis [62–64]. Additionally, *H. lippii*'s anti-inflammatory properties suppress cytokine production, further protecting renal tissues from inflammatory damage.

In Group 6 (Ag NPs after $CdCl_2$ exposure), there were no signs of inflammatory infiltration, tubular dilation, or destroyed glomeruli observed, indicating a protective effect against cadmium-induced histological alterations. Ag NPs exert multifaceted protective mechanisms, including antioxidant, anti-inflammatory, cytoprotective, and detoxifying actions [65,66]. These nanoparticles mitigate oxidative stress and inflammation, reduce apoptosis, and promote tissue repair and regeneration [67]. Moreover, Ag NPs enhance angiogenesis, improving blood flow to damaged areas and facilitating tissue recovery, thereby preserving normal kidney architecture despite cadmium exposure [62,67,68]. The comprehensive protective effects of Ag NPs underscore their potential therapeutic value in preventing and treating Cd-induced nephrotoxicity.

Finally, in Group 7 (*H. lippii* + Ag NPs after $CdCl_2$ exposure), the architectural damage parameters were restored to near-normal levels, compared to Group 2. No inflammatory infiltration, tubular dilation, or destroyed glomeruli were observed, highlighting the synergistic effects of combining *H. lippii* extract with Ag NPs. The antioxidants and anti-inflammatory compounds in *H. lippii* complement the unique properties of Ag NPs, enhancing the overall therapeutic efficacy against cadmium toxicity. This combination strategy may offer a comprehensive defense against Cd-induced cellular damage by leveraging antioxidant pathways from *H. lippii* and multifunctional protective mechanisms from Ag NPs. These findings support the therapeutic potential of combining natural plant extracts with nanotechnology-derived nanoparticles for the effective and safe treatment of kidney damage induced by heavy metals like cadmium.

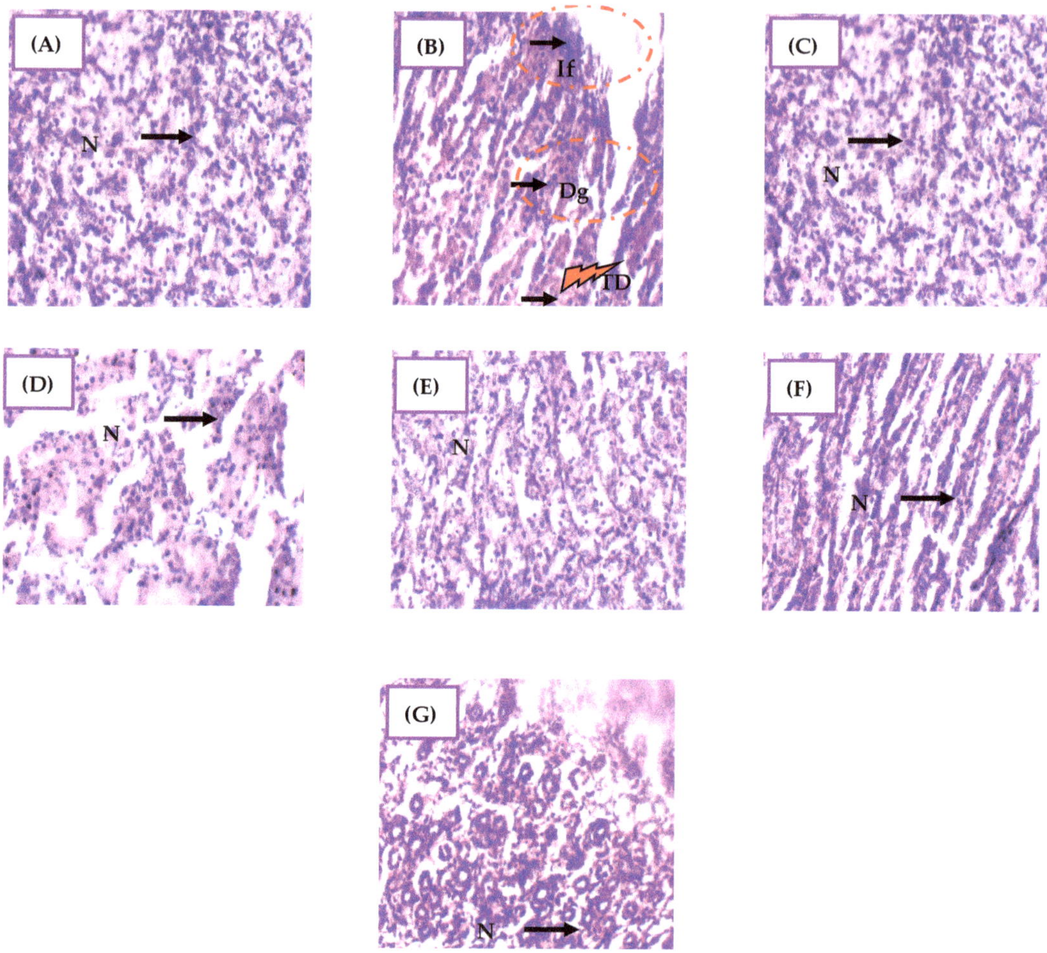

Figure 7. Micrographs of representative kidney tissue sections from rats in the different experimental groups, showing the effect of $CdCl_2$ exposure and the mitigating effect of *H. lippii* and Ag NPs. (**A**) Group 1 (control); (**B**) Group 2 ($CdCl_2$ exposure); (**C**) Group 3 (*H. lippii* extract alone); (**D**) Group 4 (*H. lippii* after $CdCl_2$ exposure); (**E**) Group 5 (Ag NPs); (**F**) Group 6 (Ag NPs after $CdCl_2$ exposure); (**G**) Group 7 (*H. lippii* and Ag NPs after $CdCl_2$ exposure). N, normal cell; IF, inflammatory cells; DG, destroyed glomeruli. TD, Tubular dilatation; 40×.

3. Material and Methods

3.1. Chemicals and Reagents

The cadmium chloride ($CdCl_2$, 99%), silver nitrate ($AgNO_3$, 99.9%), potassium dihydrogen phosphate (KH_2PO_4, 99.5%), dibasic potassium phosphate (K_2HPO_4, 99.95%), ascorbic acid (vitamin C, 99.9%), ethylenediaminetetraacetic acid (EDTA, 99.0%), 2-thiobarbituric acid (TBA, 97.0%), salicylic acid ($C_7H_6O_3$, 95.5%), 5,5′-dithiobis-2-nitrobenzoic acid (DTNB,

98.28%), 4-nitro blue tetrazolium chloride (NBT, 99.9%), ethanolamine (C_2H_7NO, 99%), O-cresolphthalein ($C_{22}H_{18}O_4$, 95%,), 8-hydroxyquinoline (C_9H_7NO, 99.99%), Tris pH 7.8 ($(HOCH_2)_3CNH_2$, 99.9%), α-ketoglutaric acid ($C_5H_6O_5$, 99.5%), 2-4 dichlorophenol ($(CH3)_2C6H3OH$, 99%), sodium hydroxide (NaOH, 99%), picric acid ($C_6H_3N_3O_7$, 99.8%), 4–aminophenazone (4-AP) ($C_{13}H_{17}N_3O$, 98%), thiobarbituric acid ($C_4H_4N_2O_2S$, 99%), sodium chloride (NaCl, 99%), methionine ($C_5H_{11}NO_2S$, 99.3%), riboflavin ($C_{17}H_{20}N_4O_6$, 98%), hydrogen peroxide (H_2O_2, 99.9%), ethanol (CH_3CH_2OH, 99.5%), hematoxylin ($C_{16}H_{14}O_6$, 85%), eosin ($C_{20}H_6Br_4Na_2O_5$, 90%), potassium mercuric iodide ($HgI_2 \cdot KI$, >98%), ferric chloride (FeCl3, 98%), acetic anhydride ($(CH3CO)_2O$, 99%), sulfuric acid (H_2SO_4, 98%), ammonia (NH_4OH, 99%), hydrochloric acid (HCl, 99%), and chloroform ($CHCl_3$, 94%) were obtained from Sigma-Aldrich (St. Louis, MO, USA). In March 2022, the aerial parts of *H. lippii* were collected in the Elhamadin region, El-Oued province, Algeria (33° 35′ 00″ N 6° 56′ 33″ E). These specimens were identified by a botany specialist. Following identification, the aerial parts were carefully stored in dry, cool conditions away from light at room temperature.

3.2. Preparation the H. lippii Aqueous Extract

The *H. lippii* aerial parts (10 g) were infused in 100 mL of distilled water and left at room temperature in the dark for 24 h. Then, the mixture was filtered using paper filters and the filtrate dried completely at 40 °C. The resulting extract was weighed and stored at 4 °C [69].

3.3. Phytochemical Screening

The phytochemical screening of the *H. lippii* extracts involved specific qualitative tests to identify its chemical constituents, each using standardized reagents and volumes. Alkaloids were detected using two different reagents: Mayer's reagent (potassium mercuric iodide), and Wagner's reagent (iodine in potassium iodide). Each reagent (1 mL) was added separately to 1 mL of the extract. The presence of alkaloids was indicated by the formation of a cream-colored precipitate with the Mayer's reagent, and a brown or reddish brown precipitate with the Wagner's reagent [70]. Additionally, tannins were identified by adding 2–3 drops of 5% ferric chloride solution to 1 mL of the extract. The presence of catechic tannins was indicated by a blue–black coloration, while gallic tannins produced a greenish black coloration [71]. To detect terpenes and sterols, 1–2 mL of a Liebermann –Burchard reagent (a mixture of acetic anhydride and concentrated sulfuric acid) was added to 1 mL of the extract, followed by gentle heating. The presence of terpenes and sterols was confirmed by the formation of a blue–green coloration [72]. Saponins were identified by their ability to form stable foam. One milliliter of the extract was mixed with 10 mL of distilled water and shaken vigorously. The formation of stable foam indicated the presence of saponins [73]. Additionally, mucilage was detected by adding 10 mL of absolute ethanol to 1 mL of the extract, resulting in a gelatinous mass [74]. Moreover, polyphenolic compounds were identified by adding 2–3 drops of 5% ferric chloride solution to 1 mL of the extract, with colored complexes indicating their presence [75]. Additionally, flavonoids were detected by adding 1 mL of dilute ammonia solution to 1 mL of the extract, followed by 1 mL of concentrated sulfuric acid. The presence of flavonoids was indicated by the formation of a yellow coloration, which disappeared upon standing [76]. Finally, anthocyanins were detected by adding a small amount of hydrochloric acid followed by a small amount of ammonia. If anthocyanins are present, the color will change, showing red [77]. Each method utilized these reagents and volumes to qualitatively assess the presence or absence of specific phytochemicals in the *H. lippii* extract. A positive sign (+) indicated the presence of the phytochemical, whereas a negative sign (−) indicated its absence.

3.4. High-Performance Liquid Chromatography (HPLC) Analysis

The phenolic compounds present in the crude extract were identified using HPLC equipped with a UV-Vis type Shimadzu LC20 AL system. The analytical Shim-pack VP-

ODSC18 column (4.6 mm × 250 mm, 5 μm) was coupled with a UV-VIS detector SPD 20A (Shimadzu, Kyoto, Japan) and a universal injector (Hamilton 25 μL). The reverse-phase chromatography was performed with non-polar aliphatic residues and with acetonitrile and 0.1% acetic acid as the mobile phase and gradient elution. The flow rate was set at 1 mL/min, and the injection volume was set at 0.45 μL. The injection volumes for standard and sample were 20 μL, and the monitoring wavelength was 268 nm. To identify and confirm the retention times of the compounds, we used nine standards of known compounds, including caffeic acid (Retention time (min): 16.27), p-Coumaric acid (Retention time (min): 23.81), gallic acid (Retention time (min): 5.29), vanillic acid (Retention time (min): 15.53), chlorogenic acid (Retention time (min): 13.39), naringin (Retention time (min): 34.78), rutin (Retention time (min): 28.37), quercetin (Retention time (min): 45.04), and vanillin (Retention time (min): 21.46). These standards were run under the same HPLC conditions as the sample extracts to establish baseline retention times.

3.5. Ag NPs Synthesis and Characterization

For the Ag NP synthesis, 90 mL of a 1 mM $AgNO_3$ solution was mixed with 10 mL of the *H. lippii* extract, resulting in the appearance of a brownish tinge, indicative of Ag NP synthesis. Then, the mixture was heated to 60 °C and incubated in the dark for 24 h. Ag NP formation was confirmed by UV-vis analysis, followed by centrifugation to ensure complete separation and washed with ethanol and distilled water. The resulting Ag NPs were carefully collected from the final precipitate and dried [21]. To evaluate the Ag NP's crystallinity and crystal structure, an X-ray diffraction (XRD) analysis was performed using CuKα radiation (30 kV and 20 mA), with a wavelength of 0.154281 Å and a scanning speed of 0.05°. Scanning electron microscopy (SEM) (Thermo Scientific, Quatro, Thermo Fisher Scientific, Dreieich, Germany) was used to assess the Ag NP size and morphology.

3.6. Animal Procurement and Housing

A total of 53 adult male Wistar albino rats, with an average weight of 232.36 ± 3.81 g, were bought from the Pasteur Institute Animal Facility, Algiers, Algeria. Upon arrival, rats were acclimated to the controlled laboratory environment at the Department of Molecular and Cellular Biology, University of El-Oued, Algeria, for 2 weeks. The housing conditions were 19 °C, a relative humidity of 64%, and a 12-h light/12-h dark cycle. Throughout the study, rats had ad libitum access to tap water and standard rat chow. Ethical approval for the animal experiments and protocols was obtained from the Institutional Animal Ethical Committee (IAEC), University of El Oued, Algeria.

3.7. Cadmium Toxicity Experiment Design

After acclimatization, the rats were randomly allocated into seven groups (n = 5 animals/group). The doses of $CdCl_2$, Ag NPs, and *H. lippii* were determined based on previous studies and $CdCl_2$ LD_{50} [11,27,78], to ensure optimal exposure and treatment durations. The experimental groups were as follows:

- Group 1: control group (normal water throughout the study period).
- Group 2: exposure to 50 mg/kg body weight/day $CdCl_2$ dissolved in drinking water for 5 weeks.
- Group 3: 100 mg/kg body weight/day *H. lippii* aqueous extract by oral gavage for 5 weeks.
- Group 4: exposure to $CdCl_2$ for 5 weeks, followed by treatment with 100 mg/kg body weight/day *H. lippii* (by oral gavage) for the last 15 days.
- Group 5: 0.1 mg/kg body weight/day Ag NPs by intraperitoneal injection for 5 weeks.
- Group 6: $CdCl_2$ exposure for 5 weeks, followed by treatment with 0.1 mg/kg body weight/day of Ag NPs (intraperitoneal injection) for the last 15 days.
- Group 7: $CdCl_2$ exposure for 5 weeks and then treatment with 100 mg/kg body weight/day *H. lippii* (oral gavage) and 0.1 mg/kg body weight/day Ag NPs (intraperitoneal injection) for the last 15 days.

The study meticulously monitored the welfare of the rats, with regular recording of their body weights. Established protocols were followed to minimize rat movement and ensure humane procedures. The chloroform was used solely for anesthesia, not euthanasia, in accordance with the intended protocol. A low dose of 94% chloroform in cotton was administered via inhalation to induce dizziness in the rats. Subsequently, euthanasia was conducted via decapitation to ensure swift and humane termination. Blood collection was then performed from the severed neck, adhering to the ethical standards that were thoroughly confirmed [79,80].

3.8. Sub-Acute Toxicity Study

The acute toxicity of Ag NPs and *H. lippii* aqueous extract was investigated following the guidelines established by the Organization for Economic Cooperation and Development (OECD) 425. Six groups, each comprising three male Wistar albino rats, were established as follows:

- Group 1 (control group): normal water.
- Groups 2 to 4: administration by oral gavage of one dose of *H. lippii* aqueous extract (100, 1000, 4000 mg/kg)
- Groups 5 and 6: one intraperitoneal injection of Ag NPs (2, 10 mg/kg).

The sub-acute toxicity was evaluated by monitoring various parameters at different time intervals until day 14: symptoms of toxicity, body weight changes, side effects, movement patterns, diarrhea, ocular abnormalities, and death.

3.9. Body Weight

The rats were weighed regularly. The mean body weight was calculated by summing the body weight of each mouse and dividing this number by the number of rats. The body weight changes (%) from baseline were computed using the following formula:

$$\text{Body Weight Change (\%)} = (\text{Final Body Weight} - \text{Baseline Body Weight}/\text{Baseline Body Weight}) \times 100$$

3.10. Relative Kidney Weight

The kidneys were weighed after sacrifice and the relative weight was calculated as follows:

$$\text{Relative kidney weight} = (\text{kidney weight}/\text{final body weight}) \times 100$$

3.11. Renal Function Biomarkers

The renal function was evaluated by measuring key serum biomarkers (urea, uric acid, creatinine, glucose, albumin, cholesterol, and triglycerides) using the appropriate Spinreact kits (Barcelona, Spain), following the manufacturer's instructions.

3.12. Oxidative Stress Markers

To determine the malondialdehyde (MDA) level, 200 μL of kidney tissue and 800 μL of the TBA reagent were combined in glass test tubes that were tightly capped and heated at 100 °C in a water bath for 15 min. After 30 min of cooling in a cold-water bath, the tubes were left open to allow the reaction gas escape. The supernatant absorbance at 532 nm was measured using a spectrophotometer after centrifugation at 3000 rpm for 5 min [81].

To determine the GSH level, 200 μL of salicylic acid (0.25%) was mixed with 800 μL of kidney tissue, followed by centrifugation at 1000 rpm for 5 min. Then, 25 μL of DTNB (0.01 mol/L) and 500 μL of the supernatant were added to 1000 μL of tris buffer (0.4 M tris, 0.02M NaCl, pH = 8.9). After 5 min of incubation, the absorbance was measured at 412 nm [82].

To determine the SOD activity, 50 μL of each kidney tissue was mixed with 1000 μL of 0.1 mM EDTA/13 mM methionine, followed by the addition of 1800 μL of 50 mM phosphate buffer, and then 85 μL of NBT and 22.6 μL of riboflavin. Absorption was measured at

560 nm. The same protocol was used for the blank where 50 µL of the phosphate buffer was added instead of the sample [82].

The catalase activity was determined as previously described [40]. The reaction was initiated by combining 200 µL of 0.030 M H_2O_2 with 20 µL of each kidney tissue and 780 µL of 0.1 M phosphate buffer (pH 7.5). H_2O_2 decomposition was tracked by measuring the decrease in absorbance at 240 nm every 30 s for 2 min. The enzymatic activity was quantified as international units per minute per gram of protein (IU/min/g of protein).

3.13. Histopathological Analysis of Kidney Tissues

The kidneys were isolated from the euthanized rats and immediately fixed in a 10% formaldehyde solution. Then, they were dehydrated in ethanol at increasing concentrations (60%, 70%, 80%, and 100%), followed by clearing with xylene and embedding in paraffin. Sections (4~6 µm thickness) were cut from the paraffin-embedded blocks using a Histoline rotary microtome (Thermo Scientific Micron HM 325, Histoline, Milan, Italy). The tissue sections were stained with hematoxylin and eosin and examined under a light microscope to detect morphological changes or abnormalities.

4. Statistical Analysis

Data were expressed as mean ± standard error of the mean (SEM). Groups were compared using Student's *t*-test. Statistical analysis was carried out using Minitab (Version 13Fr) and Excel (version 2007).

5. Conclusions

This study investigated the therapeutic potential of *Helianthemum lippii* (*H. lippii*) extract and silver nanoparticles (Ag NPs) synthesized using *H. lippii* extract in mitigating cadmium (Cd)-induced nephrotoxicity in adult Wistar rats (n = 5/group). The experimental groups included untreated controls, rats exposed to $CdCl_2$ for 35 days, and those treated with *H. lippii* or Ag NPs alone post-Cd exposure, as well as combinations of both treatments. Initial sub-acute toxicity assessments confirmed the safety of *H. lippii* and Ag NPs across various doses, establishing their suitability for therapeutic use. Comprehensive analyses of kidney function parameters, oxidative stress markers, histopathological features, and body weight changes revealed significant improvements following treatment with *H. lippii* and Ag NPs after Cd exposure. Both treatments effectively restored kidney function by reducing creatinine and blood urea nitrogen levels, indicative of improved renal health. Furthermore, *H. lippii* extract and Ag NPs exhibited potent antioxidant properties, enhancing activities of superoxide dismutase (SOD), catalase, and glutathione (GSH), while reducing malondialdehyde (MDA) levels, thus mitigating Cd-induced oxidative stress. Histopathological evaluations demonstrated preserved kidney architecture, reduced inflammatory responses, and minimized tubular dilation and fibrosis in treated groups compared to Cd-exposed controls. Importantly, the combined treatment of the *H. lippii* extract and Ag NPs showed synergistic effects, highlighting enhanced therapeutic efficacy in alleviating Cd-induced nephrotoxicity. These findings underscore the potential of *H. lippii*-based nanoparticles as novel therapeutic agents for managing heavy-metal toxicity, encouraging further research and clinical applications to optimize their use in medical practice.

Supplementary Materials: The following supporting information can be downloaded at: https://www.mdpi.com/article/10.3390/ph17080982/s1, Table S1. Baseline body weight, body weight changes between baseline and the study end, and relative kidney weight at the study end in the seven rat groups. Table S2. Serum biochemical markers in the different rat groups at the study end. Table S3. Kidney function markers in the seven rat groups. Table S4. Kidney oxidative stress markers in the seven rat groups. Table S5. Semi-quantitative results of the histological analysis of the kidney architecture in the different rat groups.

Author Contributions: Conceptualization, I.L., B.D.A. and A.B.; Methodology, I.L., B.D.A. and A.B.; Software, I.L., B.D.A. and A.B.; Validation, I.L., B.D.A. and A.B.; Formal analysis, I.L., B.D.A. and

A.B.; Investigation, I.L., B.D.A. and A.B.; Resources, I.L., B.D.A. and A.B.; Data curation, I.L., D.C. and A.B.; Writing—original draft, I.L., M.B. and A.B.; Writing—review & editing, A.A., M.B. and A.B.; Visualization, A.A., D.C., M.B. and A.B.; Supervision, M.B. and A.B.; Project administration, A.A., D.C., M.B. and A.B.; Funding acquisition, A.A., D.C., M.B. and A.B. All authors have read and agreed to the published version of the manuscript.

Funding: The author(s) declare financial support was received for the research, authorship, and/or publication of this article from the Researchers Supporting Project number (RSP-2024R78) at King Saud University, Riyadh, Saudi Arabia for their funding.

Institutional Review Board Statement: Not applicable.

Informed Consent Statement: Not applicable.

Data Availability Statement: The original contributions presented in the study are included in the article/Supplementary material, further inquiries can be directed to the corresponding author.

Conflicts of Interest: The authors declare that the research was conducted in the absence of any commercial or financial relationships that could be construed as a potential conflict of interest. The author(s) declared that they were an editorial board member of Frontiers at the time of submission.

References

1. Ye, X.; Qian, H.; Xu, P.; Zhu, L.; Longnecker, M.P.; Fu, H. Nephrotoxicity, neurotoxicity, and mercury exposure among children with and without dental amalgam fillings. *Int. J. Hyg. Environ. Health* **2009**, *212*, 378–386. [CrossRef]
2. Satarug, S.; Gobe, G.C.; Vesey, D.A. Multiple targets of toxicity in environmental exposure to low-dose cadmium. *Toxics* **2022**, *10*, 472. [CrossRef]
3. Satarug, S.; Vesey, D.A.; Gobe, G.C.; Đorđević, A.B. The validity of benchmark dose limit analysis for estimating permissible accumulation of cadmium. *Int. J. Environ. Res. Public Health* **2022**, *19*, 15697. [CrossRef]
4. Monsefi, M.; Fereydouni, B. The effects of cadmium pollution on female rat reproductive system. *J. Infertil. Reprod. Biol.* **2013**, *1*, 1–6. [CrossRef]
5. Rana, M.N.; Tangpong, J.; Rahman, M.M. Toxicodynamics of lead, cadmium, mercury and arsenic-induced kidney toxicity and treatment strategy: A mini review. *Toxicol. Rep.* **2018**, *5*, 704–713. [CrossRef]
6. Chen, M.; Li, X.; Fan, R.; Yang, J.; Jin, X.; Hamid, S.; Xu, S. Cadmium induces BNIP3-dependent autophagy in chicken spleen by modulating miR-33-AMPK axis. *Chemosphere* **2018**, *194*, 396–402. [CrossRef]
7. So, K.-Y.; Lee, B.-H.; Oh, S.-H. The critical role of autophagy in cadmium-induced immunosuppression regulated by endoplasmic reticulum stress-mediated calpain activation in RAW264. 7 mouse monocytes. *Toxicology* **2018**, *393*, 15–25. [CrossRef]
8. Liu, Q.; Zhang, R.; Wang, X.; Shen, X.; Wang, P.; Sun, N.; Li, X.; Li, X.; Hai, C. Effects of sub-chronic, low-dose cadmium exposure on kidney damage and potential mechanisms. *Ann. Transl. Med.* **2019**, *7*. [CrossRef]
9. Seif, M.M.; Madboli, A.-N.; Marrez, D.A.; Aboulthana, W.M. Hepato-renal protective effects of Egyptian purslane extract against experimental cadmium toxicity in rats with special emphasis on the functional and histopathological changes. *Toxicol. Rep.* **2019**, *6*, 625–631. [CrossRef]
10. Ibrahim, M.A.; Almaeen, A.H.; Abd El Moneim, M.; Tammam, H.G.; Khalifa, A.M.; Nasibe, M.N. Cadmium-Induced Hematological, Renal, and Hepatic Toxicity: The Amelioration by: Spirulina platensis. *Saudi J. Forensic Med. Sci.* **2018**, *1*, 5–13. [CrossRef]
11. Ijaz, M.U.; Shahzadi, S.; Hamza, A.; Azmat, R.; Anwar, H.; Afsar, T.; Shafique, H.; Bhat, M.A.; Naglah, A.M.; Al-Omar, M.A. Alleviative effects of pinostrobin against cadmium-induced renal toxicity in rats by reducing oxidative stress, apoptosis, inflammation, and mitochondrial dysfunction. *Front. Nutr.* **2013**, *10*, 1175008. [CrossRef]
12. Smereczański, N.M.; Brzóska, M.M. Current levels of environmental exposure to cadmium in industrialized countries as a risk factor for kidney damage in the general population: A comprehensive review of available data. *Int. J. Mol. Sci.* **2023**, *24*, 8413. [CrossRef]
13. Mitra, S.; Chakraborty, A.J.; Tareq, A.M.; Emran, T.B.; Nainu, F.; Khusro, A.; Idris, A.M.; Khandaker, M.U.; Osman, H.; Alhumaydhi, F.A. Impact of heavy metals on the environment and human health: Novel therapeutic insights to counter the toxicity. *J. King Saud Univ.-Sci.* **2022**, *34*, 101865. [CrossRef]
14. Hashim, M.; Arif, H.; Tabassum, B. An overview of the ameliorative efficacy of Catharanthus roseus extract against Cd2+ toxicity: Implications for human health and remediation strategies. *Front. Public Health* **2024**, *12*, 1327611. [CrossRef]
15. Çavuşoğlu, D.; Macar, O.; Kalefetoğlu Macar, T.; Çavuşoğlu, K.; Yalçın, E. Mitigative effect of green tea extract against mercury (II) chloride toxicity in Allium cepa L. model. *Environ. Sci. Pollut. Res.* **2022**, *29*, 27862–27874. [CrossRef]
16. Aghababaei, F.; Hadidi, M. Recent advances in potential health benefits of quercetin. *Pharmaceuticals* **2023**, *16*, 1020. [CrossRef]
17. El-Saadony, M.T.; Yang, T.; Korma, S.A.; Sitohy, M.; Abd El-Mageed, T.A.; Selim, S.; Al Jaouni, S.K.; Salem, H.M.; Mahmmod, Y.; Soliman, S.M. Impacts of turmeric and its principal bioactive curcumin on human health: Pharmaceutical, medicinal, and food applications: A comprehensive review. *Front. Nutr.* **2023**, *9*, 1040259. [CrossRef]

18. Kumari, A.; Kumar, D. Evaluation of antioxidant and cytotoxic activity of herbal teas from Western Himalayan region: A comparison with green tea (Camellia sinensis) and black tea. *Chem. Biol. Technol. Agric.* **2022**, *9*, 33. [CrossRef]
19. Burdușel, A.-C.; Gherasim, O.; Grumezescu, A.M.; Mogoantă, L.; Ficai, A.; Andronescu, E. Biomedical applications of silver nanoparticles: An up-to-date overview. *Nanomaterials* **2018**, *8*, 681. [CrossRef]
20. Zidane, Y.; Laouini, S.E.; Bouafia, A.; Meneceur, S.; Tedjani, M.L.; Alshareef, S.A.; Almukhlifi, H.A.; Al-Essa, K.; Al-Essa, E.M.; Rahman, M.M. Green synthesis of multifunctional MgO@ AgO/Ag_2O nanocomposite for photocatalytic degradation of methylene blue and toluidine blue. *Front. Chem.* **2022**, *10*, 1083596. [CrossRef]
21. Laib, I.; Ali, B.D.; Boudebia, O. Green synthesis of silver nanoparticles using Helianthemum lippii extracts (Hl-NPs): Characterization, antioxidant and antibacterial activities, and study of interaction with DNA. *J. Organomet. Chem.* **2023**, *986*, 122619. [CrossRef]
22. Laib, I.; Ali, B.D.; Alsalme, A.; Croun, D.; Bechelany, M.; Barhoum, A. Therapeutic potential of silver nanoparticles from Helianthemum lippii extract for mitigating cadmium-induced hepatotoxicity: Liver function parameters, oxidative stress, and histopathology in wistar rats. *Front. Bioeng. Biotechnol.* **2024**, *12*, 1400542. [CrossRef]
23. Plescia, F.; Venturella, F.; D'Anneo, A.; Catania, V.; Gargano, M.L.; Polito, G.; Schillaci, D.; Palumbo Piccionello, A.; Lauricella, M.; Venturella, G. Phytochemical-rich extracts of Helianthemum lippii possess antimicrobial, anticancer, and anti-biofilm activities. *Plant Biosyst.-Int. J. Deal. All Asp. Plant Biol.* **2022**, *156*, 1314–1324. [CrossRef]
24. Ibtissam, L.; Djahra, A.B. Phytochemical investigation of Helianthemum lippii l. aerial Dum. Cours part and evaluation for its antioxidant activities. *Int. J. Second. Metab.* **2022**, *9*, 229–237. [CrossRef]
25. Mahmoud, S.Y.; Alshammari, S.O. Bioactive compounds of methanolic extract of Helianthemum lippii grows in Hafr Al-Batin region, northeastern Saudi Arabia. *Acta Fytotech. Et Zootech.* **2022**, *25*, 60–66. [CrossRef]
26. Mouffouk, S.; Mouffouk, C.; Mouffouk, S.; Haba, H. Medicinal, Pharmacological and Biochemical Progress on the Study of Genus Helianthemum: A Review. *Curr. Chem. Biol.* **2023**, *17*, 147–159. [CrossRef]
27. Boutlelis, D.A.; Mounia, B.; Salah, B.; Hakim, B.; Rebiai, A.; Laib, I.; Chaima, B.; Djemaa, F.; Islam, R. Bio-Synthesis of Zinc Nanoparticle Using Helianthemum Lippii L. Extract and Improving in Rats Their Hepatoprotective Effects against Carbon Tetrachloride Induced Liver Damage. *Ann. Rom. Soc. Cell Biol.* **2022**, *26*, 1949–1963.
28. Ahmed, S.; Ahmad, M.; Swami, B.L.; Ikram, S. Green synthesis of silver nanoparticles using Azadirachta indica aqueous leaf extract. *J. Radiat. Res. Appl. Sci.* **2016**, *9*, 1–7. [CrossRef]
29. Mittal, A.K.; Kaler, A.; Banerjee, U.C. Free Radical Scavenging and Antioxidant Activity of Silver Nanoparticles Synthesized from Flower Extract of Rhododendron dauricum. *Nano Biomed. Eng.* **2012**, *4*, 118–124. [CrossRef]
30. Kılınçarslan Aksoy, Ö.; Seçme, M.; Mammadov, R. Antioxidant, cytotoxicity, apoptotic properties of extracts of andricus sternlichti galls and their phenolic characterisation by HPLC. *Chem. Biodivers.* **2023**, *20*, e202200742. [CrossRef]
31. Zielińska, D.; Zieliński, H.; Laparra-Llopis, J.M.; Szawara-Nowak, D.; Honke, J.; Giménez-Bastida, J.A. Caffeic acid modulates processes associated with intestinal inflammation. *Nutrients* **2021**, *13*, 554. [CrossRef]
32. Carrillo-Martinez, E.J.; Flores-Hernández, F.Y.; Salazar-Montes, A.M.; Nario-Chaidez, H.F.; Hernández-Ortega, L.D. Quercetin, a flavonoid with great pharmacological capacity. *Molecules* **2024**, *29*, 1000. [CrossRef]
33. Barhoum, A.; Van Assche, G.; Makhlouf, A.S.H.; Terryn, H.; Baert, K.; Delplancke, M.-P.; El-Sheikh, S.M.; Rahier, H. A green, simple chemical route for the synthesis of pure nanocalcite crystals. *Cryst. Growth Desig.* **2015**, *15*, 573–580. [CrossRef]
34. Ghasemi, S.; Dabirian, S.; Kariminejad, F.; Koohi, D.E.; Nemattalab, M.; Majidimoghadam, S.; Zamani, E.; Yousefbeyk, F. Process optimization for green synthesis of silver nanoparticles using Rubus discolor leaves extract and its biological activities against multi-drug resistant bacteria and cancer cells. *Sci. Rep.* **2024**, *14*, 4130. [CrossRef]
35. Khanal, L.N.; Sharma, K.R.; Paudyal, H.; Parajuli, K.; Dahal, B.; Ganga, G.; Pokharel, Y.R.; Kalauni, S.K. Green synthesis of silver nanoparticles from root extracts of Rubus ellipticus Sm. and comparison of antioxidant and antibacterial activity. *J. Nanomater.* **2022**, *2022*, 1832587. [CrossRef]
36. Asefian, S.; Ghavam, M. Green and environmentally friendly synthesis of silver nanoparticles with antibacterial properties from some medicinal plants. *BMC Biotechnol.* **2024**, *24*, 5. [CrossRef]
37. Poli, V.; Madduru, R.; Aparna, Y.; Kandukuri, V.; Motireddy, S.R. Amelioration of cadmium-induced oxidative damage in wistar rats by Vitamin C, zinc and N-acetylcysteine. *Med. Sci.* **2022**, *10*, 7. [CrossRef]
38. Pyatha, S.; Kim, H.; Lee, D.; Kim, K. Co-exposure to lead, mercury, and cadmium induces neurobehavioral impairments in mice by interfering with dopaminergic and serotonergic neurotransmission in the striatum. *Front. Public Health* **2023**, *11*, 1265864. [CrossRef]
39. Wu, Y.; Tian, W.; Cheng, C.; Yang, L.; Ye, Q.; Li, W.; Jiang, J. Effects of cadmium exposure on metabolism, antioxidant defense, immune function, and the hepatopancreas transcriptome of Cipangopaludina cathayensis. *Ecotoxicol. Environ. Saf.* **2023**, *264*, 115416. [CrossRef]
40. Liu, X.; Deng, Q.; Yang, H.; Wang, J.; Wang, M. Oxidative stress of Cadmium and Lead at environmentally relevant concentrations on hepatopancreas of macrobrachium nipponensis and their mixture interactivity: Implications for water quality criteria amendment. *Int. J. Environ. Res. Public Health* **2022**, *20*, 360. [CrossRef]
41. Winiarska-Mieczan, A. Protective effect of tannic acid on the brain of adult rats exposed to cadmium and lead. *Environ. Toxicol. Pharmacol.* **2013**, *36*, 9–18. [CrossRef]

42. Winiarska-Mieczan, A.; Krusiński, R.; Kwiecień, M. Tannic acid influence on lead and cadmium accumulation in the hearts and lungs of rats. *Adv. Clin. Exp. Med.* **2013**, *22*, 615–620.
43. Bem, E.M.; Piotrowski, J.K.; Sobczak-Kozlowska, M.; Dmuchowski, C. Cadmium, zinc, copper and metallothionein levels in human liver. *Int. Arch. Occup. Environ. Health* **1988**, *60*, 413–417. [CrossRef]
44. Sainath, S.; Meena, R.; Supriya, C.; Reddy, K.P.; Reddy, P.S. Protective role of Centella asiatica on lead-induced oxidative stress and suppressed reproductive health in male rats. *Environ. Toxicol. Pharmacol.* **2011**, *32*, 146–154. [CrossRef]
45. BarathManiKanth, S.; Kalishwaralal, K.; Sriram, M.; Pandian, S.R.K.; Youn, H.-s.; Eom, S.; Gurunathan, S. Anti-oxidant effect of gold nanoparticles restrains hyperglycemic conditions in diabetic mice. *J. Nanobiotechnol.* **2010**, *8*, 16. [CrossRef]
46. Majeed, M.; Hakeem, K.R.; Rehman, R.U. Synergistic effect of plant extract coupled silver nanoparticles in various therapeutic applications-present insights and bottlenecks. *Chemosphere* **2022**, *288*, 132527. [CrossRef]
47. Rehman, G.; Umar, M.; Shah, N.; Hamayun, M.; Ali, A.; Khan, W.; Khan, A.; Ahmad, S.; Alrefaei, A.F.; Almutairi, M.H. Green synthesis and characterization of silver nanoparticles using Azadirachta indica seeds extract: In vitro and in vivo evaluation of anti-diabetic activity. *Pharmaceuticals* **2023**, *16*, 1677. [CrossRef]
48. El-Baz, Y.G.; Moustafa, A.; Ali, M.A.; El-Desoky, G.E.; Wabaidur, S.M.; Iqbal, A. Green synthesized silver nanoparticles for the treatment of diabetes and the related complications of hyperlipidemia and oxidative stress in diabetic rats. *Exp. Biol. Med.* **2023**, *248*, 2237–2248. [CrossRef]
49. Liu, J.; Habeebu, S.S.; Liu, Y.; Klaassen, C.D. Acute CdMT Injection Is Not a Good Model to Study Chronic Cd Nephropathy: Comparison of Chronic CdCl2and CdMT Exposure with Acute CdMT Injection in Rats. *Toxicol. Appl. Pharmacol.* **1998**, *153*, 48–58. [CrossRef]
50. Uchida, N.S.; Silva-Filho, S.E.; Cardia, G.F.E.; Cremer, E.; Silva-Comar, F.M.d.S.; Silva, E.L.; Bersani-Amado, C.A.; Cuman, R.K.N. Hepatoprotective effect of citral on acetaminophen-induced liver toxicity in mice. *Evid.-Based Complement. Altern. Med.* **2017**, *2017*, 1796209. [CrossRef]
51. González-Gallego, J.; García-Mediavilla, M.V.; Sánchez-Campos, S.; Tuñón, M.J. Anti-inflammatory and immunomodulatory properties of dietary flavonoids. In *Polyphenols in Human Health and Disease*; Elsevier: Amsterdam, The Netherlands, 2014; pp. 435–452. [CrossRef]
52. Ozkan, G.; Ceyhan, T.; Çatalkaya, G.; Rajan, L.; Ullah, H.; Daglia, M.; Capanoglu, E. Encapsulated phenolic compounds: Clinical efficacy of a novel delivery method. *Phytochem. Rev.* **2024**, *23*, 1–39. [CrossRef]
53. Carmo de Carvalho e Martins, M.d.; da Silva Santos Oliveira, A.S.M.; da Silva, L.A.A.; Primo, M.G.S.; de Carvalho Lira, V.B. Biological indicators of oxidative stress [malondialdehyde, catalase, glutathione peroxidase, and superoxide dismutase] and their application in nutrition. In *Biomarkers in Nutrition*; Springer: Cham, Switzerland, 2022; pp. 1–25. [CrossRef]
54. Ebhohon, S.O.; Asoya, E.V.; Okwor, L.O.; Ezeokeke, C. Nephroprotective Effects of Aqueous Extract of Loranthus micranthus Linn Leaf Against Cadmium-Induced Kidney Toxicity in Male Rats. *J. Basics Appl. Sci. Res.* **2023**, *1*, 16–26. [CrossRef]
55. Albasher, G.; Albrahim, T.; Aljarba, N.; Alharbi, R.I.; Alsultan, N.; Alsaiari, J.; Rizwana, H. Involvement of redox status and the nuclear-related factor 2 in protecting against cadmium-induced renal injury with Sana Makki (*Cassia senna* L.) pre-treatment in male rats. *An. Acad. Bras. Cienc.* **2020**, *92*, e20191237. [CrossRef]
56. Laib, I.; Djahra, A.B. Phenolic Compound Profile And Evaluation Of Biological Activities Of The Crude Extract and Some Bioactive Compounds of *Helianthemum lippii* AERIAL PARTS. *Ann. Oradea Univ. Biol. Fascicle/Analele Univ. Din Oradea Fasc. Biologie.* **2023**, *30*, 117–124.
57. Abdallah, E.A.; Almilaibary, A.; El-Refaei, M.F. Fagonia indica ameliorates chromium-induced nephrotoxicity: Role of antioxidant activity and pro-inflammatory cytokines in in-vivo renoprotection. *Arch. Environ. Occup. Health* **2023**, *78*, 289–303. [CrossRef]
58. Salama, B.; Alzahrani, K.J.; Alghamdi, K.S.; Al-Amer, O.; Hassan, K.E.; Elhefny, M.A.; Albarakati, A.J.A.; Alharthi, F.; Althagafi, H.A.; Al Sberi, H. Silver nanoparticles enhance oxidative stress, inflammation, and apoptosis in liver and kidney tissues: Potential protective role of thymoquinone. *Biol. Trace Elem. Res.* **2023**, *201*, 2942–2954. [CrossRef]
59. Guo, A.H.; Kumar, S.; Lombard, D.B. Epigenetic mechanisms of cadmium-induced nephrotoxicity. *Curr. Opin. Toxicol.* **2022**, *32*, 100372. [CrossRef]
60. Karami, E.; Goodarzi, Z.; Ghanbari, A.; Bandegi, A.R.; Yosefi, S.; Dehdashti, A. In vivo antioxidant and kidney protective potential of Atorvastatin against cadmium chloride-induced kidney injury in male Wistar rat. *All Life* **2022**, *15*, 1025–1036. [CrossRef]
61. Dkhil, M.A.; Diab, M.S.; Lokman, M.S.; El-Sayed, H.; Bauomy, A.A.; Al-Shaebi, E.M.; Al-Quraishy, S. Nephroprotective effect of Pleurotus ostreatus extract against cadmium chloride toxicity in rats. *An. Acad. Bras. Ciências* **2020**, *92*, e20191121. [CrossRef]
62. Djahra, A.B.; Lmhanat, I.; Benkaddour, M.; Benkherara, S.; Laib, I.; Benine, C. Traditional Herbal Remedies from Algeria for Treating Digestive Disorders. *J. Drug Deliv. Ther.* **2023**, *13*, 84–92. [CrossRef]
63. Kukreti, N.; Chitme, H.R.; Varshney, V.K.; Abdel-Wahab, B.A.; Khateeb, M.M.; Habeeb, M.S. Antioxidant properties mediate nephroprotective and hepatoprotective activity of essential oil and hydro-alcoholic extract of the high-altitude plant Skimmia anquetilia. *Antioxidants* **2023**, *12*, 1167. [CrossRef]
64. Gao, C.; Liu, C.; Chen, Y.; Wang, Q.; Hao, Z. Protective effects of natural products against drug-induced nephrotoxicity: A review in recent years. *Food Chem. Toxicol.* **2021**, *153*, 112255. [CrossRef]
65. Kotcherlakota, R.; Das, S.; Patra, C.R. Therapeutic applications of green-synthesized silver nanoparticles. In *Green Synthesis, Characterization and Applications of Nanoparticles*; Elsevier: Amsterdam, The Netherlands, 2019; pp. 389–428. [CrossRef]

66. Zhang, L.; Wu, L.; Mi, Y.; Si, Y. Silver nanoparticles induced cell apoptosis, membrane damage of Azotobacter vinelandii and Nitrosomonas europaea via generation of reactive oxygen species. *Bull. Environ. Contam. Toxicol.* **2019**, *103*, 181–186. [CrossRef]
67. Ibtissam, L.; Boutlilis, D.A. Interaction Study of Greenly Synthesized Silver Nanoparticles with Bovine Serum Albumin (BSA) Using Spectrophotometric and Voltammetric Assays. *Curr. Trends Biotechnol. Pharm.* **2023**, *17*, 1013–1019. [CrossRef]
68. Wei, L.; Lu, J.; Xu, H.; Patel, A.; Chen, Z.-S.; Chen, G. Silver nanoparticles: Synthesis, properties, and therapeutic applications. *Drug Discov. Today* **2015**, *20*, 595–601. [CrossRef] [PubMed]
69. Budha Magar, A.; Shrestha, D.; Pakka, S.; Sharma, K.R. Phytochemistry, biological, and toxicity study on aqueous and methanol extracts of Chromolaena odorata. *Sci. World J.* **2023**, *2023*, 6689271. [CrossRef]
70. Ouandaogo, H.S.; Diallo, S.; Odari, E.; Kinyua, J. Phytochemical Screening and GC-MS Analysis of Methanolic and Aqueous Extracts of Ocimum kilimandscharicum Leaves. *ACS Omega* **2023**, *8*, 47560–47572. [CrossRef] [PubMed]
71. Nhon Hoang, T.N.; Phan, T.T.; Lien Phan, T.K.; Van Nguyen, N.H.; Dao Dong, T.A.; Anh Le, T.H. Phytochemical Screening, Extraction, and Determination of the Bioactivities of the Extract-Enriched Polyphenols and Saponins from Musa balbisiana Fruit. *J. Food Process. Preserv.* **2023**, *2023*, 2581641. [CrossRef]
72. Mokhtar, L.M.; Salim, I.A.; Alotaibi, S.N.; Awaji, E.A.; Alotaibi, M.M.; Doman, A.O. Phytochemical Screening and Antimicrobial Activity of Methanolic Extract of *Cymbopogon schoenanthus* (L.)(azkhar) Collected from Afif City, Saudi Arabia. *Life* **2023**, *13*, 1451. [CrossRef]
73. Sadeq, O.; Mechchate, H.; Es-Safi, I.; Bouhrim, M.; Jawhari, F.; Ouassou, H.; Kharchoufa, L.; AlZain, M.; Alzamel, N.; Al Kamaly, O.M. Phytochemical Screening, Antioxidant and Antibacterial Activities of Pollen Extracts from Micromeria Fruticosa, Achillea Fragrantissima, and Phoenix Dactylifera. *Plants* **2021**, *10*, 676. [CrossRef]
74. Gacem, M.A.; Telli, A.; Gacem, H.; Ould-El-Hadj-Khelil, A. Phytochemical screening, antifungal and antioxidant activities of three medicinal plants from Algerian steppe and Sahara (preliminary screening studies). *SN Appl. Sci.* **2019**, *1*, 1721. [CrossRef]
75. Nisa, H.; Kamili, A.N.; Bandh, S.A.; Lone, B.A.; Parray, J.A. Phytochemical screening, antimicrobial and antioxidant efficacy of different extracts of Rumex dentatus L.–a locally used medicinal herb of Kashmir Himalaya. *Asian Pac. J. Trop. Dis.* **2013**, *3*, 434–440. [CrossRef]
76. María, R.; Shirley, M.; Xavier, C.; Jaime, S.; David, V.; Rosa, S.; Jodie, D. Preliminary phytochemical screening, total phenolic content and antibacterial activity of thirteen native species from Guayas province Ecuador. *J. King Saud Univ.-Sci.* **2018**, *30*, 500–505. [CrossRef]
77. Saeed, R.A.; Khan, M.I.; Butt, M.S.; Faisal, M.N. Phytochemical screening of Prunus avium for its antioxidative and anti-mutagenic potential against DMBA-induced hepatocarcinogenesis. *Front. Nutr.* **2023**, *10*, 1132356. [CrossRef]
78. Singh, A.; Dar, M.Y.; Joshi, B.; Sharma, B.; Shrivastava, S.; Shukla, S. Phytofabrication of silver nanoparticles: Novel drug to overcome hepatocellular ailments. *Toxicol. Rep.* **2018**, *5*, 333–342. [CrossRef]
79. Aguwa, U.; Eze, C.; Obinwa, B.; Okeke, S.; Onwuelingo, S.; Okonkwo, D.; Ogbuokiri, D.; Agulanna, A.; Obiesie, I.; Umezulike, A. Comparing the effect of methods of rat euthanasia on the brain of Wistar rats: Cervical dislocation, chloroform inhalation, diethyl ether inhalation and formalin inhalation. *J. Adv. Med. Med. Res.* **2020**, *32*, 8–16. [CrossRef]
80. Kongara, K.; McIlhone, A.; Kells, N.; Johnson, C. Electroencephalographic evaluation of decapitation of the anaesthetized rat. *Lab. Anim.* **2014**, *48*, 15–19. [CrossRef]
81. Lee, W.-K.; Probst, S.; Scharner, B.; Deba, T.; Dahdouh, F.; Thévenod, F. Distinct concentration-dependent oxidative stress profiles by cadmium in a rat kidney proximal tubule cell line. *Arch. Toxicol.* **2024**, *98*, 1043–1059. [CrossRef]
82. Ma, Y.; Su, Q.; Yue, C.; Zou, H.; Zhu, J.; Zhao, H.; Song, R.; Liu, Z. The effect of oxidative stress-induced autophagy by cadmium exposure in kidney, liver, and bone damage, and neurotoxicity. *Int. J. Mol. Sci.* **2022**, *23*, 13491. [CrossRef]

pharmaceuticals

MDPI

Article

The Impact of Silver Nanoparticles Functionalized with Spirulina Protein Extract on Rats

Ludmila Rudi [1,*], Inga Zinicovscaia [2,3], Liliana Cepoi [1], Tatiana Chiriac [1], Dmitrii Grozdov [2] and Alexandra Kravtsova [2]

1 Institute of Microbiology and Biotechnology, Technical University of Moldova, MD 2028 Chisinau, Moldova; liliana.cepoi@imb.utm.md (L.C.); tatiana.chiriac@imb.utm.md (T.C.)
2 Joint Institute for Nuclear Research, Joliot-Curie 6, 141980 Dubna, Russia; zinikovskaia@mail.ru (I.Z.); dsgrozdov@rambler.ru (D.G.); alexkravtsova@yandex.ru (A.K.)
3 Horia Hulubei National Institute for RD in Physics and Nuclear Engineering, 30, Str. Reactorului, 077125 Magurele, Romania
* Correspondence: ludmila.rudi@imb.utm.md

Abstract: Background/Objectives: This study investigates the biocompatibility and physiological impacts of silver nanoparticles (AgNPs) functionalized with Spirulina protein extract (SPE) on laboratory rats. The objective was to assess and compare the systemic distribution, organ accumulation, and changes in hematological and biochemical parameters between biofunctionalized and non-functionalized silver nanoparticles. **Methods:** AgNPs were functionalized with SPE. Adult Wistar rats were administered these nanoparticles to assess their distribution across various organs using ICP-MS analysis. Hematological and biochemical markers were measured to evaluate systemic effects. **Results**: Functionalized silver nanoparticles demonstrated preferential accumulation in the brain, liver, and testicles, with significant clearance observed post-administration. The persistence of AgNPs SPE in reproductive organs was established. Hematological analysis revealed moderate changes, suggesting mild immune activation. Biochemical tests indicated transient increases in liver enzymes, signaling reversible hepatic stress. **Conclusions**: The biofunctionalization of AgNPs with Spirulina protein extract modifies the nanoparticles' systemic behavior and organ distribution, enhancing their biocompatibility while inducing minimal physiological stress. These findings support the potential of Spirulina-based coatings to mitigate the toxicity and enhance the therapeutic efficacy of nanomedical agents.

Keywords: silver nanoparticles; biofunctionalization; Spirulina protein extract; rats; organ accumulation; hematological indicators; biochemical indicators

1. Introduction

Silver nanoparticles have become an increasingly widespread area of research and application due to their essential capabilities in medicine, industry, and consumer products. Due to their antimicrobial efficacy, AgNPs are widely used in various products such as toothbrushes and toothpaste, food packaging, and others [1,2]. Additionally, AgNPs have shown potential as vaccine adjuvants, enhancing their effectiveness [3].

AgNPs, with their antibacterial, anti-inflammatory, and potential anticancer activities, are integrated into numerous medical fields [4]. Their role in combating multidrug-resistant bacteria is particularly noteworthy [5]. In wound treatment, AgNPs are a valuable tool used in dressings and gels to prevent infections and accelerate healing [6].

Due to their unique contrast properties, AgNPs are being explored in oncology as therapeutic agents for destroying cancer cells through cytotoxic mechanisms and medical imaging [7,8]. Additionally, in medical diagnostics, AgNPs are used in biosensors and diagnostic platforms to rapidly and precisely detect pathogens or specific biomarkers [7].

The therapeutic properties of AgNPs are influenced by their physicochemical characteristics, such as size, shape, size distribution, dose, origin, mode of administration, and specific surface area [9]. These characteristics determine their biological activity, stability in different environments, and ability to interact with molecules and cells. The functionalization of nanoparticles plays a crucial role in optimizing these properties, influencing their reactivity, stability, aggregation, bioavailability, and toxicity. For example, nanoparticles functionalized with thiobarbituric acid exhibit improved dispersibility and increased stability in aqueous solutions, while those functionalized with 11-mercaptoundecanoic acid and chitosan modify protein interactions and have slightly reduced toxicity [10,11].

By adjusting the size and coating of nanoparticles, it is possible to develop AgNPs that are optimized for specific applications [12]. Controlled surface functionalization of nanoparticles with various biomolecules, such as peptides or proteins, can prevent aggregation and enhance antimicrobial effects [13,14]. An effective method of biofunctionalizing silver nanoparticles is their synthesis using biological materials, where the reducing substrate largely determines the final properties of the AgNPs [15]. Different biological substrates can serve as matrices for synthesizing AgNPs with valuable properties. For example, nanoparticles synthesized using extracts from *Cuminum cyminum* L. seeds have shown reduced toxicity and anticancer properties [16]. Silver nanoparticles synthesized using extracts from the cyanobacterium *Spirulina platensis* have demonstrated antibacterial effects against *S. aureus* and *E. coli* [17]. Similarly, nanoparticles synthesized with aloe vera gel extract have exhibited antifungal effects and 100% inhibition of mice's B16F10 melanoma cell line [18]. Silver nanoparticles obtained using flavonoid extracts from *Perilla frutescens* have significantly inhibited Gram-positive and Gram-negative bacterial pathogens and anticancer effects in colon cancer [19]. Nanoparticles synthesized using *Solanum nigrum* and *Pouteria sapota* extracts have shown potential for reducing blood sugar levels in diabetic animals [20]. The variability in the antibacterial effect of AgNPs is attributed to the biological components on the surface of the nanoparticles, which can influence their antibacterial mechanisms [5].

Conjugating AgNPs with bioactive molecules such as peptides, antibodies, or drugs is another crucial aspect of functionalization, essential for developing targeted delivery systems or enhancing therapeutic efficacy [21,22]. For example, conjugating AgNPs with Amoxicillin offers a promising strategy for combating antibiotic-resistant bacterial strains [23]. Silver nanoparticles conjugated with C-phycocyanin have shown effectiveness in healing dermal wounds, reducing erythrocyte toxicity, and benefiting from antibacterial properties [24].

Spirulina platensis, a cyanobacterium known for its antioxidant, anti-inflammatory, and immunomodulatory properties, is used in multiple biomedical applications [25,26]. Due to its rich composition of proteins, polysaccharides, and pigments, Spirulina reduces support for functionalizing and conjugating nanoparticles [27,28]. The interaction with nanoparticles allows Spirulina's biological components to provide stability and biocompatibility while simultaneously reducing the potential toxicity of the nanoparticles [17].

This study investigated the accumulation characteristics and the changes in hematological and biochemical parameters in laboratory rats resulting from administering citrate-stabilized silver nanoparticles biofunctionalized with Spirulina protein extract, compared to non-functionalized citrate-stabilized nanoparticles.

2. Results

2.1. Composition of Spirulina Protein Extract (SPE)

Table 1 presents the amino acid composition of the Spirulina protein extract (SPE). The extract contains a variety of essential amino acids (histidine, isoleucine, leucine, lysine, methionine, phenylalanine, threonine, tryptophan, and valine) and non-essential amino acids (alanine, arginine, aspartic acid, cysteine, glutamic acid, glycine, proline, serine, and tyrosine). The total extracted protein content was 52%. Non-essential amino acids constitute 68.68% (35.71 mg/100 mg extract), while essential amino acids comprise 31.32% (16.28 mg/100 mg extract).

Table 1. Amino acids composition of the Spirulina protein extract (SPE).

Amino Acid	Protein Extract from Spirulina (SPE)	
	mg/100 mg Extract	% Total Extract
Alanine	4.28	8.23
Arginine	5.58	10.73
Asparagine	0.00	0.00
Aspartic acid	5.02	9.66
Cysteine	1.14	2.19
Glutamic acid	9.04	17.39
Glutamine	0.00	0.00
Glycine	2.88	5.54
Histidine *	0.81	1.56
Isoleucine *	0.08	0.15
Leucine *	5.12	9.85
Lysine *	3.16	6.08
Methionine *	0.15	0.29
Phenylalanine *	2.27	4.37
Proline	2.03	3.90
Threonine *	2.59	4.98
Tryptophan *	0.19	0.37
Serine	3.06	5.89
Tyrosine	2.68	5.15
Valine *	1.91	3.67
Total	51.99	100.00

* Essential amino acids.

Glutamic acid is the most abundant non-essential amino acid, at 9.04 mg/100 mg extract (17.39% of the total amino acids). The extract also contains significant amounts of arginine (5.58 mg/100 mg extract or 10.77%) and aspartic acid (5.02 mg/100 mg extract or 9.66%). Among the essential amino acids, leucine is in the highest concentration (5.12 mg/100 mg extract or 9.85%). Lysine (3.16 mg/100 mg extract or 6.08%) and threonine (2.59 mg/100 mg extract or 4.98%) were also detected in substantial amounts. Methionine (0.15 mg/100 mg extract or 0.29%) and tryptophan (0.19 mg/100 mg extract or 0.37%) were the least concentrated among the essential amino acids. Asparagine and glutamine were not detected in the SPE.

2.2. *Characteristics of Silver Nanoparticles Biofunctionalized with Spirulina Protein Extract*

2.2.1. FTIR Spectra

Figure 1 presents FTIR spectra for the Spirulina protein extract (SPE) and the suspension formed from silver nanoparticles functionalized with this extract (AgNPs-SPE). These spectra highlight the complex interactions between the nanoparticles and protein components through shifts and changes in the intensities of specific bands.

Both spectra exhibit several characteristic bands. The bands at 3138 cm^{-1} and 3050 cm^{-1}, specific to the SPE spectrum, correspond to the stretching vibrations of O-H and N-H bonds found in proteins. The band at 2853 cm^{-1} corresponds to the stretching vibrations of C-H bonds from alkyl groups and is common in aliphatic side chains of proteins. The bands at 1657 cm^{-1} and 1618 cm^{-1} are crucial for characterizing the secondary structure of proteins. They are specific to Amide I and Amide II, corresponding to the stretching vibrations of C=O and N-H bonds in peptide structures. The band at 1403 cm^{-1} corresponds to the symmetric stretching vibrations of the COO^- group in amino acids.

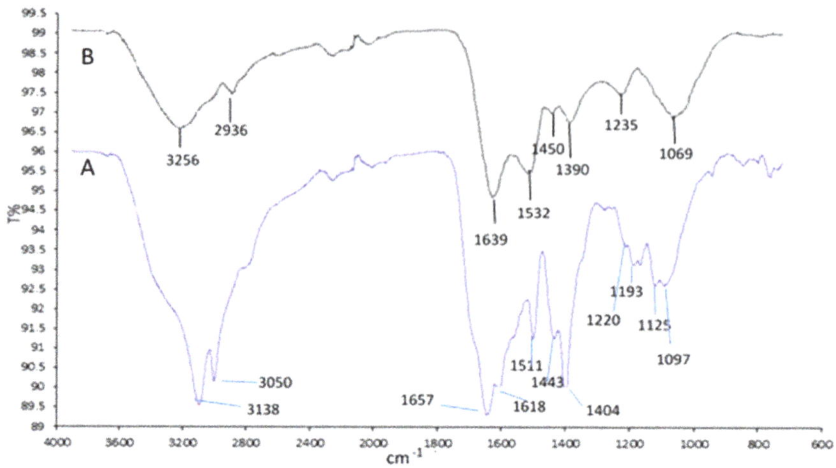

Figure 1. FTIR spectra of (A) Spirulina protein extract (SPE) and (B) the functional mixture AgNPs-SPE.

In the "fingerprint" region, the band at 1284 cm^{-1} is typically associated with C-N stretching vibrations in amines or Amide III. In the frequency range of 1218–1125 cm^{-1}, functional groups are often associated with the stretching vibrations of C-O or C-N bonds, which appear in amide groups or etheric and alcoholic structures within proteins. Bands in the 1200–1000 cm^{-1} range are associated with C-O and C-N vibrations within the protein structure. This region provides specific details about the chemical composition of the analyzed protein extract.

The FTIR spectrum of the AgNPs-SPE mixture recorded a shift in bands in the 3200–2800 cm^{-1} region compared to the protein extract SPE. The addition of citrate-stabilized AgNPs caused a change in -OH and -NH bands, possibly due to the formation of hydrogen bonds and electrostatic interactions between proteins and nanoparticles. As a result, characteristic SPE bands, such as those at 3138 cm^{-1} and 3050 cm^{-1}, were shifted or reduced in intensity in the case of AgNPs-SPE. Additionally, new bands appeared at 2920 cm^{-1} and 2936 cm^{-1} in the AgNPs-SPE spectrum, indicating interactions between Ag nanoparticles and the aliphatic side chains of the protein. This may suggest a rearrangement of C-H structures in the presence of nanoparticles.

The shift of bands from 1637 to 1639 cm^{-1} and 1532 to 1534 cm^{-1} represents changes in the Amide I and II regions, suggesting a direct interaction between AgNPs and the protein backbone. The stabilizing citrate may bind proteins through electrostatic interactions, altering C=O and N-H bonds.

The "fingerprint" region was entirely altered. For instance, the peak at 1403 cm^{-1}, characteristic of the COO^- group in proteins, diminished in the presence of nanoparticles, suggesting interactions with citrate. The band at 1390 cm^{-1}, which could be attributed to O-H interactions, reflects a modification in protein structure after interaction with citrate-stabilized nanoparticles. The band at 1235 cm^{-1}, corresponding to N-H vibrations, may indicate changes in the amide bonds of the protein due to the formation of the complex with nanoparticles.

In the presence of silver nanoparticles, the bands at 1284 cm^{-1} and 1218–1125 cm^{-1} changed in intensity due to the formation of electrostatic and/or hydrogen bonds between AgNPs and the protein substrate, which altered the initial vibrations of the C-N or C-O bonds.

In the 1062–1069 cm^{-1} region, associated with the S=O group in proteins, the peak at 1069 cm^{-1} was accentuated, suggesting the binding of nanoparticles to sulfate functional groups in Spirulina proteins.

2.2.2. UV-VIS

The UV-Vis spectra presented in Figure 2 display characteristic maxima for protein extract obtained from Spirulina biomass (SPE) and highlight the alteration (deformation) of the spectrum in the functional mixture AgNP-SPE. The peaks identified at 230 nm and 280 nm (Figure 2A) are characteristic of proteins derived from Spirulina biomass, with the peak at 280 nm attributed to the presence of aromatic amino acids, reflecting the presence of these structures in the tested protein extract. The deformation of the absorption spectrum, with variations appearing in the 340–400 nm range (Figure 2B), can be attributed to interactions between the silver nanoparticles and the protein components in the Spirulina extract. The UV-Vis spectrum is crucial for characterizing the specific plasmon resonance of silver nanoparticles. These small fluctuations suggest interactions between the nanoparticles and the biological matrix.

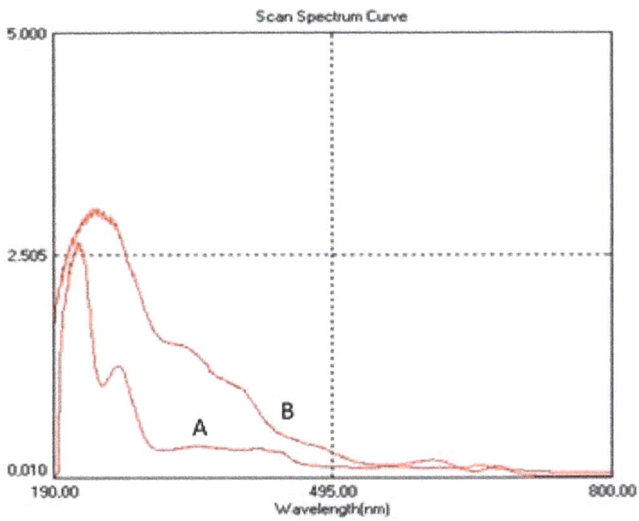

Figure 2. UV-Vis absorption spectra of (A) Spirulina protein extract (SPE) and (B) functional mixture AgNPs-SPE.

2.2.3. Antioxidant Activity Stability of SPE and AgNPs-SPE

The antioxidant activity of the SPE and the AgNPs-SPE mixture was monitored over 30 days from the preparation of the mixture. It was established that the functional mixture underwent a stabilization period lasting 5 days. Initially, the mixture exhibited antioxidant values 47.7% higher than the protein matrix. On the third day, the reduction capacity of AgNPs-SPE was 82.6% above the value of SPE. By the fifth day, the antioxidant activity had decreased and was 27.3% higher. Subsequently, monitoring of antioxidant activity showed stability in the DPPH test values. The DPPH reduction capacity of AgNPs-SPE was 34.4–42% higher than the antioxidant activity of SPE (Figure 3).

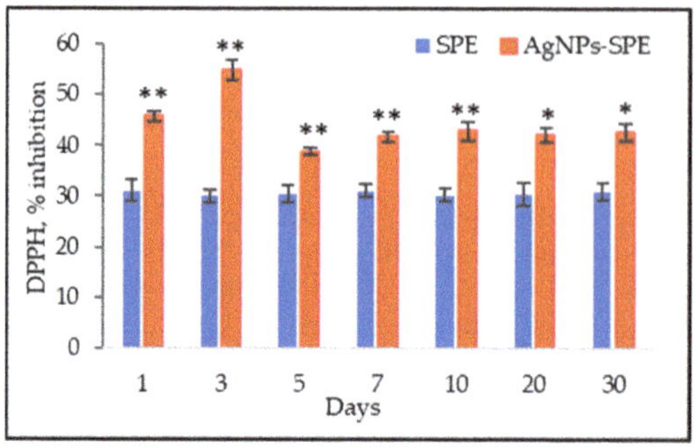

Figure 3. Antioxidant activity (DPPH, % inhibition) of Spirulina protein extract (SPE) and functional mixture (AgNPs-SPE) monitored over 30 days. * $p < 0.05$ and ** $p < 0.01$ indicate a significant difference between adjacent groups.

2.3. Silver Accumulation in Animal Organs

The content of silver in animal organs following administration of AgNPs and AgNP-SPE is presented in Figure 4.

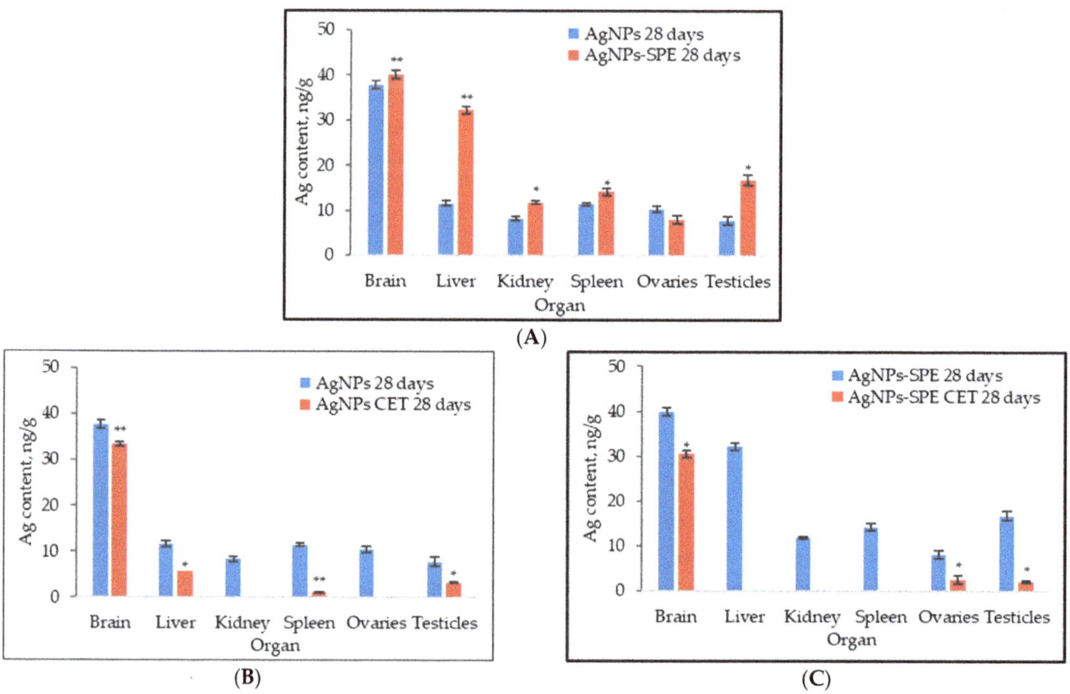

Figure 4. The content of silver in rats' organs: (**A**) animals administered AgNPs and AgNPs-SPE for 28 days, measured immediately after the end of the experiment; (**B**) animals administered AgNPs for 28 days with measurements taken after a clearance expiration time (CET, 28 days); (**C**) animals administered AgNPs-SPE for 28 days with measurements taken after a clearance expiration time (CET, 28 days). * $p < 0.05$ and ** $p < 0.01$ indicate a significant difference between adjacent groups.

Silver was detected in all examined organs of the laboratory animals. As observed in Figure 4A, the metal from AgNP-SPE accumulated in organs in larger quantities. The highest silver content was found in brain tissue, followed by the liver, testes, spleen, kidneys, and ovaries. Similarly, silver from non-functionalized nanoparticles also accumulated significantly in brain tissue, followed by the liver, spleen, ovaries, kidneys, and testes. In the case of nanoparticles functionalized with Spirulina protein extract, the silver detected in the liver was 2.76 times higher ($p < 0.01$) compared to the silver content from non-functionalized nanoparticles in the same organ. A similar effect was observed for the amount of metal accumulated in the testes, which was 2.12 times higher ($p < 0.05$) following the administration of AgNP-SPE. The kidneys ranked second to last in silver accumulation in both groups.

Figure 4B presents the results of eliminating non-functionalized AgNPs from organs at the end of the 28-day clearance period. Minimal amounts of silver were eliminated from brain tissue. Although the difference in silver content before and after the clearance period was statistically significant, only 10.7% of the accumulated silver was eliminated from the brain. The amount of metal in the liver decreased by 51.2% and in the testes by 57.3%. Silver was eliminated from the kidneys and ovaries.

Figure 4C shows the results obtained after the clearance period following the administration of AgNP-SPE. Silver was eliminated from the liver, kidneys, and spleen. In the brain, 24% of the silver was eliminated ($p < 0.05$). In the ovaries, 24.3% ($p < 0.05$) of the accumulated metal remained, and in the testes, 12.3% ($p < 0.05$) remained.

2.4. Hematological and Biochemical Indicators in Animals

2.4.1. Hematological Indicators

Table 2 shows the results of hematological tests conducted on animals from the four groups after 28 days of nanoparticle administration. The tests were performed immediately after the animals were sacrificed.

Table 2. Hematological indices in rats.

Experimental Group	C (−)		AgNPs	
Animal Sex	Male	Female	Male	Female
HB g/L	153.25 ± 5.32	160.67 ± 4.04	155.0 ± 1.15	152.30 ± 2.31 *
RBC, 10^{12}/L	8.73 ± 0.34	8.83 ± 0.28	8.58 ± 0.21	8.14 ± 0.09 *
WBC, 10^{9}/L	18.07 ± 2.41	15.76 ± 2.51	16.75 ± 3.12	13.56 ± 0.84
PLT, 10^{9}/L	505.0 ± 101.22	626.0 ± 232.0	613.50 ± 32.21 *	633.0 ± 43.30
PMN, %	31.79 ± 6.80	24.33 ± 4.15	22.08 ± 6.17 *	24.0 ± 0.17
LY, %	56.30 ± 8.12	58.87 ± 3.35	60.68 ± 3.99	61.2 ± 5.02
MON, %	6.03 ± 1.84	9.50 ± 0.46	8.38 ± 0.61 *	6.20 ± 1.25 *
EOS, %	4.45 ± 0.30	6.73 ± 1.50	8.3 ± 2.55 *	8.07 ± 1.95 *
BAS, %	0.58 ± 0.33	0.47 ± 0.38	3.83 ± 0.60 **	0.64 ± 0.23 *
RET, %	3.35 ± 0.37	3.35 ± 1.81	2.92 ± 0.13 *	4.03 ± 0.44
Experimental Group	**C (+)**		**AgNPs-SPE**	
Animal Sex	**Male**	**Female**	**Male**	**Female**
HB g/L	151.25 ± 5.50	151.33 ± 4.51	152.75 ± 3.50	138.0 ± 10.39 *
RBC, 10^{12}/L	8.11 ± 0.43	8.19 ± 0.41	8.41 ± 0.13	7.87 ± 0.31 *
WBC, 10^{9}/L	12.59 ± 3.69	12.92 ± 4.08	14.24 ± 3.19	12.02 ± 2.23
PLT, 10^{9}/L	523.25 ± 116.25	672.0 ± 77.09	490.75 ± 125.65	643.33 ± 198.94
PMN, %	25.08 ± 9.41	24.77 ± 1.46	26.63 ± 2.55	35.67 ± 9.58 *
LY, %	56.40 ± 11.97	62.47 ± 2.63	53.83 ± 1.99	52.17 ± 5.83
MON, %	6.70 ± 3.11	8.23 ± 1.75	7.62 ± 1.60	8.70 ± 1.73
EOS, %	5.56 ± 0.82	7.23 ± 2.29	5.38 ± 0.37	5.10 ± 0.52
BAS, %	0.68 ± 0.10	0.30 ± 0.10	3.30 ± 1.41 *	0.67 ± 0.29 *
RET, %	3.43 ± 0.45	3.97 ± 1.19	4.13 ± 0.25 *	7.54 ± 0.76 *

C (−)—negative control; C (+)—positive control (Spirulina protein extract); AgNPs—experimental group administered with silver nanoparticles; AgNPs-SPE—experimental group administered with silver nanoparticles functionalized with Spirulina protein extract; HB—hemoglobin; RBC—erythrocytes; WBC—leukocytes; PLT—platelets; PMN—polymorphomultinuclear neutrophil granulocytes; LY—lymphocytes; EOS—eosinophils; BAS—basophils; MON—monocytes; RET—reticulocyte; $n = 4$ for male; $n = 3$ for female; * $p < 0.05$; ** $p < 0.01$.

Table 2 indicates that, in the group of female rats administered AgNPs, hematological indicators showed a slight decrease in hemoglobin levels and erythrocyte (RBC) count ($p < 0.05$). A 33.0% increase in monocyte (MON) count ($p < 0.05$) and a 12.8% decrease in reticulocyte (RET) count ($p < 0.05$) were observed. In male rats, a 21.5% increase in platelet (PLT) count ($p < 0.05$) and a 30.5% reduction in polymorphonuclear neutrophils (PMN) ($p < 0.05$) were recorded. Both male and female rats showed an increase in eosinophil (EOS) and basophil (BAS) counts. In males, the EOS count increased by 86.52% ($p < 0.05$) and the BAS count increased 6.6-fold ($p < 0.01$), while in females, the EOS count increased by 19.9% and the BAS count by 36.3%. In the female group, the monocyte count was 34.7% lower ($p < 0.05$) compared to the control group, while in males, this indicator was 39% higher. In males, the reticulocyte count decreased by 22% ($p < 0.05$), whereas in females, it increased by 20%. In the female rats administered the AgNP-SPE, hematological indicators showed a slight reduction in hemoglobin levels and erythrocyte count ($p < 0.05$). A 44.0% increase in PMN count was observed ($p < 0.05$). An increase in BAS and RET counts was noted in both male and female rats. In males, the BAS count increased 4.84-fold ($p < 0.05$), while in females, it doubled ($p < 0.05$). The reticulocyte count showed a 20.4% increase ($p < 0.05$) in the male group and a 90% increase ($p < 0.05$) in the female group.

2.4.2. Biochemical Indicators

Table 3 shows the biochemical test results for animals from the four groups after 28 days of nanoparticle administration. The tests were performed immediately after the animals were sacrificed.

Table 3. Biochemical indices in rats.

Experiment Group	**C (−)**		**AgNPs**	
Animal Sex	**Male**	**Female**	**Male**	**Female**
Prot, g/L	58.55 ± 7.09	59.53 ± 4.51	60.75 ± 3.72	57.43 ± 3.27
Glu, mmol/L	4.93 ± 0.35	6.22 ± 0.40	5.26 ± 0.64	5.76 ± 0.75
CREA, μM/L	92.76 ± 20.03	84.97 ± 4.04	161.40 ± 19.13 *	170.30 ± 16.8 **
Urea mg/dL	29.35 ± 8.76	28.62 ± 6.81	28.91 ± 4.69	26.57 ± 4.41
ALT, U/L	173.6 ± 9.08	103.45 ± 8.60	237.45 ± 25.63 *	201.83 ± 47.89 *
AST, U/L	3.57 ± 0.86	3.57 ± 0.12	4.63 ± 0.13 *	7.23 ± 1.79 *
Experiment Group	**C (+)**		**AgNPs-SPE**	
Animal Sex	**Male**	**Female**	**Male**	**Female**
Prot, g/L	66.13 ± 2.29	61.57 ± 9.74	60.73 ± 3.55	57.33 ± 9.67
Glu, mmol/L	6.33 ± 0.51	5.26 ± 0.91	5.86 ± 0.76	3.76 ± 1.22 *
CREA, μM/L	105.60 ± 4.16	94.60 ± 4.30	176.4 ± 4.16 **	168.90 ± 4.21 **
Urea mg/dL	24.75 ± 6.95	26.57 ± 5.63	27.60 ± 4.61	27.16 ± 5.33
ALT, U/L	197.45 ± 39.07	168.07 ± 67.32	178,68 ± 12.23	227.50 ± 1.66 **
AST, U/L	3.07 ± 2.22	2.53 ± 1.79	4.83 ± 5.24 *	5.13 ± 1.01 *

C (−)—negative control; C (+)—positive control (Spirulina protein extract); AgNPs—experimental group administered silver nanoparticles; AgNPs-SPE—experimental group administered silver nanoparticles functionalized with Spirulina protein extract; Prot—total protein; Glu—glucose; CREA—creatinine; ALT—alanine aminotransferase; AST—aspartate aminotransferase; $n = 4$ for male; $n = 3$ for female; * $p < 0.05$; ** $p < 0.01$.

An increase in blood creatinine levels was observed in the experimental animal group. In males, the increase was 34% ($p < 0.05$), while in the female group, it was 2.5 times higher ($p < 0.05$). Elevated liver function indicators were also recorded (Table 3). ALT levels in males were 36.8% higher ($p < 0.05$) and 95% higher ($p < 0.05$) in females compared to the control group. AST levels increased by 29.7% ($p < 0.05$) in males and by 2.2 times ($p < 0.05$) in females.

A rise in blood creatinine levels was also observed in the rats administered AgNPs functionalized with Spirulina protein extract. In males, creatinine levels were 67% higher ($p < 0.01$), and in females, it was 78.5% higher ($p < 0.05$). In the female group, blood glucose levels were reduced, which remained within normal limits. Additionally, elevated liver function indicators were determined. In males, ALT levels did not change. In females, ALT increased by 35.4% ($p < 0.01$). AST levels increased by 57.3% ($p < 0.05$) in males and by 2.2 times ($p < 0.05$) in females.

2.4.3. Hematological and Biochemical Indices in Animals after 28 Days of AgNPs Administration and Following the 28-Day Clearance Period

Calculations were performed for the entire group, which consisted of three males and two females, to analyze the changes in hematological and biochemical indices in animals. For an appropriate comparison, values were also calculated for the experimental group of four males and three females, sacrificed 28 days after nanoparticle administration. The results of these calculations are presented in Tables 4 and 5.

Table 4. Hematological indices in rats after 28 days of AgNPs and AgNPs-SPE administration and a 28-day clearance period.

Indices	C (−)	AgNPs	AgNPs CET	C (+)	AgNPs-SPE	AgNPs-SPE CET
HB g/L	156.43 ± 5.94	153.86 ± 2.11	154.00 ± 1.87	145.57 ± 7.14	146.43 ± 10.2	150.0 ± 1.41
RBC, 10^{12}/L	8.77 ± 0.30	8.39 ± 0.28	8.41 ± 0.29	8.15 ± 0.38	8.18 ± 0.35	8.05 ± 0.50
WBC, 10^9/L	17.08 ± 2.55	15.38 ± 2.83 *	14.84 ± 2.68	12.73 ± 3.52	13.29 ± 2.86	15.70 ± 2.08
PLT, 10^9/L	556.8 ± 165.6	623.5 ± 37.7	621.4 ± 35.5	587.0 ± 122.7	556.1 ± 163.0	472.0 ± 159.8
PMN, %	28.59 ± 6.69	23.0 ± 3.18 *	23.66 ± 4.84	22.37 ± 7.51	30.5 ± 7.56 *	23.36 ± 4.20 *
LY, %	57.40 ± 6.21	60.9 ± 4.06	59.80 ± 4.40	62.00 ± 9.19	53.11 ± 3.76	58.74 ± 4.82
MON, %	7.56 ± 2.33	7.44 ± 1.42	8.04 ± 1.61	7.36 ± 2.55	8.08 ± 1.62	8.01 ± 2.02
EOS, %	5.43 ± 1.61	8.20 ± 2.23 *	7.85 ± 2.42	6.33 ± 1.67	5.24 ± 0.44	7.07 ± 1.23
BAS, %	0.53 ± 0.33	2.23 ± 0.42 *	0.64 ± 0.42	0.51 ± 0.22	2.17 ± 1.73 *	0.8 ± 0.77
RET, %	3.35 ± 1.08	3.39 ± 0.65	3.33 ± 0.60	3.66 ± 0.81	5.84 ± 0.50 *	4.26 ± 0.17

C (−)—negative control; C (+)—positive control (Spirulina protein extract); AgNPs—experimental group administered with silver nanoparticles; AgNPs-SPE—experimental group administered with silver nanoparticles functionalized with Spirulina protein extract; $n = 7$ for C (−), C (+), AgNPs, and AgNPs-SPE; $n = 5$ for AgNPs CET, and AgNPs-SPE CET; * $p < 0.05$ for the differences between the groups AgNPs/C (−), AgNPs CET/AgNPs, AgNPs-SPE/C (+), and AgNPs-SPE CET/AgNPs-SPE.

Table 5. Biochemical indices in rats after 28 days of AgNPs and AgNPs-SPE administration and a 28-day clearance period.

Indices	C (−)	AgNPs	AgNPs CET	C (+)	AgNPs-SPE	AgNPs-SPE CET
Prot, g/L	58.97 ± 5.68	59.34 ± 3.70	68.87 ± 3.50	64.17 ± 6.47	59.27 ± 6.38	62.46 ± 4.04
Glu, mmol/L	5.49 ± 0.77	5.47 ± 0.68	5.49 ± 0.41	5.87 ± 0.86	4.96 ± 1.34	5.65 ± 0.47
CREA, μM/L	86.43 ± 14.9	165.2 ± 17.10 **	69.33 ± 3.71 **	100.93 ± 7.77	172.77 ± 5.92 *	68.04 ± 3.92 *
Urea, mg/dL	29.03 ± 5.69	27.01 ± 4.36	31.17 ± 0.36	25.53 ± 5.97	27.41 ± 4.49	33.72 ± 0.36
ALT, U/L	162.4 ± 39.6	222.0 ± 45.0 **	188.2 ± 13.5 *	184.9 ± 50.2	199.6 ± 27.0 *	208.6 ± 10.6
AST, U/L	3.57 ± 2.31	5.74 ± 1.74 *	5.43 ± 0.80	2.84 ± 1.90	4.96 ± 2.56	7.03 ± 0.68 *

C (−)—negative control; C (+)—positive control (Spirulina protein extract); AgNPs—experimental group administered with silver nanoparticles; AgNPs-SPE—experimental group administered with silver nanoparticles functionalized with Spirulina protein extract; $n = 7$ for C (−), C (+), AgNPs, and AgNPs-SPE; $n = 5$ for AgNPs CET and AgNPs-SPE CET; * $p < 0.05$ and ** $p < 0.01$ for the differences between the groups AgNPs/C (−), AgNPs CET/AgNPs, AgNPs-SPE/C (+), and AgNPs-SPE CET/AgNPs-SPE.

Hematological tests performed on rats treated with citrate-stabilized AgNPs confirmed the persistence of changes observed during nanoparticle treatment: decreased levels of leukocytes and polymorphonuclear cells, and increased eosinophil levels. Basophil levels returned to those of the negative control group. In animals treated with AgNPs functionalized with Spirulina protein extract, the number of polymorphonuclear cells, basophils, and reticulocytes was restored after the clearance period. A moderate increase in leukocyte count was also observed, a process that began during the administration period, leading to a 23.3% increase compared to the positive control group (Table 4).

After the clearance period, biochemical indicators evaluated in animals showed restoration of renal and hepatic parameters. In animals treated with citrate-stabilized AgNPs, clearance results indicated normal creatinine and alanine aminotransferase levels, similar to those in the negative control group. However, AST levels remained elevated among the liver enzymes. Except for AST, all other biochemical indicators returned to normal values, comparable to those in the control group (Table 5).

The clearance period normalized creatinine levels in animals treated with AgNPs functionalized with Spirulina protein extract. However, aminotransferase levels did not fully recover, with ALT remaining relatively elevated by 12.8% compared to the animals in the C (+) group. AST levels showed a continuous and significant increase of 41.7% ($p < 0.05$) compared to AST levels in animals treated for 28 days, which is 2.47 times higher than the positive control group (Table 5).

3. Discussion

The concept of nanoparticle functionalization is not new, with extensive research documenting the synthesis of nanoparticles using reducing substrates of plant or microbial origin, as well as their functionalization through accumulation in the structure of microorganisms during the growth cycle.

Additionally, the functionalization of nanoparticles with organic or bioactive compounds to reduce toxicity and increase their bioavailability is well known [29]. Moreover, recent studies have shown that biologically active substances are conjugated with nanoparticles to facilitate their targeted delivery to specific organs while maintaining the desired therapeutic effect [30].

Previous research achieved the biofunctionalization of AgNPs within Spirulina biomass by cultivating the cyanobacteria in a mineral medium supplemented with AgNPs [27]. This method led to the integration of nanoparticles into the biomass structures, providing insights into the bioaccumulation and potential toxicity of AgNPs when internalized by Spirulina during growth. The biomass administered to rats resulted in the accumulation of nanoparticles in different organs and their complete elimination, except for the brain [27].

Spirulina is well known for its numerous health benefits, and extracts from the biomass of this cyanobacterium have been extensively studied as nutraceuticals and in other applications. For example, organic solvent extracts from Spirulina biomass have demonstrated antibacterial, antioxidant, anti-inflammatory, and antidiabetic effects [31]. Protein extracts from Spirulina can be utilized in clinical applications to harness their immunomodulatory, antioxidant, and anti-inflammatory properties [17,32]. The protein compounds in Spirulina positively influence endothelial function and are recognized for their effectiveness in preventing and managing cardiovascular diseases [25]. The ability of Spirulina protein extract to influence nanoparticle accumulation in various tissues and enhance their elimination depends on the structural stability of the functional mixture formed. The stability of the bonds between the proteins in the protein extract and silver nanoparticles is crucial, as these bonds can impart new properties to the nanoparticles, distinct from those of synthetic AgNPs [33]. In this study, the experimental conditions used to obtain the functional mixture favored the formation of electrostatic and hydrogen bonds between the protein structures and citrate-stabilized silver nanoparticles, as evidenced by the changes observed in the UV-Vis and FTIR spectra. Additionally, the AgNPs-SPE functional mixture demonstrated a stable antioxidant activity. In a protein mixture, proteins interact with AgNPs, stabilizing them and preventing their aggregation. This stabilization reduces the likelihood of undesired redox reactions, thereby maintaining consistent values obtained in the antioxidant assay with DPPH.

The most conclusive evidence of the functional mixture's efficacy was observed in the differential accumulation of silver in the tested organs, compared to the values obtained for simple silver nanoparticles.

In the present study, after the functionalization of silver nanoparticles with Spirulina protein extract and the characterization of their properties, these nanoparticles were administered to rats as a functional mixture with the synthesis matrix. The dosage of nanoparticles administered to the rats was 1 μg per animal, which was selected based on previous studies [27]. Higher doses of silver nanoparticles are inherently toxic, and their adverse effects have been well documented. This low dose was chosen to replicate levels similar to those used in medical applications or encountered in consumer products. The accumulation of unmodified silver nanoparticles and those in the mix with Spirulina protein extract was evaluated in various organs, including reproductive tissues. Both types of nanoparticles accumulated significantly in brain tissue, quickly crossing the blood–brain barrier. The amount of silver collected in the brain was substantial, which is highly concerning, indicating a potential risk for humans, particularly in AgNPs' use in cosmetics and food packaging. After a 28-day clearance period, 11.4% to 24% of the accumulated silver was eliminated from the brains of the animals. The remaining silver content in the brain was approximately equal for both types of nanoparticles. Other researchers have also reported the persistence of accumulated silver in the brain even after a clearance period, highlighting its slow elimination from this organ [34]. Even with low concentrations, the maximum amount of nanoparticles was detected in brain tissue. It has been demonstrated that AgNPs administered via subcutaneous injection penetrate the rat brain and accumulate as nanoparticles [35].

Citrate-stabilized AgNPs accumulated in all organs, liver, spleen, ovaries, kidneys, and testes, with concentrations ranging between 7.9 and 11.63 ng/g. This effect is supported by other studies, which have established that regardless of the administration route—oral, intravenous, inhalation, intranasal application, or absorption through the skin—once AgNPs enter the body, they are distributed through the systemic circulation to organs such as the liver, kidneys, lungs, spleen, heart, gonads, and brain [34,36,37]. In the case of oral administration, nanoparticles cross the intestinal barrier and are absorbed from the gastrointestinal tract either as nanoparticles or in ionic form [38].

AgNPs functionalized with Spirulina protein extract exhibited specific affinity (tropism) for liver tissue, where they accumulated in amounts similar to those in the brain, three times higher than the accumulation of silver from engineered AgNPs, followed by the testes and spleen. Proteins bound to nanoparticles may interact with specific receptors on liver, kidney, and spleen cells, thereby facilitating their accumulation in these excretory organs. Regarding the route of NP administration, the oral pathway involves the capture of NPs by the reticuloendothelial system of the liver, leading to their retention for eventual elimination [14].

Due to their small size and protein functionalization, silver nanoparticles of 10 nm accompanied by Spirulina protein components could induce a tolerogenic immune response through specific interaction with liver cells. Functionalization with Spirulina protein components might enhance the specificity of these nanoparticles for immune cells and help modulate the immune response. However, potential toxicity risks associated with the small size must be considered, and safety and biodistribution studies should be conducted to ensure their safe use in therapeutic applications [39].

This study observed that the testes accumulated significant concentrations of silver from the functionalized AgNPs-SPE mixture. This suggests a possible increase in nanoparticle affinity for the functionalized mixture's protein component. In the literature, some authors have attempted to mitigate this effect of AgNPs by biofunctionalizing them with plant extracts, but the results were contrary. Silver nanoparticles continued accumulating in the testes even after a post-administration period, thus confirming their toxicity to testicular tissue, regardless of their origin [40]. Some authors have concluded that in the brain and testes, unlike other organs, AgNPs are prone to persistence [34,41].

However, it has been demonstrated that the coating of nanoparticles can influence their tropism for the testes. For example, silver nanoparticles coated with polyethylene glycol did not exhibit affinity for the testes when administered in similar doses. On the other hand, AgNPs functionalized with live Spirulina platensis culture, orally administered to rats, significantly accumulated in the testes but were eliminated entirely over time [27].

In the case of AgNPs-SPE administration, complete elimination of silver from the testes was not observed, suggesting an increased affinity for the protein component of the functional mixture. The affinity of testicular tissue for AgNPs functionalized with Spirulina protein extract is determined by its components and can be explored for targeted drug delivery.

In the current study, it appears that the clearance period was insufficient for eliminating silver from the testes in the case of AgNPs-SPE. During the 28-day observation period, 87.7% ($p < 0.05$) of the accumulated metal was eliminated. It is possible that extending the clearance period could lead to the complete elimination of silver from testicular tissues. A similar increased affinity was observed for ovarian tissue. Once again, the silver that accumulated through the administration of citrate-stabilized AgNPs was eliminated entirely from ovarian tissue, while in the case of AgNPs-SPE, 68.7% ($p < 0.05$) was eliminated.

The silver from AgNPs-SPE was completely eliminated from the liver, spleen, and kidneys, demonstrating their stability within the protein extract structure and in the circulatory system. This allowed for more efficient transport to excretory organs, in contrast to non-functionalized AgNPs, which are less likely to be quickly recognized and captured by the reticuloendothelial system, allowing them to circulate longer in the bloodstream and be eliminated more slowly. Another hypothesis is that the protein material may be metabolized and eliminated more rapidly, reducing the potential for long-term toxicity [42].

In the case of citrate-stabilized AgNPs, elimination from the liver was not complete. This could be due to the formation of Ag ions, which are more challenging to eliminate from excretory organs [3].

Eliminating silver nanoparticles through the liver and kidneys was associated with increased levels of specific markers, indicating compromised function of these organs. In the present study, a significant increase in blood creatinine levels was observed after the administration of both AgNPs, with the highest values, and AgNP-SPE, with toxicity being more pronounced in female rats. Another study established the dependence of nanoparticle elimination from the kidneys on ovarian hormonal activity [43].

Significant increases in hepatic indicators were observed. ALT levels increased significantly in females, while in males treated with AgNPs-SPE, the values were similar to those of the control group. AST levels were elevated in males and extremely high in females. It can be noted that hepatic indicators were affected by the gender of the rats rather than by the amount of silver accumulated in the liver.

The clearance period restored ALT values in both experimental groups, but this was not the case for AST, which remained elevated. This marker remained high even in the rats treated with the AgNPs-SPE, which may indicate delayed or long-term effects.

In this study on rats treated with AgNPs, hematological indicators showed a significant increase in eosinophils and basophils, suggesting a marked inflammatory response. In females, a slight reduction in hemoglobin levels and erythrocyte count was observed, along with a significant increase in monocyte count and a decrease in reticulocytes. In the group treated with AgNPs-SPE, the changes were even more pronounced, with significant increases in the number of polymorphonuclear cells, basophils, and reticulocytes, indicating the potential effects of the treatment on the maturation and function of blood cells. After the clearance period, an increase in lymphocyte count was observed in females, which may be attributed to a persistent inflammatory process [44]. These changes highlight the potential impact of silver nanoparticles on the hematological system, requiring further evaluation to fully understand their mechanisms and implications. A similar response was observed in laboratory animals treated with AgNPs (PEG) and AgNPs functionalized with Spirulina biomass [27]. It is important to note that this immune system response is reversible, with the restoration of hematological indicators.

4. Materials and Methods

4.1. Preparation of Spirulina Protein Extract

The cyanobacterium strain *Spirulina platensis* CNMN-CB-02 biomass was used to obtain the protein extract. This strain is stored in the National Collection of Non-Pathogenic

Microorganisms at the Institute of Microbiology and Biotechnology, Technical University of Moldova. Spirulina was cultivated under photoautotrophic conditions in a mineral medium containing the necessary macro- and microelements for growth and biomass accumulation in 1000 mL Erlenmeyer flasks with a suspension volume of 500 mL for 6 days. After separating the biomass from the culture medium, it was demineralized with a 1.5% ammonium acetate solution (Sigma-Aldrich Chemie GmbH, Taufkirchen, Germany) and standardized to a concentration of 100 mg/mL. The protein content in the biomass was 68–72%.

For protein extraction, the biomass was mixed with a 0.45% sodium hydroxide solution (Sigma-Aldrich Chemie GmbH, Taufkirchen, Germany) at a ratio of 1 g of biomass to 0.5 L of solution (g/L). Protein extraction was performed at 25 ± 1 °C with continuous stirring for 60 min. The supernatant was separated by centrifugation. A second extraction was performed with 200 mL of 0.45% sodium hydroxide solution for 30 min at the same temperature. The first and second extracts were combined, and the final mixture was dialyzed to a pH of 7.0–7.2. The final protein extract (SPE) was standardized to a concentration of 1% dry substance, with a protein content of 52%.

4.2. Functionalization of AgNPs with the Formation of the AgNPs-SPE Functional Mixture

To prepare the functional mixture of SPE and AgNPs, 10 nm silver nanoparticles stabilized in citrate, 0.02 mg/mL (Sigma-Aldrich Chemie GmbH, Taufkirchen, Germany), were used. Specification for AgNPs: 10 ± 0.2 nm particle size TEM (730786, Lot # MKCK8345). A total of 20 mL of AgNP suspension was added to 200 mL of 1% SPE solution. The mixture was stirred slowly at 200 rpm at 25 ± 1 °C for 120 min. The resulting AgNPs-SPE functional mixture contained 1.0 mg/mL SPE and 1 μg/mL AgNPs.

4.3. Animals and Experimental Design

The animal experiments were conducted in the Vivarium of the Laboratory of Stress Physiology, Adaptation, and General Sanocreatology at the Institute of Physiology and Sanocreatology in Moldova, in compliance with Law No. 211/2017 of the Parliament of the Republic of Moldova on the protection of animals used for experimental or scientific purposes (published in the Official Gazette No. 1–6, Article 02 on 5 January 2018), which transposes Directive 2010/63/EU of the European Parliament and of the Council of 22 September 2010 on the protection of animals used for scientific research, published in the Official Journal of the European Union L 276 on 20 October 2010. The Institute of Physiology and Sanocreatology Ethics Committee in Moldova (IREC) approved the experiments (approval IREC No. IREC/26/06.02.2023).

In the experiment, 48 Wistar albino rats (28 males and 20 females) were used, divided into four groups, each consisting of 7 males and 5 females, housed in separate cages. The animals were acclimatized under standard conditions (temperature of 22 ± 2 °C, relative humidity of 55 ± 5%, 12 h light/12 h dark photoperiod). Throughout the experiment, all animals were maintained under standard conditions with free access to water and a regular diet. The experimental groups received the following supplements: C (−)—negative control group with regular diet; C (+) positive control group with regular diet mixed with Spirulina protein extract; experimental group 1 (AgNPs)—regular diet mixed with silver nanoparticles; experimental group 2 (AgNPs-SPE)—regular diet supplemented with the mixture of silver nanoparticles functionalized with Spirulina protein extract.

The animals were fed according to these dietary regimens for 28 days in the institute's vivarium. After this period, four males and three females from each group were sacrificed to collect blood for hematological and biochemical analyses and to harvest organs (brain, liver, spleen, kidneys, testes, and ovaries) for ICP-MS analysis. The remaining animals were maintained under optimal conditions with a regular diet for an additional 28 days (clearance period), after which they were sacrificed according to the described procedure.

The amount of AgNPs administered to the animals in experimental groups 3 and 4 was 1 μg of silver per day per animal. The positive control group received the same amount of Spirulina protein extract as the experimental group 4. The non-functionalized nanoparticle suspension and the AgNPs-SPE mixture were incorporated into whole rye flour breadcrumbs and administered to the rats as their first meal.

4.4. Methods for Characterizing AgNPs-SPE and Detecting Silver

4.4.1. UV-Vis Spectra Recording

Samples of Spirulina protein extract and AgNPs mixture with Spirulina protein extract were prepared by dilution with distilled water. The spectra were recorded using a UV-Vis Spectrophotometer 80T (PG Instruments Ltd., Lutterworth, UK) within the wavelength range of 190–800 nm, with a spectral resolution of 1 nm.

4.4.2. Fourier Transform Infrared (FTIR) Analysis

The analyzed samples were dehydrated at 40 °C. The IR spectra in the region of 4000–400 cm^{-1} were recorded at room temperature using a Perkin-Elmer FTIR spectrometer (PerkinElmer Inc., Waltham, MA, USA) equipped with an air-cooled DTGS (Deuterated Triglycine Sulfate) detector.

4.4.3. ICP-MS Analysis

Before analysis, organs were dried at 70 °C until a constant weight. Next, 0.1 g of each sample were mixed with 3 mL of HNO_3 (Sigma-Aldrich, Taufkirchen, Germany) and 1 mL of H_2O_2 (Sigma-Aldrich, Germany). Sample digestion was performed in an ETAS-6 analytical autoclave with resistive heating at 180 °C, pressure at 20 bar, power at 400 W, during 1.5 h. After cooling, samples were quantitatively transferred into 20 mL flasks and diluted to volume with deionized water. Silver content in samples was measured by ICP-MS using XSeries II (Thermo Scientific, Waltham, MA, USA). The uncertainty of measurements varied from 5 to 10%.

4.4.4. Determination of Antioxidant Activity

The non-biological DPPH (1,1-diphenyl-2-picrylhydrazyl) radical reduction method was used. A 0.05 mM DPPH solution was prepared in 55% ethyl alcohol. The reaction mixture contained 2.9 mL DPPH solution and 0.1 mL sample. The incubation duration was 30 min. The absorbance of the samples was recorded at 517 nm. The value of the antioxidant activity was reported as % inhibition of DPPH [45].

4.5. Blood Hematology and Biochemistry

Hematology was evaluated using a Sysmex XT-2000i automated hematology analyzer (GMI Inc., Ramsey, MN, USA) with preset settings for analysis. Blood biochemistry was performed using a semi-automatic photometer, StarDust MC15 (DiaSys Diagnostic Systems, Holzheim, Germany).

4.6. Statistical Analysis

All experiments were conducted in triplicate. The results in all tables and histograms are presented as mean values ± standard deviations. Statistical differences between the values were evaluated using Student's *t*-tests.

5. Conclusions

This study's conclusions on the impact of silver nanoparticles functionalized with Spirulina protein extract (AgNPs-SPE) on rat health include significant observations related to their distribution, accumulation, and biological effects. The nanoparticles showed variable distribution across organs, including the brain and reproductive organs, demonstrating their ability to cross biological barriers such as the blood–brain barrier. Significant accumulation and persistence of silver in reproductive organs suggest potential long-term toxicity. The functionalization process influences the rates of nanoparticle accumulation and elimination. Thus, biofunctionalized silver nanoparticles accumulate in significantly higher amounts in the brain, liver, spleen, kidneys, and testes and are completely eliminated from the liver and spleen, unlike non-functionalized nanoparticles. The persistence of both types of nanoparticles in the sexual glands after a 28-day clearance period raises reasonable concerns regarding the health of the offspring of animals exposed to low levels of nanoparticles.

Both AgNPs and AgNPs-SPE affected hematological parameters, indicating possible inflammatory reactions and changes in cell maturation processes.

The administration of AgNP-SPE induced moderate changes in hematological parameters, as evidenced by increased polymorphonuclear cells and reticulocytes in females. Additionally, the significant increase in eosinophils and basophils indicates an inflammatory response and activation of the immune system, suggesting that the body recognized the functionalized nanoparticles as foreign agents. After the 28-day clearance period, these hematological indicators returned to normal levels, indicating that the immune and inflammatory effects of AgNP-SPE are transient and reversible. Thus, eliminating the nanoparticles from the body appears to restore immune balance.

The administration of AgNP-SPE also induced transient biochemical changes, particularly related to liver and kidney function. After the clearance period, most indicators returned to normal levels, except for AST, suggesting potential residual effects on the liver.

The impact of AgNPs on the liver and kidney and their persistence in these vital organs requires further evaluation to determine the safety and appropriate dosing of AgNPs-SPE. Specifically, studies should investigate the long-term effects on hepatic and renal tissue, the exact localization of AgNPs within reproductive tissues, their impact on reproductive function, and the duration of their persistence in these organs.

Author Contributions: Conceptualization, L.R., T.C. and L.C.; methodology, L.R., D.G. and A.K.; software, D.G.; validation, I.Z. and L.C.; investigation, T.C., L.R. and A.K.; data curation, L.R.; writing—original draft preparation, L.R., T.C. and L.C.; writing—review and editing, L.R. and L.C. All authors have read and agreed to the published version of the manuscript.

Funding: This research was funded by the Government of the Republic of Moldova—National Agency for Research and Development, Project 20.80009.5007.05 "Biofunctionalized metal nanoparticles—obtaining using cyanobacteria and microalgae".

Institutional Review Board Statement: The Ethics Committee of Institute of Physiology and Sanocreatology, R. Moldova (protocol code IREC No. IREC/26/06.02.2023) approved the animal study protocol.

Informed Consent Statement: The study was approved by the Institute of Physiology and Sanocreatology Animal Ethics Committee in Moldova (IREC), and all procedures followed the relevant guidelines for the care and use of laboratory animals.

Data Availability Statement: Data are contained within the article.

Conflicts of Interest: The authors declare no conflicts of interest. The funders had no role in the design of this study, the collection, analysis, or interpretation of data, the writing of the manuscript, or the decision to publish the results.

References

1. Calderón-Jiménez, B.; Johnson, M.E.; Montoro Bustos, A.R.; Murphy, K.E.; Winchester, M.R.; Vega Baudrit, J.R. Silver Nanoparticles: Technological Advances, Societal Impacts, and Metrological Challenges. *Front. Chem.* **2017**, *5*, 6. [CrossRef] [PubMed]
2. Keat, C.L.; Aziz, A.; Eid, A.M.; Elmarzugi, N.A. Biosynthesis of nanoparticles and silver nanoparticles. *Bioresour. Bioprocess.* **2015**, *2*, 47. [CrossRef]
3. Liu, S.; Hu, M.; Liu, X.; Liu, X.; Chen, T.; Zhu, Y.; Liang, T.; Xiao, S.; Li, P.; Ma, X. Nanoparticles and Antiviral Vaccines. *Vaccines* **2024**, *12*, 30. [CrossRef]
4. Jangid, H.; Singh, S.; Kashyap, P.; Singh, A.; Kumar, G. Advancing biomedical applications: An in-depth analysis of silver nanoparticles in antimicrobial, anticancer, and wound healing roles. *Front. Pharmacol.* **2024**, *15*, 1438227. [CrossRef]
5. Bruna, T.; Maldonado-Bravo, F.; Jara, P.; Caro, N. Silver Nanoparticles and Their Antibacterial Applications. *Int. J. Mol. Sci.* **2021**, *22*, 7202. [CrossRef]

6. Tian, J.; Wong, K.K.; Ho, C.M.; Lok, C.N.; Yu, W.Y.; Che, C.M.; Chiu, J.F.; Tam, P.K. Topical Delivery of Silver Nanoparticles Promotes Wound Healing. *ChemMedChem Chem. Enabling Drug Discov.* **2007**, *2*, 129–136. [CrossRef] [PubMed]
7. Miranda, R.R.; Sampaio, I.; Zucolotto, V. Exploring silver nanoparticles for cancer therapy and diagnosis. *Colloids Surf. B Biointerfaces* **2022**, *210*, 112254. [CrossRef]
8. Takáč, P.; Michalková, R.; Čižmáriková, M.; Bedlovičová, Z.; Balážová, L'.; Takáčová, G. The Role of Silver Nanoparticles in the Diagnosis and Treatment of Cancer: Are There Any Perspectives for the Future? *Life* **2023**, *13*, 466. [CrossRef] [PubMed]
9. Burdus, A.C.; Gherasim, O.; Grumezescu, A.M.; Mogoantă, L.; Ficai, A.; Andronescu, E. Biomedical applications of silver nanoparticles: An up-to-date overview. *Nanomaterials* **2018**, *8*, 681. [CrossRef]
10. Borowik, A.; Butowska, K.; Konkel, K.; Banasiuk, R.; Derewonko, N.; Wyrzykowski, D.; Davydenko, M.; Cherepanov, V.; Styopkin, V.; Prylutskyy, Y.; et al. The Impact of Surface Functionalization on the Biophysical Properties of Silver Nanoparticles. *Nanomaterials* **2019**, *9*, 973. [CrossRef]
11. Hassanen, E.I.; Khalaf, A.A.; Tohamy, A.F.; Mohammed, E.R.; Farroh, K.Y. Toxicopathological and immunological studies on different concentrations of chitosan-coated silver nanoparticles in rats. *Int. J. Nanomed.* **2019**, *14*, 4723–4739. [CrossRef] [PubMed]
12. Menichetti, A.; Mavridi-Printezi, A.; Mordini, D.; Montalti, M. Effect of Size, Shape and Surface Functionalization on the Antibacterial Activity of Silver Nanoparticles. *J. Funct. Biomater.* **2023**, *14*, 244. [CrossRef] [PubMed]
13. Le Ouay, B.; Stellacci, F. Antibacterial activity of silver nanoparticles: A surface science insight. *Nanotoday* **2015**, *10*, 339–354. [CrossRef]
14. Ravindran, A.; Chandran, P.; Khan, S.S. Biofunctionalized silver nanoparticles: Advances and prospects. *Colloids Surf. B Biointerfaces* **2013**, *105*, 342–352. [CrossRef] [PubMed]
15. Hussein, H.A.; Abdullah, M.A. Biosynthesis, Mechanisms, and Biomedical Applications of Silver Nanoparticles. In *Functional Bionanomaterials—Nanotechnology in the Life Sciences*; Thangadurai, D., Sangeetha, J., Prasad, R., Eds.; Springer International Publishing: Cham, Switzerland, 2020. [CrossRef]
16. Dinparvar, S.; Bagirova, M.; Allahverdiyev, A.M.; Abamor, E.S.; Safarov, T.; Aydogdu, M.; Aktas, D.J. A nanotechnology-based new approach in the treatment of breast cancer: Biosynthesized silver nanoparticles using *Cuminum cyminum* L. seed extract. *Photochem. Photobiol. B* **2020**, *208*, 111902. [CrossRef]
17. Gul, A.; Baig, M.N.; Ahmed, D.; Najam, Z.; Aslam, T.; Ali, S. Green synthesis of silver nanoparticles from *Spirulina platensis* extract: Antibacterial and antioxidant potential. *BioNanoScience* **2024**. [CrossRef]
18. Alwhibi, M.S.; Soliman, D.A.; Awad, M.A.; Alangery, A.B.; Al Dehaish, H.; Alwasel, Y.A. Green synthesis of silver nanoparticles: Characterization and its potential biomedical applications. *Green Process. Synth.* **2021**, *10*, 412–420. [CrossRef]
19. Hou, T.; Guo, Y.; Han, W.; Zhou, Y.; Netala, V.R.; Li, H.; Li, H.; Zhang, Z. Exploring the Biomedical Applications of Biosynthesized Silver Nanoparticles Using *Perilla frutescens* Flavonoid Extract: Antibacterial, Antioxidant, and Cell Toxicity Properties against Colon Cancer Cells. *Molecules* **2023**, *28*, 6431. [CrossRef]
20. Torabian, F.; Rezayat, A.A.; Nour, M.G.; Ghorbanzadeh, A.; Najafi, S.; Sahebkar, A.; Sabouri, Z.; Darroudi, M. Administration of Silver Nanoparticles in Diabetes Mellitus: A Systematic Review and Meta-analysis on Animal Studies. *Biol. Trace Elem. Res.* **2022**, *200*, 1699–1709. [CrossRef]
21. Prasher, P.; Sharma, M.; Mudila, H.; Gupta, G.; Sharma, A.K.; Kumar, D.; Bakshi, H.A.; Negi, P.; Kapoor, D.N.; Chellappan, D.K.; et al. Emerging trends in clinical implications of bio-conjugated silver nanoparticles in drug delivery. *Colloid Interface Sci. Commun.* **2020**, *35*, 100244. [CrossRef]
22. Ahumada, M.; Suuronen, E.J.; Alarcon, E.I. Biomolecule Silver Nanoparticle-Based Materials for Biomedical Applications. In *Handbook of Ecomaterials*; Martínez, L., Kharissova, O., Kharisov, B., Eds.; Springer International Publishing: Cham, Switzerland, 2019. [CrossRef]
23. Buthenia, A.; Hasoon, K.H.; Jawad, I.S.; Mohammed, N.N.; Hussein, K.F.; Al-azawi, M.S.J. Silver nanoparticles conjugated amoxicillin: A promising nano-suspension for overcoming multidrug resistance bacteria and preservation of endotracheal tube. *Inorg. Chem. Commun.* **2024**, *165*, 112456. [CrossRef]
24. Madhyastha, H.; Madhyastha, R.; Thakur, A.; Kentaro, S.; Dev, A.; Singh, S.; Chandrashekharappa, R.B.; Kumar, H.; Acevedo, O.; Nakajima, Y.; et al. c-Phycocyanin primed silver nano conjugates: Studies on red blood cell stress resilience mechanism. *Colloids Surf. B Biointerfaces* **2020**, *94*, 111211. [CrossRef] [PubMed]
25. Prete, V.; Abate, A.C.; Di Pietro, P.; De Lucia, M.; Vecchione, C.; Carrizzo, A. Beneficial Effects of Spirulina Supplementation in the Management of Cardiovascular Diseases. *Nutrients* **2024**, *16*, 642. [CrossRef] [PubMed]
26. Fais, G.; Manca, A.; Bolognesi, F.; Borselli, M.; Concas, A.; Busutti, M.; Broggi, G.; Sanna, P.; Castillo-Aleman, Y.M.; Rivero-Jiménez, R.A.; et al. Wide Range Applications of Spirulina: From Earth to Space Missions. *Mar. Drugs* **2022**, *20*, 299. [CrossRef]
27. Rudi, L.; Zinicovscaia, I.; Cepoi, L.; Chiriac, T.; Peshkova, A.; Cepoi, A.; Grozdov, D. Accumulation and Effect of Silver Nanoparticles Functionalized with *Spirulina platensis* on Rats. *Nanomaterials* **2021**, *11*, 2992. [CrossRef]
28. Muthusamy, G.; Thangasamy, S.; Raja, M.; Chinnappan, S.; Kandasamy, S. Biosynthesis of silver nanoparticles from Spirulina microalgae and its antibacterial activity. *Environ. Sci. Pollut. Res. Int.* **2017**, *24*, 19459–19464. [CrossRef]
29. Das, B.; Tripathy, S.; Adhikary, J.; Chattopadhyay, S.M.; Debasis, D.; Sandeep, K.D.; Sabyasachi, D.; Aditi, D.; Sankar, K.; Das, D.; et al. Surface modification minimizes the toxicity of silver nanoparticles: An in vitro and in vivo study. *J. Biol. Inorg. Chem.* **2017**, *22*, 893–918. [CrossRef]

30. Meena, J.; Gupta, A.; Ahuja, R.; Singh, M.; Bhaskar, S. Inorganic nanoparticles for natural product delivery: A review. *Environ. Chem. Lett.* **2020**, *18*, 2107–2118. [CrossRef]
31. Sowmya, S.; Suba Sri, M.; Dineshkumar, R. In vitro Therapeutic Effect of Spirulina Extract. *Asian J. Biol. Life Sci.* **2021**, *10*, 582–589. [CrossRef]
32. Karkos, P.D.; Leong, S.C.; Karkos, C.D.; Sivaji, N.; Assimakopoulos, D.A. Spirulina in Clinical Practice: Evidence-Based Human Applications. *Evid. Based Complement. Alternat. Med.* **2011**, *2011*, 531053. [CrossRef]
33. Goel, M.; Sharma, A.; Sharma, B. Recent Advances in Biogenic Silver Nanoparticles for Their Biomedical Applications. *Sustain. Chem.* **2023**, *4*, 61–94. [CrossRef]
34. Lee, J.H.; Kim, Y.S.; Song, K.S.; Ryu, H.R.; Sung, J.H.; Park, J.D.; Park, H.M.; Song, N.W.; Shin, B.S.; Marshak, D.; et al. Biopersistence of silver nanoparticles in tissues from Sprague-Dawley rats. *Part. Fibre Toxicol.* **2013**, *10*, 36. [CrossRef] [PubMed]
35. Tang, J.; Xiong, L.; Wang, S.; Wang, J.; Liu, L.; Li, J.; Wan, Z.; Xi, T. Influence of silver nanoparticles on neurons and blood-brain barrier via subcutaneous injection in rats. *Appl. Surf. Sci.* **2008**, *255*, 502–504. [CrossRef]
36. Loeschner, K.; Hadrup, N.; Qvortrup, K.; Larsen, A.; Gao, X.; Vogel, U.; Mortensen, A.; Lam, H.R.; Larsen, E.H. Distribution of silver in rats following 28 days of repeated oral exposure to silver nanoparticles or silver acetate. *Part. Fibre Toxicol.* **2011**, *8*, 18. [CrossRef]
37. Sung, J.H.; Ji, J.H.; Park, J.D.; Yoon, J.U.; Kim, D.S.; Jeon, K.S.; Song, M.Y.; Jeong, J.; Han, B.S.; Han, J.H.; et al. Subchronic inhalation toxicity of silver nanoparticles. *Toxicol. Sci.* **2009**, *108*, 452–461. [CrossRef] [PubMed]
38. Park, M.V.; Neigh, A.M.; Vermeulen, J.P.; de la Fonteyne, L.J.; Verharen, H.W.; Briedé, J.J.; van Loveren, H.; de Jong, W.H. The effect of particle size on the cytotoxicity, inflammation, developmental toxicity and genotoxicity of silver nanoparticles. *Biomaterials* **2011**, *32*, 9810–9817. [CrossRef] [PubMed]
39. Yang, L.; Kuang, H.; Zhang, W.; Aguilar, Z.P.; Wei, H.; Xu, H. Comparisons of the biodistribution and toxicological examinations after repeated intravenous administration of silver and gold nanoparticles in mice. *Sci. Rep.* **2017**, *7*, 3303. [CrossRef]
40. Opris, R.; Toma, V.; Olteanu, D.; Baldea, I.; Baciu, A.M.; Lucaci, F.I.; Filip, G.A. Effects of Silver Nanoparticles Functionalized with *Cornus Mas* L. Extract on Architecture and Apoptosis in Rat Testicle. *Nanomedicine* **2019**, *14*, 275–299. [CrossRef]
41. van der Zande, M.; Vandebriel, R.J.; Van Doren, E.; Kramer, E.; Herrera Rivera, Z.; Serrano-Rojero, C.S.; Gremmer, E.R.; Mast, J.; Peters, R.J.; Hollman, P.C.; et al. Distribution, elimination, and toxicity of silver nanoparticles and silver ions in rats after 28-day oral exposure. *ACS Nano* **2012**, *6*, 7427–7442. [CrossRef]
42. Wei, Y.; Quan, L.; Zhou, C.; Zhan, Q. Factors relating to the biodistribution & clearance of nanoparticles & their effects on in vivo application. *Nanomedicine* **2018**, *13*, 1495–1512. [CrossRef]
43. Kim, Y.S.; Song, M.Y.; Park, J.D.; Song, K.S.; Ryu, H.R.; Chung, Y.H.; Chang, H.K.; Lee, J.H.; Oh, K.H.; Kelman, B.J.; et al. Subchronic oral toxicity of silver nanoparticles. *Part. Fibre Toxicol.* **2010**, *7*, 20. [CrossRef] [PubMed]
44. Qin, G.; Tang, S.; Li, S.; Lu, H.; Wang, Y.; Zhao, P.; Li, B.; Zhang, J.; Peng, L. Toxicological evaluation of silver nanoparticles and silver nitrate in rats following 28 days of repeated oral exposure. *Environ. Toxicol.* **2017**, *32*, 609–618. [CrossRef] [PubMed]
45. Gulcin, İ.; Alwasel, S.H. DPPH Radical Scavenging Assay. *Processes* **2023**, *11*, 2248. [CrossRef]

pharmaceuticals

MDPI

Article

Evaluation of Hippocampal Microanatomy and Neuro-Biomarkers Following Administration of Silver Nanoparticles Conjugated with Tenofovir Disoproxil Fumarate in Experimental Diabetic Rats

Sodiq Kolawole Lawal [1,2,*], Samuel Oluwaseun Olojede [3], Babatunde Adebola Alabi [4], Kafalotse Sylvia Dithole [1], Samuel Thopho Matula [1], Edwin Coleridge Naidu [2], Carmen Olivia Rennie [2] and Onyemaechi Okpara Azu [5]

1 School of Nursing, Faculty of Health Sciences, University of Botswana, Private Bag UB 0022, Plot 4775, Notwane Road, Gaborone, Botswana; ditholek@ub.ac.bw (K.S.D.); matulast@ub.ac.bw (S.T.M.)

2 Discipline of Clinical Anatomy, School of Laboratory Medicine & Medical Sciences, Nelson R Mandela School of Medicine, University of KwaZulu-Natal, Durban 3629, South Africa; naidue@ukzn.ac.za (E.C.N.); rennie@ukzn.ac.za (C.O.R.)

3 Division of Human Anatomy, Department of Human Biology, Faculty of Medicine and Health Sciences, Walter Sisulu University, Nelson Mandela Drive, Mthatha 5117, South Africa; solojede@wsu.ac.za

4 Department of Pharmacology and Therapeutics, Bowen University, Iwo P.O. Box 284, Nigeria; babatunde.alabi@bowen.edu.ng

5 Department of Medical Biosciences, University of the Western Cape, Bellville 7535, South Africa; oazu@uwc.ac.za

* Correspondence: lawals@ub.ac.bw; Tel.: +267-78200847

Abstract: Adverse complications like metabolic disorders, neurotoxicity, and low central nervous system (CNS) penetration are associated with the long-term use of tenofovir disoproxil fumarate (TDF). Therefore, some modifications are required to enhance neurological functions using silver nanoparticles (AgNPs). This study aimed to evaluate the neuroprotective impact of silver nanoparticles (AgNPs)-conjugated TDF as AgNPs-TDF on the hippocampal microanatomy and some neuro-biomarkers of diabetic rats. Forty-two male Sprague-Dawley rats, with an average weight of 250 ± 13 g, were divided into non-diabetic and diabetic groups. They were further divided into 3 groups each ($n = 7$): non-diabetic control (NC), non-diabetic + TDF (NTF), and non-diabetic + TDF + silver nanoparticles (NTS), as well as diabetic control (DC), diabetic + TDF (DTF), and diabetic + TDF + silver nanoparticles (DTS). The characterization of AgNPs-TDF was assessed, and the conjugates were administered to the diabetic rats, followed by behavioral testing and biochemical, immunohistochemical, and microanatomy analyses of the hippocampus. The results showed that the administration of AgNPs-TDF significantly reduced the blood glucose level, malondialdehyde (MDA), and inflammatory biomarker concentrations in DTS compared with the DTF and DC groups. Furthermore, AgNPs-TDF administration significantly increased the levels of tissue superoxide dismutase (SOD), reduced glutathione (GSH), and insulin-like growth factor-1 in DTS compared with the DTF and DC groups. In addition, the DTS group revealed a monomorphic pattern of dark-stained neuronal nuclei similar to the control group and showed neuroprotective effects on hippocampal microanatomy compared with the DTF group. This study shows that AgNPs-TDF restores various alterations in the hippocampus and improves cognitive functions in diabetic rats.

Keywords: tenofovir; silver nanoparticles; neurotoxicity; metabolic disorder; microanatomy; diabetes

1. Introduction

The inception of combined antiretroviral therapy (cART) has benefited people living with HIV, and such benefits achieved with prolonged administration of cART include reduced mortality, morbidity, and opportunistic infection, immune system enhancement, viral load suppression, and cluster of differentiation 4 cell count (CD4 count) improvement [1,2]. Despite these better outcomes, long-term administration of cART has been linked with severe metabolic disorders and neurotoxicity [3,4]. Especially, some antiretroviral drugs belonging to nucleoside reverse transcriptase inhibitors (NRTIs), such as abacavir, stavudine, emtricitabine, lamivudine, and tenofovir disoproxil fumarate (TDF), have been linked with neurotoxicity [5].

Tenofovir disoproxil fumarate is a widely used drug either alone or in combination with other antiretroviral drugs as a cocktail known as highly active antiretroviral therapy (HAART) for managing HIV and AIDS [6,7]. TDF alone is often used as pre-exposure prophylaxis (PrEP) by HIV-negative individuals and sex workers because it is highly effective at reducing the risk of sexual acquisition or transmission of HIV [7,8]. A study has reported that TDF's oral administration in combination with emtricitabine (FTC) is the most effective PrEP for HIV prevention compared with other combinations [9]. Furthermore, statistics have shown that about 1.5 million people were placed on TDF-based oral prophylaxis therapy in 2021, leading to the global decline in the spread of HIV [8]. Despite the advantages of TDF, studies have associated TDF with severe metabolic disturbances, neurotoxicity, and mitochondrial dysfunction [3,4,6]. Several studies have reported the association of long-term exposure to TDF with glucose metabolism disorders, such as insulin resistance and diabetes mellitus [10,11]. The mechanism of TDF-induced neurotoxicity has been linked to mitochondrial toxicity and inhibition of DNA polymerase γ resulting from increased oxidase stress [12,13].

In addition to the neurotoxicity associated with TDF, empirical evidence has described TDF as having low CNS penetration amongst the NRTIs [14]. In addition, a similar study has reported only a low concentration of tenofovir in the cerebrospinal fluid (CSF), among other antiretroviral drugs [15]. Thus, the quantity of TDF in the CNS may not be sufficient to reduce the viral loads but enough to cause neurotoxicity [14,16].

Recently, attention has been drawn to the use of nanoparticle drug delivery vehicles to navigate biological barriers and deliver antiretroviral drugs to anatomical sanctuary sites, such as the CNS, testicular tissue, and lymphoid organs, which harbor HIV [17]. Among several nanoparticles that have been widely employed, silver nanoparticles are currently receiving attention as potential agents in delivering cART to nervous tissues owing to their tunable shape ability [16,18,19]. In addition, silver nanoparticles are utilized in biomedical research to deliver therapeutic agents across the CNS due to their unique properties, such as anti-inflammatory, antidiabetic, antiviral, and antioxidant, which are vital to the alleviation of HIV-associated neurocognitive disorders and toxicity associated with antiretroviral drugs [19–22]. Based on these reports, we speculated that silver nanoparticle–TDF conjugates could protect the hippocampus against TDF-associated neurotoxicity via inhibition of inflammatory mediator release, oxidative stress, hippocampal neuronal cell membrane integrity alteration, hippocampal nerve organelle disintegration, hippocampal astrocytes, and glial cell degeneration.

As illustrated in Figure 1, HIV has the ability to cross the blood–brain barrier (A), but a combined therapy of antiretroviral drugs (C) has been reported with low CNS-penetrating power. Similarly, all nanoparticles, including the silver nanoparticle (B), have higher penetrating power to the biological barriers. Hence, we hypothesized that combining silver nanoparticles (AgNP) with antiretroviral drugs (ARDs) would solve the issue of CNS penetration. We also hypothesized that silver nanoparticle-conjugated TDF can decrease the blood glucose level in STZ-induced hyperglycemic rats and improve cognitive functions due to the antidiabetic and antioxidant properties of silver nanoparticles. Therefore, the current study evaluated the consequences of the interaction of silver nanoparticles conjugated with tenofovir disoproxil fumarate on the hippocampal microanatomy and neuro-biomarkers in diabetic rats.

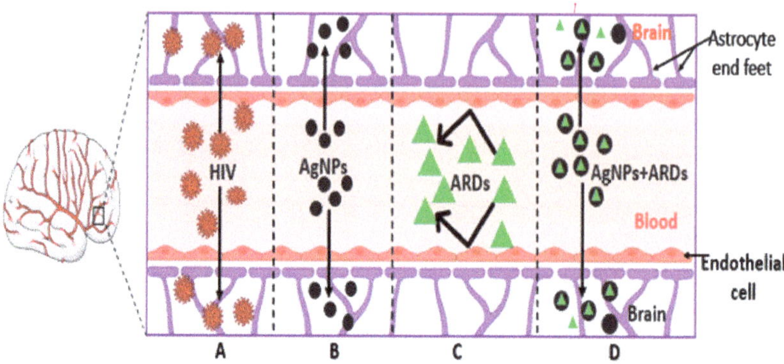

Figure 1. Illustration of the permeability of the blood–brain barrier to (**A**) HIV, (**B**) silver nanoparticles, (**C**) ARDs/TDF, and (**D**) AgNPs + ARDs. HIV (**A**) penetrates the BBB by infected monocytes, and in most cases, the infected monocytes travel via the astrocytes, leading to neuroinflammation. AgNPs (**B**) have the potential to pass through the BBB due to their unique properties, such as their tunable size and shape. However, most antiretroviral drugs (**C**) have meager CNS-penetrating power. The conjugated AgNPs + ARDs navigate the BBB and interact with nervous tissues (**D**).

2. Results

2.1. The Results of AgNPs-TDF Characterisation

The AgNPs-TDF conjugate was investigated using ultraviolet–visible spectroscopy (UV–vis Spec), a transmission electron microscope of a high-resolution type (HR-TEM), and an energy-dispersive X-ray spectroscopic machine (EDX spec), respectively.

2.2. Ultraviolet–Visible Spectroscopy Analysis

Figure 2: The UV–vis absorbance peaked at the range of 325–328 nm for the nanoconjugates (AgNPs-TDF) for the four concentrations (0.5 M, 1 M, 1.5 M, and 2 M) in this study, as shown in Figure 2. Additionally, Figure 2 shows that the conjugated AgNPs-TDF displayed absorbance peaks in two areas, found at 250 nm and between 325 and 328 nm. The observed absorbance peak values between 325 and 328 nm for the AgNPs-TDF are attributed to the localized surface plasmon resonance (SPR).

2.3. Transmission Electron Microscopy (TEM) Analysis

Figure 3: The size and shape of the AgNPs-TDF were analyzed using TEM, as shown in Figure 1. The size of the nanoconjugated drug for a 0.5 M concentration ranged from 12 to 22 nm, and a concentration of 0.5 M exhibited a size range of 3–4 nm, with an average of 7 nm, while the 1 M concentration had an average particle size of 20 nm, although their sizes were within 13–32 nm. In addition, the concentrations of 1.5 M and 2 M showed sizes ranging from 13 to 32 nm (7 nm on average) and 5 to 23 nm (12 nm on average), respectively. The AgNPs-TDF of 1 M and 2 M concentration showed spherical shapes, while 0.5 M and 1.5 M displayed a mixture of spherical and hexagonal shapes.

2.4. Energy Dispersive X-Ray (EDX) Analysis

Figure 4: The elemental constituents of the formulated nanodrug were revealed by the energy-dispersive X-ray analysis, as shown in Figure 2. The results show that the AgNPs peaked at 3 keV. In addition, it was observed that the AgNPs were constituted with different percentages per weight. The weight of Ag in the AgNPs-TDF increased from 5.45% for 0.5 M to 38.59%, which is 1.5 M to 42.70% for 2 M and 43.03% for 1 M. The presence of elements including phosphorus, oxygen, and carbon signifies the proper conjugation of AgNPs and TDF.

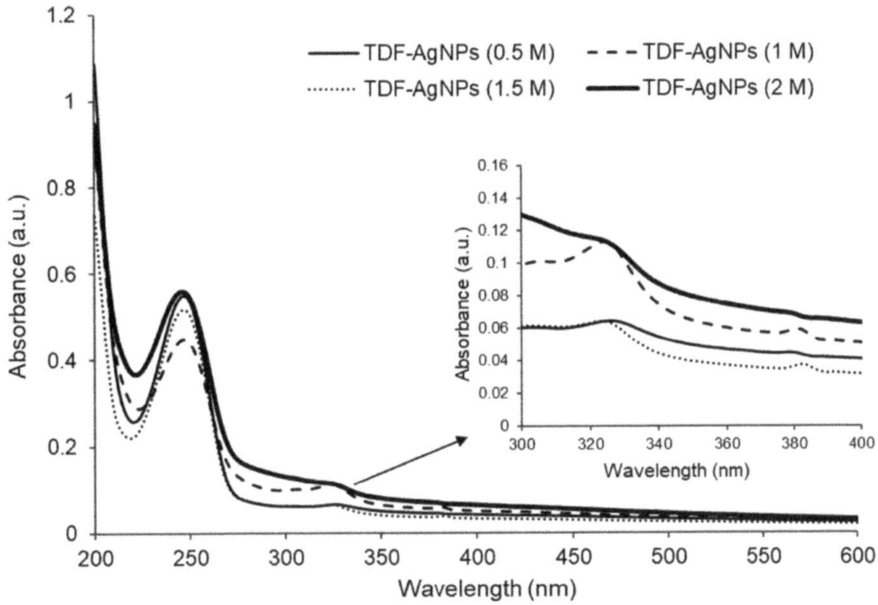

Figure 2. The ultraviolet-visible spectrum of the AgNPs-TDF at various concentrations. Adapted from a previous publication by Olojede et al. [23].

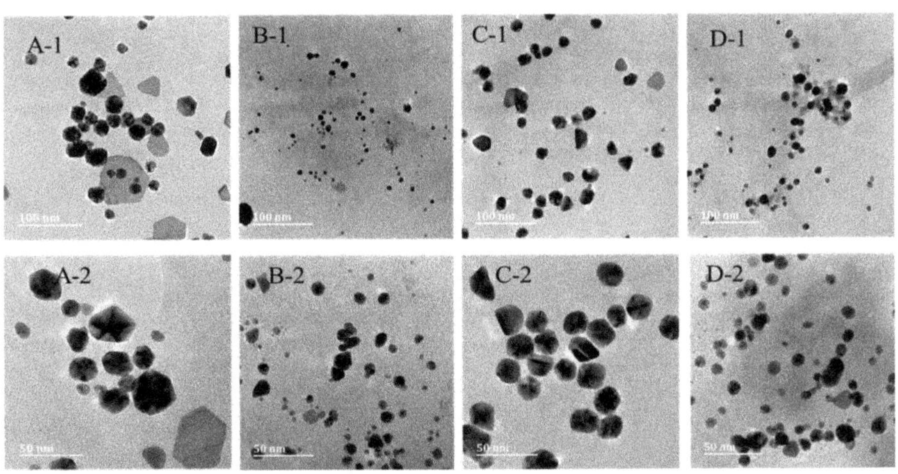

Figure 3. HR-TEM images of AgNPs-TDF (0.5 M) (**A**), AgNPs-TDF (1 M) (**B**), AgNPs-TDF (1.5 M) (**C**), and AgNPs-TDF (2 M) (**D**). (**A-1**) denotes 100 nm, (**A-2**) denotes 50 nm (0.5 M), (**B-1**) represents 100 nm, (**B-2**) represents 50 nm (1.0 M), (**C-1**) depicts 100 nm, (**C-2**) depicts 50 nm (1.5 M), (**D-1**) illustrates 100 nm, (**D-2**) illustrates 50 nm (2.0 M). Adapted from a previous publication by Olojede et al. [23].

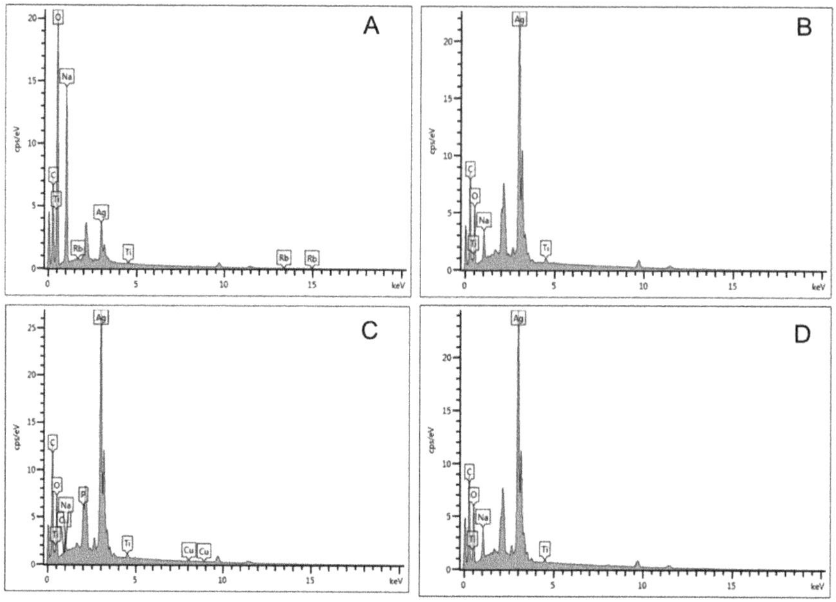

Figure 4. EDX spectra of AgNPs-TDF (0.5 M) (**A**), AgNPs-TDF (1 M) (**B**), AgNPs-TDF (1.5 M) (**C**), and AgNPs-TDF (2 M) (**D**). Adapted from a previous publication by Olojede et al. [23].

Table 1: EDX analysis showing the elemental components of various concentrations of the AgNPs-TDF conjugate.

Table 1. Energy dispersive X-ray analysis shows elemental components of the various concentrations of AgNPs-TDF conjugate. C = carbon, O = oxygen, Na = sodium, Ti = titanium, Ag = silver, Rb = rubidium, Cu = copper, and P = phosphorus.

Elements	Sample 0.5 M (Wt%)	Sample 1.0 M (Wt%)	Sample 1.5 M (Wt%)	Sample 2.0 M (Wt%)
C	30.64	25.32	30.76	25.51
O	49.76	27.63	27.51	27.76
Na	13.95	3.40	0.47	3.69
Ti	0.09	0.62	0.52	0.34
Ag	5.45	43.03	38.59	42.70
Rb	0.11	00.00	00.00	0.00
Cu	00.00	00.00	0.30	0.00
P	00.00	00.00	1.85	0.00
Total	100	100	100	100

2.5. Effects of AgNPs-TDF on Bodyweight Difference and Blood Glucose Levels

Figure 5a,b: There was a significant reduction in body weight of all the treated animals in the non-diabetic and diabetic groups when compared with non-diabetic control (NC). The diabetic control group (DC) had a significant reduction in body weight compared to the normal control and other treated groups. Interestingly, the group treated with AgNPs-TDF (DTS) showed a significant improvement in body weight compared with all the diabetic-treated groups (DC and DTF) (Figure 5a). The weekly weight difference (dynamics of the animals) was measured and recorded during the experiment but there was no significant difference. Thus, the initial and final weight difference is discussed in this manuscript.

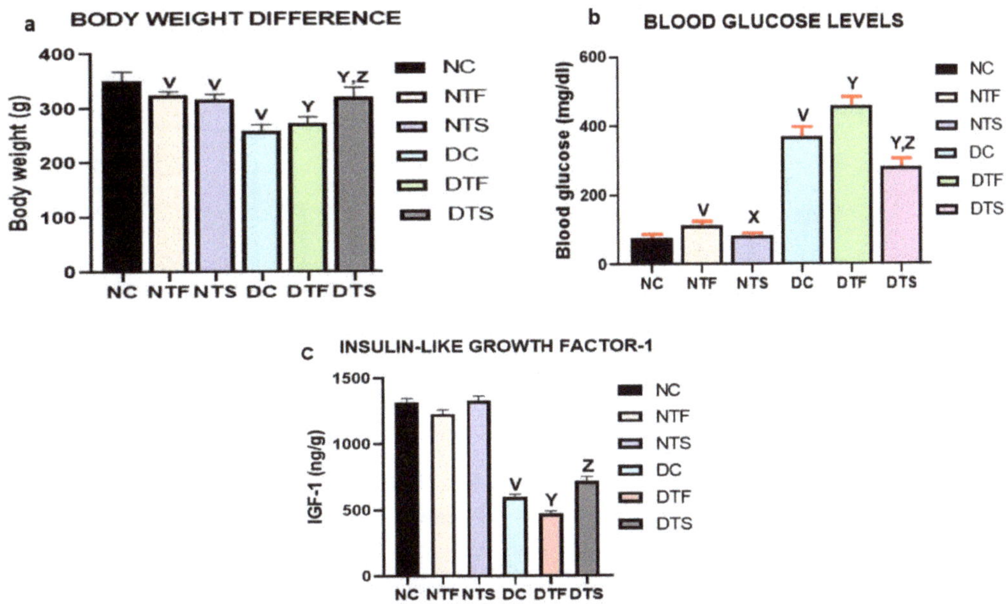

Figure 5. (**a**–**c**) Effects of AgNPs-TDF on bodyweight difference, blood glucose levels, and insulin-like growth factor-1 (IGF-1): ^{V} $p < 0.05$ vs. NC, ^{X} $p < 0.05$ vs. NTF, ^{Y} $p < 0.05$ vs. DC, ^{Z} $p < 0.05$ vs. DTF. NC = nondiabetic control, NTF = non-diabetic + TDF, NTS = non-diabetic + silver nanoparticles + TDF, DC = diabetic control, DTF = diabetic + TDF, DTS = diabetic + silver nanoparticles + TDF. Data are presented as mean ± SEM and are significant at $p < 0.05$. (n = 7).

Similarly, the blood glucose level was significantly higher in the diabetic control (DC) compared with the other diabetic-treated groups (DTF and DTS). However, DTS had significantly reduced blood glucose levels compared with DC and DTF. Notably, there was a statistically significant decrease in the blood glucose level of NTS compared with the non-diabetic treated NTF (Figure 5b).

There was no significant difference in the concentration of IGF-1 in all the non-diabetic groups (NC, NTF, and NTS). The IGF-1 was significantly reduced in the diabetic control group (DC) compared with the normal control group (NC). There was a significant increase in the concentration of IGF-1 in group DTS compared with group DTF (Figure 5c).

2.6. Effects of AgNPs-TDF on Spatial Working Memory

Figure 6: The cognitive functions of the experimental animals were assessed using Morris water maze escape latency. In training and testing, all the diabetic groups performed poorly compared with the non-diabetic groups. The test showed no difference between the TDF-treated and AgNPs-TDF-treated groups. However, the AgNPs-TDF-treated group spent more time in the quadrant previously containing the platform than the TDF-treated group and spent a significant amount of time in the quadrant compared with the diabetic control.

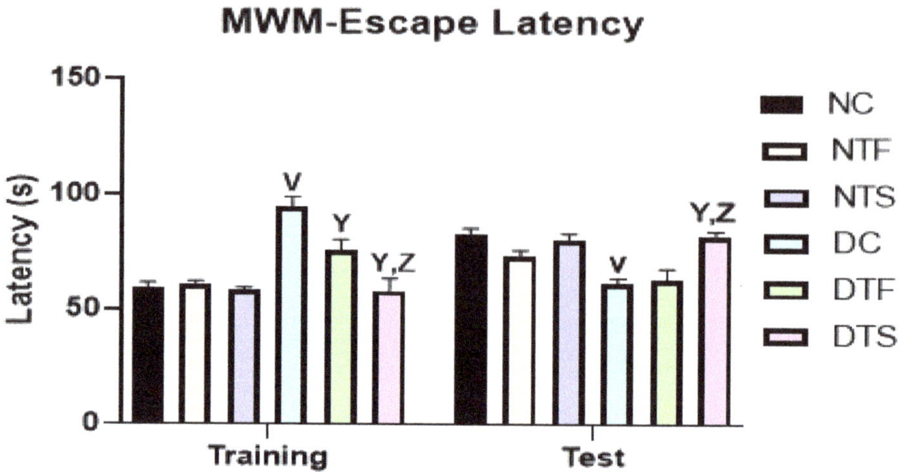

Figure 6. Effects of AgNPs-TDF on spatial working memory: ^{V} $p < 0.001$ vs. NC, ^{Y} $p < 0.001$ vs. DC, ^{Z} $p < 0.001$ vs. DTF. NC = nondiabetic control, NTF = non-diabetic + TDF, NTS = non-diabetic + silver nanoparticles + TDF, DC = diabetic control, DTF = diabetic + TDF, DTS = diabetic + silver nanoparticles + TDF. Data are presented as mean ± SEM and are significant at $p < 0.001$. (n = 7).

2.7. Effects of AgNPs-TDF on Locomotion and Explorative Behavior

Figure 7: The locomotion and explorative behavior of the experimental animals were assessed using an open-field test. The center line crossing, total line crossing, and rearing were used to examine the explorative and anxiety-like behavior. All the diabetic groups had a reduction in locomotion and explorative behaviors compared to the non-diabetic groups. Interestingly, the group treated with AgNPs-TDF significantly improved locomotion and exploration compared to the diabetic control and TDF-treated group.

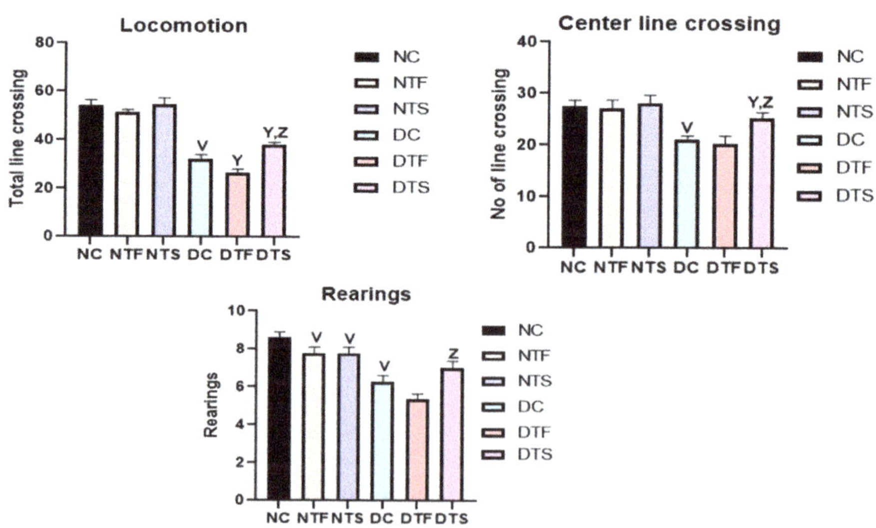

Figure 7. Effects of AgNPs-TDF on locomotion and explorative behavior: ^{V} $p < 0.05$ vs. NC, ^{Y} $p < 0.05$ vs. DC, ^{Z} $p < 0.05$ vs. DTF. NC = nondiabetic control, NTF = non-diabetic + TDF, NTS = non-diabetic + silver nanoparticles + TDF, DC = diabetic control, DTF = diabetic + TDF, DTS = diabetic + silver nanoparticles + TDF. Data are presented as mean ± SEM and are significant at $p < 0.05$.

2.8. Effects of AgNPs-TDF on Hippocampal Oxidative Stress Markers

Table 2: This table shows the results for the antioxidant parameters in the experimental animals. MDA was significantly higher in the diabetic rats and diabetic TDF-treated rats than in the other groups. The AgNPs-TDF-treated rats showed a significant decrease in MDA compared to the diabetic and diabetic TDF-treated rats. Similarly, the antioxidant parameters (SOD and GSH) were significantly increased in the diabetic AgNPs-TDF-treated rats compared to diabetic TDF-treated only.

Table 2. Effects of AgNPs-TDF on hippocampal oxidative stress markers: ^{V} $p < 0.05$ vs. NC, ^{X} $p < 0.05$ vs. NTF, ^{Y} $p < 0.05$ vs. DC, ^{Z} $p < 0.05$ vs. DTF. NC = nondiabetic control, NTF = non-diabetic + TDF, NTS = non-diabetic + silver nanoparticles + TDF, DC = diabetic control, DTF = diabetic + TDF, DTS = diabetic + silver nanoparticles + TDF. Data are presented as mean ± SEM and are significant at $p < 0.05$. (n = 5).

Hippocampal Oxidative Markers	Animal Grouping					
	NC	NTF	NTS	DC	DTF	DTS
MDA (nmol/mg)	30 ± 1.34	41.42 ± 1.57 ^{V}	30.46 ± 1.71 ^{X}	65.73 ± 1.79 ^{V}	72.64 ± 1.47 ^{Y}	45.30 ± 0.97 ^{Y,Z}
SOD (u/mg)	10.06 ± 0.23	9.26 ± 0.22	9.19 ± 0.39	4.87 ± 0.17 ^{V}	3.54 ± 0.32 ^{Y}	6.29 ± 0.18 ^{Y,Z}
CAT (nmol/mg)	16.50 ± 0.70	12.83 ± 0.78	14.12 ± 0.56 ^{X}	7.51 ± 0.36 ^{V}	7.70 ± 0.59	9.93 ± 0.42 ^{Y}
GSH (nmol/mg)	91.26 ± 3.12	76.38 ± 3.92	86.23 ± 3.30 ^{V}	49.02 ± 1.77 ^{V}	37.34 ± 1.03 ^{Y}	62.85 ± 2.16 ^{Y,Z}

2.9. Effects of AgNPs-TDF on Hippocampal Inflammatory Markers

Table 3: Neuroinflammation was assessed using TNF-α and IL-1β. The non-diabetic rats treated with TDF showed a significant increase in TNF-α compared to the control group. Similarly, the diabetic TDF-treated rats had a high-level TNF-α concentration compared to the diabetic control and AgNPs-TDF-treated rats. Interestingly, there was a significant decrease in the IL-1β and TNF-α concentrations in the AgNPs-TDF-treated rats compared to the diabetic control and TDF-treated only.

Table 3. Effects of AgNPs-TDF on hippocampal inflammatory markers: ^{V} $p < 0.05$ vs. NC, ^{Y} $p < 0.05$ vs. DC, ^{Z} $p < 0.05$ vs. DTF. NC = nondiabetic control, NTF = non-diabetic + TDF, NTS = non-diabetic + silver nanoparticles + TDF, DC = diabetic control, DTF = diabetic + TDF, DTS = diabetic + silver nanoparticles + TDF. Data are presented as mean ± SEM and are significant at $p < 0.05$. (n = 5).

Groups/Parameters	TNF-α (pg/mL)	IL-1β (pg/mL) (n = 5)
NC	185.4 ± 4.71	35.19 ± 1.00
NTF	234.50 ± 6.29 ^{V}	43.48 ± 2.83
NTS	204.60 ± 6.09	40.55 ± 2.52
DC	339.90 ± 13.85 ^{V}	72.84 ± 1.98 ^{V}
DTF	412.30 ± 14.14 ^{Y}	88.96 ± 1.76 ^{Y}
DTS	309.50 ± 4.908 ^{Y,Z}	55.13 ± 1.53 ^{Y,Z}

2.10. Effects of AgNPs-TDF on Hippocampal Ultrastructure—Neuronal Nuclear Membrane

Figure 8: The ultrastructure of the hippocampus was processed using TEM, and the results were analyzed. The nuclear membranes of the non-diabetic groups (NC, NTF, and NTS) showed a distinct oval-shaped nuclear membrane (NM) covering the nucleolus. The nuclear membrane (NM) was affected in all the diabetic groups (DC, DTF and DTS), showing a distorted and irregular-shaped membrane. However, the DTF group showed a similar oval-shaped nuclear membrane with vacuolating neoplasms.

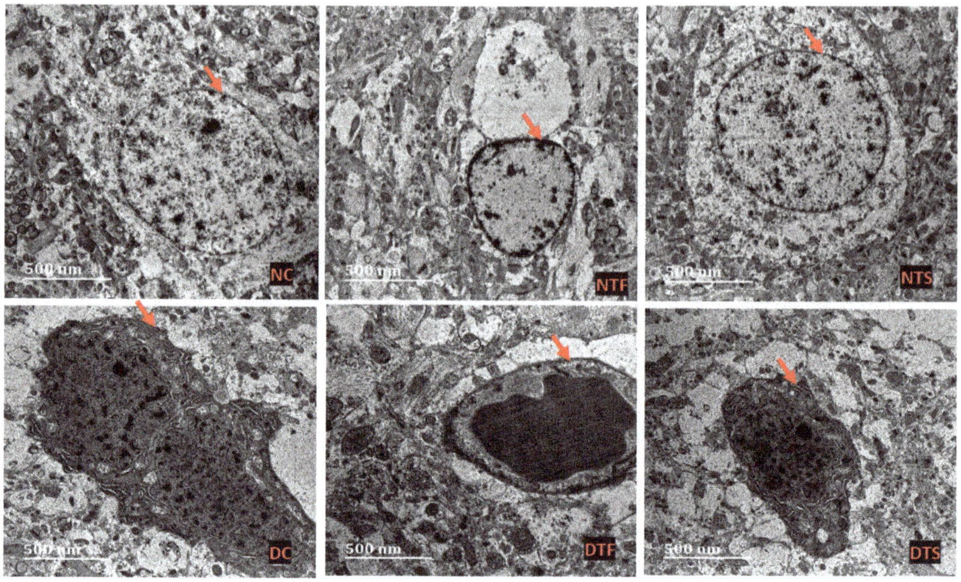

Figure 8. Effects of AgNPs-TDF on hippocampal ultrastructure neuronal nuclear membrane. NC = nondiabetic control, NTF = non-diabetic + TDF, NTS = non-diabetic + silver nanoparticles + TDF, DC = diabetic control, DTF = diabetic + TDF, DTS = diabetic + silver nanoparticles + TDF, red arrow = nuclear membrane. (n = 2).

2.11. Effects of AgNPs-TDF on Hippocampal Neuronal Nissl Bodies

Figure 9: Cresyl violet was used to stain the neuronal cell. The neurons of all the diabetic-treated rats showed chromophobic and pyknotic neuronal nuclei compared with the non-diabetic rats. Interestingly, the AgNPs-TDF showed a monomorphic pattern of dark-stained neuronal nuclei similar to the control group.

2.12. Effects of AgNPs-TDF on Hippocampal GFAP-Astrocytic Cells

Figure 10: This shows the hippocampal-astrocytic cells in all the experimental rats. The normal control (NC) showed distinct astrocytes interconnected with the neighboring cells compared to the diabetic control (DC). There was a loss of distinct astrocytic cells in the diabetic rats treated with TDF compared to the rats treated with AgNPs-TDF.

2.13. Effects of AgNPs-TDF on Hippocampal Astrogliosis

Figure 11 shows the hippocampal astrogliosis in all the experimental rats. There was a significant increase in GFAP-positive astrocytic cells in all the diabetic-treated groups (DC, DTF, and DTS). Notably, the diabetic rats treated with TDF (DTF) significantly increased the number of activated astrocytes compared with the diabetic control (DC). However, in group DTS, the AgNPs-TDF significantly reduced the activation of GFAP-positive cells compared to the other diabetic groups.

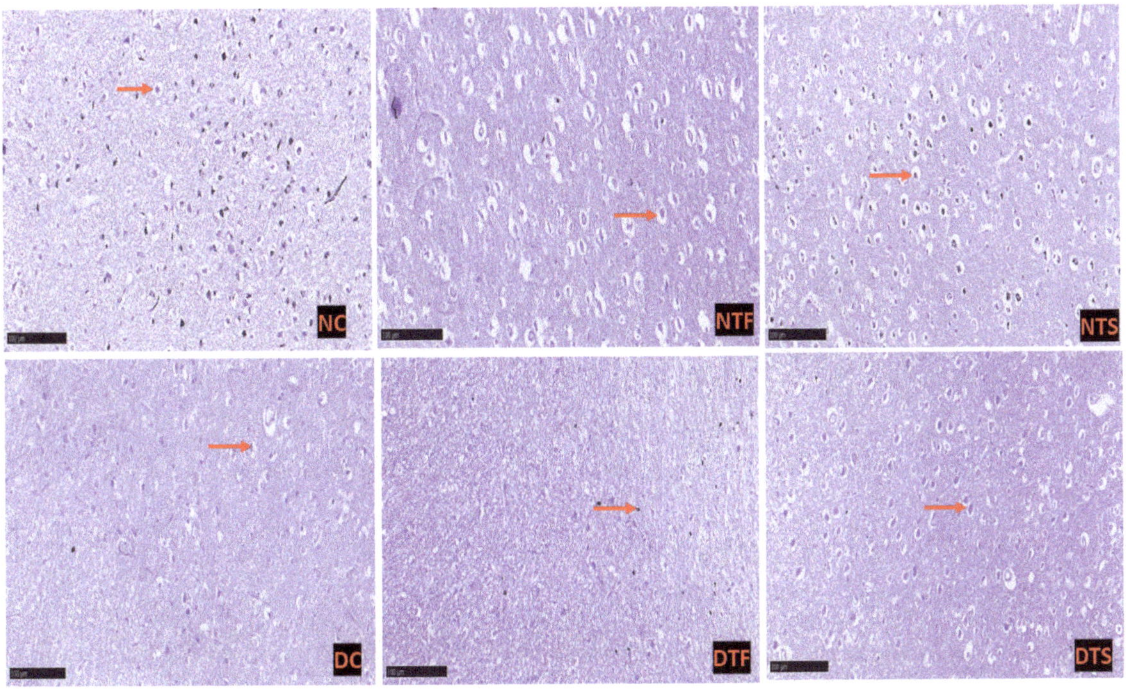

Figure 9. Effects of AgNPs-TDF on hippocampal neuronal Nissl bodies: NC = nondiabetic control, NTF = non-diabetic + TDF, NTS = non-diabetic + silver nanoparticles + TDF, DC = diabetic control, DTF = diabetic + TDF, DTS = diabetic + silver nanoparticles + TDF, red arrow = neurons. (n = 2).

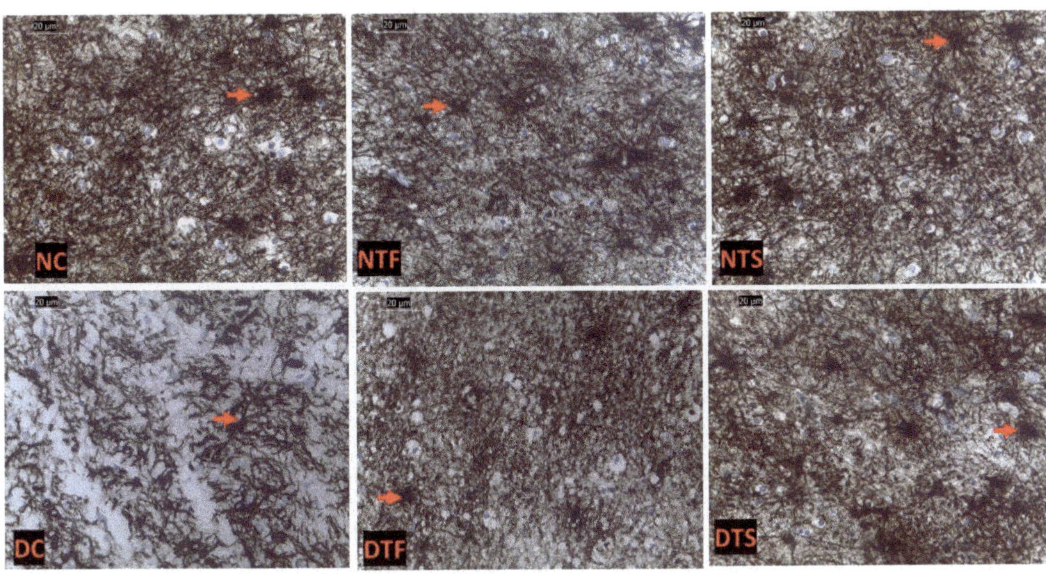

Figure 10. Effects of AgNPs-TDF on hippocampal GFAP-astrocytic cells: NC = nondiabetic control, NTF = non-diabetic + TDF, NTS = non-diabetic + silver nanoparticles + TDF, DC = diabetic control, DTF = diabetic + TDF, DTS = diabetic + silver nanoparticles + TDF, red arrow = astrocytic cell. (n = 2).

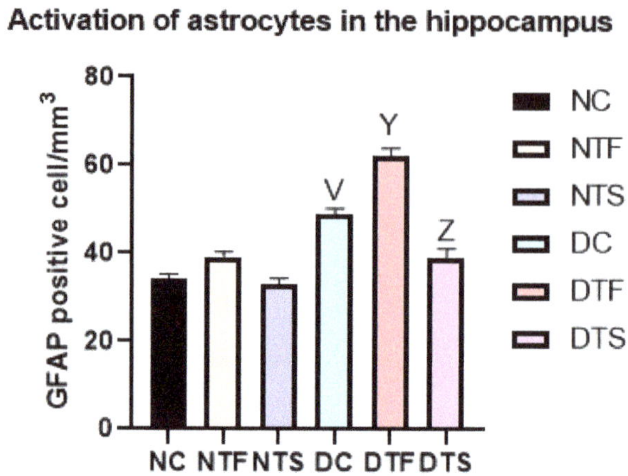

Figure 11. Effects of AgNPs-TDF on hippocampal GFAP-astrocytic cells: NC = nondiabetic control, NTF = non-diabetic + TDF, NTS = non-diabetic + silver nanoparticles + TDF, DC = diabetic control, DTF = diabetic + TDF, DTS = diabetic + silver nanoparticles + TDF. ^{V} $p < 0.05$ vs. NC, ^{Y} $p < 0.05$ vs. DC, ^{Z} $p < 0.05$ vs. DTF (n = 2).

3. Discussion

The nanoparticle drug delivery system has been viewed as an emerging field of nanomedicine that addresses issues related to biological penetration, challenges of targeted delivery, and therapeutic-associated toxicities. These functions have been ascribed to the properties of nanoparticles, which include tunable shape and size, as well as targeted and controlled release [23]. However, ample amounts of these nanoparticles have been loaded with several therapeutic agents and evaluated in vitro and in vivo with promising results. However, there is a dearth of information on the utilization of silver nanoparticles with proven anti-inflammatory, antidiabetic, antiviral, and antioxidant activities for their potential management of TDF-induced neurotoxicity. Hence, this study was conceived to unravel the mechanisms underlying the neuroprotective effects of silver nanoparticle-conjugated tenofovir disoproxil fumarate on the hippocampal microanatomy and neuro-biomarkers in diabetic rats.

Characterization represents an essential process to examine the peak value, size, shape, and elemental constituents of nanoparticles and conjugates. The observed absorbance peak values within two regions (between 325 and 328 nm and at 250 nm) for the AgNPs-TDF may be attributed to the localized surface plasmon resonance (SPR). Previously, Menon et al. [24] revealed that variations in the absorption peak and color changes are mostly determined by the SPR around the region of the electromagnetic spectrum. This indicates that the wavelength in the regions reported in this study was absorbed. Similarly, previous research has described the effect of the sensitivity of SPR to the shape and size changes of nanoparticles [25]. More so, both spherical and hexagonal nanoparticles were obtained in this investigation, which may be another factor for the absorption peak value noticed. Therefore, the SPR region was observed at 325 to 328 nm, possibly because of a combination of hexagonal and spherical-shaped nanoparticles, which agrees with a previous investigation [26]. In addition, the absorption peak of 250 nm recorded in this study has been previously documented in a similar spectrophotometric study that shows an absorption peak value of 259 nm for TDF, which signifies the proper conjugation of TDF to AgNPs [27].

The observed nanoparticle size ranging from 3 nm to 32 nm is similar to Van Dong and colleagues' findings [28], who documented spherical-shaped AgNPs of sizes ranging between 4 and 40 nm. However, a mixture of hexagonal, rod, and spherical-shaped particles was observed in this study. However, the results acquired with 1 M and 2 M of AgNPs-TDF were predominantly spherical-shaped particles, which concurs with an investigation by Yang and co-workers [29], who documented spherical-shaped AgNPs of sizes within 30 nm. With an increased interest in AgNPs, experts have described particle size, especially within 30 nm, and shape, especially spherical-shaped, as important factors to consider when using AgNPs for pharmaceutical and biological uses [30].

The appropriate peak of AgNPs was noticed in this study, which aligns with the investigation performed by Mukherji and colleagues [31], who documented a peak of 3 keV for the AgNPs. In addition, the presence of the elemental constituents present in the TDF and AgNPs, such as phosphorus, carbon, and oxygen, signifies the proper conjugation of TDF with AgNPs. The remaining elements present in the results of the EDX were obtained from a reducing agent (trisodium citrate), while the copper grid employed to mount the samples gives copper, titanium, and rubidium, as found in the sample.

This study observed an elevated blood glucose level in diabetic rats treated with tenofovir disoproxil fumarate, confirming its metabolic disturbances reported in the literature [11,32]. Insulin resistance is common among HIV-positive people under antiretroviral treatment due to certain factors, including weight gain [32,33]. However, the moderate weight loss observed in this study suggests that other factors may play a role in metabolic disturbance rather than body weight gain, which is in line with other studies [33,34]. The silver nanoparticles possess antidiabetic effects, as reported by Alkaladi et al. [19]; in this study, the animals treated with the silver nanoparticles–TDF conjugate showed a consistent decrease in blood glucose level with improved body weight gain compared to the diabetic TDF-treated group.

This suggests that the silver nanoparticles improved glucose uptake and muscle cell sensitivity to blood glucose, thereby reducing blood glucose levels, similar to previous studies [35]. This effect was attributed to the special characteristics of silver nanoparticles, like large ratio of surface area to volume and antidiabetic properties, which act to inhibit carbohydrate metabolic enzymes (alpha-amylase and alpha-glucosidase) to reduce blood glucose levels [19,36].

Insulin-like growth factor systems and signaling pathways are involved in the differentiation, growth, and maintenance of neurons and supporting cells of the brain, as well as the prevention of neuronal apoptosis. However, damage to these systems is involved in neurodegenerative disorders like dementia and Alzheimer's and metabolic dysfunctions [37,38]. The significant increase in IGF-1 levels in diabetes treatment suggests the capability of AgNP to enhance insulin secretion. This finding agrees with previous investigations that revealed the activities of AgNPs to lower blood sugar levels and enhance the secretion and sensitivity of insulin, which increase the level of IGF-1 in diabetic rats [13,39]. These findings altogether suggest that an increase in the IGF-1 level is responsible for the decrease in blood glucose level observed in this experiment.

The prevalence of neurocognitive disorders is still high in HIV-positive people despite the numerous benefits of combined therapy, including TDF [3]. The current study showed an extent of neurocognitive dysfunction in the tenofovir-treated group. However, the animals treated with the AgNPs-TDF conjugate showed improved neurocognitive function through restoring various alterations in the hippocampal ultrastructure and improving memory assessment in diabetic rats. This observation could be attributed to the ability of silver nanoparticles to deliver a low-dose and effective drug release, reducing TDF's neurotoxic effect [40,41].

Further investigation in this current study revealed the metabolic disturbance of TDF via oxidative stress markers. Glutathione, which is involved in tissue repair and combating stress-induced tissue damage, was depleted in the diabetic TDF-treated animals with increased lipid peroxidation. This result correlates with a previous study [42]. However, the silver nanoparticles ameliorated the oxidative effects by blocking TDF's excessive reactive oxygen species (ROS) production via increased antioxidant glutathione [43].

In the present study, the neurotoxic effect was evidenced by the high concentration of neuroinflammatory markers (IL-1β and TNF-α) in the hippocampus of the TDF-treated animals. Several studies have reported the neuroinflammatory effects of TDF [44,45]. However, the conjugated silver nanoparticles with tenofovir drastically reduced the concentration of neuroinflammatory markers. Studies have reported the anti-inflammatory properties of silver nanoparticles with green synthesis [38,46], and the mechanism of these anti-inflammatory activities has been linked with the ability of silver nanoparticles to inhibit some selected cytokine agents, such as IL-6 and IL-1β [47]. More evidence has emerged that AgNPs lower the initiation of transcription pathways involving TNFR1/NF-KB, directly reducing TNF-α's inflammatory response [48].

The observed distorted neuronal nuclear membrane and astrocytic cells in the hippocampus of diabetic rats, as seen in the results of this study, could suggest a deleterious effect of diabetes mellitus on hippocampus cytoarchitecture. Empirical evidence has indicated that the hippocampus is one of the most essential parts of the brain susceptible to metabolic dysfunction like diabetes mellitus [49]. A similar in vivo study on an animal model revealed diabetic-induced neuronal nuclear membrane alterations, reduction in cell body diameter, neuronal nuclear reduction, and decreased neuronal density in the hippocampus [50]. In addition, the loss of connection between the surrounding neuroglia and neurons in diabetic rats indicates hippocampal injury, which is consistent with a previous study that documented neuroglia degeneration and detachment in an experimental diabetic rat model [51,52]. Consequently, it leads to neuronal death because the function of the neuroglia is to support and insulate neurons; once the connection is lost, the neurons are susceptible to death [52]. This diabetic-induced hippocampal damage and neuronal cell death were attributed to insulin resistance, chronic hyperglycemia, and deficits in hippocampal insulin signaling, which leads to cognitive and behavioral [53]

Furthermore, alteration to the neuronal cell membrane in diabetic rats treated with tenofovir disoproxil fumarate indicates damage to the hippocampus.

An investigation by Fields, Swinton [3] documented alterations to the hippocampal structures in an in vivo mice model, similar to the result of this present study, although not in a diabetic condition. Several studies have attributed mitochondrial dysfunction and accumulation of reactive oxygen species as mechanisms responsible for tenofovir-induced hippocampal neuronal alteration and, consequently, neurocognitive impairments [54–56]. Additionally, the chromophobic and pyknotic neuronal cells' hippocampal neurons noticed with tenofovir administration in this study concur with a similar investigation that reported negative Nissl-stained hippocampal neuronal cells following administration of an antiretroviral combination containing tenofovir in diabetic rats [57]. In addition, the loss of GFAP-astrocytic cells in the TDF-treated rats observed indicates astrogliosis, as reported by previous studies [58,59]. These reports, together, suggest a hippocampal neuron distortion with the administration of tenofovir in diabetic or non-diabetic conditions.

Interestingly, a monomorphic pattern of dark-stained neuronal nuclei and restoration in the loss of astrocytic cells following administration of AgNPs-TDF in this study indicates some neuroprotective impact of nanoparticles synthesized from silver. Although many studies have suggested that silver nanoparticles are neurotoxic in vitro and in vivo [60–62], this is on account that smaller particle sizes like silver nanoparticles can easily navigate the blood–brain barrier to gain access to and interact with brain tissue [63]. However, emerging evidence has revealed that the neurotoxicity of silver nanoparticles largely depends on several factors, such as the concentration of silver nitrate, surface coating, reducing agent, particle size, particle shape, level of exposure, agglomeration, and method of preparation [64]. The neuroprotective impact obtained may be attributed to the smaller size and spherical shape of silver nanoparticles used in this study, which elicits its antioxidant, antidiabetic, and anti-inflammatory properties to restore some hippocampal alterations. This study agrees with Lawal et al. [13] findings, who reported improved neurocognitive deficits through silver nanoparticles' antioxidant, antidiabetic, and anti-inflammatory properties loaded with antiretroviral drugs. This finding suggests that the biological activities of silver nanoparticles could be effectively exploited in the delivery of antiretroviral drugs by taking care of factors associated with its toxicity profile to enhance the efficacy of these agents in managing neurocognitive deficits.

4. Materials and Methods

4.1. Material

The TDF (300 mg) was purchased at the Dis-Chem pharmacy in Durban, South Africa. Streptozotocin (STZ), trisodium citrate, sodium hydroxide, and silver nitrate ($AgNO_3$) were purchased from Sigma-Aldrich Company, Johannesburg, South Africa. Enzyme-linked immunosorbent assay (ELISA) kits, TNF-α (cat no: E-EL-R0019), interleukin (IL)-1β (cat no: E-EL-R0012), and primary antibody (Anti-GFAP: AB10062) and secondary antibody (Goat Anti-mouse IGg: AB150113) (Elab Science Biotechnology Co., Ltd., Houston, TX, USA) were sourced from BIOCOM Africa (pty), Ltd., Centurion, South Africa.

4.2. Animal

Forty-two (42) adult male Sprague-Dawley rats weighing between (250 ± 13 g) were acquired from the Biomedical Research Unit of the University of KwaZulu-Natal (UKZN-BRU). All the animals were kept in the animal laboratory in highly ventilated plastic cages 24 cm in height, 36 cm wide, and 52 cm in length. They were allowed to feed (standard rat pellets) and drink freely. The room temperature was maintained at 24–26 °C with a 12:12 light:dark cycle.

4.3. Ethical Approval

The animal laboratory procedures and study protocol were approved by the Research Ethical Committee of the University of KwaZulu-Natal with AREC number (AREC/044/19D). All the procedures were carried out at the Biomedical Research Unit (BRU) and overseen by a certified veterinarian (SAVC registration number SAVC D14/11254).

The animals received humane care based on the Care and Use of Laboratory Animals guide provided by the National Institute of Health (NIH Publications No. 80-23).

4.4. Experimental Design

The rats were left to acclimatize for seven (7) days; after that, they were divided randomly into diabetic and non-diabetic groups. Both the non-diabetic and diabetic groups were further divided into three (3) subgroups (n = 7). The non-diabetic groups 1–3 (designated as non-diabetic control (NC)) received 0.5 mL/100 g distilled water per os (p.o.), non-diabetic + tenofovir (NTF) were administered 26.8 mg/kg/bw TDF p.o., and non-diabetic + tenofovir + silver nanoparticles (NTS) were administered 6.7 mg/kg AgNPs-TDF intraperitoneally (i.p.), respectively.

Similarly, the diabetic groups 4–6 (designated as diabetic control (DC)) were administered 0.5 mL/100 g distilled water per os (p.o.), diabetic + tenofovir (DTF) received 26.8 mg/kg/bw TDF p.o., and diabetic + tenofovir + silver nanoparticles (DTS) received 6.7 mg/kg AgNPs-TDF intraperitoneally (i.p.), respectively.

The given dose was determined by our previous studies [42,65], and the animal dose for TDF was estimated from the human equivalent dose (HED), as described by the United States Food and Drug Administration (FDA) [66]. The administration of the testing agents began after diabetes induction. Oral administration was given daily for eight weeks, and intraperitoneal injection was completed 5/7 days for 8 weeks. The TDF was administered orally, while the AgNPs-TDF was administered intraperitoneally. The reason for administering AgNPs-TDF intraperitoneally was informed by the need for several physiological barriers and hurdles, such as gastric mucosal composition, gastric motility, and gastric pH, before the loaded drug can reach the target cell.

Moreover, under the 3 Rs and 5 Freedom of Animal Research Ethics, we reduced the IP administration from 7 days a week to 5 days. Behavioral assessments were conducted on the second resting day of the animals to cater to the animals' welfare.

4.5. Induction of Type II Diabetes Mellitus in Experimental Rats

After seven (7) days of acclimatization, each rat's baseline body weight and blood glucose were measured and recorded. After that, hyperglycemia with insulin resistance was induced using the fructose–streptozotocin (STZ) rat model described by Wilson and Islam [67]. Briefly, the diabetic groups (4–6) received a fructose solution (10% fructose solution *ad libitum*) for two weeks. On the final day of administering fructose, the rats were fasted overnight, and freshly prepared 40 mg/Kg/bw STZ dissolved in 0.9% NaCl with 100 mM sodium citrate buffer (pH 4.5) was given via the intraperitoneal route. In contrast, the control rats were given the same volume of citrate buffer (vehicle). Fasting blood glucose levels $\geq$ 200 mg/dL were an indication of diabetes in the rats.

4.5.1. Synthesis of AgNPs and Formulations of AgNPs-TDF

Silver nitrate ($AgNO_3$) and trisodium citrate (TSC) were employed to synthesize the silver nanoparticles. An aqueous solution of 0.3 M $AgNO_3$ and four concentrations (0.5 M, 1 M, 1.5 M, and 2.0 M) of TSC were prepared. The silver nanoparticles were prepared by mixing the two solutions (20 mL of $AgNO_3$ and 20 mL of concentrations of TSC in a ratio of 1:1) in a beaker while continuing to stir for 5 min at 90 °C. The pH of 10.5 was adjusted using NaOH. The resultant solution was stirred continuously until the color changed from colorless to amber color. A solution of 0.35 M of tenofovir dyspraxia fumarate (TDF) was prepared by dissolving the crystal form of TDF in 1 M of NaOH. The already synthesized AgNPs were then mixed with a solution of TDF (50 mL of TDF and 100 mL of AgNPs in a ratio of 1:2) and sonicated at a frequency of 20–40 kHz for 15 min. Lastly, the AgNPs-TDF supernatant was analyzed with UV–vis spec, and the percentage incorporated was determined and calculated. The full protocol has been previously described [23]. The efficiency of the percentage of AgNPs-TDF incorporated was calculated as follows:

$$\%\,IE = \frac{Q_2 - Q_1}{Q_1} \times 100 \; = 85.00 \, \pm \, 0.0\%.$$

where Q_1 = quantity of unincorporated drug and Q_2 = total amount of drug coupled with the silver nanoparticles.

4.5.2. Characterization of AgNPs and AgNPs-TDF

The characterization of the AgNPs and AgNPs-TDF was reported previously by [23]. Briefly, the formulation of the AgNPs-TDF conjugate was confirmed with ultraviolet–visible (UV–vis) spectroscopy (Shimadzu MultSpec-1501, Shimadzu Corporation, Tokyo, Japan) at an absorption peak from 325 to 328 nm. Fourier transform infrared (FTIR) spectroscopy (Perkin-Elmer Universal ATR spectrometer, Waltham, MA, USA) was used to identify the various functional groups in the AgNPs-TDF conjugates. The presence of C-N and O-H functional groups in the AgNPs-TDF confirmed that AgNPs-TDF was conjugated. The size and morphology of the AgNPs-TDF were examined by a high-resolution transmission electron microscope (HR-TEM, JEOL 2100, Chiba, Japan) operated at a voltage of 200 kV. The HR-TEM revealed the nanoparticle shape and size of the AgNPs-TDF conjugates to be spherical, and the mean particle sizes were 12 nm to 22 nm.

A field emission scanning electron microscope (FESEM, Carl Zeiss, Oberkochen, Germany), operated at a voltage of 5 kV with energy dispersive X-ray (EDX, Aztec Analysis Software, version 6.0 Southampton, UK), was used to determine the elemental components, and this confirmed the presence of silver in the AgNPs-TDF.

4.6. Blood Glucose and Body Weight Difference Measurement

After diabetic induction and during the drug administration, fasting blood glucose was obtained using a glucometer (Sigma-Aldrich, Durban, South Africa) via the tail vein of the rats on a weekly basis. The body weight difference was measured using a sensitive weighing balance.

4.7. Behavioral Studies

4.7.1. Morris Water Maze for Spatial Working Memory

On the 7th week of administration, the spatial working memory was evaluated using the Morris water maze, as described by the previous studies of Greish et al. and Morris [68,69]. Briefly, the instrument is made up of a standard circular swimming pool 100 cm in diameter half-filled with water of about 22–25 °C. Each of the rats was assigned 120 s to locate the platform that was hidden 2 cm below the water level, and the animal that could not find the escape platform after 120 s of the trial time was calmly led to the platform and allowed to be on the platform for a few seconds. In addition, the latency was recorded.

After two days, the test was repeated on each animal, following the same procedure as the training trial. The percentage of time spent swimming in the quadrant previously containing the platform was recorded and calculated to determine the spatial working memory.

The animals that spent longer in the quadrant previously containing the platform were considered to have learned and retained memory.

4.7.2. Open Field Test for Locomotion and Explorative Behavior

The rats were assessed for locomotion and explorative behavior through the open-field test during the resting day of administration in the 7th week. The open-field apparatus was set up according to previous studies [70,71]. Briefly, using a measuring diameter 70 cm long × 70 cm wide × 35 cm high with several 15 cm × 15 cm squares, a large rectangular measuring box was used. The rats were positioned in the center of the square and examined for 5 min. Parameters like total line cross, center line cross, and rearing were obtained. The exploration of the animals was assessed using the number of times the animal stood up on its posterior limbs (rearing). This behavior imitates an activity of space exploration of a new environment [72].

4.8. Euthanasia Procedure and Tissue Harvesting

Twenty-four (24) hours after the last administration, the experimental animals were euthanized using isoflurane in a closed container. The animals were observed until signs of breathing stopped, and the animals (n = 2) were humanely euthanized according to standard protocol by the AREC-approved guidelines. Tissue samples were collected for histological and immunohistochemical analysis. Two (2) out of seven (7) animals were used for histological and immunohistochemical analysis. This was done to prevent other brain tissues used for biochemical analysis from being contaminated with fixatives.

4.9. Determination of Antioxidant Levels and Other Biochemical Analyses

The hippocampal tissue was homogenized with 0.1 M phosphate buffer (pH 7.5) using a polytron homogenizer. The homogenate was centrifuged at 15,000 rpm for 5 min in a Centrikon H-401 (Kontron, Munich, Germany) centrifuge at 4 °C. After centrifugation, the upper part was collected and analyzed. The following antioxidant superoxide dismutase (SOD) and catalase (CAT) were analyzed according to previous protocols [65,73] reduced glutathione (GSH) was determined using Ellman's protocol [66] and the malondialdehyde (MDA) level was determined using the method of Mkhwanazi et al. [67].

4.10. Determination of Inflammatory Biomarkers

The tumor necrosis factor-α (TNF-α) and interleukin (IL)-1β concentrations were quantified in the hippocampal homogenates using their specific ELISA kits (Elab Science Biotechnology Co., Ltd., Houston, TX, USA) based on the instructions and protocols of the manufacturer.

4.11. Histopathological and Immunohistological Studies

The brain was carefully removed and weighed, then post-fixed in 4% paraformaldehyde for 48 h. The hippocampus was dissected from the brain using a rat atlas and processed for histological analysis. The tissue was infiltrated with 30% sucrose for 3 days at 4 °C. The paraffin-embedded tissue was sectioned at 5 μm using a Leica RM 2255 microtome and stained according to Bancroft and Stevens protocol [74] for hematoxylin and eosin (H&E) and Nissl staining.

The remaining sections of the hippocampus used immunohistochemical analysis. Firstly, the sections were washed in PBL and pre-incubated in 5% goat serum (0.1 M with 0.4% Triton X-100, 1 M PBL and albumen) for 1 h at 4 °C, then directly incubated in the primary antibody (anti-GFAP) diluted in PBSA-Triton at a ratio of 1:5000. After that, the sections were washed in PBST (2 × 10 min) and incubated in a secondary antibody for 2 h at room temperature. They were then rinsed in PBST (2 × 10 min) and incubated with an avidin–biotin complex for 2 h, followed by several washes (1 × 10 min in PBST and 2 × 10 min in Tris buffer (0.05 M, PH 7.6)). Peroxidase activity detection was carried out with 3-3′ diaminobenzidine. The immunoreactive reaction was stopped by washing the sections once in 0.1 M Tris buffer (10 min) and twice in 0.1 M PBS (10 min). The sections were dehydrated in progressive ethanol baths, cleared in 2 successive xylene baths, mounted onto gelatin-coated slides, and coverslipped. The primary antibody (Anti-GFAP: AB10062) and secondary antibody (Goat Anti-mouse IGg: AB150113) (Elab Science Biotechnology Co., Ltd., Houston, TX, USA) were sourced from BIOCOM Africa (pty), Ltd.

4.12. *Transmission Electron Microscopic Analysis of Hippocampal Tissue*

The hippocampal tissue sectioned at 1 mm^3 was post-fixed in glutaraldehyde (12 h) and washed (3 × 10 min) in phosphate buffer. After that, it was transferred to osmium tetroxide (2 h) and washed again in phosphate buffer (3 × 5 min). The sections were dehydrated in varying degrees of acetone-containing solutions (30%, 50%, 75%, and 100% for 5 min) and embedded in Durcopan (Fluka). The hippocampal tissue was re-sectioned (1 μm in thickness) using an ultramicrotome (Leica Ultracut R), contracted by lead and uranyl acetate, and finally examined with a transmission electron microscope.

4.13. *Statistical Analysis*

All the data were analyzed using Graph Pad Prism 8 for Windows (GraphPad Software San Diego, CA, USA). $p < 0.05$ was considered statistically significant and presented as mean ± SEM. The differences between the means were compared using one-way analysis (ANOVA), followed by Tukey's multiple comparison test to determine the statistical significance between the groups.

G Power Software (Version: 3.1.9.7.) was used to calculate the number of animals based on the difference in the means between two independent groups to arrive at a total sample size of 42 animals. This was based on the literature, and the minimum number of animals per group for behavioral studies was eight (8) to have statistically significant values.

5. Conclusions

This study provides invaluable insights into the adverse effects of diabetes mellitus and tenofovir disoproxil fumarate on hippocampal microanatomy and neuro-biomarker alteration. It underscores the neuroprotective role of silver nanoparticle-capped tenofovir disoproxil fumarate, which restores various alterations on the hippocampal microstructures and cognitive functions in rats via silver nanoparticles' antioxidant and anti-inflammatory activities. In addition, the unique properties of silver nanoparticles could be effectively exploited in the delivery of antiretroviral drugs to the CNS to enhance the efficacy of these agents in managing neurocognitive deficits.

Author Contributions: Conceptualization, S.K.L. and O.O.A.; data curation, K.S.D.; formal analysis, S.K.L.; funding acquisition, C.O.R. and O.O.A.; investigation, S.O.O. and S.T.M.; methodology, S.K.L., S.O.O., B.A.A., S.T.M. and C.O.R.; project administration, E.C.N. and O.O.A.; supervision, K.S.D., ECSN, C.O.R. and O.O.A.; validation, S.O.O., B.A.A. and ECSN; visualization, C.O.R.; writing—original draft, S.K.L. and B.A.A.; writing—review and editing, S.K.L., S.O.O., K.S.D., S.T.M. and C.O.R. All authors have read and agreed to the published version of the manuscript.

Funding: This research work was partially supported by the College of Health Sciences, University of KwaZulu-Natal. A grant was awarded to the lead author (640967).

Institutional Review Board Statement: This study was conducted in accordance with the Declaration of Helsinki and approved by the Institutional Review Board (or Ethics Committee) of the University of KwaZulu-Natal (AREC/044/19D). The animal study protocol was approved by the Institutional Ethics Committee of the University of KwaZulu-Natal (AREC/044/19D).

Informed Consent Statement: Not applicable.

Data Availability Statement: The raw data supporting the conclusions of this article will be made available by the authors upon request.

Acknowledgments: The authors appreciate the technical support of the staff of the Biomedical Research Unit (BRU) and the School of Chemistry and Physics, Natural Product Laboratory from the University of KwaZulu-Natal.

Conflicts of Interest: None of the authors has conflicts of interest to disclose.

References

1. Chan, P.; Yoon, B.; Colby, D.; Kroon, E.; Sacdalan, C.; Sriplienchan, S.; Pinyakorn, S.; Ananworanich, J.; Valcour, V.; Vasan, S.; et al. Immunological, Cognitive, and Psychiatric Outcomes After Initiating Efavirenz- and Dolutegravir-based Antiretroviral Therapy During Acute Human Immunodeficiency Virus Infection. *Clin. Infect. Dis.* **2023**, *76*, e718–e726. [CrossRef] [PubMed]
2. Marsh, K.; Eaton, J.W.; Mahy, M.; Sabin, K.; Autenrieth, C.S.; Wanyeki, I.; Daher, J.; Ghys, P.D. Global, regional and country-level 90–90–90 estimates for 2018: Assessing progress towards the 2020 target. *Aids* **2019**, *33*, S213–S226. [CrossRef] [PubMed]
3. Fields, J.A.; Swinton, M.K.; Carson, A.; Soontornniyomkij, B.; Lindsay, C.; Han, M.M.; Frizzi, K.; Sambhwani, S.; Murphy, A.; Achim, C.L.; et al. Tenofovir disoproxil fumarate induces peripheral neuropathy and alters inflammation and mitochondrial biogenesis in the brains of mice. *Sci. Rep.* **2019**, *9*, 17158. [CrossRef]
4. Petruccelli, K.C.S.; Baía-Da-Silva, D.C.; Val, F.; Valões, M.S.; Cubas-Vega, N.; Silva-Neto, A.V.; Sampaio, V.; Alencar, A.; Pecoits-Filho, R.; Moreira, R.C.; et al. Kidney function and daily emtricitabine/tenofovir disoproxil fumarate pre-exposure prophylaxis against HIV: Results from the real-life multicentric demonstrative project PrEP Brazil. *AIDS Res. Ther.* **2022**, *19*, 12. [CrossRef] [PubMed]
5. Lanman, T.; Letendre, S.; Ma, Q.; Bang, A.; Ellis, R. CNS Neurotoxicity of Antiretrovirals. *J. Neuroimmune Pharmacol.* **2021**, *16*, 130–143. [CrossRef]
6. Turner, D.; Drak, D.; O'connor, C.C.; Templeton, D.J.; Gracey, D.M. Renal function change after switching tenofovir disoproxil fumarate for tenofovir alafenamide in the HIV-positive patients of a metropolitan sexual health service. *AIDS Res. Ther.* **2019**, *16*, 40. [CrossRef]
7. Patel, R.R.; Presti, R.; Harrison, L.C.; Powderly, W.G.; Chan, P.A. Tenofovir disoproxil fumarate as pre-exposure prophylaxis for HIV prevention in women with osteoporosis: A case report and review of the literature. *Antivir. Ther.* **2018**, *23*, 379–382. [CrossRef]
8. Abdool Karim, S.S.; Baxter, C.; Abdool Karim, Q. Advancing HIV prevention using tenofovir-based pre-exposure prophylaxis. *Antivir. Ther.* **2022**, *27*, 13596535211067589. [CrossRef]
9. Saberi, P.; Scott, H.M. On-Demand Oral Pre-exposure Prophylaxis with Tenofovir/Emtricitabine: What Every Clinician Needs to Know. *J. Gen. Intern. Med.* **2020**, *35*, 1285–1288. [CrossRef]
10. Glidden, D.V.; Mulligan, K.; McMahan, V.; Anderson, P.L.; Guanira, J.; Chariyalertsak, S.; Buchbinder, S.P.; Bekker, L.-G.; Schechter, M.; Grinsztejn, B.; et al. Metabolic Effects of Preexposure Prophylaxis with Coformulated Tenofovir Disoproxil Fumarate and Emtricitabine. *Clin. Infect. Dis.* **2018**, *67*, 411–419. [CrossRef]
11. Ozturk, N.B.; Akyuz, M.; Gulluoglu, M.; Akyuz, F. S3176° Tenofovir Disoproxil Fumarate-Related Metabolic Syndrome and Steatohepatitis in a Case of Chronic Hepatitis B. *Am. J. Gastroenterol.* **2022**, *117*, e2036. [CrossRef]
12. Zhao, X.; Sun, K.; Lan, Z.; Song, W.; Cheng, L.; Chi, W.; Chen, J.; Huo, Y.; Xu, L.; Liu, X.; et al. Tenofovir and adefovir down-regulate mitochondrial chaperone TRAP1 and succinate dehydrogenase subunit B to metabolically reprogram glucose metabolism and induce nephrotoxicity. *Sci Rep* **2017**, *7*, 46344. [CrossRef] [PubMed]
13. Lawal, S.; Olojede, S.O.; Sulaiman, S.O.; Aladeyelu, O.S.; Moodley, R.; Naidu, E.C.S.; Rennie, C.O.; Azu, O.O. Tenofovir-silver nanoparticles conjugate ameliorates neurocognitive disorders and protects ultrastructural and cytoarchitectonic properties of the prefrontal cortex in diabetic rats. *Bosn. J. Basic Med. Sci.* **2022**, *22*, 569. [CrossRef] [PubMed]
14. Best, B.M.; Letendre, S.L.; Koopmans, P.; Rossi, S.S.; Clifford, D.B.; Collier, A.C.; Gelman, B.B.; Marra, C.M.; McArthur, J.C.; McCutchan, J.A.; et al. Low cerebrospinal fluid concentrations of the nucleotide HIV reverse transcriptase inhibitor, tenofovir. *JAIDS J. Acquir. Immune Defic. Syndr.* **2012**, *59*, 376–381. [CrossRef] [PubMed]
15. Ntshangase, S.; Mdanda, S.; Naicker, T.; Kruger, H.G.; Baijnath, S.; Govender, T. Spatial distribution of elvitegravir and tenofovir in rat brain tissue: Application of matrix-assisted laser desorption/ionization mass spectrometry imaging and liquid chromatography/tandem mass spectrometry. *Rapid Commun. Mass Spectrom.* **2019**, *33*, 1643–1651. [CrossRef]

16. Lawal, S.K.; Lawal, S.K.; Olojede, S.O.; Faborode, O.S.; Aladeyelu, O.S.; Matshipi, M.N.; Sulaiman, S.O.; Naidu, E.C.S.; Rennie, C.O.; Azu, O.O. Nanodelivery of antiretroviral drugs to nervous tissues. *Front. Pharmacol.* **2022**, *3*, 1025160. [CrossRef]
17. Bowen, A.; Sweeney, E.E.; Fernandes, R. Nanoparticle-Based Immunoengineered Approaches for Combating HIV. *Front. Immunol.* **2020**, *11*, 789. [CrossRef]
18. Zhang, X.F.; Liu, Z.G.; Shen, W.; Gurunathan, S. Silver Nanoparticles: Synthesis, Characterization, Properties, Applications, and Therapeutic Approaches. *Int. J. Mol. Sci.* **2016**, *17*, 1534. [CrossRef]
19. Alkaladi, A.; Abdelazim, A.M.; Afifi, M. Antidiabetic activity of zinc oxide and silver nanoparticles on streptozotocin-induced diabetic rats. *Int. J. Mol. Sci.* **2014**, *15*, 2015–2023. [CrossRef]
20. Bedlovicova, Z.; Strapac, I.; Balaz, M.; Salayova, A. A Brief Overview on Antioxidant Activity Determination of Silver Nanoparticles. *Molecules* **2020**, *25*, 3191. [CrossRef]
21. Luceri, A.; Francese, R.; Lembo, D.; Ferraris, M.; Balagna, C. Silver Nanoparticles: Review of Antiviral Properties, Mechanism of Action and Applications. *Microorganisms* **2023**, *11*, 629. [CrossRef]
22. Khashan, A.A.; Dawood, Y.; Khalaf, Y.H. Green chemistry and anti-inflammatory activity of silver nanoparticles using an aqueous curcumin extract. *Results Chem.* **2023**, *5*, 100913. [CrossRef]
23. Olojede, S.O.; Lawal, S.K.; Mahlangeni, N.; Shelembe, B.; Matshipi, M.N.; Moodley, R.; Rennie, C.O.; Naidu, E.C.; Azu, O.O. Synthesis and characterization of a conjugate of silver nanoparticles loaded with tenofovir disoproxil fumarate. *Next Nanotechnol.* **2024**, *5*, 100058. [CrossRef]
24. Menon, S.; Kumar, V. A review on biogenic synthesis of gold nanoparticles, characterization, and its applications. *Resour.-Effic. Technol.* **2017**, *3*, 516–527. [CrossRef]
25. Kosuda, K.; Bingham, J.; Wustholz, K.; Van Duyne, R. Nanostructures and surfaceenhanced Raman spectroscopy. *Handb. Nanoscale Opt. Electron.* **2010**, *309*, 117–152.
26. Uddin, A.R.; Siddique, M.A.; Rahman, F.; Ullah, A.A.; Khan, R. Cocos nucifera Leaf Extract Mediated Green Synthesis of Silver Nanoparticles for Enhanced Antibacterial Activity. *J. Inorg. Organomet. Polym. Mater.* **2020**, *30*, 3305–3316. [CrossRef]
27. Mondal, N.; Singh, Y. Development and validation of different spectrophotometric methods for estimation of tenofovir disoproxil fumarate from bulk drug and tablets. *Int. J. Pharm. Sci. Res.* **2014**, *5*, 623.
28. Van Dong, P.; Ha, C.H.; Binh, L.T.; Kasbohm, J. Chemical synthesis and antibacterial activity of novel-shaped silver nanoparticles. *Int. Nano Lett.* **2012**, *2*, 9. [CrossRef]
29. Yang, Z.; Huck, W.T.S.; Clarke, S.M.; Tajbakhsh, A.R.; Terentjev, E.M. Shape-memory nanoparticles from inherently non-spherical polymer colloids. *Nat. Mater.* 2005. *4*, 486–490. [CrossRef]
30. Iravani, S.; Korbekandi, H.; Mirmohammadi, S.V.; Zolfaghari, B. Synthesis of silver nanoparticles: Chemical, physical and biological methods. *Res. Pharm. Sci.* **2014**, *9*, 385–406.
31. Mukherji, S.; Bharti, S.; Shukla, G.; Mukherji, S. Synthesis and characterization of size- and shape-controlled silver nanoparticles. *Phys. Sci. Rev.* **2019**, *4*, 20170082. [CrossRef]
32. Kanters, S.; Renaud, F.; Rangaraj, A.; Zhang, K.; Limbrick-Oldfield, E.; Hughes, M.; Ford, N.; Vitoria, M. Evidence synthesis evaluating body weight gain among people treating HIV with antiretroviral therapy—A systematic literature review and network meta-analysis. *EClinicalMedicine* **2022**, *48*, 101412. [CrossRef] [PubMed]
33. Hocqueloux, L.; Menard, A.; Arvieux, C.; Joly, V.; Becker, A.; Chéret, A.; Duvivier, C.; Cabié, A.; Delpierre, C.; Allavena, C.; et al. Weight gain following the single substitution of tenofovir disoproxil fumarate by tenofovir alafenamide in HIV-infected people from the French Dat'AIDS cohort: A propensity score-matched analysis. *HIV Med.* **2023**, *24*, 925–932. [CrossRef] [PubMed]
34. Bosch, B.; Akpomiemie, G.; Chandiwana, N.; Sokhela, S.; Hill, A.; McCann, K.; Qavi, A.; Mirchandani, M.; Venter, W.D. Weight and Metabolic Changes After Switching from Tenofovir Alafenamide/Emtricitabine (FTC) + Dolutegravir (DTG), Tenofovir Disoproxil Fumarate (TDF)/FTC + DTG, and TDF/FTC/Efavirenz to TDF/Lamivudine/DTG. *Clin. Infect. Dis.* **2023**, *76*, 1492–1495. [CrossRef] [PubMed]
35. Wahab, M.; Bhatti, A.; John, P. Evaluation of Antidiabetic Activity of Biogenic Silver Nanoparticles Using Thymus serpyllum on Streptozotocin-Induced Diabetic BALB/c Mice. *Polymers* **2022**, *14*, 3138. [CrossRef] [PubMed]
36. Malapermal, V.; Botha, I.; Krishna, S.B.N.; Mbatha, J.N. Enhancing antidiabetic and antimicrobial performance of *Ocimum basilicum*, and *Ocimum sanctum* (L.) using silver nanoparticles. *Saudi J. Biol. Sci.* **2017**, *24*, 1294–1305. [CrossRef] [PubMed]
37. Russo, V.; Gluckman, P.D.; Feldman, E.L.; Werther, G.A. The insulin-like growth factor system and its pleiotropic functions in brain. *Endocr. Rev.* **2005**, *26*, 916–943. [CrossRef]
38. Mikhailova, E.O. Silver nanoparticles: Mechanism of action and probable bio-application. *J. Funct. Biomater.* **2020**, *11*, 84. [CrossRef]
39. Biadgo, B.; Tamir, W.; Ambachew, S. Insulin-like Growth Factor and its Therapeutic Potential for Diabetes Complications—Mechanisms and Metabolic Links: A Review. *Rev. Diabet. Stud.* **2020**, *16*, 24–34. [CrossRef]
40. Todorova, M.; Milusheva, M.; Kaynarova, L.; Georgieva, D.; Delchev, V.; Simeonova, S.; Pilicheva, B.; Nikolova, S. Drug-Loaded Silver Nanoparticles-A Tool for Delivery of a Mebeverine Precursor in Inflammatory Bowel Diseases Treatment. *Biomedicines* **2023**, *11*, 1593. [CrossRef]
41. Gonzalez-Carter, D.A.; Leo, B.F.; Ruenraroengsak, P.; Chen, S.; Goode, A.E.; Theodorou, I.G.; Chung, K.F.; Carzaniga, R.; Shaffer, M.S.P.; Dexter, D.T.; et al. Silver nanoparticles reduce brain inflammation and related neurotoxicity through induction of H2S-synthesizing enzymes. *Sci. Rep.* **2017**, *7*, 42871. [CrossRef]

42. Olojede, S.O.; Lawal, S.K.; Dare, A.; Naidu, E.C.; Rennie, C.O.; Azu, O.O. Evaluation of tenofovir disoproxil fumarate loaded silver nanoparticle on testicular morphology in experimental type-2 diabetic rats. *Artif. Cells Nanomed. Biotechnol.* **2022**, *50*, 71–80. [CrossRef] [PubMed]
43. Keshari, A.K.; Srivastava, R.; Singh, P.; Yadav, V.B.; Nath, G. Antioxidant and antibacterial activity of silver nanoparticles synthesized by *Cestrum nocturnum*. *J. Ayurveda Integr. Med.* **2020**, *11*, 37–44. [CrossRef] [PubMed]
44. Zulu, S.S.; Simola, N.; Mabandla, M.V.; Daniels, W.M. Effect of long-term administration of antiretroviral drugs (Tenofovir and Nevirapine) on neuroinflammation and neuroplasticity in mouse hippocampi. *J. Chem. Neuroanat.* **2018**, *94*, 86–92. [CrossRef]
45. Khawaja, A.A.; Taylor, K.A.; Lovell, A.O.; Nelson, M.; Gazzard, B.; Boffito, M.; Emerson, M. HIV Antivirals Affect Endothelial Activation and Endothelial-Platelet Crosstalk. *Circ. Res.* **2020**, *127*, 1365–1380. [CrossRef]
46. Govindappa, M.; Hemashekhar, B.; Arthikala, M.-K.; Rai, V.R.; Ramachandra, Y. Characterization, antibacterial, antioxidant, antidiabetic, anti-inflammatory and antityrosinase activity of green synthesized silver nanoparticles using Calophyllum tomentosum leaves extract. *Results Phys.* **2018**, *9*, 400–408. [CrossRef]
47. Bold, B.E.; Urnukhsaikhan, E.; Mishig-Ochir, T. Biosynthesis of silver nanoparticles with antibacterial, antioxidant, anti-inflammatory properties and their burn wound healing efficacy. *Front. Chem.* **2022**, *10*, 972534. [CrossRef] [PubMed]
48. Fehaid, A.; Fujii, R.; Sato, T.; Taniguchi, A. Silver Nanoparticles Affect the Inflammatory Response in a Lung Epithelial Cell Line. *Open Biotechnol. J.* **2020**, *14*, 113–123. [CrossRef]
49. Foghi, K.; Ahmadpour, S. Diabetes mellitus type1 and neuronal degeneration in ventral and dorsal hippocampus. *Iran. J. Pathol.* **2014**, *9*, 33–37.
50. Piotrowski, P.; Wierzbicka, K.; Smialek, M. Neuronal death in the rat hippocampus in experimental diabetes and cerebral ischaemia treated with antioxidants. *Folia Neuropathol.* **2001**, *39*, 147–154.
51. Nagayach, A.; Patro, N.; Patro, I. Astrocytic and microglial response in experimentally induced diabetic rat brain. *Metab. Brain Dis.* **2014**, *29*, 747–761. [CrossRef]
52. Brown, G.C.; Neher, J.J. Inflammatory neurodegeneration and mechanisms of microglial killing of neurons. *Mol. Neurobiol.* **2010**, *41*, 242–247. [CrossRef]
53. Lizarbe, B.; Soares, A.F.; Larsson, S.; Duarte, J.M.N. Neurochemical modifications in the hippocampus, cortex and hypothalamus of mice exposed to long-term high-fat diet. *Front. Neurosci.* **2019**, *12*, 985. [CrossRef] [PubMed]
54. Xu, P.; Wang, Y.; Qin, Z.; Qiu, L.; Zhang, M.; Huang, Y.; Zheng, J.C. Combined medication of antiretroviral drugs tenofovir disoproxil fumarate, emtricitabine, and raltegravir reduces neural progenitor cell proliferation in vivo and in vitro. *J. Neuroimmune Pharmacol.* **2017**, *12*, 682–692. [CrossRef] [PubMed]
55. Akay, C.; Cooper, M.; Odeleye, A.; Jensen, B.K.; White, M.G.; Vassoler, F.; Gannon, P.J.; Mankowski, J.; Dorsey, J.L.; Buch, A.M.; et al. Antiretroviral drugs induce oxidative stress and neuronal damage in the central nervous system. *J. Neurovirology* **2014**, *20*, 39–53. [CrossRef]
56. Yin, F.; Sancheti, H.; Patil, I.; Cadenas, E. Energy metabolism and inflammation in brain aging and Alzheimer's disease. *Free Radic. Biol. Med.* **2016**, *100*, 108–122. [CrossRef] [PubMed]
57. Lawal, S.K.; Olojede, S.O.; Dare, A.; Faborode, O.S.; Naidu, E.C.S.; Rennie, C.O.; Azu, O.O. Silver nanoparticles conjugate attenuates highly active antiretroviral therapy-induced hippocampal nissl substance and cognitive deficits in diabetic rats. *J. Diabetes Res.* **2021**, *2021*, 2118538. [CrossRef]
58. VandeVord, P.J.; Leung, L.Y.; Hardy, W.; Mason, M.; Yang, K.H.; King, A.I. Up-regulation of reactivity and survival genes in astrocytes after exposure to short duration overpressure. *Neurosci. Lett.* **2008**, *434*, 247–252. [CrossRef] [PubMed]
59. Sajja, V.S.; Hlavac, N.; VandeVord, P.J. Role of glia in memory deficits following traumatic brain injury: Biomarkers of glia dysfunction. *Front. Integr. Neurosci.* **2016**, *10*, 7. [CrossRef]
60. Powers, C.M. Developmental Neurotoxicity of Silver and Silver Nanoparticles Modeled In Vitro and In Vivo. Ph.D. Thesis, Duke University, Durham, NC, USA, 2010.
61. Yin, N.; Yao, X.; Zhou, Q.; Faiola, F.; Jiang, G. Vitamin E attenuates silver nanoparticle-induced effects on body weight and neurotoxicity in rats. *Biochem. Biophys. Res. Commun.* **2015**, *458*, 405–410. [CrossRef]
62. Skalska, J.; Strużyńska, L. Toxic effects of silver nanoparticles in mammals–does a risk of neurotoxicity exist? *Folia Neuropathol.* **2015**, *53*, 281–300. [CrossRef] [PubMed]
63. Strużyńska, L.; Skalska, J. Mechanisms underlying neurotoxicity of silver nanoparticles. *Cell. Mol. Toxicol. Nanoparticles* **2018**, *1048*, 227–250.
64. Suthar, J.K.; Vaidya, A.; Ravindran, S. Toxic implications of silver nanoparticles on the central nervous system: A systematic literature review. *J. Appl. Toxicol.* **2023**, *43*, 4–21. [CrossRef]
65. Aebi, H. Catalase. In *Methods of Enzymatic Analysis*; Elsevier: Amsterdam, The Netherlands, 1974; pp. 673–684.
66. Ellman, G.L. Tissue sulfhydryl groups. *Arch. Biochem. Biophys.* **1959**, *82*, 70–77. [CrossRef]
67. Mkhwanazi, B.N.; Serumula, M.R.; Myburg, R.B.; Van Heerden, F.R.; Musabayane, C.T. Antioxidant effects of maslinic acid in livers, hearts and kidneys of streptozotocin-induced diabetic rats: Effects on kidney function. *Ren. Fail.* **2014**, *36*, 419–431. [CrossRef] [PubMed]
68. Greish, K.; Alqahtani, A.A.; Alotaibi, A.F.; Abdulla, A.M.; Bukelly, A.T.; Alsobyani, F.M.; Alharbi, G.H.; Alkiyumi, I.S.; Aldawish, M.M.; Alshahrani, T.F.; et al. The Effect of Silver Nanoparticles on Learning, Memory and Social Interaction in BALB/C Mice. *Int. J. Environ. Res. Public Health* **2019**, *16*, 148. [CrossRef]

69. Morris, R. Developments of a water-maze procedure for studying spatial learning in the rat. *J. Neurosci. Methods* **1984**, *11*, 47–60. [CrossRef] [PubMed]
70. Eilam, D. Open-field behavior withstands drastic changes in arena size. *Behav. Brain Res.* **2003**, *142*, 53–62. [CrossRef] [PubMed]
71. Bădescu, S.; Tătaru, C.; Kobylinska, L.; Georgescu, E.; Zahiu, D.; Zăgrean, A.; Zăgrean, L. Effects of caffeine on locomotor activity in streptozotocin-induced diabetic rats. *J. Med. Life* **2016**, *9*, 275.
72. Sturman, O.; Germain, P.L.; Bohacek, J. Exploratory rearing: A context- and stress-sensitive behaviour recorded in the open-field test. *Stress* **2018**, *21*, 443–452. [CrossRef]
73. Kakkar, P.; Das, B.; Viswanathan, P.N. A modified spectrophotometric assay of superoxide dismutase. *Indian J. Biochem. Biophys.* **1984**, *21*, 130–132.
74. Biancotti, J.C.; Kumar, S.; De Vellis, J.; Drapeau, V.; Després, J.P.; Bouchard, C.; Allard, L.; Fournier, G.; Leblanc, C.; Bancroft, J.D.; et al. Theory and Practice of Histological Techniques, Edinburgh: Churchill Livingstone. *Cogn. Impair. Sleep-Deprived Ovariectomized (OVX) Female Rats Volunt. Exerc.* **2020**, *11*, 2615–2628.

MDPI AG
Grosspeteranlage 5
4052 Basel
Switzerland
Tel.: +41 61 683 77 34

Pharmaceuticals Editorial Office
E-mail: pharmaceuticals@mdpi.com
www.mdpi.com/journal/pharmaceuticals

www.ingramcontent.com/pod-product-compliance
Lightning Source LLC
Chambersburg PA
CBHW061831210926
51850CB00006B/853
9783725847518